Practical Neuroophthalmology

Notice

Medicine is an ever-changing science. As new research and clinical experience broaden our knowledge, changes in treatment and drug therapy are required. The authors and the publisher of this work have checked with sources believed to be reliable in their efforts to provide information that is complete and generally in accord with the standards accepted at the time of publication. However, in view of the possibility of human error or changes in medical sciences, neither the authors nor the publisher nor any other party who has been involved in the preparation or publication of this work warrants that the information contained herein is in every respect accurate or complete, and they disclaim all responsibility for any errors or omissions or for the results obtained from use of the information contained in this work. Readers are encouraged to confirm the information contained herein with other sources. For example and in particular, readers are advised to check the product information sheet included in the package of each drug they plan to administer to be certain that the information contained in this work is accurate and that changes have not been made in the recommended dose or in the contraindications for administration. This recommendation is of particular importance in connection with new or infrequently used drugs.

Practical Neuroophthalmology

Timothy J. Martin, MD
Associate Professor of Ophthalmology and Neurology
Wake Forest School of Medicine/Wake Forest Baptist Health
Winston-Salem, North Carolina

James J. Corbett, MD
Professor of Neurology and Ophthalmology
University of Mississippi Medical Center
Jackson, Mississippi
Levitt Visiting Professor of Neuroophthalmology
University of Iowa
Iowa City, Iowa

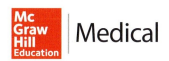

New York Chicago San Francisco Lisbon London Madrid Mexico City
Milan New Delhi San Juan Seoul Singapore Sydney Toronto

Practical Neuroophthalmology

Copyright © 2013 by McGraw-Hill Education LLC. All rights reserved. Printed in China. Except as permitted under the United States Copyright Act of 1976, no part of this publication may be reproduced or distributed in any form or by any means, or stored in a data base or retrieval system, without the prior written permission of the publisher.

1 2 3 4 5 6 7 8 9 0   CTP/CTP   18 17 16 15 14 13

ISBN 978-0-07-178187-9
MHID 0-07-178187-0

This book was set in ITC Garamond by MPS Limited.
The editors were Anne M. Sydor and Cindy Yoo.
The production supervisor was Jeffrey Herzich.
The illustration manager was Armen Ovsepyan.
Project management was provided by Charu Khanna, MPS Limited.
Cover photo ©MedicalRF.com.
China Translation & Printing Services, Ltd. was printer and binder.

This book is printed on acid-free paper.

Library of Congress Cataloging-in-Publication Data
Martin, Timothy J.
  Practical neuroophthalmology / Timothy J. Martin, James J. Corbett.
    p. ; cm.
  ISBN 978-0-07-178187-9 (book : alk. paper)
  ISBN 0-07-178187-0 (book : alk. paper)
  ISBN 0-07-178188-9 (ebook)
    I. Corbett, James J. (James John), 1940- II. Title.
    [DNLM: 1. Eye Diseases—diagnosis. 2. Eye Manifestations. 3. Nervous System Diseases—complications. 4. Vision Disorders—diagnosis. WW 141]
  RE75
  617.7'154—dc23
                                                            2013009821

McGraw-Hill Education LLC books are available at special quantity discounts to use as premiums and sales promotions, or for use in corporate training programs. To contact a representative please e-mail us at bulksales@mcgraw-hill.com.

To Faye, Elizabeth, Matthew, and Hannah
— T.J.M. —

To Joyce, John, Jillian, and Jennifer
—J.J.C. —

CONTENTS

Preface ix

Acknowledgments xi

SECTION I: NEURO-OPHTHALMIC HISTORY AND EXAMINATION

Chapter 1. Neuro-Ophthalmic History and Examination 3

SECTION II: THE SENSORY VISUAL SYSTEM

Chapter 2. Testing Sensory Visual Function 31

Chapter 3. Understanding Visual Field Defects 59

Chapter 4. Optic Nerve Disorders 85

Chapter 5. Disorders of the Chiasm and Retrochiasmal Visual Pathways 139

Chapter 6. Unexplained Visual Loss: Anterior Segment, Retinal, and Nonorganic Disorders 161

SECTION III: THE VISUAL MOTOR SYSTEM

Chapter 7. Examination of the Visual Motor System 185

Chapter 8. Ocular Motility Disorders: Extraocular Muscles and the Neuromuscular Junction ... 201

Chapter 9. Ocular Motility Disorders: Cranial Nerve Palsies 217

Chapter 10. Supranuclear Visual Motor System and Nystagmus 239

Chapter 11. The Pupil 261

Chapter 12. The Facial Nerve 287

SECTION IV: ADDITIONAL TOPICS

Chapter 13. Pain and Sensation 303

Chapter 14. Neurovascular and Neurocutaneous Diseases 319

Index 335

PREFACE

The intent of *Practical Neuroophthalmology* is to present the basic principles of clinical neuroophthalmology in a readable, user-friendly format. Rather than present a list of facts, the authors ask "why" at every opportunity to demonstrate that the myriad of complex neuro-ophthalmic signs and symptoms are often a logical consequence of anatomy and pathophysiology. The textbook is not meant to be a reference only, but invites the reader to sit down and read through a chapter or two.

Practical Neuroophthalmology is the rebirth of *Neuro-ophthalmology: The Requisites in Ophthalmology* (Martin TJ, Corbett J: Mosby, 2000), which was written in a logical, cause-and-effect manner with neuroanatomical correlation whenever possible, and was a favorite particularly of residents in ophthalmology, neurology, and neurosurgery. The authors are pleased to present this new, up-to-date work, keeping the popular presentation style of the first textbook.

Significant features of *Practical Neuroophthalmology* include the following:

- *Comprehensive coverage of the subject matter for clinical use or review.* The text is designed to encompass material likely to be needed for board examinations, but is clinically oriented to be useful for the practitioner.
- *Neuro-anatomic approach, with anatomy discussed in the context of disease states.* With this approach, the consequences of disease can be more readily understood, rather than simply memorized.
- *Discussion of neuroophthalmology from the perspective of an ophthalmologist and a neurologist.* The text addresses the unique abilities (and limitations) that each specialty has in the evaluation and management of patients with neuro-ophthalmic disorders.
- *Summary of the neuro-ophthalmic history and examination in Section I.* This allows a comprehensive overview of the history and examination initially (Chapter 1), further explored in detail in the sections devoted to afferent disorders (Chapter 2) and efferent disorders (Chapter 7).
- *A chapter devoted to interpreting visual fields.* Chapter 3 provides a basic understanding of visual field interpretation, which is reinforced when specific diseases are discussed in Chapters 4–6.
- *A chapter aimed at the problem of unexplained visual loss.* Chapter 6 discusses and illustrates elusive and commonly misdiagnosed disorders.
- *Figures and clinical photographs in full color, with many original illustrations.* For example, the supranuclear pathways are illustrated from the *examiner's perspective* (Figures 10–3, 10–6, and 10–8).
- *Original clinical case profiles.* Optic disc photographs, visual fields, magnetic resonance imaging or computed tomography scans, clinical course, and other data from an illustrative case are presented together in a single figure to give the reader a visual summary of the disease (Figures 4–10 and 4–15).
- *Photographic surveys of disease manifestations.* Clinical photographs from different patients with the same disease are presented together in a single figure to show the spectrum of disease presentation (Figures 14–6 and 14–10).
- *Composite figures (tables within illustrations).* Complex information is visualized as well as described. Examples include sixth cranial nerve syndromes (Figure 9–11) and causes of intracranial hypertension (Figure 4–17).
- *Many tables and boxes devoted to differential diagnosis.* Important clinical decision-making information discussed in the text is synthesized and reinforced in outline form.
- *Text boxes that provide additional insight without disturbing the flow of the main text.* A number of text boxes are devoted to clarifying otherwise confusing information, such as a glossary of perimetric terms (Box 3–1) and discussion of Wilbrand knee (Box 3–2).
- *Key points summarized at the end of each chapter.* A concise list of the most salient points from each chapter is provided so the reader can review the teaching goals of the chapter.
- *Suggested reading at the end of each chapter.* Books, chapters, and journal articles that provide further detail are listed in each chapter. Classic works as well as major current references are provided. The listing is not meant to be exhaustive,

but to provide a short list of important or resourceful references.

A number of excellent neuroophthalmology textbooks are currently available. The books listed below are sources that the authors have found particularly useful, each filling a unique role as a resource for neuroophthalmology.

Walsh and Hoyts' Clinical Neuro-ophthalmology, Vols 1–3, 6th ed (Miller NR, Newman NJ, Biousse V, Kerrison JB, eds: Philadelphia, Pa; London: Lippincott Willliams & Wilkins; 2005). *This three-volume set is the exhaustive, authoritative "bible" of neuroophthalmology.*

Neuro-ophthalmology: Diagnosis and Management, 2d ed (Liu GT, Volpe NJ, Galetta SL: Philadelphia: Saunders Elsevier; 2010). *An in-depth, single-volume text, well written and beautifully illustrated.*

The Neurology of Eye Movements, 4th ed (Leigh RJ, Zee DS: New York, NY; 2006). *The encyclopedic final authority on ocular motility disorders.*

Neuro-ophthalmology Review Manual, 7th ed (Kline LB: Thorofare, NJ; SLACK; 2013). *A well-organized classic review text, written in outline form, that condenses neuro-ophthalmic pearls into a reader-friendly paperback.*

We hope that the reader will find that *Practical Neuroophthalmology* has a unique place among the many excellent textbooks of neuroophthalmology: a direct approach that is clinically oriented and covers the breadth of this fascinating field of study, and one that seeks to not only to inform, but to explain.

Timothy J. Martin, MD

Winston-Salem, North Carolina

James J. Corbett, MD

Jackson, Mississippi

February 2013

ACKNOWLEDGMENTS

The authors are indebted to the talented illustrators and photographers who have helped produce the figures that are the heart of this book. The clinical photographs and photo-illustrations are the work of current and previous ophthalmic photographers at the Wake Forest University Eye Center: Mark D. Clark, MFA, CRA; David T. Miller, CRA; Shannon Josey, BFA; Charita Petree Hill; Richard E. Hackel, CRA; and Marshall E. Tyler, CRA. At the University of Mississippi Medical Center we wish to thank ophthalmic photographers Matthew Olsen, CRA; Jody Watkins; and Elizabeth Smith, CRA. Medical illustrator Annemarie Johnson, CMI, Wake Forest School of Medicine, has had a role in most of the drawings in this book: She produced new and unique illustrations for this book, and her original illustrations for our previous book were the foundation for most of the others.

Our thanks to the Department of Ophthalmology, Wake Forest School of Medicine, for the use of departmental resources to produce this book, and for the encouragement and support of the chairman, Craig Greven, MD.

The authors are also grateful for the teaching and inspiration of their many neuroophthalmology mentors, most notably H. Stanley Thompson, MD, and William F. Hoyt, MD.

SECTION I

Neuro-Ophthalmic History and Examination

Section I contains a single chapter that discusses the neuro-ophthalmic history, outlines the components of the neuro-ophthalmic examination, and introduces the important high-tech tools that have become a standard part of the examination.

The goal of the discussion on taking a history is to convince the reader of a truth that most of us learn the hard way: *The few extra minutes it takes to complete a thorough history and examination on the first encounter often spares both the patient and physician hours of frustration.* The ophthalmologist will need to venture beyond asking questions specifically about the eye, as the signs and symptoms that confirm the diagnosis are frequently outside the bounds of vision alone. The neurologist will need to be familiar with questions regarding the eye and visual disturbances.

The discourse on the neuro-ophthalmic examination in this section is brief, only because the bulk of the discussion on examination technique is in later chapters (comprising a sizable percentage of this book), where they are discussed in the context of related anatomy and disease. However, a logical order and flow of the examination is presented here, with reference to the more detailed material elsewhere in the book.

High-tech tools have become commonplace and are an indispensible part of the neuro-ophthalmic examination. Clinical testing devices and neuroimaging are discussed in Chapter 1 because they are truly an extension of the examination, and because many of the clinical examples in the chapters that follow assume a basic understanding of these imaging techniques.

CHAPTER 1

Neuro-Ophthalmic History and Examination

- ▶ INTRODUCTION 3
- ▶ CHIEF COMPLAINT AND HISTORY OF PRESENT ILLNESS 3
  - Visual loss 4
  - Positive visual phenomena and hallucinations 5
  - Diplopia 8
  - Ptosis (blepharoptosis) 9
  - Anisocoria 9
  - Pain and photophobia 10
- ▶ REVIEW OF SYSTEMS AND OTHER HISTORY 11
- ▶ EXAMINATION OVERVIEW 11
  - Function 11
  - Structure 11
  - Putting it all together 11
- ▶ EXAMINING THE EYE AND ORBIT 12
- ▶ CLINICAL ANCILLARY TESTS 13
  - Photography 14
  - Intravenous fluorescein angiography 14
  - Optical coherence tomography 15
  - Ultrasonography 19
- ▶ NEUROIMAGING 19
  - Computed tomography 20
  - Magnetic resonance imaging 20
  - Imaging the orbit 21
  - Imaging the brain 24
  - Cerebral angiography 24
  - Functional neuroimaging 26
- ▶ KEY POINTS 27

▶ INTRODUCTION

The art and science of obtaining a meaningful history is the keystone of neuroophthalmology. Some may doubt the importance of the history in ophthalmology—because the examiner has the unique ability to actually see the organ of interest inside and out in vivo (unlike the cardiologist or nephrologist)—but a single day in a busy neuroophthalmology clinic will put that notion to rest.

We do not wish to imply that neuro-ophthalmic history-taking should be a lengthy, memorized barrage of questions relating to every system in the body. Instead, the effective examiner is similar to a mechanic with a large chest of tools, carefully selecting the correct instruments for the task at hand. Because effective history-taking depends on a thorough knowledge of the many manifestations of disease in the visual system, it is truly the most complex "procedure" a physician can perform on a patient. A guide, outlining the components of the neuro-ophthalmic history, is provided in Table 1–1.

▶ CHIEF COMPLAINT AND HISTORY OF PRESENT ILLNESS

Neuro-ophthalmic *chief complaints* usually concern visual loss, positive visual phenomena, diplopia, ptosis, anisocoria, pain, and photophobia. Vision complaints are often difficult for patients to articulate. In addition, neuro-ophthalmic patients commonly present with an array of seemingly disjointed complaints, offering a considerable challenge to even to the most determined historian. For this reason, crystallizing the patient's concerns into a list of individual complaints, prioritized by the *patient's* degree of concern, is vital. Information concerning each complaint can then be gathered logically. At the end of the history and examination, the physician can then return to this list to form an assessment and devise a plan that specifically addresses the patient's reason for seeing the physician. Even if the examination reveals more serious concerns, the patient's original complaints should not be ignored. Even if you have made a life-saving discovery in your history and examination, the patient is unlikely to be

▶ TABLE 1-1. ELEMENTS AND RATIONALE OF THE HISTORY

Components of History	Comments
Chief complaint(s)	List the patient's current concerns in order of importance.
History of present illness	Explore details of each complaint.
Review of systems	Inquire about specific symptoms. Include pertinent ophthalmic, neurological, and medical system reviews.
Past history	Identify known ophthalmic, neurological, and medical disorders; previous surgeries; and medical or radiation therapies.
Medications	List all prescription medicines, eye drops, vitamins, over-the-counter drugs, birth control pills, injections, and home remedies.
Other drugs	Inquire about the use of illegal drugs, alcohol, and tobacco.
Allergies	Note drug or environmental allergies. Try to distinguish true allergic reactions from side effects.
Social/sexual	Assess risks of HIV and other sexually transmitted diseases.
Occupational/recreational	Evaluate potential exposure to toxins, trauma, as well as the affect of the disorder on the patient's ability to work safely.
Family history	Explore ophthalmic, neurological, and medical disorders that may be hereditary.

Abbreviation: HIV, human immunodeficiency virus.

satisfied until you have also addressed the patient's initial concerns.

The *history of present illness* is an expanded description of each complaint, exploring characteristics such as those listed in Table 1–2. In this era of the electronic medical record (EMR), the patient's history is expected to fit into convenient "one-size-fits-all" drop-down menus. Even if EMR limits how the history is officially *recorded*, physicians should not be limited in how they *collect* and *think* about the patient's history. Complex histories are often best assessed by plotting the patient's progression of symptoms, treatments, and associated factors over time. This process is especially helpful when the patient can see a plot in progress (eg, sketched on paper or on a dry-erase board in the examination room) as the history is being collected (Figure 1–1).

In the first half of this chapter, important elements in the history of present illness (see Table 1–2) are used to illustrate common neuro-ophthalmic histories. The examples given are not all-inclusive, and will make more sense when specific disorders are covered in detail in later chapters. The intent here is to convince the reader that the *details of the patient's history are important*, and that they are often crucial to determining the diagnosis.

VISUAL LOSS

The sensory experience that we call vision is not easily described. "Vision" includes the complexities of shape, color, contrast, stereopsis, and movement across the

▶ TABLE 1-2. HISTORY OF PRESENT ILLNESS: CHARACTERISTICS THAT HELP DEFINE THE CHIEF COMPLAINT

Location
Quality
Severity
Timing
Duration
Context
Modifying factors
Associated symptoms

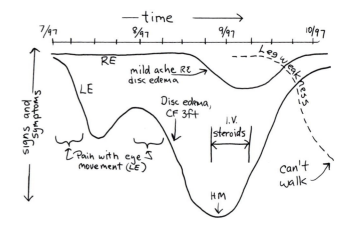

Figure 1-1. Time course "plot" of a complex history.
A 51-year-old man presented with a history of visual loss in each eye, followed by lower extremity weakness (neuromyelitis optica). The temporal relationships of the patient's visual loss and recovery, eye pain, lower extremity weakness, and treatment are evident when the events are diagramed with the assistance of the patient. Information from previous examinations (such as visual acuities) can be incorporated. Documenting the time course of events in this manner allows understanding of complex events at a glance (and can be scanned into electronic medical records).

vast visual fields of both eyes. Not surprisingly, patients may have difficulty finding precise words to describe abnormalities in the quality of their visual experience.

Visual loss may be described by patients as blindness, blurriness, or dimness; a skim, cloud, curtain, or screen covering vision; washed-out color; or broken, twisted vision (metamorphopsia). The descriptions patients choose are helpful. For example, patients with optic neuropathies often describe their vision as dim or dark, whereas patients with cataract are more likely to report blurriness. Complaints of poor color vision are common with optic neuritis. Metamorphopsia is almost always the result of macular disease.

Patients may be able to localize their visual disturbance to one eye, or to a portion of the visual field. Patients typically have difficulty understanding *homonymous* (see Box 3–1) visual field loss, ascribing the problem exclusively to the eye on the side of the visual field loss. Visual loss may be global, affecting the entire visual field of one or both eyes, or may be confined to a specific area of the visual field. Patients with anterior ischemic optic neuropathy frequently describe loss of the lower or upper half of their visual field. Patients with central visual field loss may report that objects seem to disappear into a central cloud when they try to look at them, but are made clearer when they look to the side. Formal perimetry provides a more quantitative assessment of a visual field defect, but much can be learned by listening to the patient's qualitative description.

The severity of visual loss can be assessed by what a patients could or could not do with their degree of visual loss. For example, a patient with a scintillating scotoma from migraine may continue to work at the computer during an episode; a patient with progressing cataract may have given up playing cards or driving.

The time course of visual loss is often the most important diagnostic clue in the history (Figure 1–2). Visual loss may be unchanging, improving, worsening, fluctuating, or transient. The time course in *transient visual loss* is particularly important, because no signs or symptoms may be apparent at the time of the examination (Table 1–3).

In some cases, it may be difficult to ascertain if monocular visual loss truly occurred suddenly, or if it is a problem of long duration that was *discovered suddenly* when the normal-seeing eye was incidentally covered. For example, a patient may discover poor vision in his right eye when using a rifle site at the start of hunting season.

The context of visual loss—the surrounding circumstances of the event—provides many diagnostic clues that are usually self-evident, such as traumatic optic neuropathy in the setting of a blow to the brow, or retinal emboli after carotid endarterectomy or cardiac surgery.

Patients should be asked about what may modify the symptoms—circumstances that make their vision better or worse. In transient visual loss, particular precipitating factors should be sought. Increased body temperature from a hot shower or sauna may cause blurring of vision in patients who have had optic neuritis (Uhthoff phenomenon). Transient visual obscurations frequently occur with postural changes in patients with papilledema.

Associated symptoms may also provide major diagnostic clues, such as scalp tenderness and jaw claudication with visual loss from giant cell arteritis, or pain with eye movement associated with optic neuritis.

POSITIVE VISUAL PHENOMENA AND HALLUCINATIONS

Aberrations of vision may be negative or positive. Visual loss—defects or deficiencies in the sensory visual experience—is a negative visual symptom. Positive visual symptoms involve seeing things that are not images of the real world, described by patients as flashes, lightning streaks, jagged lines, complex patterns of color and form, or formed hallucinations and illusions (Box 1–1). Patients are often reluctant to tell their physician if they are "seeing things," and may need to be specifically asked. The source of positive visual phenomena may be the eye itself (entoptic phenomena such as flashes from retinal traction or detachment), "release phenomena" generated by the

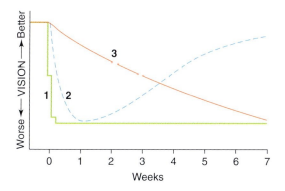

Figure 1–2. Time course of visual loss. Visual loss in anterior ischemic optic neuropathy is usually sudden in onset, without much change over time **(1)**. Optic neuritis causes a decline in vision over days, followed by a slower recovery over months **(2)**. A slow, progressive decline is characteristic of compressive optic neuropathies **(3)**.

> ▶ **BOX 1-1. HALLUCINATIONS, ILLUSIONS, AND DELUSIONS**
>
> *Hallucinations* are sensory perceptions when no corresponding sensory stimulus is present. Visual hallucinations are images perceived in the absence of a visual stimulus from the environment.
>
> *Illusions* are the misperception of a stimulus present in the external environment
>
> *Delusions* are the elaboration of illusions or hallucinations into a series of fixed, false beliefs.

▶ TABLE 1-3. DURATION, ETIOLOGY, AND CHARACTERISTICS OF TRANSIENT VISUAL LOSS

Duration	Etiology	Characteristics	Associated Factors	Comments
Seconds (usually less than 1 minute)	Papilledema (rarely with optic disc drusen or anomaly)	One or both eyes	Often related to postural changes, Valsalva	Called TVOs
Seconds to minutes	Vasculitis (giant cell arteritis in patients older than 60 years)	Usually monocular	Headache, scalp tenderness	May signal impending arteritic ischemic optic neuropathy
Less than 1 minute	VBI	Bilateral dimming, blurring, and loss of focus	Dizziness, slurred speech, perioral numbness, or "drop attack"	Usually briefer than retinal embolic events
3–5 minutes	Retinal embolic disease (*amaurosis fugax*)	Monocular, described as a "curtain coming down over vision" or "Swiss cheese" vision	Atherosclerotic carotid artery disease, cardiac or other embolic sources, hyperviscosity, hypercoagulable states	Retinal emboli may be seen on fundus examination
5–45 minutes	Migraine aura (occipital lobe)	Binocular and homonymous, often alternating sides	Progressing scintillations (iridescent jagged edge) with scotoma in its wake	Headache usually follows, or may be acephalgic
	Occipital lobe lesion (rarely)	Binocular and homonymous, always same side		Arteriovenous malformation or other lesion
	Retinal migraine (retinal artery vasospasm)	Monocular	Transient visual loss without scintillations	A diagnosis of exclusion, even when patients have a convincing history of migraine
Variable duration, possibly hours	Uhthoff phenomenon in multiple sclerosis	Blurring with increased body temperature (exercise, hot shower)		Occurs in an eye with current or previous optic neuritis
	Dry eye syndrome or other external ocular disease	May clear with blinking, worsen with reading		Ocular irritation, red eye, tearing; findings may be subtle
	Other ocular causes	Angle closure, retinal vein occlusion, ocular ischemia, recurrent hyphema		Usually evident on ocular examination
		Orbital mass with gaze-evoked optic nerve compression		

Abbreviations: TVOs, transient visual obscurations; VBI, vertebrobasilar insufficiency.

central nervous system (CNS) in blind areas of the visual field, or true hallucinations from CNS disease (Table 1–4).

Localization may be helpful: bright, brief flashes from a vitreous or retinal detachment are typically seen in the temporal visual field; migraine aura are homonymous. The formed hallucinations of Charles Bonnet syndrome (Box 1–2) are visualized in the nonseeing portion of the visual field: central in macular degeneration, in a homonymous pattern in occipital disease.

As with other symptomatology, the time course is often diagnostic. The scintillating scotoma of migraine starts small and expands over 15 to 45 minutes. Flashes

▶ **TABLE 1-4. POSITIVE VISUAL PHENOMENA**

	Name	Description	Associated Disorders
Entoptic phenomena associated with disease	Photopsias, phosphenes	Brief, spontaneous "spots" of light	Optic neuritis and retinal disorders
	Moore lightning streaks	Fleeting streaks of light usually seen in the temporal visual field with eye movement	Vitreous traction, retinal detachment, or may be a normal entoptic event
	Floaters	Dark spots or squiggles that float predictably with eye movement	Shadows from vitreous condensation, or debris from vitreous detachment, hemorrhage, or inflammation
Normal entoptic phenomena	Afterimages	Complimentary-colored images fixed in the visual field after prolonged viewing or after a bright flash, caused by bleaching of retinal pigments	Normal physiologic phenomenon, but enhanced by retinal dysfunction
	Scheerer ("blue field" entoptic) phenomenon	Multitude of small, clear, "tadpoles" that move rapidly in small circles, best seen against blue sky or white clouds	Thought to represent individual white blood cells in retinal capillaries
	Purkinje images	Retinal blood vessels made visible by shifting light source	Patients often comment that they see this phenomenon when being examined at the slitlamp
CNS processes (see Box 5–2 for details)	Scintillating scotoma	Dynamic, zig-zag lines seen homonymously that progress over 5–45 minutes, usually moving from center to periphery	Migraine aura (headache may follow), or rarely occipital lobe disease
	Unformed hallucinations	Nondescript patterns and lights	Occipital/parietal lobe seizures, or same as for formed hallucinations
	Formed hallucinations	Hallucinations of very real-appearing objects, persons, or animals	Drug or disease-induced delirium, seizures involving visual association cortex, or "release" hallucinations in blind areas of the visual field (Charles Bonnet syndrome)

Abbreviation: CNS, central nervous system.

▶ **BOX 1-2. CHARLES BONNET SYNDROME (RELEASE VISUAL HALLUCINATIONS)**

In 1769 Swiss naturalist Charles Bonnet described vivid, detailed hallucinations experienced by his blind grandfather, who he observed had normal mentation. DeMorsier introduced the term "Charles Bonnet syndrome" in 1936 to describe visual hallucinations in elderly patients, not necessarily with vision loss. Thus Charles Bonnet syndrome technically includes many situations other than release hallucinations in vision loss, but popular usage typically limits the term to release hallucinations.

Release visual hallucinations are relatively common in patients with poor vision (10–40%), and are characterized by unformed or formed hallucinations, typically in the area of blindness. Patients with central scotomas from macular degeneration see the hallucinations centrally; patients with occipital stroke see them in the blind homonymous hemifields. The formed hallucinations are vivid and detailed—patients don't say "like a mouse," they describe a detailed mouse "with fur and eyes and pink ears." The hallucinations often fit into the visible surroundings: all faces have beards, rows of tiny pine trees are growing on the carpet. Unlike many other causes of hallucinations, the patient is aware that the hallucinations are not real and is not usually threatened by them. Understandably, patients are often very reluctant to discuss them, especially when family is present in the examination room.

Release hallucinations can persist for years, but usually subside over time. There is no known effective treatment, though selective serotonin reuptake inhibitor (SSRI) antidepressants have been suggested. The hallucinations may be more frequent when vision is at its poorest, so sometimes increasing the lighting in the home (such as in a dark hallway where symptoms occur) may help. The most important thing the physician can do is make the diagnosis—often a clinical diagnosis, but in some cases neuroimaging and other evaluation is needed to rule out other causes of hallucinations—and offer education and warranted assurance that patients are not "losing their mind."

from vitreous/retinal pathology are described as "like lightning." Phosphenes, lasting seconds, can occur with optic neuritis, often in response to sudden loud noises.

The context, especially with formed hallucinations, is helpful: delirium in alcohol withdrawal, hallucinations in Parkinson disease, hypnagogic and hypnopomic hallucinations seen with narcolepsy and sleep apnea.

The association of headache following a migrainous scintillating scotoma is well known, but patients can have acephalgic (no headache) migrainous visual aura.

DIPLOPIA

Technically, diplopia refers to seeing the same image twice in a given field of view. However, the main reason patients are symptomatic with diplopia is that it is accompanied by *confusion*. In confusion, two superimposed images occupy the central vision, causing confusion as to which is the real "straight ahead" image. In general, patients (and physicians) find it easier to discuss diplopia/confusion in terms of "double vision" and the separation of two identical images. Diplopic images that are minimally separated may be described as blur rather than double: the unwary examiner may be convinced that "blur" must mean an afferent disorder (cataract, optic neuritis, etc) and miss an ocular motility disorder.

Diplopia resulting from *binocular* misalignment (strabismus) typically produces double images that are equally clear. In this case, the patient's diplopia disappears when either eye is covered. *Monocular diplopia* is present even when a single eye is viewing alone, and is frequently caused by anterior segment disorders (Table 1–5). Patients with supranuclear palsies usually have vague visual complaints, and unlike other motility disturbances only occasionally describe double vision, despite an obvious misalignment of the eyes. Patients with congenital strabismus or long-standing ocular deviations often develop effective suppression of a misaligned eye and therefore may not experience diplopia.

▶ **TABLE 1–5. CAUSES OF MONOCULAR DIPLOPIA**

Common:
  Nuclear sclerotic cataract
  Ocular surface disease (dry eye)
  Corneal basement membrane disease ("map-dot-fingerprint" dystrophy)
  Irregular corneal astigmatism

Less common:
  Macular diseases with traction
  Iridectomy or atrophic iris hole
  Subluxated lens
  Functional (nonorganic) disorder

Rare:
  "Central" (cerebral) polyopia

The patient's description of the relative orientation of the two images in diplopia, and how this orientation changes in different directions of gaze, has great diagnostic value. Sixth cranial nerve palsies result in horizontal diplopia, with greatest separation of the images in the direction of the palsied lateral rectus muscle. Diplopia may not be present at near or when gaze is directed away from the palsied muscle in this condition. Vertical or diagonal diplopia may be the result of third or fourth cranial nerve palsies. A "tilt" to one of the images is typically reported with fourth cranial nerve palsies. Ocular myasthenia may cause diplopia of any orientation that may change over time. Diplopic images that are greatly separated may be better tolerated, because the second image is more easily ignored than when the competing images are close together or overlapping.

Understanding the time course and duration of diplopia is important. Transient or variable diplopia may be the result of a transient ischemic attack, vertebrobasilar insufficiency, decompensating strabismus, or myasthenia gravis. Diplopia that is abrupt in onset suggests a vascular event such as an ischemic cranial mononeuropathy (cranial nerves [CNs] III, IV, or VI) or a brainstem ischemic event. Ischemic cranial mononeuropathies typically resolve completely in 8 to 12 weeks. Gradually worsening diplopia suggests compression of CNs III, IV, or VI, or an orbital process such as orbital Graves disease. Patients with ocular myasthenia may describe a lengthy history of intermittent, variable diplopia, often worsening toward the end of the day.

Examples of the importance of the context in which diplopia occurs include post-lumbar puncture sixth cranial nerve palsies, vertical diplopia after cataract surgery, or skew deviation after brainstem stroke. Head trauma is a common cause of fourth, sixth, and occasionally third cranial nerve palsies, and may also cause diplopia from extraocular muscle injury or entrapment in an orbital fracture.

Patients should be questioned about any factors that modify their symptoms. Diplopia from myasthenia gravis is typically improved on arising in the morning and after a nap, and worsened with fatigue. As previously discussed, binocular diplopia should vanish if either eye is covered. Patients who complain of diplopia but do not spontaneously close or cover one eye likely have monocular diplopia (from cataract or other ocular cause), rather than a neurological cause.

The presence of ptosis or anisocoria is of particular importance in assessing ocular motility disturbances. Third cranial nerve palsies are usually associated with a ptosis of the involved eye. The presence of a dilated pupil in this setting may suggest a compressive, rather than ischemic, mechanism. Myasthenia may cause ptosis of either one or both eyelids, and may be associated with ocular misalignment (but not anisocoria), facial weakness, or systemic (proximal limb and bulbar) weakness. Eyelid *retraction* (with "scleral show") frequently accompanies the diplopia from orbital Graves disease. The character of the pain associated with diplopia may help differentiate possible diagnoses such as giant cell arteritis (vasculitic ischemic cranial mononeuropathy), ophthalmoplegic migraine, aneurysm (compression of the third cranial nerve), idiopathic orbital inflammatory syndrome, and other disorders.

PTOSIS (BLEPHAROPTOSIS)

Patients describe ptosis in a number of imaginative ways, including "swelling" of the eyeball or eyelid, "one eye smaller than the other," or as a "lazy eye."

Occasionally patients may complain of a droopy eyelid when the eyelid retraction of the contralateral eye is the real problem. Asymmetric bilateral ptosis may be attributed only to the worse eye by the patient. Ptosis from an oculosympathetic paresis usually only measures 1 to 2 mm, whereas ptosis from a third cranial nerve palsy can range from minimal to total. Blepharospasm is spontaneous *activation* of the orbicularis muscles (overacting eyelid *protractors*), and may occasionally be confused with ptosis—a *deficiency* of lid elevation (weak eyelid *retractors*). An apparent bilateral ptosis can occur from CNS disease causing an inability to open the eyes known as *apraxia of eyelid opening*.

Patients may not be aware how long ptosis has been present, especially a minimal ptosis that is functionally asymptomatic. Old photographs provide an objective record of the patient's appearance. A drivers' license or other photos in the patient's wallet (or on his or her cell phone) are immediate sources, or the patient may need to bring other photographs from home on subsequent visits (Box 1–3). Variability of ptosis with fatigue and ptosis that "switches eyes" over time are hallmarks of ocular myasthenia.

The history may place ptosis in the context of trauma, contact lens wear, topical ocular medications, ocular surgeries, or neurosurgical procedures, narrowing the differential diagnosis.

A smaller pupil associated with a ptotic lid may represent an oculosympathetic paresis, whereas a larger pupil with ptosis suggests the possibility of a third cranial nerve palsy. Disorders that cause ocular pain may be the source of a "protective ptosis."

ANISOCORIA

Patients may discover pupillary inequality themselves, especially when they have lightly colored irides. More frequently, it is someone else—a family member, friend, or physician—who notes a difference in pupil size between the two eyes, sending an otherwise asymptomatic patient for further evaluation. Thus, patients with anisocoria usually have fewer observations to volunteer than those with diplopia or visual loss.

Which pupil is the abnormal one is not always obvious. Although patients are quick to ascribe pupillary inequality to a "bad eye," the examiner will need to wait for the pupillary examination to determine which pupil—the smaller or the larger of the two—is the abnormal one.

Although certain conditions cause intermittent pupillary dilation, the variability of anisocoria reported by the patient is most likely the result of changes in lighting conditions and accommodation. Interestingly, patients who examine their own pupils in the mirror will only observe the pupil size in an accommodative state, typically in a bright light—minimizing the anisocoria in Adie pupil and Horner syndrome. As with ptosis, examination of the patient's driver's license or

▶ BOX 1-3. "FAT SCAN"

A valuable yet underutilized diagnostic resource is the patient's photo album (sometimes called "family album tomography" or FAT scan). Old photographs are particularly helpful in demonstrating that certain signs have been present for years—ptosis, anisocoria, strabismus, head position, or facial asymmetry—simplifying the differential diagnosis or evaluation. For example, new diplopia may indeed be from a decompensated congenital superior oblique palsy when a life-long head tilt is demonstrated in photographs through the years (see Figure 9–9). A Horner syndrome that is evident in photographs from 5 years previous may not need an extensive evaluation.

In this digital age, patients may not need to actually bring in a photo album—more often than not, patients have access to many photographs on their smartphones, which can zoom in to see the area in question (though it's still helpful to know how to look at a printed photograph with an indirect lens or the slitlamp). In any case, most patients are very motivated and only too happy to pour through old photographs when instructed what to look for. Whenever possible, it is important keep a copy of old photographs that have influenced your clinical decision making for the patient's chart.

With digital photograph and video capability on most cell phones, it is very easy for patients to get photographs or videos of transient signs, such as variable ptosis or strabismus, intermittent anisocoria, or other signs. It is worth asking if patients have taken photographs or videos during transient events (especially "tech savvy" patients), as they may not volunteer this information to the physician. This is also an opportunity to instruct the patient that such photographs or videos can be helpful in recording future transient events for the physician.

other photographs (with magnification provided by the slitlamp or an indirect ophthalmoscopy lens) may establish the duration of anisocoria. The importance of the pupil size and its association with ptosis and diplopia has been discussed. Adie pupil is usually associated with transient blurred vision when accommodation is changed from near to distance, because of tonicity of accommodation.

PAIN AND PHOTOPHOBIA

Pain around the face and eyes can be difficult to assess for several reasons: pain is difficult for patients to describe, tolerance of pain differs widely among individuals, a "secondary gain" agenda may be present, and pain cannot be objectively measured. Patients often have their own diagnosis for chronic or recurrent pain, such as blaming "sinus disease" for migraine headaches.

The location, quality, and severity of pain offer important clinical clues. The gritty foreign-body sensation typical of dry eye or other external ocular disease is described quite differently from the continuous "toothache" quality of idiopathic orbital inflammatory syndrome, or the excruciating "ice pick" of cluster headache. It is helpful to have patients grade the intensity of their pain on a scale of 1 (mild) to 10 (worst pain imaginable). Pain from a rupturing posterior communicating artery aneurysm causing a third cranial nerve palsy may be a 10 ("the worst headache of my life"), whereas the pain associated with an ischemic mononeuropathy of the third cranial nerve is usually low on the pain scale.

The time course of pain may be the most important characteristic to explore in the history. Cluster headaches, as the name implies, occur in "clusters" that may only happen over several months of the year. The pain of trigeminal neuralgia is exceedingly severe, but lasts only seconds at a time. Migraine headache in women is often synchronous with the menstrual cycle.

The context of head and eye pain may offer an obvious explanation, such as pain associated with herpes zoster ophthalmicus, ophthalmic surgery, or trauma, or in intraocular inflammatory disorders.

Avoidance behavior reveals important modifying factors. Patients with trigeminal neuralgia intermittently lightly touch but fiercely protect the "trigger area." Giant cell arteritis may cause pain when wearing a hat, combing hair, or even placing the head on a pillow. In contrast, patients may find themselves massaging and pushing on their head to help relieve migraine or other headaches. Associated symptoms, such as a scintillating scotoma preceding a migraine headache, may point to the diagnosis.

▶ **TABLE 1–6. CONDITIONS ASSOCIATED WITH PHOTOPHOBIA**

Ocular disease
Anterior segment
- Dry eyes (common)
- Corneal diseases (corneal ulcers, keratitis, pterygium)
- Iritis

Posterior segment
- Vitritis, retinitis
- Retinal disorders
- Cone dystrophies, retinitis pigmentosa, albinism, cancer-associated retinopathy

Neurological conditions
- Migraine (common)
- Blepharospasm
- Progressive supranuclear palsy
- Head injury
- Meningeal irritation (meningitis, subarachnoid hemorrhage)

Psychiatric conditions
- Depression (common)
- Anxiety disorder, panic disorder

Other
- Hangover headache
- Medications: barbiturates, benzodiazepines, chloroquine, methylphenidate, haloperidol, zoledronate
- Fibromyalgia, chronic fatigue

Essential photophobia

Adapted with permission from Digre KD, Brennan KC. Shedding light on photophobia. *Neuro-Ophthalmol* 2012;32: 69, Table 1.

Photophobia, literally "fear" or avoidance of light, has several distinct forms (Table 1–6). First, this term describes patients who experience eye pain with light exposure from eye disease, such as from the pupillary light reaction pulling on an inflamed iris in iritis. Light may also cause pain because the light is too bright relative to the sensitivity of a dark-adapted retina, such as the physiologic photosensitivity experienced when walking out into bright sunlight from a dark movie theater. However, other forms of photophobia are more difficult to understand: photophobia with migraine, or CNS diseases such as meningitis, encephalitis, and subarachnoid hemorrhage; and particularly patients with photophobia without evident ocular or CNS disease. These mysterious forms of photophobia may be mediated by pathways other than the classic retino-geniculate-calcarine pathway that serves vision. One potential pathway that may mediate photophobia involves melanopsin-containing *intrinsically photosensitive retinal ganglion cells* (IPRGCs)—light-sensitive ganglion cells (which do not need photoreceptor input) that connect through nonvisual pathways to the brain.

Photophobia can also describe situations where individuals avoid light not because of pain, but because of visual loss. For example, patients with cone dystrophy or primary cone dysfunction (achromatopsia) see less well in the light-adapted state (when cone function predominates) than in the dark, and avoid daylight (hemeralopia). Patients with ocular surface disease or cataract lose contrast because of light scattering in bright light and may prefer mesopic conditions. Some disorders such as ocular surface disease (dry eye syndrome) seem to have both components of photophobia: pain with light exposure and poorer vision with bright light.

▶ REVIEW OF SYSTEMS AND OTHER HISTORY

After the details of the current problem have been understood, the patient should be asked about ophthalmic problems not mentioned in the present history, such as transient or lasting visual changes, positive visual phenomena, diplopia, ptosis, eye pain or irritation, or "red" eyes (see Table 1–1). For many patients, a neurological system review is also appropriate (eg, when optic neuritis, stroke, transient ischemic attack [TIA], or myasthenia gravis are suspected) and should include questions about headache, weakness, numbness, clumsiness, vertigo, slurred speech, confusion, and forgetfulness. In some patients general medical questions including the presence of fever, chills, myalgias, arthralgias, skin rashes, nausea, vomiting, malaise, palpitations, and chest pain are required.

A complete listing of the patient's known medical, neurological, and ophthalmic disorders is necessary, because the visual complaint may be a manifestation of a known diagnosis. Specific inquiry should be made about any trauma, surgery, radiation treatment, or chemotherapy. The medication history often suggests diseases that the patient did not reveal in the medical history. Patients may not mention vitamins and nutritional supplements, birth control pills, daily aspirin, hormonal supplements, or other over-the-counter medications, and may need to be specifically asked. Allergies to medications, foods, diagnostic contrast agents, or environmental factors should be listed. The family history is important, especially with ocular disorders such as retinitis pigmentosa, glaucoma, or hereditary optic neuropathies, and systemic disorders including neurofibromatosis, diabetes mellitus, systemic hypertension, early cardiovascular disease, or early death from stroke or myocardial infarction.

The social history should address alcohol, tobacco, and illegal drug use. Assessment of the patient's risk factors for human immunodeficiency virus (HIV) or other sexually transmitted diseases may change the physician's developing differential diagnosis. The occupational history will reveal not only exposure to potential toxins, but also allow the physician to understand the impact of the patient's visual complaint in his or her workplace.

▶ EXAMINATION OVERVIEW

The neuro-ophthalmic examination evaluates the *function* of the afferent and efferent visual systems, and the *structure* of the eye and orbit (and brain, with neuroimaging). Not uncommonly the examiner may need to venture beyond the eye, and should be comfortable with elements of a neurological or general medical examination.

FUNCTION

Testing visual function is limited in that it is a *sensory* examination, and as such is largely reliant on the subjective responses of the patient. Therefore, tests of visual function are as much an art as a science. Examination of the sensory and motor systems is given a great deal of attention in this book in separate chapters (Table 1–7), grouped with the discussion of related anatomy and disease. This division of the component parts of the examination into separate chapters is somewhat artificial, but allows a unified discussion of specific neuro-ophthalmic disorders and relevant examination techniques.

STRUCTURE

Ophthalmology is unique among medical subspecialties in that (eg, unlike the kidney or liver) the eye can be examined and directly visualized inside and out by the physician in the clinic. Thus, mastering the techniques to examine the eye and related structures is of obvious importance. This aspect of the examination is far more objective than testing visual function, but is dependent on the skill and knowledge of the examiner. Clinical ancillary tests and neuroimaging (discussed later in this chapter) greatly extend the physician's ability to evaluate the anatomic structures of the visual system.

PUTTING IT ALL TOGETHER

Table 1–7 shows the general flow of the component parts of the examination as one would perform them in evaluating a patient. Detailed discussions of specific neuro-ophthalmic examination techniques are presented in chapters throughout this volume, as designated in this table.

TABLE 1-7. NEURO-OPHTHALMIC EXAMINATION GUIDE

Examination Components (in Suggested Sequence)	Chapters With More Detailed Discussion	Comments
General observation		The patient's eye movements, visual behavior, facial movements, physical appearance, and demeanor should be assessed throughout the history and examination.
Visual acuity	2	Vision tests should be completed early in the examination, as bright lights, eye drops, and applanation tonometry may affect results.
Refraction	2, 6	Obtaining the *best corrected* visual acuity is important; "pinhole" acuity is helpful when equipment and expertise to perform a refraction are not available.
Tests of stereopsis	2	Technically, should be done before testing visual acuity, because occlusion of one eye may break fragile fusion.
Color vision	2	Color plates, D-15, FM 100, or other color vision tests should be performed undilated, and before the patient is exposed to bright examination lights.
Confrontation perimetry	2	Should be performed on all patients (even when formal perimetry is anticipated).
Pupil	11	Determine RAPD, record pupil size in light and dark, note any anisocoria. Note pupil response to accommodation at near if reaction to light is poor.
Motility	7	Observe fixation. Observe how the eyes move (ocular versions and ductions, convergence, pursuits, and saccades). Measure eye alignment (alternate cover testing and other tests).
Eyelids	7	Evaluate ptosis, retraction, levator function, lid crease.
Other cranial nerves	7, 12, 13	Test facial motor function (CN VII) and sensory (CN V). But do not test corneal sensitivity until the cornea has been inspected at the slitlamp. Corneal sensitivity cannot be tested after topical anesthetic. Asking the patient to compare the irritation of topical drops between the two eyes allows a rough comparison of ocular sensation (CN V).
Orbit/adnexa	7, 12	Inspection, palpation, exophthalmometry.
Slitlamp examination, tonometry	6	If the slitlamp examination is done only after dilation, details such as rubeosis, Lisch nodules, chamber anatomy, and others may be missed. Do not do tonometry or touch the cornea if pharmacologic pupil tests are anticipated.
Automated or Goldmann perimetry	2, 3	Ideally, visual fields should be performed very early in the examination (see confrontation perimetry above). However, the need for formal perimetry may not be established until this point in the examination. Young patients do best if they are not cyclopleged before perimetry. Dilation (and cycloplegia) of patients older than 40 years has a negligible effect on perimetry (if accounted for by the testing lens) and saves time. Pupils less than 3 mm should be dilated prior to perimetry.
Dilated slitlamp examination		Lens, anterior vitreous, and fundus (90-diopter lens) can now be optimally visualized.
Direct and indirect ophthalmoscopy		Visualizing the optic nerve, vasculature, macula, and retinal periphery determines the diagnosis in the majority of cases of afferent visual loss.
Other examinations		Elements of a neurological or general physical examination are often necessary. Measuring the blood pressure, palpating the pulse, auscultating (heart, carotids, and cranium), and examining the ears with an otoscope are simple but effective diagnostic tools when indicated.

Abbreviations: CN, cranial nerve; RAPD, relative afferent pupillary defect.

► EXAMINING THE EYE AND ORBIT

A basic, standard eye examination should be performed on every new neuroophthalmology patient, regardless of the complaint (Box 1–4). The time it takes to perform a basic ocular examination is minimal and the returns are frequently great—saving the patient (and physician) much frustration. The "routine" eye examination may unexpectedly reveal the diagnosis after a complex history, such as the discovery of Lisch nodules on the

▶ BOX 1-4. NEUROLOGISTS AND THE EYE EXAMINATION

The neuroophthalmology examination, as outlined in Table 1-4, is obviously designed from an ophthalmic perspective. However, most of the examination can be performed equally well in the neurology or ophthalmology clinic, with the exception of the slitlamp examination, tonometry, and some forms of dilated ophthalmoscopy.

When an ocular disorder is suspected, there should be no hesitation for the neurologist to obtain an ophthalmology consultation. Otherwise, a penlight examination is performed, looking for a crisp light reflex from the cornea and tear film, visualizing the bulbar conjunctiva, and in some cases, illuminating the anterior chamber from the side to gauge anterior chamber depth in suspected angle closure. Evaluating the red reflex with the direct ophthalmoscope at arm's length before ophthalmoscopy reveals media opacities such as cataract, with lack of red reflex suggesting vitreous hemorrhage or dense cataract.

In the past, measuring intraocular pressure required significant skills and experience with applanation tonometry and the slitlamp; now simple handheld devices such as the Tono-Pen permit easy bedside or in-office measurements. However, if a neurologist suspects elevated intraocular pressure, an ophthalmologist will still need to evaluate the patient.

The neurologist is usually confined to using the direct ophthalmoscope, with a limited view of the fundus through an undilated pupil. Obviously, evaluating the optic disc and macula is a vital part of every complete neurological examination, even when conditions are not ideal. It is not unreasonable for the neurologist to dilate the eyes for a better examination (rare cases of inducing angle-closure glaucoma notwithstanding)—but if the fundus is thought to harbor important clues to the diagnosis, the ophthalmologist's full armamentarium for viewing, photographing, and imaging the fundus should be sought. It is therefore important for the clinical neurologist to establish a professional relationship with an ophthalmology neighbor (and vice versa), as so many neuro-ophthalmic disorders require (at least) this team of two specialists.

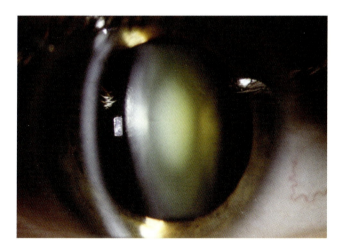

Figure 1-3. Not all patients with multiple sclerosis and visual loss have optic neuritis. A 38-year-old woman with a long history of multiple sclerosis complained of a gradual decline in the vision of both eyes. This complaint prompted an admission to the hospital and an extensive evaluation including a computed tomography (CT) scan of the head, magnetic resonance imaging (MRI) of brain and orbits, a lumbar puncture, and numerous laboratory studies for presumed optic neuritis. After high-dose intravenous steroids did not help, the patient was referred for neuro-ophthalmic consultation. The *basic, routine examination* revealed the culprit: bilateral "opalescent" nuclear sclerotic cataract, pictured in this slitlamp photograph. The history and other examination findings supported this diagnosis (myopic shift on refraction, mild diffuse visual field loss). Cataract surgery resulted in 20/20 visual acuity and normalization of a diffusely depressed visual field.

iris (diagnostic of neurofibromatosis type 1). Structural abnormalities of the iris may provide an explanation for anisocoria. Corneal basement membrane disease, dry eye, or cataract may be identified with the slitlamp, offering a potential cause for "unexplained" visual loss (Figure 1-3). Anterior segment disorders that masquerade as neurological visual loss are discussed in Chapter 6.

Techniques for examination of the fundus—optic disc, macula, vasculature, retina—are beyond the scope of this volume, but are obviously important. *The optic disc appearance is often the most important diagnostic clue in the examination of patients with afferent visual disorders.* Different perspectives can be obtained by observing the disc and retina with the direct ophthalmoscope, indirect ophthalmoscope, and indirect slitlamp examination (with the 90-diopter or similar lens).

Careful examination of the macula and retina may narrow the differential diagnosis in optic nerve or intracranial disorders (eg, the presence of hypertensive vascular changes or diabetic retinopathy in the setting of anterior ischemic optic neuropathy, or a macular star in an infectious neuroretinitis). More importantly, retinal disorders may masquerade as optic neuropathies (more on this subject in Chapter 6). The neuro-ophthalmologist must be prepared to look for subtle retinal changes and be familiar with the use and interpretation of fluorescein angiography, optical coherence tomography (OCT), electroretinography, and other clinical ancillary methods.

▶ CLINICAL ANCILLARY TESTS

Ophthalmologists have access to an increasing array of technologically advanced tools. The physician cannot possibly perform every examination technique and test on every patient. A careful, guided history and an understanding of the pathologic disorders affecting vision are required to select the right diagnostic tools. With limitations of time and resources, the ability to discern which clinical tests are appropriate is a valuable skill.

PHOTOGRAPHY

Clinical photography is an important tool in ophthalmology, perhaps more than in any other medical subspecialty. Photographs provide the ultimate documentation for following pathology of the fundus, ocular media, ocular surface, adnexa, and associated systemic manifestations.

Clinical photographs document what the physician sees on the examination, providing a visual comparison for future visits. For example, an optic disc photograph from a previous visit is often a picture "worth a thousand words" when trying to decide if there is any change in optic disc edema. In fact, serial photography of the optic disc is one of the most important tools in managing papilledema. *As with any test, the physician must look at all photographs ordered during the course of the examination.* Not uncommonly, a review of clinical photographs reveals pathology not seen initially during the examination, such as Hollenhorst plaques. Fundus photographs are particularly helpful when circumstances limit the clinical examination, such as nystagmus, squirming children (or adults!), or photophobic patients. Digital photographs can also be enhanced to see subtle pathology, such as using "red-free" display to see hemorrhage or nerve fiber layer loss.

Clinical ophthalmology photographs are also the foundation of teaching. Mapping photographs of the fundus can be stitched together to form a montage to see the "big picture" or be otherwise enhanced. However, scientific integrity requires that a clinical photograph should never be altered ("photoshopped") in a way that changes the basic information without clear designation. Obviously, adjusting brightness/contrast, color balancing, cropping, and other methods to present the data in the clearest form are still true to the clinical representation. However, clinical photographs that are otherwise manipulated should be labeled as "not original data." It is our practice to call any clinical photograph that has been manipulated for teaching purposes a *photo illustration*.

INTRAVENOUS FLUORESCEIN ANGIOGRAPHY

This powerful method of evaluating retinal vascular disorders is performed by taking a sequence of photographs of the fundus every few seconds after an intravenous injection of a florescent dye (Figure 1–4). Intravenous fluorescein

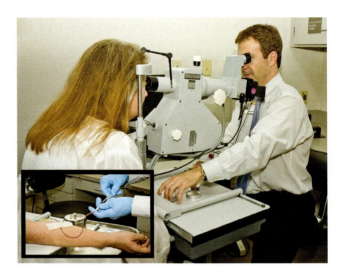

Figure 1–4. Intravenous fluorescein angiography.
Intravenous fluorescein angiography (IVFA) requires venous access, usually with a butterfly needle in an antecubital vein (inset). A series of flash photographs of the retina are taken after injection of fluorescein sodium. By using excitation and barrier photographic filters in the fundus camera, the florescent dye alone is imaged as it traverses the ocular circulation.

angiography (IVFA) is performed with a fundus camera that employs an exciter filter that insures that the flash illumination is at a wavelength of 490 nm. A blocking filter over the camera allows only reflected light at a wavelength of 525 nm to enter the camera. Thus, there is no image unless the wavelength of the light is shifted, as it is with the fluorescing intravenous dye. Therefore, the camera sees only the dye as it enters the eye and traverses the retinal arteries, capillaries, and veins. The choroidal system also fills with fluorescent dye and is visible on IVFA (Figure 1–5). Abnormal blood vessels (such as neovascularization), leakage of dye outside of vascular structures (such as in central serous retinopathy), and staining of vessel walls (as in vasculitis) are evident with this technique. As discussed in the next section, OCT has largely replaced IVFA for diagnosis of conditions such as cystoid macular edema (CME), but IVFA is still vital in the evaluation of many retinal conditions. OCT is superior to IVFA in evaluating structural abnormalities, such as macular holes and epiretinal membranes, and OCT does not require intravenous injection like IVFA. However, IVFA cannot be replaced by OCT with regard to dynamic imaging of the vascular system of the retina and choroid, and in particular, visualization of neovascularization and vascular incompetence.

IVFA has many applications in neuroophthalmology including demonstrating choroidal ischemia in giant cell arteritis (GCA), staining of the optic disc in optic disc edema and other optic neuropathies, revealing retinal arteriolar occlusions and vasculitis, and uncovering occult retinal vascular disorders in unexplained visual loss.

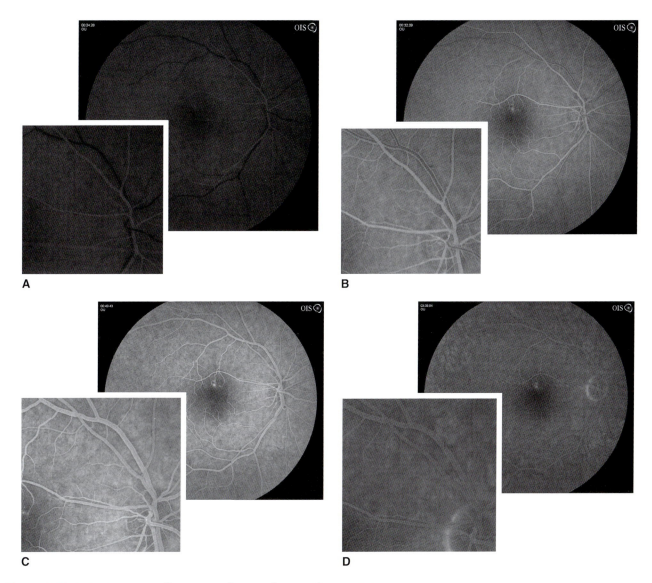

Figure 1–5. **Intravenous fluorescein angiography sequence.**
An intravenous fluorescein angiography (IVFA) study consists of a series of images of the fundus, labeled with the time in seconds after intravenous injection of fluorescein. A few selected images of an IVFA from a patient with inactive central serous chorioretinopathy are shown. (Examples of abnormal IVFAs can be found in Figures 4–12, 6–5, 6–6, 6–10, and 6–11). This sequence shows a small chorioretinal scar just superior to the fovea. The scarring produces a "window defect" in the retinal pigment epithelium (RPE), allowing the hyperfluorescence from the choroid to shine through unobstructed by the RPE. The study is otherwise normal, showing several important phases of a typical angiogram. The inset shows a magnified view of the retinal vasculature at the disc for each phase. **(A)** *Arterial phase.* The fluorescein dye quickly fills the high-flow choroid, producing a diffuse glow as the dye fills the retinal arteries. The veins remain dark. **(B)** *Early (laminar) venous phase.* The fluorescein has now traversed the retinal capillary bed, and is beginning to collect in the veins. The fluorescein arriving first to the venous system flows in a marginalized stream, producing a laminar pattern appreciated best in the inset. **(C)** *Full venous phase.* Now the arteries and veins are both filled with the fluorescent dye. **(D)** *Recirculation phase.* The dye has washed through the retinal circulation and now recirculates, much diluted. The macular scar superior to the fovea remains bright, demonstrating "staining."

OPTICAL COHERENCE TOMOGRAPHY

Optical coherence tomography (OCT) was commercially introduced in 1995, and with remarkable rapid advancements has become one of the most important innovations in diagnostic ophthalmology in the last 20 years. This technique allows rapid, noninvasive (unlike IVFA), and noncontact cross-sectional imaging of the retina and other ocular structures (Figure 1–6). Other effective methods of optically imaging the retina and optic nerve (particularly in glaucoma) include

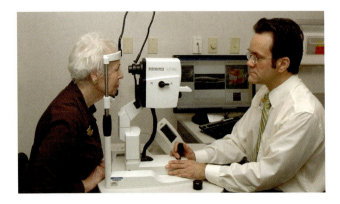

Figure 1-6. Optical coherence tomography.
The optical coherence tomography (OCT) device is noncontact and easy for the patient. Patients need to be able to fixate on a target to keep their eye from moving and degrading the image. Faster acquisition times mean that the patient does not have to keep still for long. Many devices have eye tracking capabilities to account for even the smallest of eye movements during the scan. (The Spectalis OCT from Heidelberg Engineering is pictured.)

scanning laser tomography (SLT), and scanning laser polarimetry (GDx nerve fiber analyzer). We will confine our brief discussion to OCT, which has had the broadest clinical application to neuroophthalmology.

OCT uses a beam of light to image the surface and layers beneath translucent materials. Because the retinal layers are essentially transparent (the photoreceptors are in the outer retina—light has to pass through the layers of the retina to get to the photoreceptive elements), OCT is an ideal method for imaging the layers of the retina. OCT maps the intensity of reflected light along its path in the specimen. A beam splitter sends one beam of light into the test material (test beam) and the other to a mirror (reference beam). Optical interference techniques (combining the test beam and the reference beam) allow the beam of light directly reflected from the test material to be isolated from all other scattered light. Linear movement of the beam through the retina produces a cross section, sometimes viewed in a "false color" cross-sectional display where "warm" colors (red to white) represent areas of high optical reflectivity, and "cool" colors (blue to black) represent areas of low reflectivity. Retinal thickness and other data are compared to age-matched normals to show the probability of abnormal findings. Rather than moving the sample beam through the tissue over time (called "time domain" OCT), spectral domain OCT (SD-OCT) permits rapid imaging of a 3-D "block" of the macula all at once. This block (showing surface contour) can then be displayed on a computer monitor, where it can be "sliced" by the physician to view specific cross sectional areas (Figure 1–7A). An OCT cross-section of the macula reveals more than just retinal thickness, as it distinguishes the various anatomic layers of the retina for measurement and comparison (Figure 1–7B).

The major application of OCT has been *imaging the macula*. Many maculopathies that are not readily evident on ophthalmoscopy, or even IVFA, are obvious with a simple, noninvasive OCT. The detailed cross-sectional perspective permitted by OCT has transformed our understanding and diagnosis of macular diseases such as macular holes, pseudoholes, epiretinal membranes, vitreomacular traction, cystoid macular edema, central serous retinopathy, macular degeneration, and many others. Many of the disorders just listed can be elusive and frequently masquerade as optic neuropathies (see Figures 6–7 to 6–9). OCT is therefore a valuable tool for the neuro-ophthalmologist, as it not infrequently will diagnose a macular problem early in the evaluation of unexplained visual loss, saving an extensive (and expensive) neuro-ophthalmic investigation.

OCT of the retinal nerve fiber layer looks specifically at a circular cross section of the peripapillary retina, specifically isolating and measuring the thickness of the retinal nerve fiber layer (RNFL). RNFL analysis has become a vital tool for following glaucoma, but axonal loss from any optic neuropathy can be documented and followed with this method (Figure 1–8). The thickness of the NFL varies considerably depending on the location (superior, inferior, temporal, nasal) in normal individuals, so a patient's collected data is compared to age-matched normals and presented to show probability of deviation from normal at each sector. Remember, the NFL is made up of the axons from retinal ganglion cells that converge to form the optic nerve. Diseases of the optic nerve (or even the chiasm or optic tracts) damage the axons, and retrograde degeneration causes eventual atrophy of the retinal nerve fiber layer. This can often be seen with the ophthalmoscope as optic disc pallor and nerve fiber layer dropout, but OCT measurement of the thickness of the retinal NFL provides a direct, quantitative assessment of the NFL thickness, and thus the integrity of the optic nerve. Serial measurements over time, in particular with the chronic optic atrophy of glaucoma, offer a direct objective measure of changes in the health of the optic nerve. Note, however, that axonal atrophy takes time, and optic neuropathies may not demonstrate RNFL thinning until many weeks or months after an insult, depending on the location, severity, and type of lesion. Also, optic disc edema and retinal edema may swell the RNFL, confounding the clinical meaning of the measurements. OCT of the RNFL can be helpful in neuroophthalmology in confirming or documenting suspected optic atrophy, following chronic or progressive optic neuropathies (glaucoma, compressive optic neuropathies), and identifying generalized axonal atrophy in chronic diseases such as multiple sclerosis.

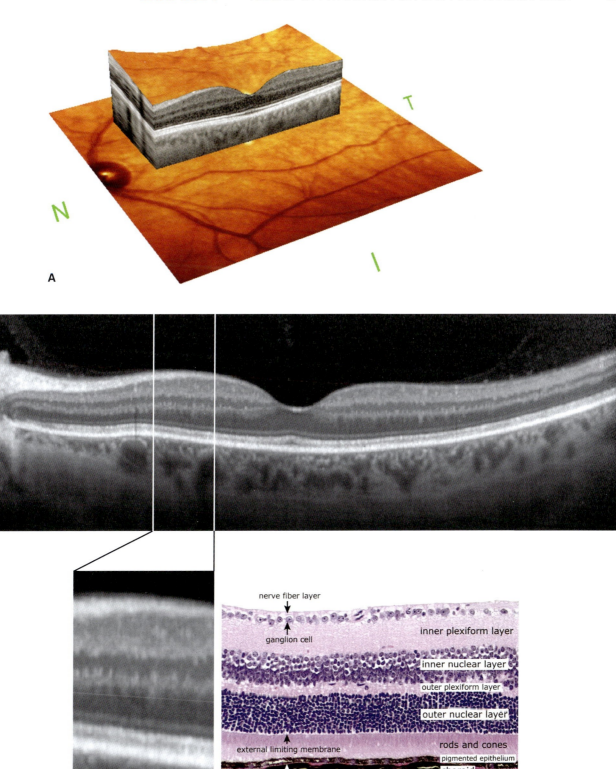

Figure 1-7. **Spectral domain optical coherence tomography of the macula.**
(A) This 3-dimensional (3-D) optical coherence tomography (OCT) map of the retina shows how a "block" of the macula can be evaluated in cross section. The operator can select the slice for visualization. The contour of the fovea and anatomic layers of the retina are evident in this normal study. (Examples of abnormal macular OCTs can be seen in Figures 6–7 to 6–9). **(B)** A segment of a normal OCT is compared to the layers of a histologic hematoxylin and eosin (H and E) stain of the retina, showing the amazing in vivo resolution—at a histologic level—of OCT in macular imaging. (Histologic section used with permission from Deltagen, Inc., San Mateo, CA).

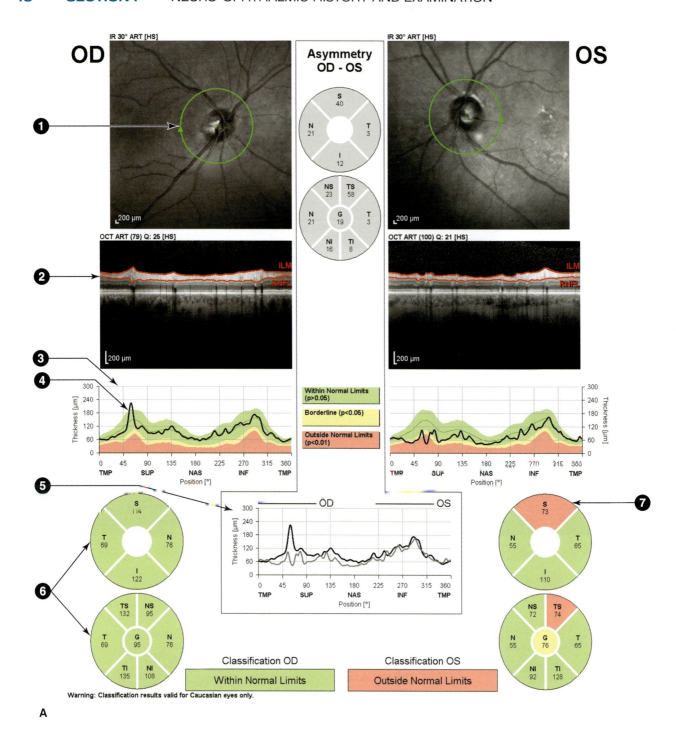

Figure 1-8. **Retinal nerve fiber layer analysis.**
(A) Optical coherence tomography (OCT) retinal nerve fiber layer (RNFL) analysis provides a circular cross section around the optic nerve (1), and selects out the RNFL (2). The thickness of the RNFL for each eye is displayed and compared to age-matched controls with color-coded statistical analysis (3). Note that the normal RNFL thickness changes depending on the orientation around the optic nerve. Showing each step of the analysis in this way allows the physician to observe any noise or inaccuracies in the measurement, such as the artifactual spike in the plot of the right eye (4), likely from the overlying superotemporal blood vessels. The RNFL thickness from the two eyes are then plotted together, here showing that the superior RNFL in the left eye is much thinner than that in the right eye (5). The average thickness for quadrants and smaller segments is displayed and color-coded, with green designating normal thickness, as seen in the right eye (6), and yellow and red corresponding to areas of abnormal thinning, as seen in the left eye superiorly (7). This patient has a normal right eye; the left eye has glaucoma, with thinning of the superior neuroretinal rim and superior RNFL.

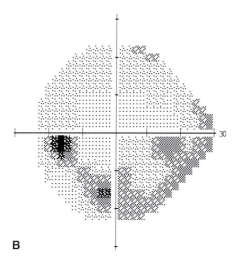

Figure 1–8. (Continued)
(B) The Humphrey 24-2 visual field of this patient's left eye shows an inferior arcuate scotoma, corresponding to the superior thinning of the RNFL demonstrated by OCT.

OCT of the optic disc permits imaging and measurement of the architecture of the optic disc to compare changes in optic disc cupping and optic disc edema over time. OCT of the optic disc may also be helpful in distinguishing true optic disc edema from pseudopapilledema, and identifying optic disc drusen.

As discussed above, OCT has many clinical applications, but the research applications of this tool may be the most important contribution to neuroophthalmology. The ability to see and measure individual retinal layers and the structure of the optic disc will allow a better understanding of the relationship between structure and function in many neuro-ophthalmic disorders.

ULTRASONOGRAPHY

Ultrasonography is ubiquitous in medicine. This technology is used in virtually every specialty, from imaging the fetus in utero to evaluating cardiac function. This noninvasive technology uses reflected sound waves to produce an acoustical cross section of soft tissue (B scan). The image produced is real time, allowing dynamic visualization of tissue. In addition, Doppler modalities permit measurement of blood flow velocity as in carotid duplex studies or Doppler imaging of orbital blood flow.

Ultrasound provides a noninvasive way to look at the eye and orbit, but its usefulness depends on the skill of the ultrasonographer (Figure 1–9). B-scan ultrasound produces cross-sectional images of the eye, allowing visualization of the retina and vitreous behind opaque media, such as with a mature white cataract (Figure 1–10). The A-scan mode measures acoustic reflectivity along a line, and is used primarily in measuring the axial length of the eye for intraocular lens calculations in cataract surgery. Both A- and B-scan modes are used to evaluate chorioretinal lesions as

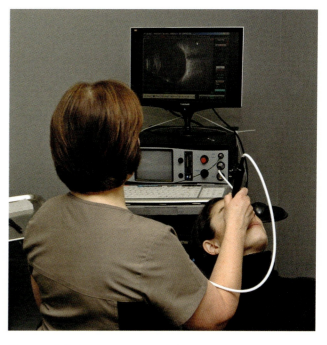

Figure 1–9. Ultrasound of the globe.
After a topical anesthetic is applied to the eye, the ultrasound probe is placed directly on the cornea to produce the best images, but the test can be done through the eyelids. A skilled ultrasonographer will produce a systematic survey of the eye in a variety of B-scan planes, with labeled printouts to document the examination. However, this is a dynamic real-time test, and much information is gained by watching the how the intraocular structures change with eye movement.

in suspected choroidal tumors, permitting measurement of a lesion's thickness and internal acoustical characteristics. Ultrasonography of the optic nerve is the gold standard for identifying optic nerve drusen, which have high acoustical reflectivity that produces a very bright signal on a B-scan image (see Figure 4–40). Ultrasound can also be used to image the orbit, allowing dynamic visualization of the extraocular muscles and orbital tissue in motion, which is particularly useful in diagnosing restrictive orbitopathies such as orbital Graves disease. The resolution of ultrasound is dependent on the frequency of the transducer and acoustic properties of the tissue examined. Lower frequencies are required to penetrate deep into tissue, so ultrasound of the orbit is a relatively low resolution. In contrast, more superficial structures such as the anterior segment can take advantage of higher frequencies: ultrasound biomicroscopy (UBM) is a specialized high-frequency ultrasound that can produce high-resolution images of the anterior segment of the eye.

▶ NEUROIMAGING

As the structure of the eye is investigated with the slitlamp and ophthalmoscope, the structure of the brain and orbit can be investigated with neuroimaging.

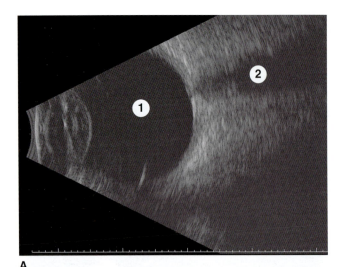

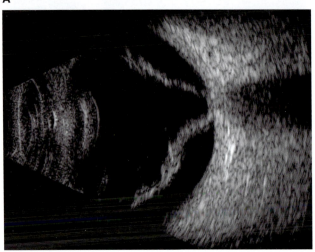

Figure 1-10. **B-scan ultrasound.**
(A) B-scan ultrasound of a normal eye. The vitreous cavity is "acoustically empty" (1). The optic nerve casts an acoustic shadow (2), as the high tissue density of the optic nerve does not allow the sound waves to readily penetrate. **(B)** This B-scan shows a chronic funnel-shaped retinal detachment—otherwise not visible behind a dense cataract.

Computed tomography (CT) and magnetic resonance imaging (MRI) allow in vivo visualization of the orbits and intracranial contents. The continued rapid advancement of CT and MRI technologies has yielded greater anatomic resolution, specialized imaging of the intracranial vasculature, and techniques that can image both structure *and function*.

COMPUTED TOMOGRAPHY

CT uses x-ray and computer-based technology to image 3-dimensional (3-D) objects as individual "slices." Intravenous injection of a radiopaque contrast material provides enhancement of vascular structures and many pathologic lesions. Since its introduction, CT technology has improved significantly, allowing greater resolution with less x-ray exposure and faster scan times (Figure 1–11). The high attenuation of x-rays by bone makes identification of structures at the skull base (such as the posterior fossa and brainstem) less satisfactory than with MRI. The orientation of the image slice was previously limited to the plane of the machine's circling x-ray/detector array ring, making axial images the easiest to obtain. Earlier-generation CT scanners would image an axial slice, then move the patient a few millimeters and image the next. The "thickness" (separation) of the slices determined the resolution of reconstructed views in other planes, which was typically poor. Newer-generation CT scanners move the patient continuously through the plane of the circling x-ray/detector array (thus sampling/slicing a spiral or helix through the patient, rather than discrete axial slices). The machines are faster and slices are thinner, and improved software allows the data to be displayed in the coronal or other orientations, with much-improved resolution (Figure 1–11B). Disadvantages of CT imaging include radiation exposure and potential adverse effects of iodinated contrast.

MAGNETIC RESONANCE IMAGING

MRI employs a powerful magnet to force the alignment of protons in hydrogen atoms, and a radio frequency pulse signal (RF pulse) to disturb this magnetically induced alignment. These protons emit their own radio frequency signal as they realign. The detection of this signal allows imaging of the density of hydrogen protons in tissue. The location of the emitted signal within three-dimensional space is made possible by using magnetic fields that form a gradient, as protons at a specific magnetic strength will produce a corresponding unique frequency response.

The echo time (TE) and repetition time (TR) are parameters of the radio frequency pulse signal that can be tailored to change the way the MRI depicts tissues. When TE and TR are set to short times (lower values) "T1-weighted" images are obtained. T1 images are also called longitudinal or spin-lattice relaxation time images. Long TE and TR times (higher values) produce "T2-weighted" images, also called transverse or spin-spin relation time images. T1 sequences show exquisite detail and anatomy. T2 sequences emphasize pathologic lesions. The cerebrospinal fluid (CSF) and the vitreous appear dark in T1 sequences (Figure 1–12A) and bright on T2 sequences (Figure 1–12B). Gadolinium (GTPA) is an intravenous contrast agent that provides enhancement of vascular structures, blood-brain barrier disruptions, and other lesions. Other specialized MRI techniques

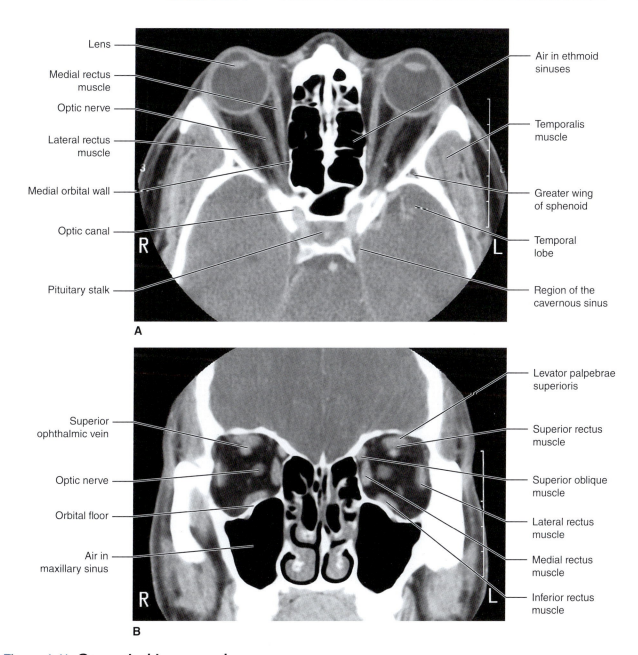

Figure 1–11. Computed tomography.
Important anatomic structures in these normal computed tomography (CT) images are labeled. Observe that CT (and magnetic resonance imaging [MRI]) images are presented with the patient's right side (R) on the viewer's left (just as if the patient were sitting in your examination chair, facing you). Examples of abnormal CT images can be found in Figures 4–36, 4–41, and 5–12. **(A)** Cranial CT, axial plane, In this soft-tissue window, bones appear bright, and air (as in the ethmoid sinuses) is black. **(B)** Cranial CT of the orbits, coronal plane. The coronal view is usually the best plane for visualizing the orbit and its contents.

can improve resolution and contrast (Table 1–8), and even reveal the *function* as well as the structure of the brain (discussed below).

IMAGING THE ORBIT

With *CT scanning*, the orbital structures are easily visualized even without contrast because the bone provides a high attenuation of x-rays (seen bright on CT images), and orbital fat and air in the sinuses offers the least attenuation (dark on CT images). The intermediate attenuation of the extraocular muscles, blood vessels, and optic nerve provides excellent natural contrast for visualization of orbital anatomy and pathology with CT (see Figure 1–11B). Coronal slices offer the best orientation for examining the orbital contents, for example, patterns of extraocular muscle enlargement help distinguish orbital Graves disease from idiopathic orbital inflammatory syndrome, cross sections of the optic nerve complex reveal enlargement from glioma or optic

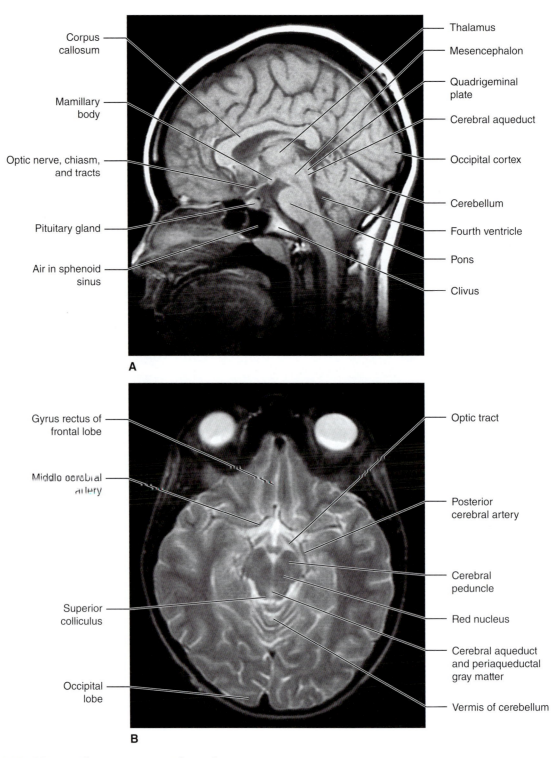

Figure 1–12. **Magnetic resonance imaging.**
Important anatomic structures are identified in these normal magnetic resonance imaging (MRI) scans. Examples of abnormal MRI images can be found in Figures 3–16, 3–22 to 3–24, 4–22, 4–23, 4–26, 4–27, 4–39, 5–5 to 5–9, 5–14, and 5–17. **(A)** T1-weighted MRI, mid-sagittal plane. T1 images usually reveal more anatomic detail of the normal brain than standard T2, and this same sequence is usually used to image with intravenous contrast. In T1 images, the cerebrospinal fluid (CSF) and vitreous appear dark. Sagittal images are particularly helpful in evaluating disorders affecting the chiasm, such as pituitary tumors. **(B)** T2-weighted MRI, axial plane at the level of the superior colliculus. Note that the vitreous and CSF appear bright on T2-weighted images. T2 images are usually better at showing disease states in the brain than T1 images. Much can be gained by comparing the signal characteristics between T1, T2, and contrast-enhanced images.

▶ TABLE 1-8. MAGNETIC RESONANCE IMAGING TECHNIQUES

MRI Modality	TR	TE	Technical/Imaging Characteristics	Advantages	Disadvantages
T1-weighted MRI	Short	Short	CSF (and vitreous) is dark and orbital fat is bright. Sequences can be run very fast—therefore has highest resolution.	High anatomic resolution; gadolinium contrast agent is used with this sequence to reveal disease states.	Bright signal from orbital fat obscures orbital details. See STIR sequence below.
T2-weighted MRI	Long	Long	Orbital fat is dark, and CSF/vitreous is bright. Maximizes differences in water content/state, thus is more sensitive to showing disease states.	Best sequence for showing edema resulting from inflammation, ischemia, demyelination.	Bright signal from CSF obscures periventricular details. See FLAIR sequence below.
Diffusion-weighted imaging (DWI)			Bright signal where there is apparent poor or limited diffusion of water, such as in cytotoxic edema.	Abnormal signal appears within 5-10 minutes of the onset of stroke.	Poorer resolution.
Short T1 inversion recovery (STIR)			Inversion-recovery pulse sequences suppress unwanted high signal from certain tissues.	A T1-weighted image but with suppression of bright signal from orbital fat to reveal orbital details.	
Fluid attenuated inversion recovery (FLAIR)	Very long	Long		A T2-weighted image but with suppression of bright signal from CSF to increase sensitivity for periventricular MS plaques.	
Magnetic resonance angiography (MRA)			Images blood flow with or without contrast agent.	Noninvasive, noncontrast method of evaluating intracranial vasculature (stenosis, aneurysms).	May not show all aneurysms or "the whole picture" since it only sees moving blood in the vessels.

Abbreviations: CSF, cerebrospinal fluid; MRI, magnetic resonance imaging; MS, multiple sclerosis; TE, time to echo; TR, time to repetition.

nerve sheath meningioma, enlargement of the superior ophthalmic vein is evident in some arteriovenous shunts, and the relationship of orbital masses to normal structures can be evaluated. The coronal views also offer the best perspective for trauma, visualizing orbital wall fractures (and soft tissue entrapment) or optic canal fractures. In the past, marked neck extension was required to obtain "true" coronal CT images—not practical in many acute trauma cases because of possible cervical vertebral instability—but high-quality reconstructed coronal views are now possible with the advent of spiral CT imaging. Imaging characteristics of lesions after giving iodinated contrast may further define the disease process. Orbital imaging (thin slice, coronal views) must be specifically requested when orbital disease is suspected, because a standard CT of the brain does not have adequate views of the orbit.

With standard T1 MRI sequences, orbital fat is very bright, obscuring anatomic detail. Special orbital fat–suppression pulse sequences reduce the overwhelming bright signal from the orbital fat to provide orbital detail that rivals CT imaging. With the use of a surface coil over the eye, the resolution of the orbit with MRI is greatly enhanced, but this technique does not allow simultaneous imaging of the brain. Unlike CT, MRI does not image bone (or fractures) or calcifications (which may be important in characterizing lesions such as meningiomas).

Overall, CT is preferred for imaging the orbit in most situations, showing bone and soft tissues well, even without contrast. However, when both the brain and the orbits need to be imaged, MRI is favored since it is superior to CT in imaging the intracranial contents in most cases, and is adequate in resolving orbital structures. Not uncommonly, both modalities may be needed to characterize an orbital lesion.

IMAGING THE BRAIN

MRI has clear advantages over CT in imaging of the intracranial contents: bony structures at the skull base limit CT resolution of the sella and posterior fossa, but are not a factor with MRI; white and gray matter have similar x-ray attenuation, but MRI easily distinguishes between these tissues. MRI has traditionally had an advantage over CT in that MRI can be viewed equally well in any orientation, but spiral CT is closing the gap in permitting viewing of data in any plane.

Cortical infarcts are not evident on CT scanning until 1 to 2 days after an event. They initially appear darker than normal brain, and eventually enhance with contrast at 3 to 7 days. MRI usually shows an infarct within several hours as a dark area on T1 and bright area on T2, with special sequences that can reveal ischemia even earlier.

Hemorrhage is easy to see immediately on CT as a bright signal, fading in intensity over 4 to 6 weeks. This characteristic makes CT ideal for evaluating patients with acute stroke who are being considered for urgent thrombolytics, because intracranial hemorrhage is a contraindication. With MRI, the changing signal characteristics of free blood offer information on the timing of a hemorrhagic event: initially hyper dense centrally and dark peripherally on T2 images, they become darker centrally and brighter peripherally over time.

Despite the clear advantages of MRI in intracranial imaging, CT imaging of the brain remains an important tool for the following reasons: CT is best for visualizing acute hemorrhage in the brain; patients with metal from injury or surgery may not be able to have an MRI; CT imaging is less expensive than MRI; the CT scanning apparatus is less claustrophobic and intimidating to the patient than MRI; some obese patients who are too heavy or too large for the MRI can have CT scans. MRI machines with "open magnets" may be an alternative for claustrophobic or heavy patients, but are limited in their magnetic strength, and therefore have less resolution than standard "closed" MRI.

CEREBRAL ANGIOGRAPHY

Imaging of the cerebral vasculature is important in many diseases of interest to neuro-ophthalmologists, such as aneurysms, vascular occlusions, arteriovenous malformations, dural sinus thrombosis, arterial dissections, and vasculitis.

Magnetic resonance angiography (MRA) takes advantage of the unique signal characteristics from the moving bloodstream to provide clear views of the intracranial vascular structures with *or without* intravenous contrast material (Figure 1–13). The sequences may also be tailored to emphasize the venous structures (magnetic resonance venography [MRV]). These techniques currently lack the detail and dynamic properties of conventional angiography, and are thus less sensitive. However, since MRA and MRV are noninvasive tests, they are very useful diagnostic tools.

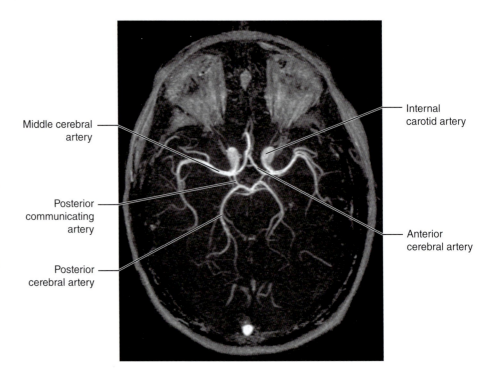

Figure 1-13. **Magnetic resonance angiography.** Specialized magnetic resonance imaging (MRI) sequences can be used to selectively view the intracranial arterial structures. This image from a magnetic resonance angiogram (MRA) shows the circle of Willis in detail. An example of magnetic resonance venography (MRV) can be seen in Figure 4–23.

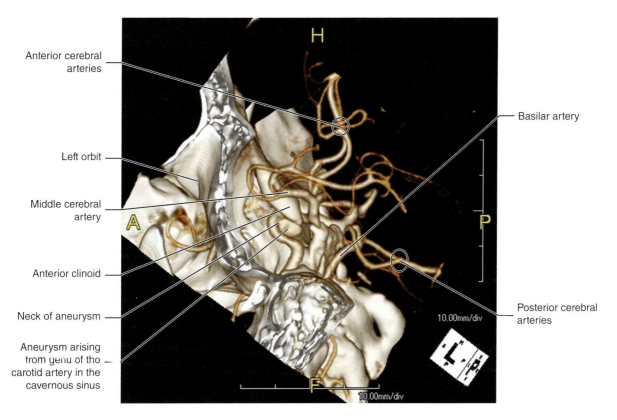

Figure 1-14. **Computed tomographic angiography of an intracavernous carotid aneurysm.** A 45-year-old woman presented with pain and a right third cranial nerve palsy. The computed tomography angiography (CTA) study did not show the expected posterior communicating aneurysm, but instead showed a right intracavernous carotid aneurysm compressing the third cranial nerve in the cavernous sinus. This CTA is presented as a 3-dimensional image of the intracranial arteries and the aneurysm as well as surrounding structures. The software allows control over the viewing angle, as well as the degree of transparency of the nonvascular structures.

CT angiography (CTA) combines traditional methods of intravascular contrast injection with 3-D imaging (spiral or helical CT). This permits a 3-D reconstruction of the data, not only detailing the vasculature, but also showing surrounding anatomy (Figure 1–14). With rapid advances in the quality and acquisition time of CT imaging, CTA and CTV (CT venography) have rivaled MRI techniques for diagnosing entities such as posterior communicating aneurysms or venous sinus stenosis.

Despite the excellent vascular imaging from both MRA and CTA, catheter angiography remains the gold standard in most vascular imaging, particularly when looking for aneurysms and arteriovenous malformations. *Catheter angiography* employs x-rays images with the injection of iodinated contrast into the vessels by way of intravascular catheters that enter vascular spaces, usually via the femoral artery or vein *Digital subtraction angiography (DSA)* uses images obtained before the contrast is introduced to digitally subtract unwanted structures in the contrasted study, increasing image quality and reducing the amount of contrast needed. By carefully advancing the catheters under fluoroscopic guidance, specific vessels can be injected and imaged. Unlike MRA and CTA, catheter angiography is a dynamic study—the neuroradiologist can see the sequence of flow as the study is being performed (Figure 1–15A). This technique allows for therapeutic intervention as well as diagnosis in some conditions: the interventional neuroradiologist can directly treat some aneurysms (Figure 1–15B), arteriovenous malformations, and fistulas with injectable thrombotic coils and glue; stenotic vessels with stents, and thrombosed vessels with thrombolytic agents delivered intravascularly at the site. Three-dimensional DSA (3-D DSA) provides an additional level of visualizing vascular structures, which is of particular value in evaluating cerebral aneurysms. 3-D DSA images can be merged with other 3-D imaging modalities to reveal the precise location of vascular structures to surrounding anatomy not typically visible on DSA. DSA remains the gold standard at present, but CT and MRI neurovascular imaging techniques are improving rapidly. DSA is an invasive technique, and the risk of stroke and other potential complications must be considered.

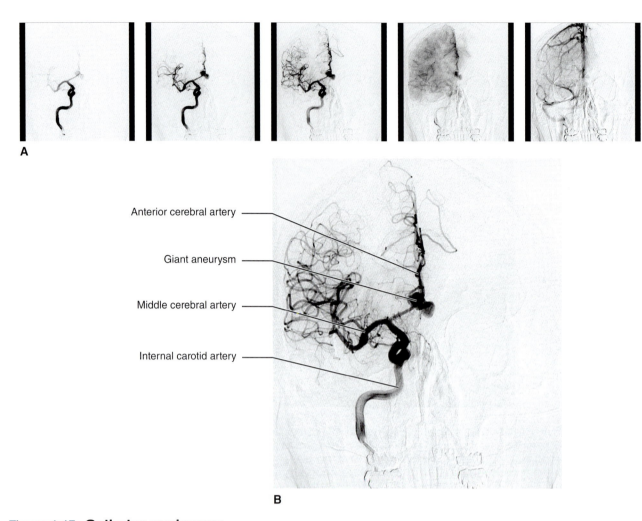

Figure 1–15. **Catheter angiogram.**
By controlling the position of an intravascular catheter (via fluoroscopy) the interventional radiologist can inject and visualize selected vascular structures. The fact that this is a dynamic study is often not appreciated, as the study is usually documented with selected still images. **(A)** This sequence of images (from a right internal carotid injection, anteroposterior view) shows flow from the internal carotid into the middle and anterior cerebral arteries, and in the last frame, venous drainage through dural venous sinuses. **(B)** This patient has a giant aneurysm at the junction of the right A1 segment and anterior communicating artery.

FUNCTIONAL NEUROIMAGING

Neuroimaging technology has come a long way since plain film x-ray and pneumoencephalography. Not only can we see the form and structure of the brain in greater detail, it is now possible to create images and maps of brain *function*.

Functional MRI maps changing neural activity by measuring (imaging) the ratio of oxygenated hemoglobin to deoxygenated hemoglobin. The technique produces low-resolution images, but permits real-time monitoring of the brain's response to various experimental stimuli. Functional MRI is also sensitive for ischemic processes at the earliest stages.

Magnetic resonance spectroscopy can detect and measure levels of a variety of metabolites in body tissues. It can be used to diagnose CNS metabolic disorders and evaluate tumor metabolism. This technique produces a spectroscopy signal, not an image. *Magnetic resonance spectroscopic imaging (MRSI)* combines both spectroscopic and imaging methods to produce a low-spatial-resolution image map of selected metabolites.

Positron emission tomography (PET) maps emissions from radiotracer accumulation in the brain and body, producing 2-D or 3-D images. The radiotracer (or ligand) is a radioactively labeled metabolic compound injected intravenously; many different ligands are available to look for specific metabolic activities. PET-CT simultaneously performs a PET scan and CT imaging, superimposing the low-resolution PET scan images on high-resolution CT images (Figure 1–16). PET and PET-CT scans are used for diagnosis of brain tumors, strokes, and dementia (particularly Alzheimer disease and Pick disease).

Single photon emission computed tomography (SPECT) is similar to PET scanning but uses gamma

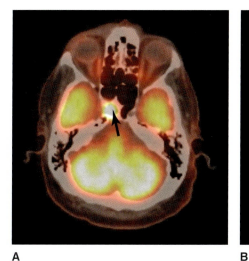
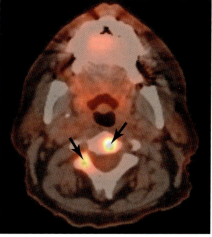
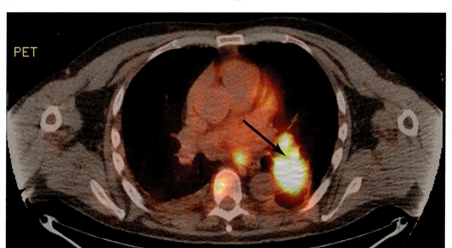

Figure 1-16. **Positron emission tomography-computed tomography.** A 62-year-old man presented with a progressive right abduction deficit. Magnetic resonance imaging (MRI) showed a right cavernous sinus mass, suspected to be metastatic. Positron emission tomography-computed tomography (PET-CT) revealed the right cavernous sinus lesion and multiple metastases (*short arrows*), with a lung mass presumed to be the primary neoplasm (*long arrow*), shown in these images through the brain (**A** and **B**) and chest (**C**). Note the normal high metabolic activity of the brain (**A**).

ray–emitting radioisotopes and a gamma camera to image. Tracer uptake and detection is much quicker than PET, thus it has higher temporal resolution (useful in epilepsy) but similar low spatial resolution.

Magnetoencephalography (MEG) uses an array of very sensitive superconducting quantum interference devices (SQUIDs) to measure the magnetic fields that are produced by electrical neural activity in the brain. This technique produces a real-time map of brain activity (high temporal resolution), but with poor spatial resolution. It is useful primarily as a research tool to map brain function, but can be used to localize the source of pathological brain activity.

► KEY POINTS

- The patient's complaints should be listed and prioritized by the *patient's* degree of concern. This list should then be the basis for the assessment and plan discussed with the patient at the conclusion of the consultation.
- Important characteristics of symptoms include location, quality, severity, timing, duration, context, modifying factors, and associated symptoms.
- For patients with visual loss, the time course (unchanging, improving, worsening, fluctuating, or transient) is often the most important diagnostic clue in the history.
- Positive visual disturbances—flashes, spots of light, iridescent zig-zags, formed hallucinations—have a myriad of causes, and a skillful history is the most productive diagnostic "procedure."
- "Blurry vision" is not always a problem with the afferent visual system—ocular misalignment (efferent visual system dysfunction) is sometimes described as blurry, rather than double.
- Diplopia resulting from binocular misalignment (strabismus) disappears when either eye is covered.
- Monocular diplopia is most commonly caused by cataract or cornea/ocular surface disease.
- Photographs of the patient (driver's license, etc) often help determine the duration of ptosis, anisocoria, or strabismus.

- Occasionally patients may complain of a droopy eyelid when the eyelid retraction of the contralateral eye is the real problem.
- Patients are quick to ascribe pupillary inequality to a "bad eye," but the examiner will need to wait for the pupillary examination to determine which pupil—the smaller or the larger of the two—is the abnormal one.
- Patients often have a self-diagnosis for chronic or recurrent pain, such as blaming "sinus disease" for migraine headaches.
- Photophobia can be caused by ocular disease (ie, ocular surface disease, iritis) or CNS disease (eg, meningitis, migraine). Photophobia without evident eye or brain disease ("essential photophobia") may have an organic basis.
- The medication history often suggests diseases that the patient did not reveal in the medical history.
- Patients may not consider vitamins, birth control pills, daily aspirin, hormonal supplements, or "prn" medications in their medication list, and may need to be specifically asked.
- A careful history is time well invested, because the history and basic examination determine which of many specialized examination techniques will lead to a diagnosis.
- Ophthalmic clinical photography often provides the best documentation for following pathology of the fundus, ocular media, ocular surface, and adnexa, and associated systemic manifestations.
- IVTA is a method of imaging the vascular system of the retina and choroid, and is particularly helpful in revealing neovascularization and vascular leakage.
- OCT is a noninvasive method for imaging the layers of the retina and optic disc, permitting rapid diagnosis of previously elusive macular disorders and providing an objective measure of optic nerve health by measuring the thickness of the peripapillary retinal nerve fiber layer.
- CT (even without contrast) is an excellent method for imaging the orbit.
- A variety of MRI sequences permit tailoring of image acquisition and presentation to accentuate certain imaging characteristics (such as inversion recovery for suppressing unwanted high signal in some tissues, DWI to see early stroke).
- When both the brain and the orbits need to be imaged, MRI is favored because it is superior to CT in imaging the intracranial contents and can also image the orbits.
- Cerebral (catheter) angiography is the gold standard at present for neurovascular imaging (aneurysm, AVM, etc); CT angiography is "high yield," but requires iodinated contrast. MRA is noninvasive and convenient to do concomitantly with MRI, but is less sensitive than CTA in some cases.

SUGGESTED READING

Books

Bose, S, Bubin R: Principles of imaging in neuro-ophthalmology, in Yanoff M, Duker JS (eds): *Ophthalmology*, 3d ed. Edinburgh: Mosby Elsevier; 2009:943ff.

Coleman DJ: *Ultrasonography of the Eye and Orbit*, 2d ed. Philadelphia, PA: Lippincott Williams & Wilkins; 2006.

Digre KB, Corbett JJ: *Practical Viewing of the Optic Disc*. Boston, MA: Butterworth-Heinemann; 2003.

Dutton, JJ: *Radiology of the Orbit and Visual Pathways*. Philadelphia, PA: Saunders Elsevier; 2010.

Eustace P: Neuro-ophthalmic history and examination, in Rosen ES, Thompson HS, Cumming WJK, et al. (eds): *Neuro-ophthalmology*. London: Mosby International Limited; 1998.

Saine PJ, Tyler ME (eds): *Ophthalmic Photography: A Textbook of Retinal Photography, Angiography and Electronic Imaging*. Boston, MA: Butterworth-Heinemann; 1997:297–306.

Wall M, Johnson CA: Principles and techniques of the examination of the visual sensory system, in Miller NR, Newman NJ, Biousse V, et al (eds): *Walsh and Hoyts' Clinical Neuro-ophthalmology*, vol 1, 6th ed. Baltimore, MD: Williams and Wilkins; 2005:83ff.

Articles

Digre KD, Brennan KC: Shedding light on photophobia. *Neuro-Ophthalmol* 2012;32:68–81.

ffytche DH: Visual hallucinations in eye disease. *Curr Opin Neurol* 2009;22(1):28–35.

Hedges TR Jr: Charles Bonnet, his life, and his syndrome. *Surv Ophthalmol* 2007;52(1):111–114.

Kardon, RH: Role of the macular optical coherence tomography scan in neuro-ophthalmology. *J Neuro-Ophthalmol* 2011;31:353–361.

Subei AM, Eggenberger ER: Optical coherence tomography: another useful tool in a neuro-ophthalmologist's armamentarium. *Curr Opin Ophthalmol* 2009;20(6):462–466.

Vaphiades MS: Imaging the neurovisual system. *Ophthalmol Clin North Am* 2004;17(3):465–480.

SECTION II

The Sensory Visual System

The process of "seeing" begins with the eyes in the front of the cranium; the visual pathways then traverse the length of the brain to the occipital cortex, where visual information is then passed forward to many cortical areas. It is no surprise that in addition to ocular diseases, many intracranial disorders interrupt and damage these pathways, producing visual loss.

This section begins with a discussion of the clinical tools used to evaluate afferent visual function (Chapter 2).

In Chapter 3, patterns of visual field loss are discussed in the context of the organization of the visual system. Chapters 4 and 5 explore the neuroanatomy of the afferent visual pathways and specific disease states that can affect it. Chapter 6 discusses a common reason for neuro-ophthalmic consultation: unexplained visual loss.

CHAPTER 2

Testing Sensory Visual Function

- ▶ CLINICAL TESTS OF CENTRAL VISUAL FUNCTION 32
  - Visual acuity testing 32
  - Contrast sensitivity testing 35
  - Brightness sense testing 37
  - Photo-stress testing 38
  - Amsler grid testing 38
  - Color vision testing 39
  - Stereopsis testing 40
  - Other tests of central vision 41
- ▶ VISUAL FIELD TESTING 41
  - The visual field: size and shape 41
  - Perimetry techniques 43
  - Interpreting perimetry results 52
- ▶ PHYSIOLOGICAL AND ELECTROPHYSIOLOGICAL RESPONSES 52
  - Relative afferent pupillary defect 52
  - Electrophysiological tests 53
- ▶ KEY POINTS 56

As discussed in Chapter 1, the clinical examination evaluates the *structure* (eg, eye examination, neuroimaging) and the *function* of the visual apparatus. The structural aspects of the examination are relatively objective, but as we shall see in this chapter, evaluating *function* introduces a significant subjective component.

In order to understand, treat, and follow disorders of the visual system, it is vital to measure how well a patient sees. Although seemingly simple, this task is far more difficult than one might think. Vision is a sensory experience, and sensory examinations are inherently difficult to perform and interpret. Most tests of visual function are subjective, since the examiner depends on the patient's description of what he or she perceives in response to a test stimulus. For this reason, visual function testing suffers from the same shortcomings as all other sensory tests—testing is subjective and depends on the willingness and ability of the patient to respond. Important exceptions to this general rule include clinical tests that employ *physiological* responses (the relative afferent pupillary defect [RAPD] test and optokinetic nystagmus [OKN] test) and *electrophysiological* tests (full-field and multifocal electroretinogram [ERG] and visually evoked potential [VEP] tests). Functional neuroimaging, as discussed in Chapter 1, could also be theoretically included in this group of objective tests of visual function.

The subjective nature of visual function testing requires that clinical tests of visual function be *interpreted* by the examiner. The meaning of the test result depends on the limitations of the study, reliability of the patient's input, and correlation with the objective aspects of the examination. The results of visual function testing can be confusing in patients who cannot or will not cooperate fully, or when the subjective and objective components of the examination do not fully agree, as with nonorganic visual loss (discussed in detail in Chapter 6).

The complexity of the visual experience also makes it difficult to objectively quantify. Vision cannot be fully characterized by a number such as "20/30," as it encompasses an expansive panorama of colors, contrasts, shadows, and motion. Even the most sophisticated clinical tests provide only an estimate of a limited aspect of visual function, and the data may not correlate directly with a patient's experience in the real world. To obtain a meaningful assessment of a patient's visual function, a number of different tests may be required. Choosing the appropriate tests requires an accurate and directed history (as discussed in Chapter 1) and an understanding of the types (and limitations) of clinical tests of visual function.

The important features of clinical tests that measure central vision and the visual fields, as well as physiological and electrophysiological responses that can be used to assess visual function, are explored in this chapter. Emphasis is placed on the three tests that form the basis of all afferent vision assessments, often called the "vital signs of vision": visual acuity, visual field, and relative afferent pupillary defect (RAPD) testing.

▶ CLINICAL TESTS OF CENTRAL VISUAL FUNCTION

The visual axis of the eye is coincident with *the foveloa*. The foveola is the center of the *fovea*, a specialized area of the retina that corresponds to central vision. The unique architecture and neural circuitry of the fovea permit high resolution and sensitivity, which are vital for important visual tasks such as reading and recognizing faces. Patients are generally symptomatic from even the most minor disturbances in their central vision.

VISUAL ACUITY TESTING

Visual acuity tests are composed of lines of characters that become progressively smaller, presented as a printed wall chart or near card, or by a projector system or computer. The most common format, the *Snellen visual acuity test*, uses uppercase letters as the test characters (optotypes) (Figure 2–1A). Other optotypes are available that do not depend on alphabet recognition, such as the line pictures that are used to test young children, or Landolt rings (shaped like the letter "c") and "tumbling Es," in which patients are asked to simply identify the orientation of the character (Figure 2–2). Unlike the Snellen visual acuity chart, LogMAR acuity tests present the same number of optotypes for each acuity line. This uniformity is necessary for statistical modeling in research studies (Figure 2–3).

In almost every case, the physician is primarily interested in the patient's *best corrected* visual acuity, so the test is performed with the patient wearing his or her glasses.

Visual acuity testing is typically performed at 20 feet. At this distance, accommodation is relaxed and unlikely to interfere with measuring the patient's true distance acuity (or determining their refraction). However, near cards are far more practical for the bedside examination (Figure 2–4), as long as the examiner allows for presbyopia (typically in patients older than 45 years) by having them wear their bifocals or reading glasses.

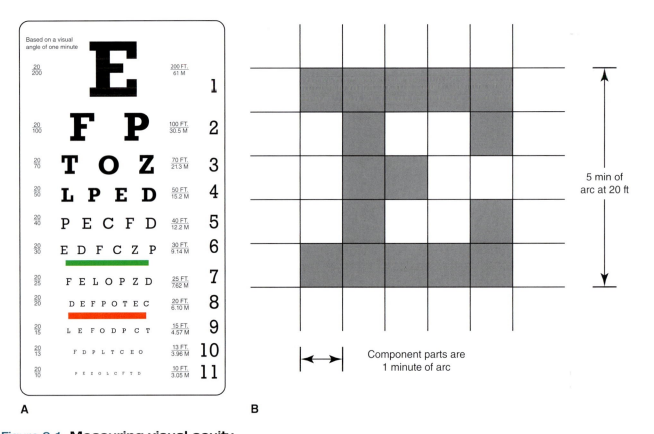

Figure 2–1. Measuring visual acuity.
(A) Snellen visual acuity wall chart. **(B)** The 20/20 letters subtend 5 minutes of arc, with each component part measuring 1 minute. Thus visual resolution of at least 1 minute of arc is required to identify the characters on the 20/20 line.

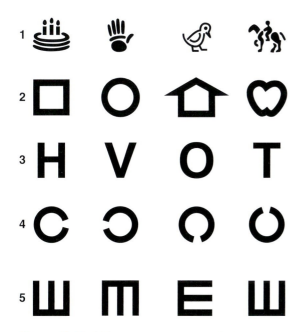

Figure 2–2. Other common optotypes used in testing visual acuity.
A variety of optotypes are available to test young children or illiterate adults. The subject may simply name the object or point to a matching picture on a control card that has large images of the symbols: Allen figures (1), Lea symbols (2), HOTV optotypes (3).

Other optotypes require the subject to say or point to show the orientation of the optotype, or to orient a symbol card he or she is holding to match the symbol on the chart: Landolt rings (4), "tumbling Es" (5).

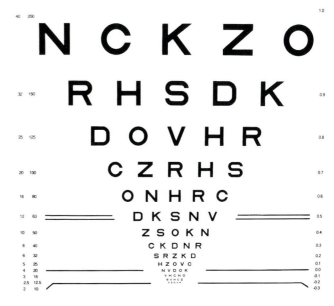

Figure 2–3. LogMAR visual acuity tests.
Snellen acuity testing has a number of shortcomings, the most obvious being that the various lines do not have the same number of test letters, ranging from one 20/400 letter to eight 20/20 letters. This causes nonuniformity of perception (crowding phenomenon) and makes statistical comparisons of changes in acuity cumbersome. LogMAR charts, such as the ETDRS (Early Treatment Diabetic Retinopathy Study) acuity chart pictured, have the same number of optotypes on each line, forming an inverted pyramid. The size of the optotype changes linearly, so visual acuities can be reported as the log of the angle of discrimination (a statistically friendly number). LogMAR acuity charts are used primarily in clinical research studies. This visual acuity chart uses Sloan letters, a letter optotype that is analogous to the Landolt C rings.

With Snellen acuity testing, the smallest line in which the patient can identify correctly more than one-half of the characters is designated as the Snellen visual acuity. A "+" modifier shows that a few characters on the next smallest line were also correctly named; a "−" modifier identifies the number of characters missed on the designated acuity line (eg, 20/30 − 2, 20/60 + 3) (Figure 2–5).

The Snellen acuity notation is expressed as a fraction, with the *numerator* identifying the standard testing distance, typically 20 feet. Characters on the 20/20 line subtend an angular size of 5 minutes of an arc. To recognize a 20/20 character, the subject must be able to resolve components of the letter that measure 1 minute of arc (Figure 2–1B). The *denominator* in the Snellen notation designates the relative size of the test character. The 20/200 E is 10 times larger than the 20/20 letters on the chart. The denominator can also be thought of as the distance at which letters on a given line would subtend 5 minutes of arc. For example, a 20/100 letter at 100 feet has the same angular size as a 20/20 letter at 20 feet: Both measure 5 minutes of an arc. A practical way of understanding Snellen notation is as follows: A

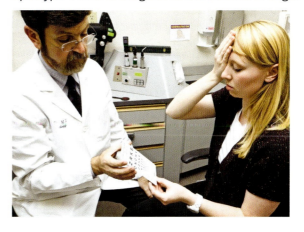

Figure 2–4. Using a near card.
There are a variety of near cards (with a selection of optotypes) available for testing visual acuity at the bedside. Important considerations include (1) patients need to wear their best correction for reading (bifocals or reading glasses); (2) testing distance should be uniform, typically 14 inches; (3) lighting should be adequate; (4) the medical record should reflect use of the near card and glasses worn.

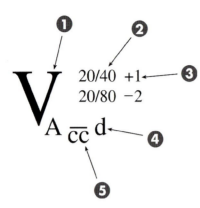

Figure 2-5. Notation of visual acuity.
"V_A" is the standard notation for visual acuity (1). The visual acuity of the right eye is written on top (2) (often designated OD or RE), and the left eye on the bottom (OS or LE). A "+" or "−" is added to the Snellen acuity (3) to note that the subject read a few letters on the following line (+), or to show the number of letters that could not be read on the designated acuity line (−). A "d" (or no designation) means that the standard 20-foot test distance was observed (4). An "n" shows that a near card (with Snellen-equivalent notation) was used to test the visual acuity (such as at the bedside). Patients who wear glasses should wear them when visual acuity is being tested (designated as "cc" for "with correction") (5). If no glasses are worn, the designation "sc" is used.

patient with 20/100 visual acuity (at 20 feet) can only distinguish what a normal-sighted person could still read from 100 feet.

The standard *metric* testing distance for Snellen visual acuity is 6 meters. Thus, the metric equivalent of 20/20 acuity is 6/6. Conversion between acuities obtained in feet or meters can be performed by treating the notation as a simple fraction: 20/40 = 6/12, 20/200 = 6/60.

Some patients may have such poor vision that they cannot see even the largest characters on the acuity chart at the standard testing distance. For these patients, the testing distance can be shortened, or methods other than Snellen acuity can be used to define the visual acuity (Box 2–1).

Visual acuity testing is performed one eye at a time. Care must be taken to fully occlude the other eye. Patients may inadvertently peek around handheld occluders with their better eye. This situation typically occurs when spectacles prevent close apposition of the occluder to the eye, or when patients insist on moving their head around to see better. In an effort to please, children frequently peek with their better eye. The patient's (or examiner's) hand may be used to cover an eye. The palm of the hand, not the fingers, should be used to insure occlusion. In patients wearing glasses, a folded tissue can be slipped behind the lens and positioned for reliable occlusion if a handheld occluder is not available or sufficient.

The measured visual acuity is severely affected by refractive errors. Thus, the visual acuity test is not a good indicator of the health of the visual pathways unless all refractive errors are accounted for. Although "pinhole acuity" can give a rough idea of true visual acuity, whenever possible, a full refraction should be obtained to determine the *best corrected visual acuity* on every patient with a complaint of visual loss (Box 2–2).

Much can be learned by simply listening to patients as they attempt to read a visual acuity chart. Patients with homonymous hemianopic visual field defects may consistently fail to see the first or last letters of a line.

▶ BOX 2-1. MEASURING AND RECORDING POOR VISUAL ACUITY

Shortening the test distance. Patients who cannot see even the largest Snellen letter can be tested by shortening the testing distance, either by bringing the patient closer to the chart or moving the acuity chart closer to the patient. At 10 feet, the test letters are twice the angular size than at 20 feet. As the numerator denotes the testing distance, a patient who could only see the 20/200 letters *at 5 feet* would be designated as 5/200. Because the Snellen notation can be treated as a simple fraction, this visual acuity would be equivalent to 20/800.

Tumbling E card. Rather than moving the chart or the patient, a 20/200 "tumbling E" card allows the examiner to test at any distance. The examiner can hold the card as close as required to the patient and vary its orientation. For example, if the patient can consistently state (or point at) which direction the 20/200 E is pointing at 5 feet, the visual acuity would be recorded as 5/200.

Counting fingers (CF). An alternative for patients whose visual acuity is "off the chart" is to record the distance at which the patient can accurately count the examiner's fingers, for example, CF 5', CF 2'. The size and spacing of an examiner's outstretched fingers is roughly the same size as the 20/200 E. Thus, CF 5' can be thought of as being (approximately) equivalent to 5/200.

Tests for very poor vision. For patients who cannot see well enough to count fingers, the ability to see *hand movement (HM)* is recorded. Patients with severe visual loss may have only *light perception (LP)*, which can be further subdivided as "LP with projection," "LP without projection," or no light perception (NLP).

▶ **BOX 2-2. PINHOLE ACUITY**

We appropriately emphasize the necessity of determining the patient's true best-corrected visual acuity. Decreased visual acuity that can be corrected with the phoropter suggests the need for eyeglasses, rather than an extensive evaluation. Conversely, vision that cannot be fully corrected with lenses suggests pathology. Pinhole acuity provides a reasonable substitute when a phoropter and refraction are not available, as may be the case in a neurology clinic. The pinhole is an optical trick that essentially serves as a universal lens, much like a pinhole camera. Visual acuity measured with a pinhole is a reasonable approximation of visual acuity at distance when a simple refractive error is the only problem. Since the pinhole eliminates optical aberrations from corneal and lenticular astigmatism, it can provide better acuity than glasses in a condition with irregular astigmatism such as keratoconus. Patients with monocular diplopia from optical media (eg, cataract, ocular surface disease) will note that their diplopia disappears with a pinhole.

Patients should have their visual acuity tested one eye at a time (first without the pinhole) in their distance glasses, if they have them. If the visual acuity is not good, then test with the pinhole (have patients keep their glasses on if they have them). It sometimes takes patients a few seconds to find a hole to look through. Significant improvement in the acuity means that the subnormal visual acuity is likely a refractive (glasses) issue, rather than pathological. However, be aware that some disorders can cause refractive changes secondarily, such as a myopic shift with cataract, or a hyperopic shift with papilledema or orbital mass.

Patients with marked constriction of the visual field, such as with retinitis pigmentosa, might have great difficulty even locating the eye chart in front of them, but may then read the smallest lines once they are "lined up."

The widespread use of Snellen visual acuity testing allows a common basis to compare visual acuities obtained almost anywhere. Unfortunately, the comparisons will be rough estimates at best, because there are so many uncontrollable variables inherent in this test method: different instruments for presenting the chart, variations in illumination of the chart, inconsistent light-adaptation of the patient, and varying examiner techniques.

CONTRAST SENSITIVITY TESTING

Visual experiences in the real world often consist of vague and subtle contrast differences, not at all like the high-contrast visual acuity letters tested in the physician's office (Figure 2–6). Contrast sensitivity testing requires the subject to try to discern the presence (or orientation) of "fuzzy bars." The test is composed of alternating bright and dark lines, where luminance varies sinusoidally (Figure 2–7A, B). By varying the spacing of the bars (spatial frequency) and amplitude of the sinusoidal wave (contrast), the data collected determine a contrast sensitivity *curve* (Figure 2–7C), rather than a single value like the Snellen visual acuity. As with visual acuity testing, a number of modalities exist for presenting contrast stimuli including wall charts, projector systems, near cards, and computer-generated tests. The Pelli-Robson Contrast Sensitivity Chart is a popular variation that combines classic optotypes with decreasing contrast (Figure 2–8).

In some cases, patients with visual complaints have relatively normal visual acuities, but abnormal contrast sensitivity curves (Box 2–3). For example, patients with multiple sclerosis may do relatively well at the high and low frequency ends of the spectrum, but may be missing a "notch" in the mid-range. Chronic papilledema and glaucoma may affect the low-frequency end of the curve, leaving the high spatial frequencies relatively unscathed. Cataract and refractive errors affect the high-frequency end far more severely than the rest of the curve.

Like most tests of central vision, the contrast sensitivity test is rarely diagnostic by itself; rather, it offers additional information regarding the nature of visual loss. Measuring contrast sensitivity is particularly

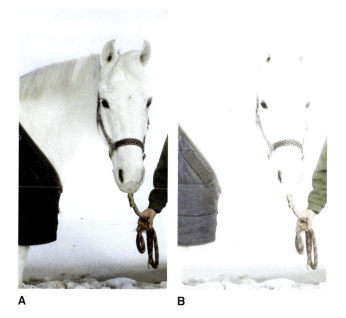

Figure 2-6. Effect of loss of contrast.
(A) Normal contrast image. **(B)** Same view with reduced contrast, as a patient with a posterior subcapsular cataract might see.

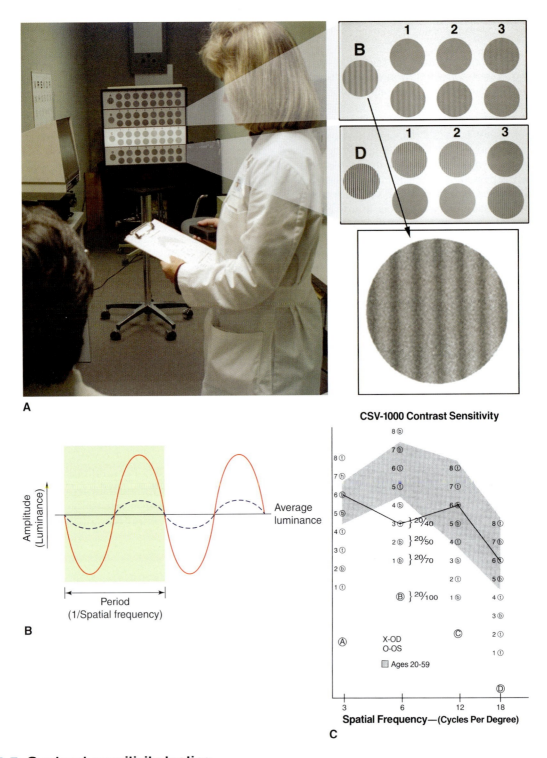

Figure 2–7. Contrast sensitivity testing.
(A) This version of a contrast sensitivity test (CSV-1000 VectorVision, Inc., Dayton, OH) uses an illuminated distance chart. This format is a "forced-choice" test, because the patient is asked to identify which of two circles contains the contrast sensitivity pattern. The gratings are in four groups of increasing spatial frequency from top to bottom. Within each group, the contrast level decreases from left to right.
(B) The gratings have a sinusoidal luminance, with the spatial frequency corresponding to the cycle of the sine wave, and contrast corresponding to the amplitude. The red curve in this diagram has the highest contrast. The dashed blue curve is lower in contrast, but both have the same spatial frequency and average luminance. **(C)** The results of the test are plotted, with spatial frequency on the horizontal axis and contrast on the vertical axis. Normal age-matched values are provided as shaded areas. This subject has an abnormal "notch" at an intermediate frequency, resulting from a previous episode of optic neuritis.

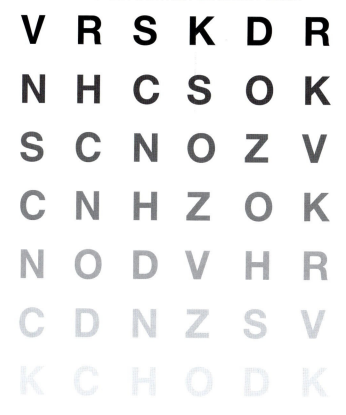

Figure 2–8. **Pelli-Robson contrast acuity chart.** Letter optotypes of the same size are presented with decreasing contrast. (Used with permission from Pelli DG, Robson JG, Wilkins AJ. The design of a new letter chart for measuring contrast sensitivity. *Clinical Vision Sciences* 1988;2(3):187–199.)

useful as part of a battery of optic nerve function tests when clinical decisions rest on subtle progression of disease (eg, optic nerve sheath meningioma, compressive orbital Graves disease, or chronic papilledema).

BRIGHTNESS SENSE TESTING

Patients with optic nerve disorders may describe their vision as dim, rather than blurry. For example, a patient who has recovered from optic neuritis may note a dramatic difference in brightness between the normal and affected eyes, even when the visual acuity and visual field in each eye are relatively normal. Such patients may volunteer that the light of the slitlamp or indirect ophthalmoscope is more tolerable in their affected eye.

> ► **BOX 2-3. PARALLEL RETINOGENICULATE PATHWAYS**
>
> There are many types of ganglion cells identified in the retina, each type coding for different kinds of information, and some projecting to destinations other than the lateral geniculate nucleus (LGN). Mammalian visual systems demonstrate (at least) two distinct projections of axons from the retina ganglion cells to the LGN, with distinct projections from the LGN to the visual cortex. These parallel pathways are most evident anatomically in the LGN, where axons from specific groups of ganglion cells synapse with specific populations of neurons in the LGN (see Figure 5–13). These anatomically distinct LGN neurons are thought to subserve different components of visual perception and define distinct "channels" of visual information processing: Small parvocellular neurons (P cells) transmit color and fine discrimination information; larger magnocellular neurons (M cells) transmit information about motion, stereopsis, and low spatial frequency contrast sensitivity. The extent to which some disorders of the visual system preferentially affect one or the other of these parallel systems can be of diagnostic help. Most physicians are more familiar with tests that predominantly evaluate the parvocellular system than with the more specialized clinical tests that examine the magnocellular system. Other than contrast sensitivity testing, M-system tests are not routinely used by most physicians, but are of value in evaluating neuro-ophthalmic disorders.
>
> **P-system tests**
>
> Visual acuity testing
> Color discrimination
> Contrast sensitivity testing (high spatial frequencies)
>
> **M-system tests**
>
> Motion discrimination tests
> Critical flicker fusion testing
> Tests of stereopsis
> Contrast sensitivity testing (low spatial frequencies)

The simplest brightness test consists of shining a bright light in each eye in turn and asking the patient to comment on the perceived brightness. Many physicians have the patient subjectively grade the brightness in the affected eye, comparing it to the normal eye at 100%. The brightness difference between the two eyes may also be measured by using neutral density filters of varying density over the normal eye, in an attempt to subjectively match the two eyes. Brightness sense testing is generally useful only in patients with monocular disorders, because a normal eye is needed for comparison.

PHOTO-STRESS TESTING

Not uncommonly, it may be difficult to determine whether central visual loss is due to pathology in the retina (macula) or the optic nerve. In the diseased macula, photoreceptors take longer to recover from a very bright light (photo-stress) than in the healthy retina. Photo-stress recovery time is not altered by optic nerve disease. The photo-stress test is performed by first identifying the smallest line on the Snellen acuity chart that the patient can read under normal testing conditions with each eye. Each eye in turn is then exposed to a bright light (such as the indirect ophthalmoscope beam) for 10 seconds to bleach the macula. The time it takes for the patient to recover the ability to read the designated Snellen acuity line is measured for each eye. Prolonged photo-stress recovery times suggest macular rather than optic nerve disease. Similar to brightness sense testing, photo-stress testing is mainly beneficial in patients with monocular complaints (who have a normal eye for comparison).

AMSLER GRID TESTING

The Amsler grid is a square containing small grid lines with a central target (Figure 2–9). This test is most useful in identifying the metamorphopsia that frequently accompanies macular disease, both as a diagnostic tool and for patient self-monitoring at home. Patients with maculopathies may report that the lines are bent, twisted, or misshapen.

The Amsler grid is also a useful test of the central visual field. When held at 33 cm, the grid covers approximately a 10° radius of the visual field from

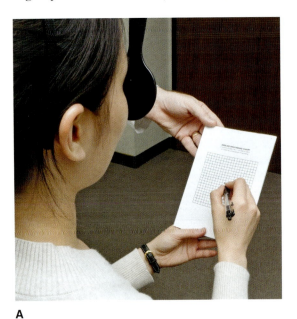

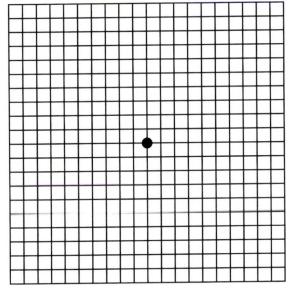

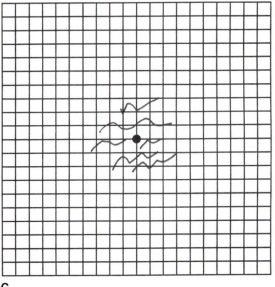

Figure 2-9. The Amsler grid test.
(A) The Amsler grid is held at reading distance (14 inches or 40 cm) and one eye is tested at a time, with best near correction (glasses used for reading). The patient is instructed to look directly at the central dot and is asked, "*Can you see all four corners of the grid? Are any of the lines blurry, wavy, distorted, bent, gray, or missing?*"
(B) Most Amsler grid scoring sheets are printed as a tablet, so the patient (with the help of the examiner) can designate abnormal portions of the grid by drawing or writing comments directly on the grid, which can then be entered into the patient's chart (or scanned into electronic medical records). **(C)** This Amsler grid is from a patient with metamorphopsia due to an epiretinal membrane. This is the same patient depicted in Figure 6–7.

fixation (each box is ~1°). Central visual field defects may make it difficult for patients to see the central dot, or they may note that some of the squares or lines are missing or are lighter than others.

Amsler grids are available in many forms: printed pads, wallet cards, online versions (recommended for the computer "home page" of patients with macular degeneration), and as smartphone apps. Variations include white lines with a black background or as a graded decrease of the contrast of the grid lines.

COLOR VISION TESTING

Color vision abnormalities may be congenital or acquired. Congenital color defects are usually caused by chromosomal abnormalities in coding for one of the three cone pigments. Defects are named by designating a prefix to describe which pigment is defective: *protan* = red, *deuteron* = green, *tritan* = blue. A suffix denotes whether there is complete absence (*-opia*), or merely a deficiency (*-anomaly*). For example, a complete lack of red pigment cones would be *protanopia*, whereas a deficiency of green cones would be *deuteranomaly*.

The presence of all three cone pigments in normal concentration is required to distinguish the entire spectrum of the color wheel. Most congenital color deficiencies are the result of chromosomal abnormalities coding for the red and green pigments on the X chromosome, and are thus manifest more commonly in men (8% of men and boys in the general population). Congenital deficiencies tend to cause "pure" red/green defects with predictable color-matching deficits.

Acquired color vision deficits may be caused by optic nerve or retinal disease (and rarely cortical disease). Optic nerve disorders reportedly tend to affect red/green color discrimination, whereas macular disorders create more blue/yellow confusion (Kollner rule). However, unlike congenital color defects, acquired disorders tend to affect the cone pathways indiscriminately. Acquired color defects are therefore more widespread in their effects on the spectrum of the color wheel, and the Kollner rule is only a rough guideline at best.

Most clinical color vision tests are specifically designed to detect and classify congenital defects, but are helpful in acquired disorders as well.

Farnsworth-Munsell 100 Hue Test

The most exhaustive (and exhausting for the patient) clinical test of color vision is the Farnsworth-Munsell 100 hue test (FM-100). This is a *just-noticeable-difference* task, which means that even normal subjects are expected to find the test difficult and to make errors.

The test involves placing 85 small tiles with subtle differences in color in rank order along the color spectrum (Figure 2–10). The FM-100 is only occasionally used in the clinical setting because it is so time-consuming and tedious. The *Farnsworth D-15* is a color-ranking test similar to the FM-100, but is much shorter (only 15 tiles) and can give information similar to that of the FM-100 (Figure 2–11).

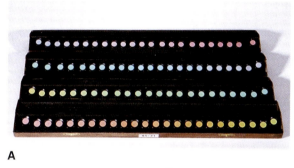

A

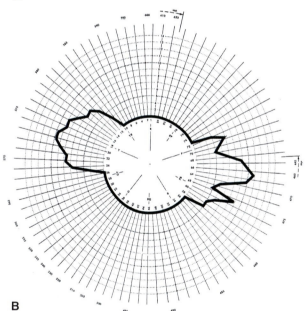

B

Figure 2–10. Farnsworth-Munsell 100 hue test.
(A) The patient is given one of four racks of removable tiles, with the first and last tiles fixed in each rack. The remaining loose tiles in the rack are removed and mixed. The patient is instructed to replace them in order, creating a color gradient from the first to the last fixed tile. The color gradients in the four trays form a continuous circle. By completing all four racks of tiles, the entire spectrum of the color wheel can be explored.
(B) The results of the Farnsworth-Munsell 100 hue test (FM-100) are presented as a circular plot, with the distance from the center circle corresponding to greater error at that point in the color wheel. In this example, the patient has an error *axis* typical for deuteranopia.

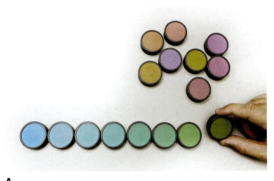

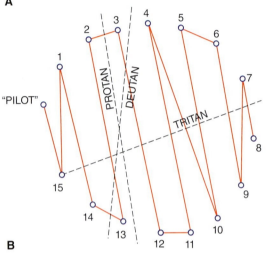

Figure 2-11. Farnsworth D15 test.
(A) Instead of 100 tiles, as in the Farnsworth-Munsell 100 hue test (FM-100), only 15 tiles are placed in order of color progression. **(B)** The result is mapped on a circular plot by connecting the numbers (on the back of each tile) in the sequence that the subject ordered the tiles. A perfect ordering of the color tiles produces a circle. This D-15 test result shows errors that align with the protanopia axis.

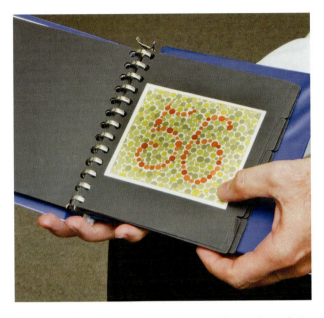

Figure 2-12. Pseudoisochromatic color plates. Color plate tests are usually in booklet form and performed at reading distance, one eye at a time (using a stick-on, clip-on, or handheld occluder to cover the nontesting eye). Obviously, patients need to be in their best glasses correction for near. The patients are asked to identify characters in a field of multicolored dots.

Pseudoisochromatic Color Plates

The Ishihara and the Hardy-Rittler-Rand color plates offer a fairly rapid assessment of color discrimination, and are routinely used clinically (unlike the FM-100). In these tests, numbers, letters, or other characters are hidden in a matrix of seemingly random dots (Figure 2–12). The shades and colors are chosen such that patients with congenital color deficits are not able to distinguish between pigments, and thus are unable to identify the hidden character. Color plate tests were originally designed for detecting congenital color deficits, but the total number of plates missed is often helpful to gauge acquired color vision defects.

Color Comparison

A simple but sensitive method of judging monocular color deficiencies consists of asking the patient to compare the color of a red bottle cap between a normal and affected eye. Similar to brightness testing, the loss of color saturation in the affected eye can be subjectively graded by the patient against the normal eye with "100%" color saturation.

STEREOPSIS TESTING

Stereopsis is the remarkable ability of the brain to synthesize the perception of depth using the images from both eyes. Each eye sees the object of regard from a slightly different angle, and these disparate images contain information that allows an awareness of depth (see Figure 3–11). Stereovision requires accurate ocular alignment and normal visual development in childhood, and tests of stereopsis are therefore primarily used to assess the ocular motor system (Figure 2–13). However, good vision in both eyes is also required, so a patient with excellent stereoacuity has at least some level of good central vision. Therefore, testing stereovision may be particularly useful in patients with nonorganic vision loss in one eye.

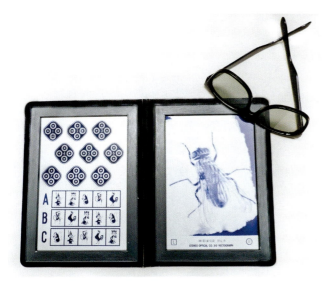

Figure 2-13. Testing stereopsis.
The Titmus Fly Stereotest is a commonly used clinical test of stereovision. Though designed for use in children, it is a useful tool for patients of all ages. This vectographic technique uses glasses with polarized lenses to present disparate images to each eye, making the images appear in three dimensions to subjects with normal stereovision. Patients are first asked to pick the fly up by a wing (patients with at least gross stereopsis will see the wings above the plane of the image and pick up a wing in the air). They are then asked to point to the animals and circles that are "sticking up" from the page. The latter two tasks have several steps requiring increasing levels stereopsis, so the patient's stereoacuity can be measured in seconds of arc.

OTHER TESTS OF CENTRAL VISION

There is an enormous number of psychophysical tests of vision in the ophthalmology, neurology, and psychology literature. This is no surprise, given the complexities of vision. Every neuro-ophthalmologist will have his or her own favorite special tests in addition to the common armamentarium of visual testing tools (Boxes 2–4, 2–5). In order for a test of visual function to be useful clinically, it must be readily understood and easily performed by the patient, and offer information that is immediately applicable in diagnosing and following visual function, and it cannot be lengthy. There are many tests that are more scientifically rigorous than the common tests we discuss in this chapter, but they are not "patient friendly" and are thus not practical as daily clinical tools.

▶ VISUAL FIELD TESTING

The tests of visual function discussed so far measure central vision, which is vital for activities requiring fine discrimination such as reading and recognizing faces.

> ▶ **BOX 2–4. PULFRICH PHENOMENON**
>
> A difference in the conduction velocity between the two optic nerves can produce erroneous perceptions of a moving object's location in space. The classic method of demonstrating this illusion is to have the patient watch a pendulum swinging in a plane perpendicular to the line of sight. Patients with unilateral optic neuritis (or normal subjects with a neutral density filter over one eye) perceive that the course of the pendulum describes an ellipse, swinging out and away from the observer when travelling toward the affected eye, and bowing toward the observer when travelling toward the normal eye. Not everyone can appreciate this illusion—only about three-quarters of normal subjects can see this phenomenon when induced with a neutral density filter over one eye. Testing for the Pulfrich phenomenon is rarely of diagnostic value, but is a fascinating observation.

> ▶ **BOX 2–5. CRITICAL FLICKER FUSION TESTING**
>
> Although fluorescent lights, television screens, and computer monitors appear to produce a constant light, they are actually emitting a rapid flicker. The limited conduction velocity of the normal optic nerve is unable to transmit the rapid undulations, giving the illusion of a steady light source. Tests of critical flicker fusion present a stimulus light whose brightness cycles sinusoidally. The frequency and amplitude of the light can be controlled. Testing algorithms attempt to find the *threshold frequency*, the lowest frequency at which the stimulus light appears to be steady. Disorders that affect conduction velocity, such as optic nerve demyelination in optic neuritis, severely lower the critical flicker fusion threshold frequency, even when visual acuity and visual fields have returned to normal. Critical flicker fusion testing is an example of a magnocellular system test (see Box 2–3).

However, it is possible to have a normal central vision but have disabling visual loss. Diseases such as retinitis pigmentosa, glaucoma, and chronic papilledema may severely affect the peripheral vision but spare the visual acuity. Because this chapter is devoted to visual sensory testing techniques, we will discuss how the visual field is measured below; however, the diagnostic interpretation of the patterns that emerge from this powerful tool is the subject of Chapter 3.

THE VISUAL FIELD: SIZE AND SHAPE

The visual field represents the extent of the visual world perceived by the eye, and includes an expansive area that

Figure 2-14. **Extent of the visual field and position of the blind spot.** Light entering the eye is focused by the cornea and lens, projecting an inverted and reversed image of the outside world on the retina. This optical system is successful in imaging a large panorama, with horizontal and vertical (*see inset*) angular dimensions as noted. Note the projection of the blind spot in the temporal visual field.

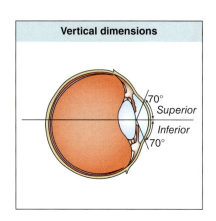
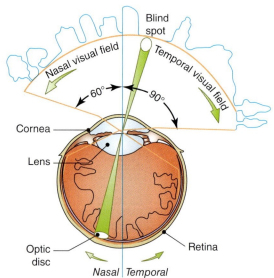

stretches from 90° temporally to 60° nasally, and approximately 70° both superiorly and inferiorly (Figure 2–14). Light entering the eye is focused by the cornea and lens to form an inverted image on the retina. Axons that convey information from the retina to the brain form the optic disc as they exit the eye, interrupting the otherwise continuous blanket of retina. The optic disc is approximately 12° to 15° on the nasal side of the visual axis and contains no photoreceptors. Thus, a blind, oval-shaped spot, measuring approximately 5° in width and 7° in height, is projected into the temporal visual field of each eye (Figure 2–14). This physiological blind spot is rarely noticed, even with monocular viewing. You can easily estimate the extent of your own visual field and the size and position of your blind spot (Box 2–6).

▶ **BOX 2-6. ESTIMATING YOUR VISUAL FIELD**

An outstretched arm (with thumb up) provides you with a ready estimate of the horizontal dimensions of your visual field. Site an object straight ahead with the right eye (left eye closed). The thumb of the right hand can be seen even when the arm is nearly 90° temporal to the line of site. In a similar fashion, the nasal field of the right eye measures about 60° nasal to the line of sight. The smaller size of the nasal visual field does not result from the nose blocking the view, but rather from the relative extent of functional temporal peripheral retina compared to the nasal peripheral retina (see Figure 2–14).

You can identify your physiological blind spot by fixating on a target with one eye and moving a small object (such as an eraser on a pencil) at arm's length approximately 15° temporal to the fixation target. The object will disappear in the blind spot and reappear when moved out of this small area.

The quality of the vision throughout the visual field is not uniform. The greatest light, color, line, and edge sensitivity is in the center of the visual field, corresponding to the tightly packed photoreceptors in the fovea. The overall density of retinal photoreceptors decreases continuously from the fovea to the peripheral retina, with a corresponding decline in the sensitivity and discrimination of the peripheral visual field. The visual field is often represented as a "hill of vision" (Figure 2–15), a three-dimensional (3-D) mountain with elevation corresponding to the sensitivity of the visual field (Box 2–7). Defects in the hill of vision from

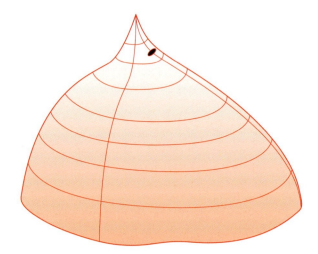

Figure 2-15. **The "hill of vision."** The size and sensitivity of the visual field are often portrayed as an island mountain in a "sea of darkness," with elevation corresponding to the sensitivity of the visual field. The tall central peak corresponds to the high sensitivity of the fovea. The height slopes steeply downward in all directions. A "bottomless well" near the peak (*small black oval*) represents the blind spot in the temporal visual field.

> **BOX 2-7. THE DYNAMIC HILL OF VISION**

The height and shape of the hill of vision is constantly changing, depending on many factors including lighting conditions, retinal adaptation, and pupil size. For example, in the dark-adapted (scotopic) retina, the densely packed cones in the fovea are much less sensitive, and the area of greatest sensitivity corresponds to the densest rod population (which is at least 10° off center). Thus, dark adaptation would significantly blunt the tip of the hill of vision.

The hill of vision concept is usually applied to retinal sensitivity tested with a white light. However, the shape of the hill of vision also depends on the type of stimulus is used to measure it. For instance, blue light stimuli that and motion-detection visual fields are more sensitive off center than centrally, and thus the hill of vision produced from these stimuli is shaped more like a volcano than a mountain peak.

disorders of the visual system may dramatically alter its contour by lopping off sections and creating precipitous cliffs, causing the island to become partially submerged and smaller, or creating deep canyons and potholes within its interior. Attempts to reliably measure and record the dimensions of the "hill of vision" in health and disease constitutes the challenging science (and art) of perimetry.

PERIMETRY TECHNIQUES

Confrontation Perimetry

Confrontation visual field testing is performed by the examiner using the examiner's hands or simple objects to compare parts of the visual field. With one eye occluded (usually covered with the palm of the patient's own hand), the patient is asked to fixate on the examiner's nose. The examiner can watch the patient's eyes to ensure compliance with fixation. Although physicians frequently test the ability of the patient to "count fingers" in the four quadrants of the visual field, this method may fail to detect all but the most dense visual field defects. Rapid finger counting, in which the fingers are extended only briefly in each quadrant, may reveal more subtle defects.

The most powerful confrontation methods require the patient to make comparisons between quadrants. In Chapter 3, it will become more evident why comparisons across the horizontal and vertical meridians of the visual field are particularly important. The simplest comparison test uses the palm side of the examiner's two hands to compare two quadrants (Figure 2–16A). For example, hands in the upper two quadrants are compared, and the patient is asked which hand looks the clearest, brightest, or sharpest. In a similar fashion, the two lower quadrants are compared. An important variation of this test includes using a red test object (eg, a mydriatic bottle cap)

to compare the color saturation (degree of redness) in different parts of the visual field. The patient is asked if two identical red test objects appear to be different shades when held in different quadrants, or is asked to compare the appearance of a single red test object as it is held in each of the four quadrants. A central scotoma can be identified by having the patient compare the color saturation of a red test object held in the peripheral visual field (usually held in the nasal visual field to avoid the physiological blind spot) to when the test object is placed on the examiner's nose (directly in the patient's visual axis).

Confrontation perimetry is performed by testing one eye at a time, but the examiner can also test the patient's field with both eyes open (unlike formal perimetry discussed below), permitting identification of overlapping homonymous visual field defects. The results of

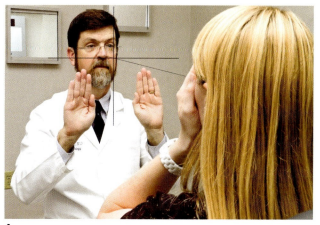
A

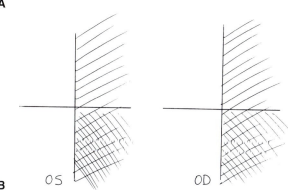
B

Figure 2–16. **Confrontation perimetry.**
(A) Simple test objects (fingers, hands, or red-topped mydriatic bottles) are used to compare the four quadrants and central area of the visual field of each eye (and both eyes together).
(B) The results of confrontation perimetry are sketched on the vertical and horizontal axes using cross-hatching, shading, or written comments. Note that the visual field results are drawn from the patient's perspective, with the visual field of the right eye (OD) on the right, and the visual field of left eye (OS) on the left (see Box 2–8). The visual field pattern depicted is a right homonymous defect, denser below than above.

confrontation perimetry are frequently sketched either by shading areas of deficiency (yet another challenge for EMR), or with brief written descriptions in each quadrant (Figure 2-16B).

Performing confrontation perimetry on every patient, even those who will have formal perimetry performed, has merit. In this way, the basic nature of the visual field defect can be characterized and the patient's ability to understand and respond can be assessed, allowing the physician to select the appropriate formal perimetric test for the patient. Since confrontation perimetry is a standard part of every neuro-ophthalmic examination, it is the most important form of perimetry to master.

Formal Perimetry

Although confrontation perimetry may be quite effective in diagnosing disorders based on the pattern of visual field loss, such testing includes too many variables to allow reliable comparisons between visits. Confrontation perimetry offers only a rough estimate of the visual field at best, and is subjective both from the perspective of the patient and the examiner. These inherent shortcomings led to the development of *formal perimetery*, in which devices are used that strive to produce quantitative, reliable, and reproducible visual fields, allowing comparison over time to follow changes in the visual field. Much of the impetus for developing visual field devices has come from the glaucoma world, as treatment of this optic neuropathy depends heavily on determining whether there is progression of visual field loss.

There are two main techniques to formally assess the shape of a patient's "hill of vision": static and kinetic. *Static* perimetry determines the sensitivity of the visual field (height/altitude of the hill of vision) at selected points in a grid pattern. This is the basis of most forms of automated (computerized) perimetry, as discussed below. In *kinetic* perimetry, a stimulus light of given size and brightness is slowly *moved* from where it is not seen, into the seeing visual field, and the patient tells the examiner as soon as the stimulus light is seen. This is repeated all around the visual field; connecting the resulting points defines an altitude line (isopter), much like the contour lines on a topographical map. Kinetic perimetry has been largely supplanted by computerized static perimetry devices, but remains an important tool for the neuro-ophthalmologist.

The retina is not flat like photographic film, but rather is hemispheric in shape, lining the inside of the eyeball. Both automated and Goldmann perimeters project the test stimuli on a corresponding hemispheric surface—the inside of a perimetry bowl. This theoretically allows testing of the entire visual field when the eye is positioned in the geometric center of the hemispheric perimeter bowl. Flat surfaces (such as the tangent screen discussed below) are limited to testing only the central visual field. The problems inherent with testing the visual field on a flat surface are most apparent the farther the stimulus is from fixation: The required size of the testing surface approaches infinity as the eccentricity of the stimulus nears 90°.

Automated (Computerized) Perimetry

Automated perimetry strategies are mostly static: Specific preselected threshold points in the visual field are tested (Figure 2-17). Determination of a threshold is performed by projecting a stimulus light of a given size and intensity

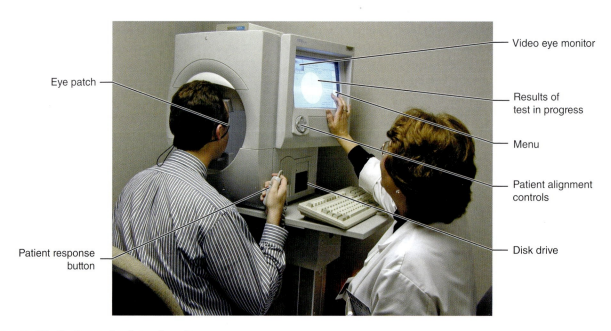

Figure 2-17. **Automated perimeter.**
The Humphrey Visual Field Analyzer II (Humphrey Instruments Inc., San Leandro, CA) is pictured.

for a brief duration, varying the intensity of the stimulus above and below the suspected threshold level to isolate the dimmest stimulus intensity that the patient can detect at a given point. Thus, a given point in the visual field receives many stimuli of varying intensities presented in a way to optimally determine the threshold. The computer tests and retests a number of points in a seemingly random fashion, until thresholds are obtained for all points.

The threshold values represent *decibels of attenuation* of the perimeter's bright stimulus light (Figure 2–18). Low threshold values mean that the stimulus light was not attenuated much and was very bright, and therefore represent points in the visual field with poor sensitivity. High threshold values correspond to more attenuation and dimmer stimuli, corresponding to greater (more normal) sensitivity. These numbers correspond to the altitude of the hill of vision at the test points (Figure 2–18, *below*). A grayscale plot is interpolated from the threshold values, with denser stippling corresponding to areas of lower sensitivity. During the test, the perimetrist watches the patient's eye on the monitor (a video camera shares the central hole for

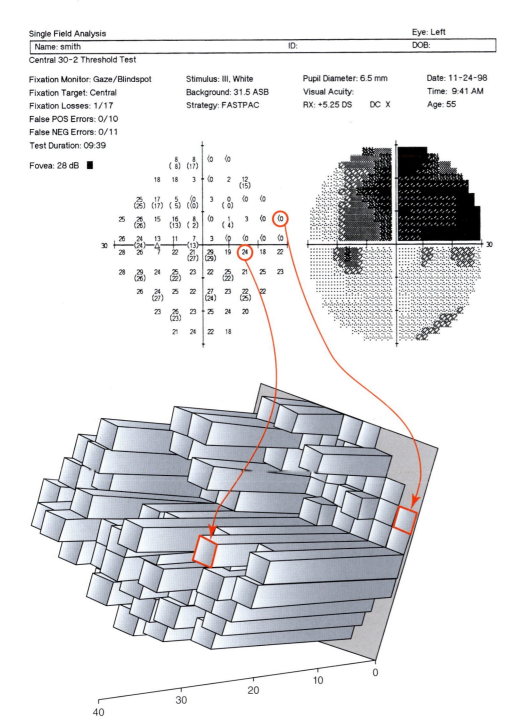

Figure 2–18. Automated visual field. This printout from the Humphrey Visual Field Analyzer shows the threshold values for each test point (*upper left*) and the gray-scale plot (*upper right*). Some points are tested twice, and the retest thresholds are shown in parentheses. A superior altitudinal visual field defect is shown. The threshold values correspond to the altitude of the hill of vision at specific test points (*below*).

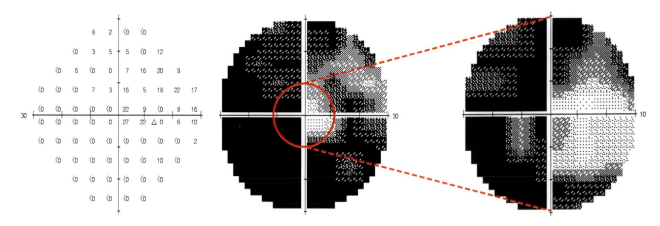

Figure 2–19. Comparing 30-2 and 10-2 automated perimetry.
A 56-year-old woman had an optic neuropathy in the right eye with severe visual field loss and a visual acuity of 20/60. This Humphrey 30-2 (*left*) shows only a small central visual field, with few responses peripherally. The 10-2 (*right*) tests the central vision only, essentially magnifying the central 10°. As opposed to the 30-2, the 10-2 concentrates on the area in which the patient has some vision, providing a more detailed map of the central island of vision. Although the 30-2 is important to show the overall state of the visual field, the 10-2 would be a better way to follow this patient over time.

fixation), and encourages the patient to maintain fixation, also observing for other irregularities in testing.

Most automated perimeters are capable of testing the full peripheral visual field, but the time-consuming nature of *threshold* perimetry often limits the test to within the central 30°. Many automated perimeters can produce a kinetic stimulus, but this modality is not commonly used. The most common and practical threshold tests on the Humphrey automated perimeter are the 30-2 threshold test (examines 76 points in a 30° radius) and the 24-2 (similar to the 30-2, but omits the most peripheral points temporally). A 10-2 examines the central vision in detail, testing 76 points in a 10° radius, which is helpful in patients with paracentral scotomas or those with marked peripheral visual field loss (Figure 2–19). The size of the stimulus light can also be increased, particularly for patients with severe visual field loss (Figure 2–20). Despite the relatively limited area of the visual field examined by

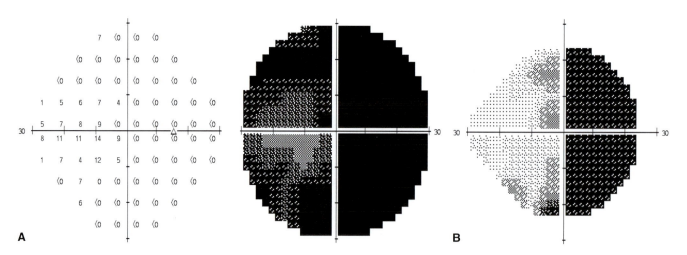

Figure 2–20. Increasing the stimulus size in computerized automated perimetry.
A 32-year-old woman had a severe meningoencephalitis resulting in bilateral optic atrophy and no light perception vision in the left eye. **(A)** Remarkably, the right eye had a visual acuity of 20/25 despite severe visual field loss, as seen in this standard Humphrey 30-2 visual field (size III, 4 mm^2 stimulus). The patient was able to see only a few of the many stimuli presented (note the <0 decibel attenuation number at most locations in the visual field). **(B)** When the patient is tested again with a *size V stimulus* setting (64 mm^2), better information emerges as the patient is now able to see more of the test stimuli. In this 24-2 visual field, a temporal visual field defect with respect of the vertical meridian emerges, consistent with a chiasmal insult. In this case, the size V stimulus gives a more revealing picture of the patient's visual field loss pattern, and would be a more effective way to follow this patient's visual field over time than the standard size III test.

the most commonly used automated threshold tests (30-2 and 24-2), these tests are successful in defining almost all common neuro-ophthalmic disorders.

Automated perimetry *screening strategies* test whether a patient can see a stimulus that would be suprathreshold in normal subjects. Screening strategies greatly shorten the testing time by not determining a threshold for every test point, but are of very limited value in following visual field defects over time. Variations include obtaining a threshold only on those points that are abnormal with suprathreshold screening.

Automated perimeters can reference a computerized database to compare the patient's performance to normal controls. This permits sophisticated statistical analysis of the visual field data and test reliability (Figure 2–21).

Patients with poor central visual acuity (20/100 or less) frequently have difficulty maintaining fixation with perimetry. On the Humphrey perimeter, an alternative fixation system can be used in which the patient is asked to look at the center of a large diamond defined by four lights in the bowl. This method is particularly useful when the patient has a discreet central scotoma.

There is a variety of automated perimetry devices. Most perform some type of static thresholding or suprathreshold (screening) tests, although there are some devices that can perform computerized kinetic techniques as well. Rather than a simple spot of light, frequency doubling technique (FDT) perimetry uses an alternating contrast sensitivity pattern as the stimulus and evaluates larger and fewer areas of the visual field, permitting testing in minutes. FDT is commonly used as a screening visual field.

Although automated perimeters, such as the Humphrey Visual Field Analyzer, are computerized and automated, they still require a responsive and cooperative patient, and thus have significant limitations as a subjective test. Even intelligent, motivated, and cooperative patients can have marked interest variability. Important clinical decisions may therefore require several visual fields to produce meaningful data.

Goldmann Perimetry

The Goldmann perimeter was one of the first perimetric devices that produced a standardized, reproducible plot of the visual field. This marvel of mechanical engineering was invented in 1945 by Hans Goldmann, and though largely supplanted by automated perimetry, still has clinical relevance for the neuro-ophthalmologist and teaching value for the student.

Goldmann perimetry is a manual, kinetic perimetric method. The operator tests the patient's visual field by moving a spot of light from nonseeing areas into seeing areas of the patient's visual field. The operator can choose from a series of standardized sizes and brightnesses. The stimulus is projected on a white perimetric bowl (with a radius of 33 cm) with carefully calibrated background illumination (Figure 2–22). The patient is positioned with the eye to be tested precisely centered within the hemispheric bowl. The patient is instructed to gaze directly at a small central hole in the perimeter bowl that contains a fixation light. The central hole is also fitted with a telescope that allows the perimetrist to monitor the patient's fixation. The examiner controls the position of the stimulus light by moving a cursor arm (over a sheet for recording the visual field) that is mechanically linked by a clever pantograph to the stimulus light projector. The brightness, size, and duration of the stimulus light are controlled by the perimetrist. For a given brightness and size, the examiner moves the stimulus from nonseeing to seeing portions of the field. The patient responds when he or she is first able to see the stimulus, and the position of the cursor can be marked directly on the record by the examiner (Figure 2–22B and Figure 2–23). This process of moving a stimulus light along a radial meridian from a nonseeing to a seeing area is repeated until sufficient points are obtained to estimate a closed circular shape. This line defines an *isopter* and represents points of equal sensitivity. The operator can then change the brightness and/or size of the stimulus light to define additional isopters. Isopter lines are analogous to contour lines on an elevation map, giving a detailed description of the contour of the "hill of vision"—complete with any craters, canyons, and lagoons that may be caused by visual system disorders (see Figure 2–23). Isopter lines tend to be spread apart for a gentle slope of the visual field, and are close together for steep changes in visual sensitivity, and coincident in the steep drop-off of absolute visual field loss.

In addition to plotting the slope of the peripheral visual field, the perimetrist can identify *scotomas*. A scotoma is a focal area of decreased sensitivity contained within the visual field, analogous to a pothole or crater in the hill of vision. A scotoma is *absolute* if the patient cannot see the largest (or brightest) possible stimulus, or it may be *relative* if some stimuli are seen. Scotomas (technically the plural of scotoma is scotomata, but convention allows the use of "scotomas") are mapped by placing the stimulus within a scotoma where it cannot be seen, and then moving the stimulus outwardly to define the edges of the scotoma. The physiological blind spot is an absolute scotoma and can be defined the same way. In fact, plotting the blind spot is usually the first task of the perimetrist because this well-defined absolute scotoma provides good practice for the patient, and allows the perimetrist an opportunity to assess the patient's understanding and cooperation.

The Goldmann perimetrist always benefits from information obtained in confrontation perimetry, as well as from the specific instructions regarding the area of interest from the physician. For example, any suspicion of a retrochiasmal defect should prompt extra time defining defects that line up along the vertical meridian.

Although the background illumination, stimulus brightness, and stimulus size can be carefully calibrated

Figure 2-21. Automated perimetry: statistical analysis.
The software algorithms for determining the visual field thresholds also explore the reliability and consistency of the test, and compare the individual patient's perimetry results with age-matched control data.

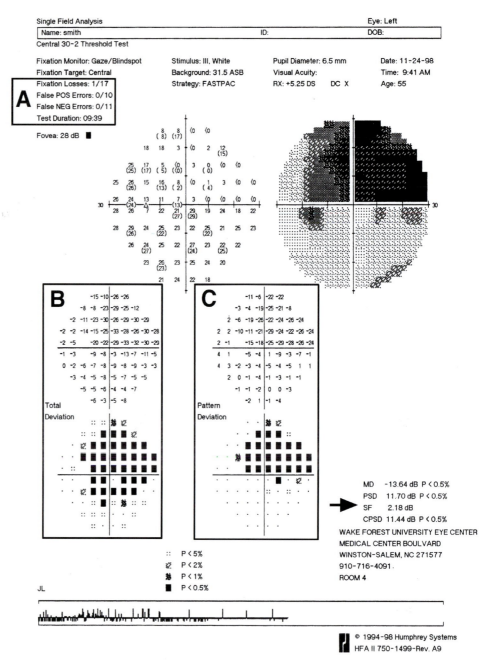

(A) Reliability data. The data is presented as a fraction: The numerator is the number of errors and the denominator is the number of times this parameter was checked.
Fixation losses: The blind spot is plotted first. Sporadically throughout the test, stimuli are placed in the blind spot where they should not been seen. If the patient responds, this suggests that the eye (and the blind spot) has moved, and a fixation loss is recorded. Fixation compliance may also be measured by tracking the image of the pupil from the video camera; this information is displayed as a graph at the bottom of the page.
False-positive errors: Some patients may anticipate the stimulus, expecting a stimulus at a regular interval. The test strategy will occasionally "skip a beat" and give an interval without a stimulus. A response during this time is a false-positive error (see Figure 6-16D).
False-negative errors: Failure to respond to a bright stimulus in an area that has been determined to be adequately sensitive generates a false-negative error.
Short-term fluctuation (SF, see arrow bottom right): This is the average difference in points tested twice, and is a measure of test consistency.

(B) Total deviation. The computer compares the threshold at each point to age-matched controls, producing the total deviation plot. A negative number means the patient had a lower sensitivity at that point than normal controls in the database. The computer then plots probability symbols for each point. Darker squares indicate greater statistical confidence that the threshold at that point is abnormal. The total deviation often shows abnormalities that are not evident on the grayscale plot (see Figures 3-14, 4-33, and 4-34). The mean deviation (MD, located above the short-term fluctuation) is essentially an average of the total deviation scores.

(C) Pattern deviation. The pattern deviation adjusts for conditions that may cause a diffuse or overall depression of the visual field (such as cataract) by adding sensitivity uniformly to the whole field. When the "corrected" visual field data are compared with the normal database, patterns emerge in the statistical plot that may have been lost in the total deviation data (where every point may have been statistically depressed). In this example, the altitudinal nature of the visual field defect is more evident in the pattern deviation than in the total deviation, because the presence of mild cataract caused a superimposed depression of the visual field as a whole (see Figure 3-3).

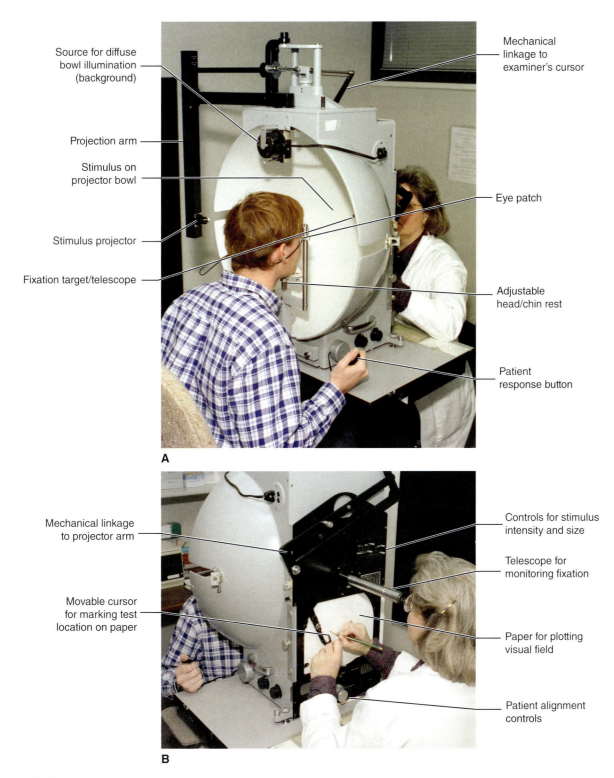

Figure 2-22. **The Goldmann perimeter.**
(A) The patient's side of the Goldmann perimeter. (B) The examiner's perspective.

and standardized, like confrontation perimetry, *the test is still subjective.* Successful Goldmann perimetry relies on the patient's ability to maintain fixation and understand the basic instructions. In addition, the test depends on the skill and strategy of the perimetrist to effectively plot the visual field before the patient becomes too fatigued to perform reliably.

Computerized automated perimetry has replaced Goldmann perimetry in many clinical arenas for a number of reasons: The manual techniques and strategies

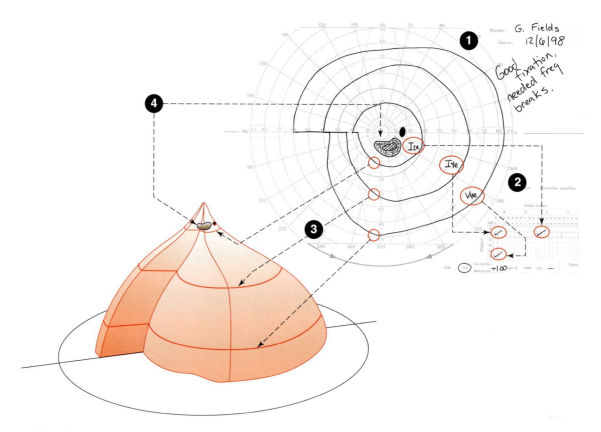

Figure 2-23. **Goldmann visual field.**
This abnormal Goldmann visual field shows a nasal step, which is a defect in the inferior nasal visual field. A small scotoma in the inferior arcuate area is also present. Corresponding defects in the hill of vision are also shown. Note the following: (1) Written reliability comments. (2) Designation of isopter lines. The Roman numeral designation denotes the size of light stimulus, and the Arabic numerals and letters show the brightness. Usually a different-colored pencil is used to plot each isopter and mark the stimulus parameters in the box. (3) An isopter can be thought of as an elevation line on a contour map of the hill of vision. The steepness of the defect is evident by the spacing of the isopters: very steep where they nearly coincide, and sloping where they are separate. (4) The scotoma does not connect to the periphery and was found by the perimetrist by spot-checking the interior of the visual field after plotting peripheral isopters.

Figure 2-24. **Comparing standard computerized automated perimetry and Goldmann perimetry.**
A patient with an anterior ischemic optic neuropathy has an inferior arcuate visual field defect and is tested with both Goldmann and Humphrey 30-2 perimetry. Observe how the visual field defect extends all the way to the limits of the visual field by Goldmann perimetry (*left*), with an altitudinal pattern beyond 30°. The Humphrey 30-2 (*right*) only looks at the central visual field (30° radius), but is usually sufficient to recognize most diagnostic patterns and effectively follow the clinical course of visual field loss over time.

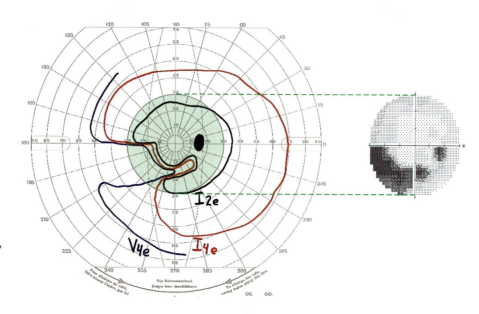

required to perform accurate Goldmann perimetry takes years to master, and are quickly becoming a lost art; and the computer provides a standardized test that does not suffer from the variability inherent with human operators. However, some patients simply do much better when a human operator is directing the test and interacting with the patient. (Theoretically, an operator should be present and interacting with the patient even with automated perimetry, but that is often not the case in a busy clinic.) The Goldmann perimeter remains useful for testing the far periphery of the visual field (Figure 2–24), testing patients with dense central scotomas (a large "x" made with black electrical tape can provide for good fixation), and patients who need a lot of instruction ("hand-holding") to perform formal perimetry.

Tangent Screen

Although some might consider a discussion of the tangent screen of historical interest only, an understanding of the principles and potential uses of this "low-tech" perimetric technique is important for the modern perimetrist to understand. Tangent screen testing is a kinetic method that uses a *flat* perimetric surface (Figure 2–25A), so it is limited to testing the central 30° of the visual field. The stimulus is a disc (which comes in standard sizes), manually moved by the examiner

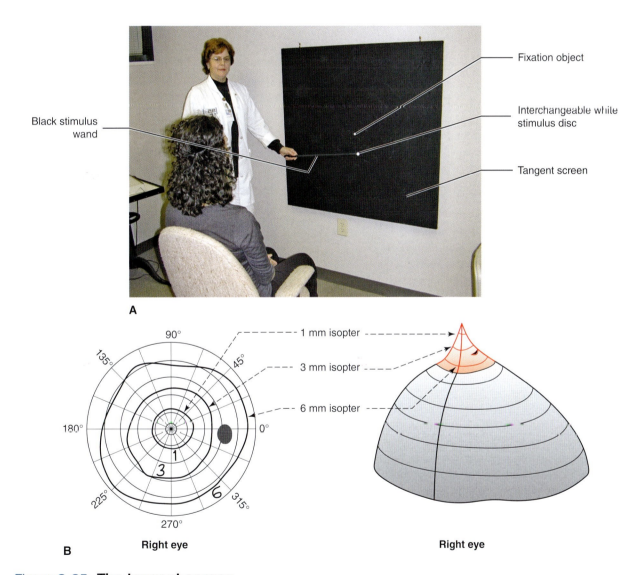

Figure 2–25. The tangent screen.
(A) The patient sits 1 meter from a black wall chart. The chart appears uniformly black to the patient, but has subtle markings for the benefit the examiner: concentric circles showing degrees from fixation and important radii. White discs of various sizes can be placed on a black wand to provide the visual stimulus.
(B) Like Goldmann perimetry, the result is plotted, determining isopters that correspond to the size of the stimulus used (*left*). Note that in the case of tangent screen testing, only the central visual field is measured, corresponding to the top of the hill of vision (*right*).

> **BOX 2–8. ORIENTING VISUAL FIELD RESULTS**
>
> Visual field results are always presented from the patient's perspective, with the right visual field on the right and the left visual field on the left (see Figures 3–6C, 3–13 to 3–15). Orienting the visual fields in this manner correctly places the blind spots in the temporal (outside) field in each eye. This convention for presenting the right and left visual fields is opposite of most every other presentation of clinical information (ie, fundus drawings or photographs, motility examination, and other tests are written down as viewed from the examiner's perspective). It is particularly important to correctly orient and label confrontation perimetry diagrams (as in Figure 2–16B) to avoid confusion.

over a black felt wall chart. Similar to Goldmann perimetry, this process is repeated over different radii to determine isopters and plot scotomas (Figure 2–25B).

With the advent of modern formal visual field testing techniques, the tangent screen is used less frequently (though some resourceful physicians will use any convenient wall as an impromptu tangent screen). This form of perimetry still has some advantages over the Goldmann and automated visual field machines: The visual field can easily be tested with both eyes open (which is helpful in defining discreet homonymous central visual field defects), and the testing distance can easily be lengthened (increasing the size of the defect projected on the tangent screen). The latter technique can be particularly helpful in examining patients with functional (nonorganic) visual loss (discussed in Chapter 6).

INTERPRETING PERIMETRY RESULTS

To interpret visual field abnormalities it is crucial to evaluate the visual fields from *both* eyes, even if the patient complains of a problem in only one eye (Box 2–8). It may be appropriate to *follow* patients with monocular pathology by only testing the affected eye, but only after the diagnosis and state of the unaffected eye is firmly established.

Recognizing the specific patterns of visual field loss from disorders of the visual system requires an understanding of the neuro-anatomy of the visual pathways. Chapter 3 explains the interpretation of visual field defects by demonstrating how the "wiring diagram" of the visual pathways determines the patterns of visual field loss.

▶ PHYSIOLOGICAL AND ELECTROPHYSIOLOGICAL RESPONSES

Tests of visual function discussed to this point require a relatively intelligent, cooperative patient. The patient's full participation is required to measure visual acuity, color vision, and visual fields because a voluntary response from the patient is required in these and most other vision tests. Fortunately, several "objective" tests are available to physicians. These tests include *physiological responses* (the RAPD and OKN tests, discussed in Chapter 7), *electrophysiological tests* (full-field and multifocal ERG and VEP testing), and *functional neuroimaging* (functional magnetic resonance imaging [MRI] and other techniques, discussed in Chapter 1). The RAPD, ERG, and VEP tests are discussed below. The utility of these objective vision tests in testing patients with functional (nonorganic) visual loss is discussed in Chapter 6.

RELATIVE AFFERENT PUPILLARY DEFECT

The pupillary response to light forms the basis of the RAPD test (also called the Marcus-Gunn pupil test, or the swinging flashlight test). In a patient with a significant monocular visual deficit (retinal or optic nerve disease), the pupils will respond more briskly when a light is shone in the normal eye than when it is shone in the affected eye. The difference in pupillary response is most apparent when the light is briskly and completely alternated between the normal and the affected eye (Figure 2–26). The eye demonstrating the poorest pupillary response to a bright light stimulus is said to have an RAPD. In some patients, the difference between the two eyes is subtle; it may only be noted as a modestly decreased amplitude of constriction. In other patients the difference may be extreme, and the pupil in the eye with the RAPD will actually be seen to dilate when the light is swung its way. The RAPD is graded from +1 (a barely detectable RAPD) to +4 (a large, obvious RAPD). The depth of the RAPD can be quantitatively measured by placing *neutral density filters* over the unaffected eye in a graded manner until the RAPD is neutralized (Figure 2–27). When there is no pupillary response to even the brightest light in an eye, the pupil response is said to be *amaurotic*.

Because both pupils respond the same (in patients with normal *efferent* outflow), either pupil can be watched to gauge the RAPD. In clinical practice, however, looking at the pupil in the eye illuminated with the test light is simply more convenient. Patients who have damage to an iris or who have a pupil that is otherwise not visible can be tested for an RAPD by observing the intact pupil as the light is swung from eye to eye. Dim illumination directed from below may enable the examiner to watch the same pupil throughout the test cycle.

The direct ophthalmoscope can be used to evaluate for an RAPD, and is particularly helpful in patients with dark irides and in children or uncooperative patients. By viewing the red reflex through the ophthalmoscope at arm's length, the pupil is easily

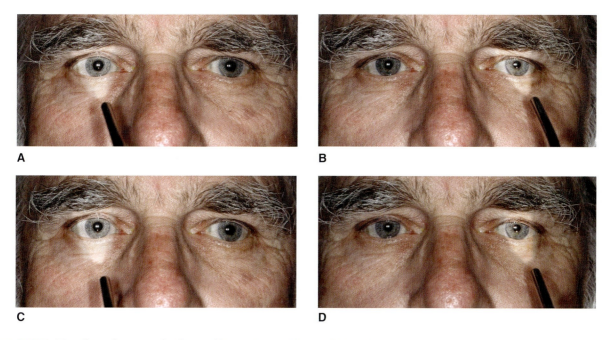

Figure 2–26. **Testing for a relative afferent pupillary defect.**
Testing for a relative afferent pupillary defect (RAPD) is performed in the dark to maximize the excursion of the pupillary response. Patients are asked to fixate on a distant target to prevent the pupillary constriction that accompanies the near reflex. A bright light (Finhoff illuminator or fresh penlight) is briskly swung from eye to eye with an interval of about one second, with careful observation of the pupillary response as each eye is stimulated. Eyes with equal afferent pupillary input produce symmetric and equal pupillary responses. Patients with monocular retinal or optic nerve disease have a less robust pupillary response in the affected eye, especially when compared to a brisk, normal response in the unaffected eye. This is a patient with an ischemic optic neuropathy in the right eye. **(A)** The pupils constrict slightly when the light is shown in the affected right eye. **(B)** The pupillary constriction is noticeably greater with the light in the unaffected left eye. Observe that both pupils are always the same the size as each other, even though an RAPD is present. **(C** and **D)** This cycle is repeated a number of times, as many factors influence pupillary reactivity; the physician continues the test until enough consistent responses are obtained to be confident of the findings.

seen. The ophthalmoscope light is shifted from eye to eye, and the pupillary response is compared as described above.

The RAPD test is most useful in patients with monocular (or asymmetric) disease, because the response of one eye is compared relative to the other eye. In the case of bilateral disease, an RAPD that has lessened might mean improvement in the poorer eye, but it can also mean worsening of the disease in the better eye.

Because the RAPD test is one of the few tests of visual function that does not depend on the cooperation of the patient, its usefulness cannot be overemphasized.

ELECTROPHYSIOLOGICAL TESTS

The neural signals that transmit visual information from the photoreceptors to the brain consist of electrical potentials. Computer technology permits measurement of these faint electrical signals generated by the retina and the brain. By repeating the stimulus and response measurement many times, low-voltage electrical responses can be extracted from the surrounding electrical noise by computerized signal averaging.

Electroretinogram

A flash of light on the retina initiates a cascade of electrical responses in the retina's neural circuitry. These changes in cellular polarity make tiny but measurable changes in the electrical potential of the eye, as measured by a corneal electrode referenced to an electrode on the skin (Figure 2–28A). With signal averaging, a predictable series of waveforms emerge, with a downward deflection corresponding to the outer retinal (photoreceptor) response (the a-wave) followed by an upward signal corresponding to inner retinal processing (the b-wave, Figure 2–28B). By varying the background, intensity, color, and timing of the stimulus light, the response of the rods and the cones can be separately evaluated.

The ERG plays an important role in the evaluation of patients with unexplained visual loss (discussed in Chapter 6). For example, some forms of retinitis pigmentosa can have a relatively normal retinal appearance, but always show marked abnormalities on ERG

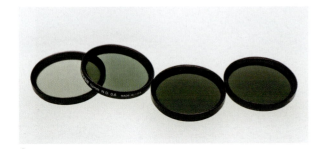

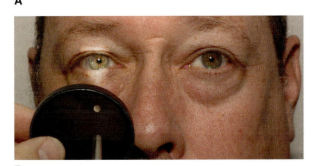

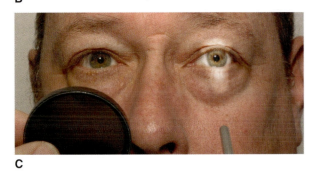

Figure 2-27. **Using neutral density filters.** To grade the relative afferent pupillary defect (RAPD), neutral density filters of increasing density are placed in front of the unaffected eye to dim the light stimulus sufficiently to neutralize the RAPD. **(A)** Set of neutral density filters. The neutral density filters are standard equipment for photographers, so they are commercially available. It is useful to have 0.3, 0.6, and 0.9 log unit (LU) values. Two 0.9 LU filters are helpful, as filters can be stacked to produce additive values approximating 1.2, 1.5, and 1.8 LU values. **(B)** The filter is held in front of the light source when the light is swung to the unaffected eye (the right eye in this patient), as the light is alternated between the right and left eyes. Note that the filter is held so that the examiner looks above the filter for an unobstructed view of the pupillary response. **(C)** After several trials, a 0.6 LU filter was found to equalize the pupillary responses in this patient. The patient therefore has a 0.6 LU RAPD in the *left* eye.

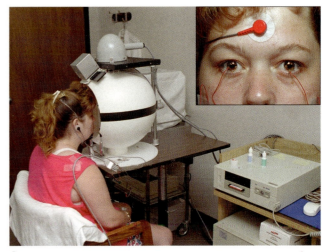

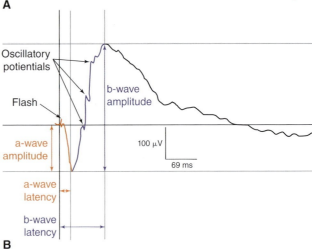

Figure 2-28. **Electroretinogram.** **(A)** A specialized contact lens electrode is placed on the patient's cornea, with a ground lead on the skin (*inset*). A Ganzfield bowl (*upper left*) allows even illumination of the retina with stimuli of various colors and intensities. The computer (*lower right*) collects the data, and using signal averaging is able to detect the low-voltage electrical waveform (UTAS-E 2000, LKC Technologies, Gaithersburg, MD). **(B)** The waveform consists of an a-wave generated by the outer retina and a b-wave from the inner retina. The oscillatory potentials are higher-frequency oscillations superimposed on the rising b-wave complex, and are also a measure of inner retinal function.

testing (see Figure 3–6). Cancer-associated retinopathy (CAR) usually produces an abnormal ERG, even when few diagnostic retinal signs are present. Central retinal arterial occlusions may leave only scant retinal clues, but an ERG is diagnostic, demonstrating an intact a-wave (from the unaffected outer retinal layer) and an absent or markedly diminished b-wave (from an ischemic insult of the inner retina; see Figure 6–4B).

The ERG measures the function of the retina, but does not include the responses from the ganglion cell layer or more distal structures. Thus, the ERG would be expected to be normal in patients with isolated optic nerve disease.

Further variations of ERG testing include using an alternating checkerboard grid as the stimulus (pattern ERG). The complex signal obtained from this stimulus is thought to primarily reflect ganglion cell layer function.

Multifocal ERG

The standard ERG employs a bright flash designed to illuminate the entire retina. This mass response may appear normal if disease is confined to a small area, such as the macula. The multifocal ERG measures the retinal response from discrete areas of the retina, much like a visual field test, producing a map of focal retinal function. The test is performed by having the patient view a grid of hexagons generated by a computer—typically 61 or 103 scaled hexagons (smaller in the center and larger in the periphery) in an interlocking grid. Each hexagon turns on and off in a seemingly random but predetermined pattern. At any given moment, one-half of the hexagons will be bright and one-half will be dark so that the overall luminance remains the same (Figure 2–29A, B). As with standard full-field ERG, a corneal or inferior fornix electrode collects the electrical signal generated by the retina. This complex signal, collected over 20 to 30 minutes, is analyzed by the computer to extrapolate an ERG signal representing the individual areas of the retina corresponding to each hexagon (Figure 2–29C). This produces an array of ERG signals, which are compared to age-matched normals. The data is usually displayed as a 3-D contour map, as the shape (values relative to each other) is more meaningful than the actual amplitude of the signals.

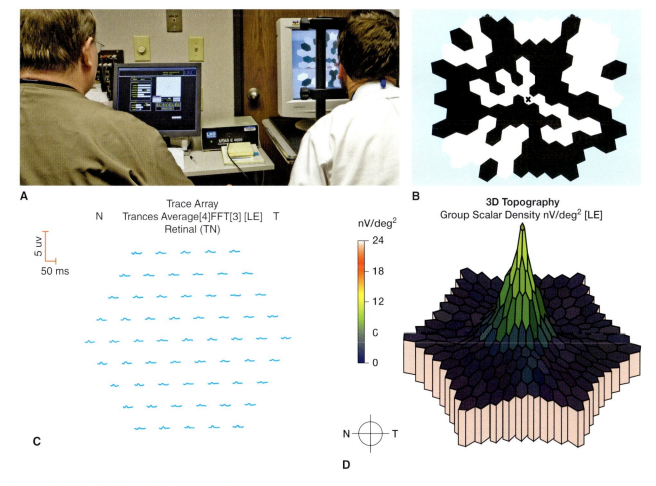

Figure 2-29. **Multifocal electroretinogram.**
(A) Multifocal electroretinogram (ERG) (LKC Technologies, Gaithersburg, MD) is pictured. The patient has an electrode in the inferior fornix of the test eye (not visible). **(B)** Multifocal ERG test pattern. The hexagons alternate black and white in a seemingly random pattern. **(C)** After many cycles, an ERG waveform can be extracted from the summated signal for the retinal areas that correspond to each specific hexagon. **(D)** Analysis of the signal can provide a three-dimensional plot of retinal sensitivity, with a central spike corresponding to the foveola. (C and D courtesy of David Browning MD)

Just like the "hill of vision," the multifocal ERG 3-D display shows a tall central peak with a rapid decline in signal amplitude relative to the distance from the foveola (Figure 2–29D). Similar to full-field ERG, the signal is generated by the inner retina (photoreceptors and bipolar cells), without any significant contribution by the retinal ganglion cells. Therefore, it is an excellent test to distinguish retina/macular disease from optic nerve disorders. Because the retina is mapped in discreet units, this test can localize retina pathology (both foveal and extrafoveal). Multifocal ERG is also far more sensitive for detecting macular diseases than a full-field ERG, since the full-field ERG is a summed response from the whole retina, which can mask discrete retinal defects. Multifocal ERG is particularly useful in exploring unexplained central vision loss with a normal-appearing macula, such as from a cone dystrophy, chloroquine toxicity, acute idiopathic blind spot enlargement (AIBSE), occult macular branch retinal artery occlusion, and others. The test requires a cooperative patient who can fixate.

Visual Evoked Potential

Electrodes placed over the occipital region on the scalp can register an electrical signal (with reference to a neutral body ground) with certain stimuli (Figure 2–30). Similar to the ERG, recorded signals are small, and computerized signal averaging is required. The patient is asked to look at a central fixation point on a monitor containing a computer-generated alternating checkerboard pattern. The complex signal obtained reflects the integrity of the visual pathway from the retina to the occipital cortex (Figure 2–30B). The timing and amplitude of the signals may distinguish the type or location of disease in the visual pathway in certain cases. For example, in optic neuritis, demyelination slows the conduction velocity, affecting the timing (increasing the latency) of the signal. Although this electrophysiological test does not require a voluntary response from the patient, the patient is required to fix on a central point, and to keep the alternating checkerboard pattern in focus with an appropriate accommodative effort. For this reason, the visual evoked potential (VEP) may not be the best test to "catch" patients with nonorganic visual loss, because an abnormal VEP response will be recorded even in normal patients if the patient fails to provide appropriate fixation and focus.

Rather than an alternating checkerboard stimulus, a bright diffuse flash can be used to obtain a VEP. The signal obtained in this manner is less distinct than the checkerboard pattern, and thus is both less specific and less sensitive, but this test requires only a minimal level of patient cooperation.

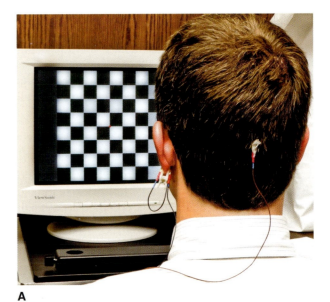

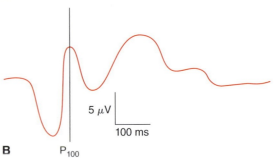

Figure 2–30. **Visual evoked potential.** **(A)** Electrodes placed over the occiput record the signals generated by an alternating checkerboard pattern. **(B)** The complex signal produced reflects the integrity of the visual pathways from the eye to the cerebral cortex. Comparison of the latency (implicit time) and amplitude of the major deflections between eyes and with an age-matched normal database allows characterization of abnormal signals.

► KEY POINTS

- Visual function cannot be fully measured by any single clinical test.
- The basic tools for evaluating all patients with (afferent) visual loss include obtaining the best-corrected visual acuity, evaluating the visual field, and looking for an RAPD.
- When the visual acuity is abnormal, the *best-corrected* visual acuity (by refraction) should be obtained. If a refraction cannot be done, the pinhole acuity may help account for uncorrected refractive errors.
- Contrast sensitivity ratings and contrast acuity tests often correlate better with a patient's "real-world"

- vision complaints than high-contrast visual acuity (eg, Snellen acuity) tests.
- Brightness sense, photo-stress, and color-comparison testing are most effective when patients have a monocular disorder because a normal eye is needed for comparison.
- The Amsler grid detects metamorphopsia, but is also an effective test of the central visual field.
- Pseudoisochromatic plates are designed for detecting congenital color defects, but are useful in obtaining some measure of acquired color defects.
- It is never sufficient to measure only central vision in patients with a visual complaint—the entire visual field must be accounted for.
- Performing confrontation perimetry helps the examiner decide what type of formal perimetry and test strategy would benefit an individual patient.
- Automated perimetry is a form of *static* perimeter: The threshold (dimmest light the patient can see) is determined for predetermined points in the visual field.
- Goldmann perimeter is a form of *kinetic* perimetry: A light of a given size and brightness is moved from the nonseeing periphery into the visual field. The series of points at which the patient first sees the light determines the isopter.
- Since the RAPD test is one of the few tests that does not depend on the cooperation of the patient, its usefulness as an objective method to follow visual loss cannot be overemphasized.
- The ERG measures global retinal function and is helpful in diagnosing retinal disorders such as retinitis pigmentosa. The ERG is normal in patients with isolated optic nerve disease.
- The multifocal ERG measures the retinal responses from discrete areas of the retina, much like a visual field test, producing a map of focal retinal function.
- A normal VEP is helpful in determining the health of the visual system, but an abnormal study may result from patient factors (eg, inattention, poor fixation or focus) other than disease.

SUGGESTED READING

Books

Barton JJS, Benatar M: *Field of Vision: A Manual and Atlas of Perimetry*. Totowa, NJ: Humana Press; 2003.

Byron LL: *Electrophysiology of Vision: Clinical Testing and Applications*. Boca Raton, FL: Taylor & Francis Group; 2005.

Frisén L: *Clinical Tests of Vision*. New York, NY: Raven Press; 1990:1–105

Glaser JS, Goodwin JA: Neuro-ophthalmic examination: the visual sensory system, in Duane TD (ed): *Duane's Clinical Ophthalmology*. Vol. 2. Philadelphia, PA: Lippincott Williams & Wilkins; 1998, Ch. 2.

Pokorny J, Smith VC, Verriest G, et al: *Congenital and Acquired Color Vision Defects*. New York, NY: Grune & Stratton; 1979.

Saunders DC: Tests of visual function, in Rosen ES, Thompson HS, Cumming WJK, et al. (eds). *Neuro-ophthalmology*. London: Mosby International Limited; 1998.

Walsh TJ (ed). *Visual Fields: Examination and Interpretation*, 2d ed. *Ophthalmology Monographs*, Vol. 3. San Francisco, CA: American Academy of Ophthalmology; 1996.

Articles

Corbett JJ: The bedside and office neuro-ophthalmology examination. *Semin Neurol* 2003;23(1):63–76.

Glaser JS, Savino PJ, Sumers KD, et al: The photostress recovery test in the clinical assessment of visual function. *Am J Ophthalmol* 1977;83:255–260.

Hart WM: Acquired dyschromatopsias. *Surv Ophthalmol* 1987;32:10–31.

Keltner JL, Johnson CA: Automated and manual perimetry. A six-year overview. Special emphasis on neuro-ophthalmic problems. *Ophthalmol* 1983;91:68.

Liu GT, Galetta SL: The neuro-ophthalmologic examination (including coma). *Ophthalmol Clin North Am* 2001;14(1):23–39.

Livingston MS, Hubel DH: Psychophysical evidence for separate channels for the perception of form, color, movement, and depth. *J Neurosci* 1987;7:3416–3468.

Thompson HS, Corbett JJ, Cox TA: How to measure the afferent pupillary defect. *Surv Ophthalmol* 1981;26:39.

Trobe JD, Acosta PC, Krischer JP, et al: Confrontation visual field techniques in detection of anterior visual pathway lesions. *Ann Neurol* 1981;10:28–34.

CHAPTER 3

Understanding Visual Field Defects

- ▶ OPTICS AND MEDIA   59
- ▶ RETINA   60
  Organization   60
  Visual field defects   61
- ▶ NERVE FIBER LAYER/OPTIC DISC   62
  Organization   62
  Visual field defects   63
- ▶ THE CHIASM   69
  Organization   69
  Visual field defects   71
- ▶ OVERVIEW OF RETROCHIASMAL DEFECTS   74
  Homonymous visual field patterns   74

- Congruous versus incongruous   76
  Effect on visual acuity   76
- ▶ OPTIC TRACT   77
- ▶ LATERAL GENICULATE NUCLEUS   78
  Organization   78
  Visual field defects   78
- ▶ OPTIC RADIATIONS   78
  Organization   78
  Visual field defects   78
- ▶ OCCIPITAL LOBE   79
  Organization   79
  Visual field defects   79
- ▶ KEY POINTS   83

This chapter explores how the *organization* of the eye and visual system dictates specific, recognizable patterns of visual field loss in disease. The principles to be discussed in this chapter generally apply to all forms of perimetry (eg, confrontation, automated perimetry, Goldmann perimetry, and other methods that were discussed in Chapter 2). In addition to the visual field examples given in this chapter, the reader is encouraged to look at additional examples of automated and Goldmann perimetry (referenced in this chapter) found throughout the book.

As discussed in Chapter 2, the visual field extends approximately 90° temporally, 60° nasally, 70° superiorly, and 70° inferiorly from the fixation point in each eye (see Figure 2–14). Thus, the area of vision in each eye is roughly oval, with more area temporal to the fixation point than nasal. Although we generally measure and display the visual field one eye at a time, it is important to remember that the visual fields from the right and left eyes actually overlap. Motor systems (discussed in Section III) keep both eyes trained on a common fixation point. Therefore, there is binocular representation of the visual field for 60° to the right and left of a common fixation point. Note that the most temporal portion of the visual field from 60° to 90° is seen by only one eye (Figure 3–1). This area of the visual field is known as the *temporal crescent*.

The afferent visual system includes the eyes (optics, media, and retina), optic nerves, chiasm, optic tracts, lateral geniculate nuclei, optic radiations, and visual (occipital) cortex (Figure 3–2). Visual information is transmitted by bundles of axons that represent specific portions of the visual field. The axonal wiring diagram seems complex on the surface, but actually follows a logical design.

In this chapter, the organization of each segment of the visual pathway is discussed, with emphasis on how the anatomic organization determines identifiable patterns of visual field loss in disease.

▶ OPTICS AND MEDIA

Although the neural pathways for vision begin in the retina, the afferent visual system begins where light rays first encounter the eye. The tear film, cornea, pupil, and lens comprise an optical system that focuses incoming light to form an image of the world on the retina. Light rays converge, forming an inverted and reversed image on the retina, with a nodal point located near the

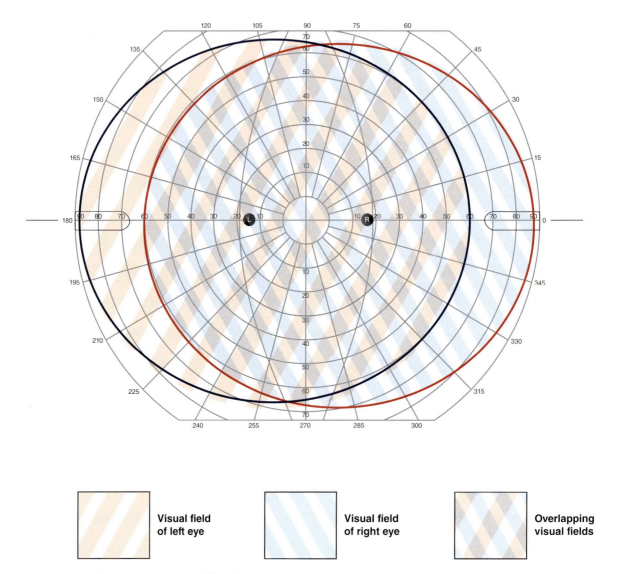

Figure 3-1. Superimposed visual fields.
The visual fields from the right and left eyes overlap with binocular viewing. The area from 60° to 90° in the temporal field of each eye is seen only by one eye (the temporal crescent). Note the position of the blind spot for each eye (L = blind spot of left eye, R = blind spot of right eye).

posterior pole of the lens. This inverted visual representation is generally maintained throughout the visual system. Therefore, lesions in *temporal* retina cause *nasal* visual field defects. Lesions that affect the *inferior* portions of the visual system (in the retina, optic nerve, or even visual cortex) cause *superior* visual field defects.

Uncorrected refractive errors or disturbances in the normally clear media (such as cataract) cause a general loss of sensitivity of the visual field. Discrete opacities in the anterior media, such as a corneal scar or cataract with a particular shape, do not create corresponding focal visual field defects. Such opacities are not "imaged" on the retina, but rather they decrease the amount of focused light reaching the retina and cause a general blur. This condition is analogous to the hill of vision remaining intact, but sinking a few feet into the "sea of darkness." Thus, anterior segment disorders cause diffuse *depression* (Box 3–1) of thresholds in static perimetry (Figure 3–3). This is analogous to *constriction* of the visual field with Goldmann testing, so called because the isopters are concentrically smaller than normal.

▶ RETINA

ORGANIZATION

The retina collects the image formed by focused light rays, translating subtle shapes, shadows, and colors into an image map of electrical impulses. Its organization

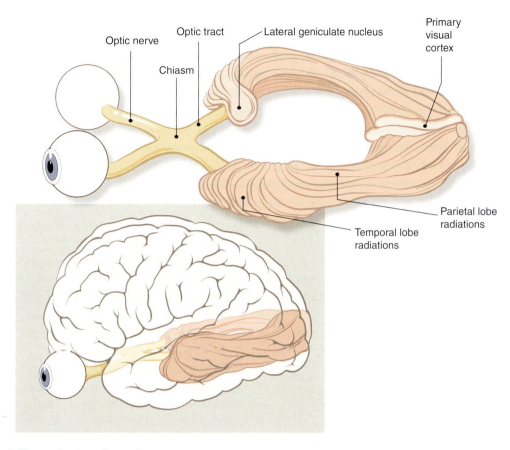

Figure 3–2. **Afferent visual system.**
The major components of the afferent visual system are identified. The *inset* shows the relative position of the visual system in the brain.

seems somewhat counterintuitive as the light-detecting cells—the photoreceptors—are buried in the deepest layers away from the incoming light (Figure 3–4). However, the photoreceptors play a metabolically demanding role in the creation of vision, and their location in the outer retina allows constant nurturing by the retinal pigment epithelium and the choroidal blood supply.

Each retina contains more than 125 million photoreceptors, but only about one million axons leave the eye. This is because neurons in the middle retinal layer process the image information from the photoreceptors, conveying a refined signal to the ganglion cells in the inner retina. Ganglion cell axons flow over the innermost layers of the retina, converging at the neuroretinal rim of the optic disc to exit the eye as the optic nerve.

In the peripheral retina, a single ganglion cell receives information from a thousand or more photoreceptor cells, whereas a ganglion cell in the fovea may receive information from only a few, or even a single photoreceptor. This ratio of photoreceptors to ganglion cells, as well as the greater concentration of ganglion cells in the macula, accounts for the much greater spatial discrimination of the fovea compared to the peripheral retina. In essence the "pixels" (receptive fields) are much finer in the center and rather coarse in the periphery. Most of the photoreceptors in the macula are cones, with cone density decreasing rapidly toward the periphery. Rod photoreceptors are virtually absent in the fovea, increasing and reaching a peak in concentration in the mid-periphery, then decreasing again more peripherally (Figure 3–5). The cone receptors are most sensitive in bright light and the rods operate best in dimmer light. Therefore, patients who depend mainly on rod function (cone dystrophies or other causes of central scotomas) avoid brightly lit conditions (hemeralopia), and those patients with rod dysfunction (retinitis pigmentosa affecting rods) have night blindness (nyctalopia).

VISUAL FIELD DEFECTS

Later in this chapter we will discuss how the organization of the visual system produces natural "straight-edged" boundaries along the vertical or horizontal

> ► **BOX 3–1. GENERAL TERMS USED TO DESCRIBE VISUAL FIELD DEFECTS**
>
> **Congruency:** The degree to which homonymous visual field defects in the right and left eyes resemble each other. The visual fields from each eye in optic tract lesions are homonymous, but tend to be incongruous (defects have different shapes and depths of visual field loss). Occipital lobe lesions cause highly congruous homonymous visual field defects.
>
> **Constriction:** In a visual field that is overall poorly sensitive, a given isopter in *kinetic perimetry* encloses a smaller area than normal. The isopter (and the visual field) is said to be constricted, analogous to the intact hill of vision partially sinking into the sea of darkness. *Concentric constriction* suggests a global, uniform effect on the visual field.
>
> **Depression:** In static perimetry, a point in the visual field is said to be depressed if the threshold is below normal. *Diffuse depression* in static perimetry is analogous to concentric constriction in kinetic perimetric terms.
>
> **Hemianopia:** (hemi = one-half + an = without + opia = vision) This term describes visual field defects that encompass half of the visual field (eg, to the right or to the left of the vertical meridian). Technically, this term could apply to a visual defect in one eye only, but it usually refers to homonymous defects (see below).
>
> **Heteronymous:** (hetero = different, opposite) This term describes defects that are present in the visual fields of both eyes but on opposite sides of the vertical meridian. This term is of little practical use, as the descriptors *bitemporal* or *binasal* are sufficient alone to designate the pattern as heteronymous.
>
> **Homonymous:** (homo = same) Defects that are present in the visual fields of both eyes and are on the same side of the vertical meridian are said to be homonymous. Use of this term implies that the defect is thought to be retrochiasmal. Homonymous defects are right or left (the side of visual space affected), may be quadrantic or hemianopic, and are usually described as congruous or incongruous (see previous definition). For example, a right optic tract lesion may cause a left incongruous homonymous defect, and a left occipital lesion may result in a right homonymous hemianopia.
>
> **Meridian:** A line that passes through the fixation point of a visual field representation. The *vertical* and *horizontal meridian*s are the most important in describing and interpreting visual field results.
>
> **Quadrantanopia:** Similar to hemianopia, except only a quadrant is affected. Suggests a homonymous defect with respect of both the horizontal and vertical meridians (see Table 3–1).
>
> **Scotoma:** (Greek, "darkness") A focal area of decreased sensitivity that is surrounded by normal visual field, analogous to a pothole or crater in the hill of vision. A scotoma is *absolute* if the patient cannot see the brightest possible stimulus (of the testing device), or may be *relative* if some stimuli are seen. *Deep* and *shallow* are also used to describe scotomas with reference to the hill of vision. Scotomas can be described by their location (*cecocentral, central, paracentral*) or shape (*arcuate, altitudinal, ring*). More than one scotoma should technically be called *scotomata*, but modern usage allows *scotomas*.
>
> **Visual field:** This term can mean one of two things: the general concept of an expanse of space that can be perceived by the eye; or an actual plot, drawing, computer readout, or map resulting from a visual field test.

meridians, or shape constraints defined by the sweeping nerve fiber layer. Lesions in the *deep (outer) retina* have no such constraints, and typically produce more nebulous shapes, defined primarily by the shape of the lesion. For example, in the predominantly rod dystrophy of retinitis pigmentosa, the central macula (mostly cones) is spared, with a donut-shaped ring scotoma in the midperiphery (Figure 3–6) that corresponds to a relatively higher density of rods (as illustrated in Figure 3–5).

In the macular area the receptive fields are small; deep retinal lesions generally produce focal visual field defects of a corresponding shape (Figure 3–7). However, outside of the macula the receptive field increases in size; focal lesions do not cause discrete corresponding scotomas, but rather a more ill-defined depression. For example, the multiple lesions produced from peripheral pan-retinal photocoagulation cause global constriction of the visual field, rather than hundreds of small scotomas. Lesions in the retina are generally visible with the ophthalmoscope, unlike lesions in the more posterior visual pathways.

► NERVE FIBER LAYER/OPTIC DISC ORGANIZATION

From ganglion cells throughout the retina, axons travel in the nerve fiber layer of the inner retina and converge to form the optic disc, positioned approximately 15° nasal to the optical center of the eye (foveola). The path from each of the ganglion cells scattered throughout the retina to the optic nerve is not necessarily a straight line; the high sensitivity and discrimination of the foveola is preserved by routing all axons around the foveola on their journey to the optic disc. Even the middle and inner retinal layers are seemingly pulled radially from the foveola to minimize any potential interference of

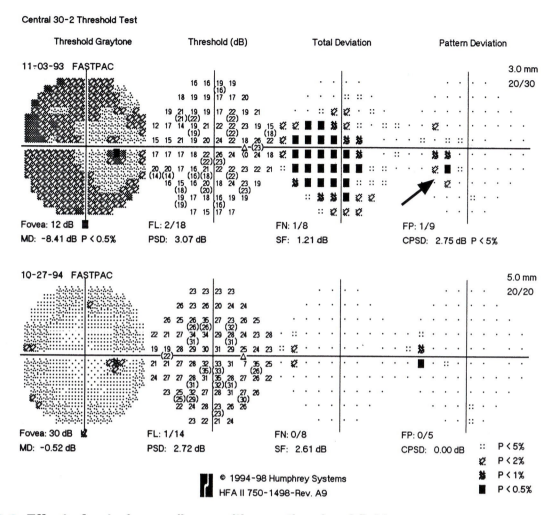

Figure 3–3. Effect of anterior media opacities on the visual field.
Opacities in the anterior segment are not imaged on the retina, but rather decrease the amount of focused light overall, causing a generalized depression. This patient with cataract and glaucoma had diffuse depression of the visual field (*upper panel*) that cleared following cataract surgery (*lower panel*). Observe that a small nasal step also present was successfully identified in the pattern deviation, even in the presence of diffuse depression (*arrow*). This printout selection from the Humphrey Visual Field Analyzer combines sequential visual fields in a format that allows easy comparison. The computer can also perform statistical comparisons of visual fields performed at different times.

a finely focused image on the sensitive foveola. This pattern of axonal routing creates a curious road map of axons in the inner retina: Axons originating temporal to the foveola must arch above or below the foveola. The horizontal *temporal raphe* is thus created because all ganglion cells above the level of the foveola send their axons arching superiorly, and those below this horizontal line send axons inferiorly. Axons from ganglion cells on the nasal side of the disc can travel directly to the optic disc, creating a radial pattern (Figure 3–8). Axons from ganglion cells between the optic disc and the foveola also have a relatively straight path. The highly concentrated ganglion cells in the macula create a concentrated sheaf of nerve fiber layer entering the temporal disc: the papillomacular bundle.

VISUAL FIELD DEFECTS

Diseases affecting axons in the optic nerve, optic disc, or nerve fiber layer (inner retina) demonstrate patterns of visual field loss that parallel the nerve fiber arrangement, frequently with sharp borders that respect the horizontal meridian (Table 3–1). Because the axons converge on the optic disc, many optic-nerve-related visual field defects connect with, or point toward, the

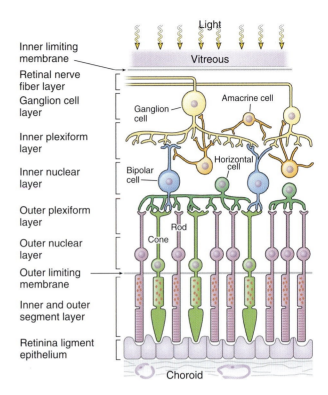

Figure 3-4. Retinal organization.
A schematic cross-section of the retina. Note that the light must pass through several layers of the retina to get to the rods and cones. This arrangement places the metabolically demanding photoreceptors in proximity to retinal pigment epithelial cells and the high-flow choroidal circulation. Ganglion cells in the inner retina receive input from a number of photoreceptors, transmitted and modulated by bipolar cells. Horizontal cells interconnect and modulate adjacent photoreceptor cells, and amacrine cells interconnect and sample groups of bipolar cells. Ganglion cell axons travel over the surface of the inner retina as the nerve fiber layer to exit the eye as the optic nerve. (Modified from Haines D: Fundamental neuroscience. Philadelphia: Churchill Livinstone, 2006.)

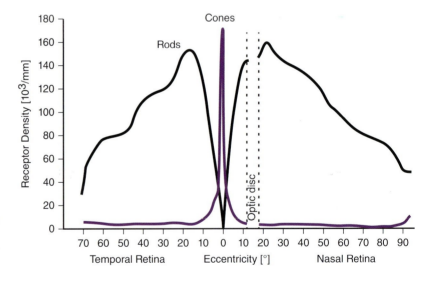

Figure 3-5. Distribution of rods and cones in the retina.
There are approximately 7 million cones in the human retina, virtually all of which are concentrated in the macula. There are about 120 million rods, in greatest concentration about 15° to 30° from the foveola. (Data from Osterberg G: Topography of the layer of rods and cones in the human retina. Acta Ophthalmol [suppl 6]:8, 1935.)

blind spot. Common patterns of optic nerve disease that reflect the organization of the nerve fiber layer include nasal steps, arcuate defects, altitudinal defects, cecocentral scotomas, and temporal wedges.

Nasal Steps

Nasal step defects are caused by optic nerve disorders that affect the long, arching axons that originate temporal to the macula, entering the disc superiorly or inferiorly. A nasal step may begin as a small depression above or below (and respecting) the horizontal meridian in the nasal visual field (see Figure 3–8A). Although a nasal step does not actually connect to the blind spot, progression of the visual field defect advances along an arcuate path that points toward the blind spot, eventually forming an arcuate scotoma. Nasal steps are so common in optic neuropathies (including glaucoma) that most visual-field testing strategies pay extra attention to the nasal visual field.

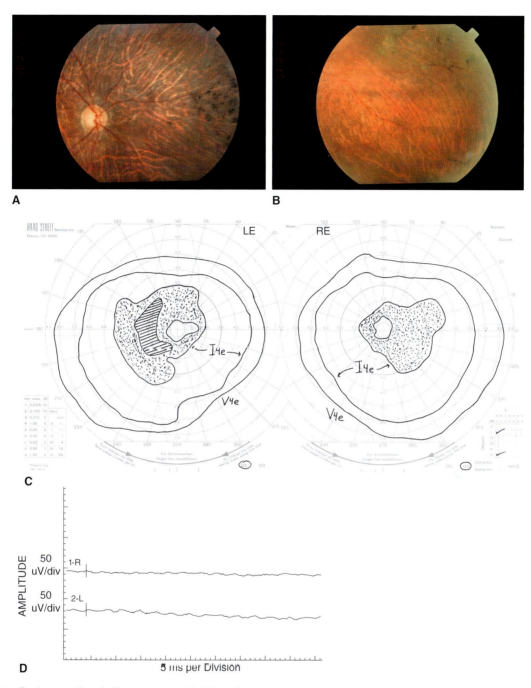

Figure 3–6. Outer retinal disease: retinitis pigmentosa.
A 75-year-old woman described a lifelong gradual decline in the vision of both eyes, saying that objects seemingly disappear and reappear from view. She was diagnosed with retinitis pigmentosa 15 years earlier—a diagnosis she shares with her mother and maternal grandfather. **(A)** Fundus photograph demonstrates slight disc pallor, arteriolar narrowing, retinal pigment epithelial (RPE) hypopigmentation, and pigment clumping. **(B)** RPE pigmentation forming "bony spicules" is seen in the retinal midperiphery. **(C)** Goldmann visual fields show a "ring scotoma" with relative sparing of the central visual field and far periphery. Objects are easily "lost" in the scotoma with movement in the visual field or with changes in fixation. No respect of the vertical or horizontal meridian is present. Because the inner retinal layers are not affected, the visual field defect does not follow patterns dictated by the nerve fiber layer. The pattern of visual field loss in this patient with disease primarily affecting the rods corresponds to the relatively greater concentration of rods in the midzone of the retina (see Figure 3–5). **(D)** The bright-flash electroretinogram (ERG) is a flat line, demonstrating that this is a disorder of photoreceptors and the outer retina (compare to normal ERG in Figure 2–28B).

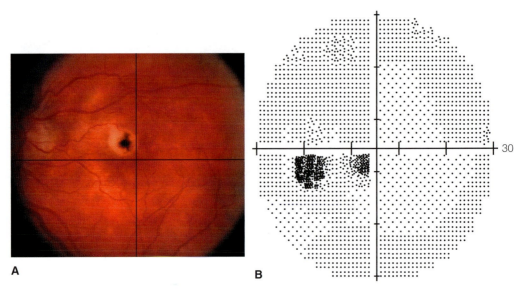

Figure 3-7. **Visual field defect with focal macular disease.**
A 45-year-old woman has reactivation of a macular histoplasmosis chorioretinal lesion. **(A)** The lesion is located just superior and nasal to the foveola (*crosshairs*) in the left eye. **(B)** The visual field defect corresponds precisely to the location and extent of the visible lesion. Observe that the visual field plot is presented as it would be seen by the patient's left eye. The optics of the eye project an inverted image of the world on the retina. Thus, the physiological blind spot is seen on the left side (in the temporal visual field), and the lesion projects a scotoma just inferior and temporal to fixation.

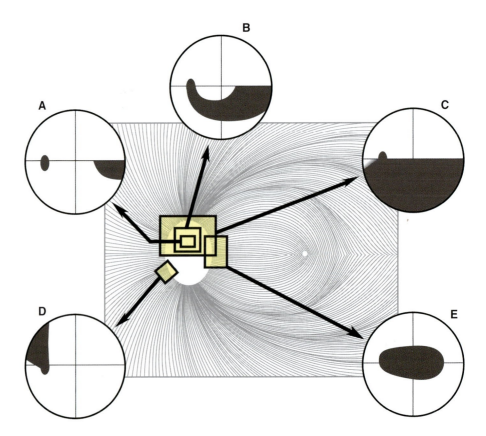

Figure 3-8. **Patterns of visual field loss: optic nerve/nerve fiber layer.** Nasally, the nerve fibers have a relatively straight course to the optic disc, but temporally, the nerve fibers arch above and below the foveola. Interruption of these axons produces distinct patterns. Note that the visual field defects in A–E can occur above or below the horizontal meridian, although only one example is shown. **(A)** Nasal step (see Figures 4–13B, 4–18D, 4–26B). **(B)** Arcuate scotoma (see Figure 3–9). **(C)** Altitudinal visual field defect (see Figures 4–10, 4–26C, 6–3A). **(D)** Temporal wedge (see Figure 3–10). **(E)** Cecocentral scotoma (see Figures 4–32 through 4–35).

TABLE 3–1. RESPECT OF THE VERTICAL AND/OR HORIZONTAL MERIDIAN

	Respect of the Vertical Meridian	
Location of Lesion	Anatomic Reason for Respect of the Vertical Meridian	Comments
Retrochiasmal lesions	Routing of axons in the posterior visual pathway is determined by an imaginary vertical line separating right and left hemifields.	Produce homonymous visual field defects.
Lesions of the body of the chiasm	Crossing fibers are affected, producing bitemporal (heteronymous) visual field defects.	Rarely "perfect," as adjacent optic nerve and tract may also be affected.
Junctional scotomas	Fibers crossing in the chiasm (from the contralateral optic nerve) are affected, in addition to the ipsilateral optic nerve.	Respect of the vertical meridian is only in the eye contralateral to the lesion. The ipsilateral eye will have an optic-nerve-related visual field defect.
	Respect of the Horizontal Meridian	
Location of Lesion	Anatomic Reason for Respect of the Horizontal Meridian	Comments
Optic nerve, optic disc, and nerve fiber layer	The peculiar routing of nerve fiber layer axons above and below the foveola forms the horizontal raphe.	Resultant visual field defects (eg, nasal steps, altitudinal) are monocular (unless the disease is bilateral).
Retina: hemiretinal artery or vein occlusion	The retinal vascular supply is divided into superior and inferior divisions, and infarction affects the corresponding ganglion cell layer and NFL.	Resultant visual defects are monocular (unless the disease is bilateral).
Central scotoma from macular degeneration or other macular or optic nerve process	Patient's fixation is by necessity at the edge of the scotoma, artifactually moving the scotoma above or below the center of visual field testing.	Produces "artificial" respect of the horizontal (and occasional vertical) meridian.
	Both Horizontal and Vertical	
Location of Lesion	Anatomic Reason for Respect of Vertical and Horizontal Meridian	Comments
Occipital lobe (most common)	Representation of the visual field above and below the horizontal meridian is separated in the primary visual cortex anantomically by the calcarine fissure, each supplied by their own branch of the posterior cerebral artery.	Infarction above or below the calcarine fissure can therefore produce a perfect quadrantanopia, respecting the vertical and horizontal meridian.
Temporal lobe	Temporal lobe fibers, representing the superior visual field, are routed around the temporal horn of the ventricular system.	Anatomic isolation of the temporal fibers provides opportunity for infarction/lesion of the temporal lobe to produce a superior quadrantanopia.
Parietal lobe	Parietal lobe fibers have a shorter course of relative separation from the temporal lobe fibers, but can rarely produce an inferior quadrantanopia.	Patients with parietal lobe lesions tend to be more severely neurologically impaired, and are thus less aware of a visual defect or less capable of voicing and documenting a visual field defect.

Abbreviation: NFL, nerve fiber layer.

Arcuate Scotomas

Arcuate scotomas reveal the sweeping path of those axons that arch around the foveola. They may be broad, as in the extension of a nasal step toward the blind spot (see Figure 3–8B), or well-defined narrow arches framing the fixation point (Bjerrum scotoma). Other variations include an extension of the blind spot (or "baring of the blind spot" in Goldmann terms) along the arcuate path (Siedel scotoma), and isolated scotomas in the arcuate bundle (Figure 3–9).

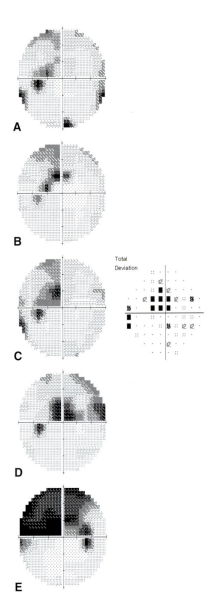

Figure 3-9. **The spectrum of arcuate scotomas.**
All of the visual fields shown are from the same patient over time, with primary open-angle glaucoma (this patient's optic discs can be seen in Figure 4-38). **(A)** October 2008: 24-2 Humphrey visual field shows an extension of the blind spot superiorly (*Seidel* scotoma).
(B) August 2009: The extension of the blind spot has extended in an arcuate fashion superior to fixation (*Bjerrum* scotoma). **(C)** November 2010: Further progression of the scotoma, now more altitudinal. The apparent respect of the vertical meridian in the grayscale presentation (*left*) is potentially misleading—the scotoma actually extends across the vertical meridian, as seen in the total deviation plot (*right*). **(D)** November 2011: The scotoma is clearly altitudinal now, with absolute respect of the horizontal meridian, extending across to the nasal visual field. **(E)** The left eye in this patient has maintained a broad arcuate scotoma, approaching a complete altitudinal defect.

Altitudinal Defects

Significant disruption of axons at the superior or inferior pole of the optic disc produces an altitudinal defect, an extensive visual field defect that lines up above or below (and respects) the horizontal meridian (see Figure 3-8C). Arcuate defects that worsen can become altitudinal visual field defects.

Cecocentral Scotomas

This defect incorporates the central visual field and blind spot, involving axons that enter the temporal margin of the disc. The defect is often oval shaped, straddling the horizontal meridian (see Figure 3-8E). Occasionally cecocentral scotomas are altitudinal, lying above or below the horizontal meridian. A distinct central scotoma (with normal field between the central defect and the blind spot) is more common in macular than optic nerve disease.

Temporal Wedge

Optic nerve disease affecting the straight radial pattern of the nerve fiber layer nasal to the disc creates a corresponding wedge-shaped defect in the temporal visual field that projects from the blind spot (see Figure 3-8D). This type of disc-related defect is uncommon, but is underappreciated because most automated strategies concentrate on the more frequently affected nasal visual field. Because no defined horizontal raphe is present in the retina nasal to the optic disc, temporal wedges are not obliged to respect the horizontal meridian.

Similar to retinal lesions, the funduscopic examination usually reveals the lesion causing optic nerve/nerve fiber layer–type visual field defects, such as optic disc edema, glaucomatous cupping, or a pale optic disc (Figure 3-10).

Because the axons maintain the same relative order throughout the optic nerve, even lesions in more posterior portions of the optic nerve may produce patterns dictated by the retinal nerve fiber layer arrangement. Such posterior lesions may not be evident on fundus examination initially, but optic disc pallor eventually develops. Destruction of axons anywhere along their course (from the inner retina to the lateral geniculate nucleus) results in retrograde atrophy and eventual loss of ganglion cells. This atrophy not only results in optic disc pallor (or cupping), but also causes loss of axons in the nerve fiber layer. This nerve fiber layer "dropout" is beautifully visualized by optical coherence tomography (OCT) nerve fiber layer imaging (see Figure 1-8A), but can also be appreciated on ophthalmoscopy, especially by using the green (red-free) light on the ophthalmoscope (see Figure 3-10B).

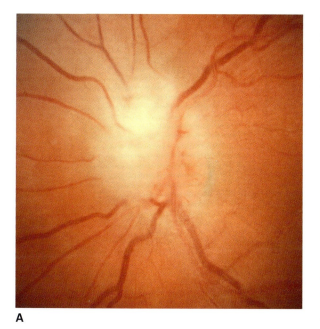
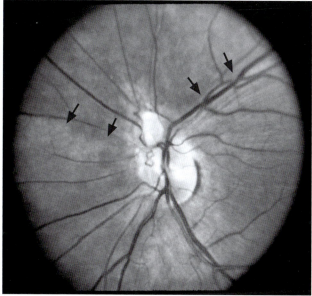
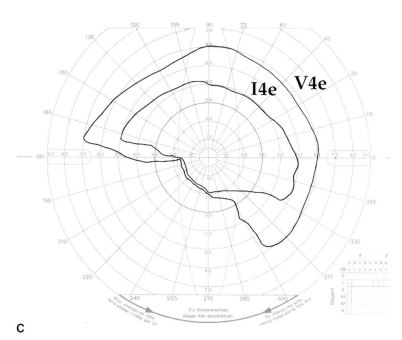

Figure 3-10. Optic disc/nerve fiber layer lesion: peripapillary toxoplasmosis chorioretinitis. A 13-year-old girl presented with decreased vision in the left eye for 1 week. **(A)** The fundus examination showed a peripapillary lesion, with vitreous cells present. An extensive work-up was remarkable only for an elevated toxoplasmosis titer. **(B)** After treatment with oral antibiotics and steroids, the lesion and associated inflammation improved significantly, but a visual field defect remained. Although the lesion was small, it affected the nerve fiber layer and adjacent area of the optic disc, causing atrophy of all axons passing through the affected area. A gap in the nerve fiber layer (*arrows*) can be seen with the ophthalmoscope, visualized best with green (red-free) light. **(C)** Goldmann perimetry shows that the visual field defect encompasses a large wedge extending both temporally and nasally from the blind spot to the periphery of the field, corresponding to the region of nerve fiber layer dropout.

▶ THE CHIASM

ORGANIZATION

The vast majority of axons originating in retinal ganglion cells are routed through the optic nerves, chiasm, and optic tracts, synapsing in the lateral geniculate nuclei (LGN). (There are subpopulations of ganglion cells that project elsewhere, as discussed in Box 2–3.) From the LGNs, axons sweep posteriorly to synapse in the primary visual cortex of the occipital lobes. Visual information from the *left* side of visual space is routed to the *right* visual cortex in the occipital lobe, with the *right* side of visual space sent to the *left* visual cortex (Figure 3–11). This re-sorting of axons occurs in the optic chiasm, where axons from the right and left eyes are rerouted into the right and left optic tracts.

The images from visual space to the left of fixation fall on the temporal half of the retina in the right eye and the nasal half of the retina in the left eye. Axons in the right optic nerve from the temporal half of the retina remain ipsilateral and travel directly into the right optic tract. Axons in the left optic nerve from the nasal half of the retina cross in the chiasm to join the right optic tract.

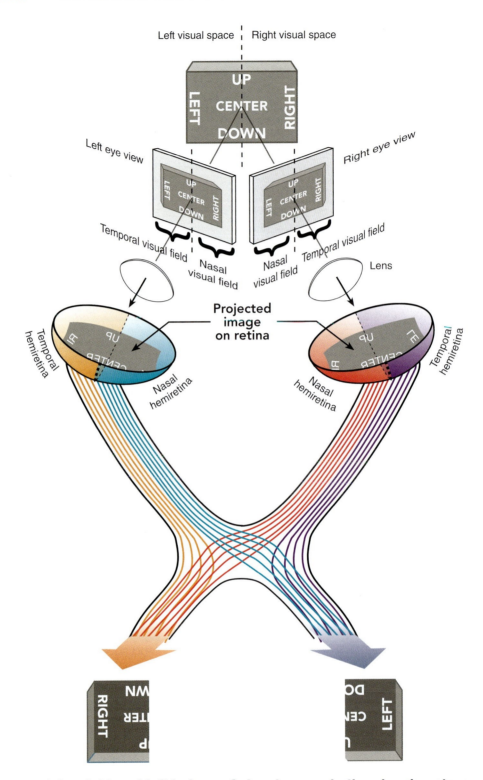

Figure 3-11. Routing of the right and left halves of visual space in the visual system.
Visual space to the right of the fixation point projects to the left visual cortex. To accomplish this, axons from the nasal hemiretina of the right eye and temporal hemiretina of the left eye are routed to the left visual cortex (and vice versa for the left half of visual space).

In a similar manner, axons forming the left optic tract correspond to the right half of visual space. Thus, axons representing the temporal visual fields (from the nasal hemiretinas) of each eye cross over to the contralateral optic tract. Axons representing the nasal visual fields (temporal hemiretina) of each eye remain ipsilateral in the chiasm (Figure 3–12). There are more axons representing the (larger) temporal field than the nasal field,

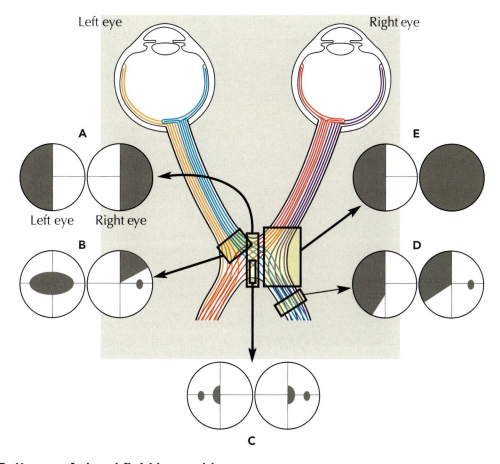

Figure 3–12. Patterns of visual field loss: chiasm.
Visual field defects from lesions affecting the chiasm have characteristic patterns. **(A)** Bitemporal visual field defect. This pattern occurs from lesions that affect the crossing axons in the body of the chiasm (see Figures 3–13, 5–4, 5–6). **(B)** Junctional scotoma. Lesions at the junction of the optic nerve and the chiasm cause an optic-nerve-related field defect in the ipsilateral eye and a superior temporal defect in the contralateral eye (see Figures 3–15, 3–16, 5–5). **(C)** Paracentral bitemporal visual field defect. A lesion affecting the central crossing fibers at the posterior notch of the chiasm causes this type of visual field loss. **(D)** Incongruous homonymous visual field defect. Optic tract lesions are homonymous (localizing the lesion to the retrochiasmal visual pathway), with greater incongruity than lesions more posterior in the visual pathway (see Figures 5–8 and 5–9). **(E)** A lesion affecting the entire hemichiasm would combine an ipsilateral optic nerve and optic tract defect, with only the nasal hemifield of the contralateral eye remaining (see Figures 3–16, 4–28, 5–7).

and thus there are slightly more crossed (53%) than uncrossed axons in the chiasm. Axons representing the central temporal visual field (crossing macular axons) are said to cross more posteriorly in the chiasm. Axons representing the superior temporal visual field (inferior nasal retinal fibers) cross more anteriorly in the chiasm.

VISUAL FIELD DEFECTS

The sorting of axons in the chiasm produces a precise segregation of retinal ganglion cell axons that can be defined by a straight (imaginary) vertical line through the foveola of each eye. For this reason visual field defects with straight boundaries along the vertical meridian are typical of lesions affecting the body of the chiasm (see Table 3–1) or more distal pathways (optic tract to occipital cortex), but would be most unusual proximal to the chiasm (optic nerve or retina). All lesions posterior to the point where the two optic nerves converge at the optic chiasm would be expected to produce visual field changes in both eyes. Therefore, *it is vital to know the status of the visual fields of both eyes in all patients with visual loss*, even when the patient's complaint is attributed to only one eye.

Bitemporal Defects

Lesions that affect the central body of the chiasm interfere primarily with the crossing axons, which

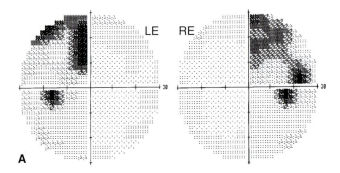

A

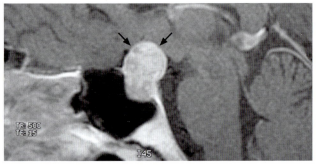

B

Figure 3-13. Visual field loss from chiasmal compression.
A 39-year-old woman complained of vague visual changes and mild, persistent headache. **(A)** Bitemporal visual field defects that respect the vertical meridian are present. The pattern suggests a lesion affecting the body of the chiasm. **(B)** Magnetic resonance imaging (midsagittal T1-weighted image with contrast) reveals an enhancing sellar/suprasellar mass consistent with a pituitary adenoma (*arrows*).

represent the temporal visual fields of each eye. The resulting bitemporal visual field abnormality is only rarely an absolute, symmetric, bilateral temporal hemifield defect (see Figure 3–12A; Figure 3–13). More commonly, conditions that affect the body of the chiasm produce field loss that is asymmetric between the two eyes, differing in the degree of temporal field loss in each eye and potential involvement of the central fields. Rarely, a lesion in the anterior chiasm can affect the crossing axons from one eye only, producing a *monocular* temporal visual field defect that must be distinguished from a nonorganic process. Lesions that involve the posterior notch of the chiasm (decussating macular fibers), may produce temporally located paracentral defects in each eye (see Figure 3–12C). Bitemporal visual field defects *that respect the vertical meridian* are virtually diagnostic of a lesion affecting the body of the chiasm, but other conditions can cause bilateral temporal visual field defects (Table 3–2, Figure 3–14).

▶ **TABLE 3-2. CAUSES OF BITEMPORAL VISUAL FIELD DEFECTS**

Disorders of the body of the chiasm. The vertical meridian is generally respected (see Figure 3-13); however, a concomitant optic-nerve-related visual field defect may be superimposed

"Big blind-spot syndromes." Examples include multiple evanescent white dot syndrome (MEWDS), acute zonular occult outer retinopathy (AZOOR), and acute idiopathic blind spot enlargement (AIBSE). Characteristics include lack of respect for the vertical meridian, paucity of fundus findings, and often an abnormal ERG (see Chapter 6).

Obliquely inserted (tilted) optic discs in myopia. A temporal peripapillary conus or retinal depression causes extension of the blind spot toward the fovea. The visual field loss may be an absolute scotoma from the conus, or refractive scotoma from depression of the retina temporal to the optic disc, and does not respect the vertical meridian. This is usually seen in patients with a long axial length (high myopia) (see Figure 3–14). However, the presence of anomalous discs does not exclude the possibility of an intracranial disorder.

Enlarged blind spots from papilledema. Expansion of the optic disc from edema causes lateral and upward displacement of peripapillary retina, producing both relative and absolute blind spot enlargement. The visual field defect is centered on the blind spot and does not extend to fixation (see Figure 4–20).

Bilateral optic neuropathies with cecocentral visual field defects. Toxic/nutritional and hereditary optic neuropathies are the most common. These scotomas include central vision and do not respect the vertical meridian (see Figures 4–33 through 4–35).

Rare causes: Sectoral retinitis pigmentosa, dermatochalasis (sagging skin of lateral upper eyelid).

Abbreviation: ERG, electroretinogram.

Binasal visual field defects could theoretically result from lateral compression on both sides of the chiasm by abnormalities of the carotid arteries or other processes, but this situation is exceedingly rare. *Binasal visual field defects are almost always the result of bilateral optic nerve disease rather than chiasmal compression.* Absolute, binasal hemianopic visual field defects (complete nasal hemifield loss) have no physiologic basis and suggest nonorganic visual loss.

Junctional Scotomas

Junctional scotomas result from lesions at the junction of the optic nerve and anterior chiasm (see Figure 3–12B).

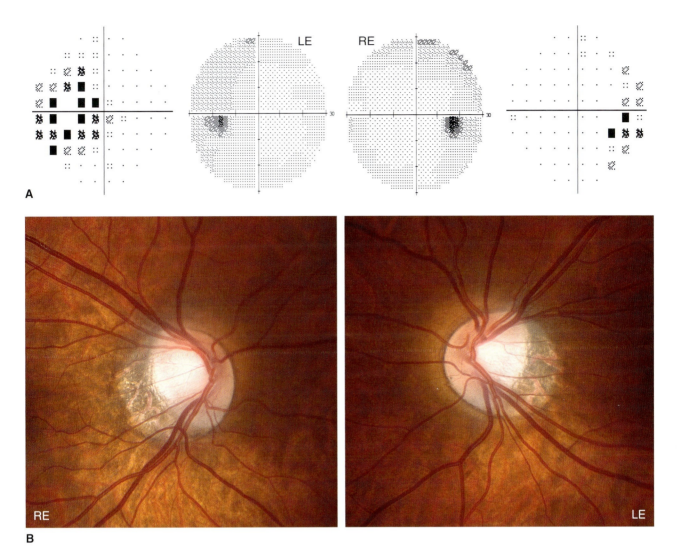

Figure 3-14. **Shallow bilateral temporal visual field loss in a patient with myopia and anomalous tilted discs.**
A 7-foot-tall, 24-year-old man was noted on a routine eye examination to have bilateral temporal visual field loss on screening frequency doubling technique (FDT) perimetry. A pituitary tumor was considered (with possible acromegaly and bitemporal visual field loss), prompting magnetic resonance imaging (MRI) of the brain that showed a normal chiasm, pituitary, and brain. **(A)** Humphrey 30-2 threshold perimetry showed shallow bilateral temporal visual field defects (most evident in the total deviation plots as shown), but without respect of the vertical meridian. **(B)** The fundus examination showed anomalous, tilted optic discs. The oblique insertion of the optic nerve is associated with a slight depression of the peripapillary retina temporal to the optic disc, which creates a "refractive scotoma" due to a poorly focused image in this area when the patient is in his best correction.

As previously discussed, axons crossing the most anteriorly in the chiasm originate from the inferior nasal retina of the contralateral eye (Box 3–2). Therefore, a lesion at the junction of the optic nerve and chiasm produces a superior temporal visual field defect in the contralateral eye, in addition to the expected visual field defect in the eye with the optic nerve lesion (Figures 3–15 and 3–16). *The temporal visual field defect is frequently asymptomatic and will not be detected unless the examiner insists on knowing the status of the visual fields of both eyes.*

Combination Defects

Mass lesions constitute the most common pathologic entity affecting the chiasm and surrounding structures (more on this topic in Chapter 5). These intracranial tumors are not precise or specific in the compressive

▶ BOX 3-2. WILBRAND KNEE?

Axons representing the superior temporal visual field (inferior nasal retinal fibers) cross anteriorly in the chiasm, and have been said to loop forward into the contralateral optic nerve before continuing as the optic tract. The concept was introduced by Hermann Wilbrand in 1904, based on the postmortem examination of the chiasm from a patient who had had an enucleation of one eye. Complete atrophy of one optic nerve provided an opportunity to see the course of the axons from the intact eye—and the axons crossing in the chiasm were seen to loop forward into the opposite atrophic optic nerve, thereafter called Wilbrand knee. This concept seemed to be validated clinically, as it is true that lesions of the anterior chiasm tend to affect the superior temporal visual field of the contralateral eye, and lesions that progress from the optic nerve into the chiasm start as a superior temporal defect, expanding into the inferior visual field (see Figure 3–16). However, in 1997 Horton showed that the "knee" was an artifact of monocular enucleation (the intact axons were pulled into the opposite optic nerve with atrophic scarring), and did not exist in postmortem specimens with intact optic nerves (Horton, 1997). Thus, there is no Wilbrand knee after all. The concept of inferior crossing axons (superior temporal visual field) being closest to the junction of the opposite optic nerve and the chiasm is true; however, they do not loop forward into the contralateral optic nerve.

damage they do to the visual system. Thus, lesions affecting the chiasm frequently produce complex visual field defects because the optic nerve(s), chiasm, and optic tract(s) may be affected in combination (see Figure 3–12E).

▶ **OVERVIEW OF RETROCHIASMAL DEFECTS**

Lesions of the posterior (retrochiasmal) visual system produce visual field defects that are *homonymous*, with varying degrees of *congruity* (see Box 3–1) that do not affect visual acuity when unilateral. These important visual field patterns will be discussed first, followed by a discussion of the peculiarities of visual field defects from lesions of the optic tract, lateral geniculate nucleus, optic radiations, and occipital lobe.

HOMONYMOUS VISUAL FIELD PATTERNS

The optic tracts contain axons from both eyes that represent the same side of visual space (see Figure 3–11). For example, the right optic tract represents left visual space, which includes all of the visual field to the left of center in both the right and left eyes. The optic tract axons synapse in the ipsilateral lateral geniculate nuclei and transfer information by way of the optic radiations to the ipsilateral occipital cortex. Therefore, lesions in the optic tracts and the posterior visual pathways produce homonymous visual field defects that are in the hemifield that is opposite the side of the lesion, respecting the vertical meridian (see Table 3–1). For example, *right* optic tract, lateral geniculate, or occipital lobe lesions will produce *left*-sided homonymous visual field defects.

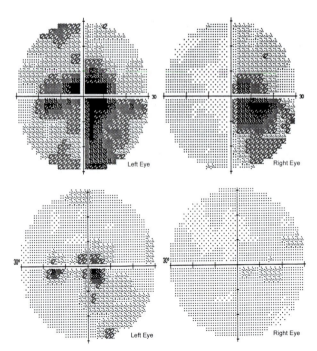

Figure 3–15. Junctional scotoma.
A 24-year-old woman with multiple sclerosis described a progressive fogginess of vision in her left eye. The visual acuity was 20/20 in the right eye and 20/200 in the left eye. The optic discs were normal in appearance. Humphrey perimetry on presentation revealed the expected central scotoma in the left eye, but also a surprising temporal visual field defect in the right eye, constituting a junctional scotoma (*top*). Magnetic resonance imaging (MRI) demonstrated demyelination at the junction of the left optic nerve and anterior chiasm, where some of the nasal fibers crossing from the right optic nerve (representing the temporal field) are also affected. The patient improved without treatment, although high-dose intravenous steroids were considered. The visual fields reveal resolution of the temporal visual defect in the right eye and marked improvement in the central scotoma in the left eye (*bottom*). The visual acuity eventually recovered to 20/30.

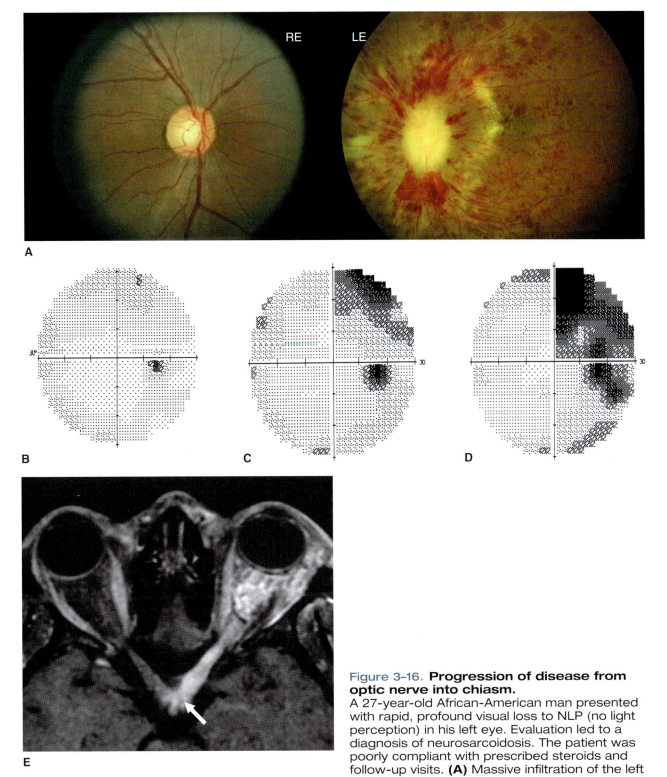

Figure 3-16. **Progression of disease from optic nerve into chiasm.**
A 27-year-old African-American man presented with rapid, profound visual loss to NLP (no light perception) in his left eye. Evaluation led to a diagnosis of neurosarcoidosis. The patient was poorly compliant with prescribed steroids and follow-up visits. **(A)** Massive infiltration of the left optic nerve is present; the right optic disc and fundus are normal. **(B)** Automated perimetry of the right eye on presentation is normal. **(C)** After 2 months a superior temporal visual field defect is present in the right eye, suggesting that the optic nerve lesion has progressed posteriorly and is now at the junction of the optic nerve and chiasm. **(D)** After 4 months, further temporal visual field loss suggests invasion of the chiasm. **(E)** Magnetic resonance imaging (axial view) reveals that the entire length of the optic nerve enhances and is enlarged, and that the chiasm is now also involved (*arrow*). This is an example of the severest form of a junctional scotoma, where optic nerve involvement results in NLP vision.

CONGRUOUS VERSUS INCONGRUOUS

There are two slightly different but overlapping views of visual space from each eye. For example, the temporal visual field of the right eye and the nasal visual field of the left eye are both images of right visual space (see Figure 3–1). In the visual cortex, slight disparities in these two views of the world are used to synthesize a sense of depth. Corresponding elements in these two pictures begin far apart (in different eyes), but end up converging toward the same anatomical point in the occipital lobe. In an optic tract, the two corresponding axonal pathways are still segregated into bundles from the right or left eyes as they go to synapse in the LGN. In the pathway from the LGN to the occipital lobes, corresponding axons become anatomically closer together as they approach a common point in the primary visual cortex of the occipital lobe. Therefore, a lesion in the occipital lobe causes homonymous visual field defects that are nearly identical in shape and depth, given the close proximity of corresponding axons and cortical neurons. Such matching visual field defects are described as highly *congruous*. Lesions in the optic tract also produce homonymous visual field defects, but they may be *incongruous* (not precisely matching in shape or depth), because corresponding axons from the right and left eye are not immediately adjacent. This concept gives rise to the general rule that between the chiasm and occipital lobe, *lesions that are more posterior (closer to the occipital lobe) tend to produce homonymous visual field defects that are more congruous*. Complete (total) homonymous hemianopic defects (which can occur from lesions anywhere from the optic tracts to the chiasm) are said to be *nonlocalizing* within the posterior visual pathway, in that the degree of congruity cannot be assessed (Figures 3–17B and 3–18).

EFFECT ON VISUAL ACUITY

A unilateral homonymous hemianopia does not affect visual acuity, even when the visual field defect is

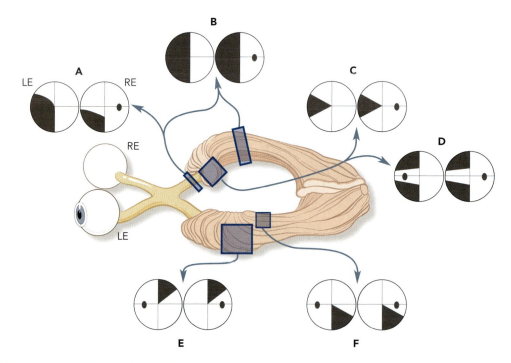

Figure 3–17. Patterns of visual field loss: optic tract, lateral geniculate nucleus, and optic radiations.
(A) A right optic tract lesion causes a left incongruous homonymous visual field defect (see Figure 5–9). **(B)** A complete left homonymous hemianopia isolates the lesion to the right retrochiasmal pathway, but is said to be "nonlocalizing" because congruity cannot be assessed to judge its precise location (see Figure 3–18). **(C, D)** A right lateral geniculate infarct may cause a left *sectoranopia*. This unusual wedge-shaped homonymous defect points to fixation and straddles the horizontal meridian. An opposite pattern, sparing the horizontal sector, can also occur. The peculiar shape and opposing patterns of these visual field defects are related to the organization of the lateral geniculate nucleus (LGN) and its dual blood supply (see Figure 5–12). **(E)** Temporal lobe lesions cause homonymous wedge-shaped superior visual field defects, or at least homonymous defects that are more dense above the horizontal meridian than below. **(F)** Parietal lobe lesions cause homonymous defects that are more dense below the horizontal meridian than above (see Figure 5–14).

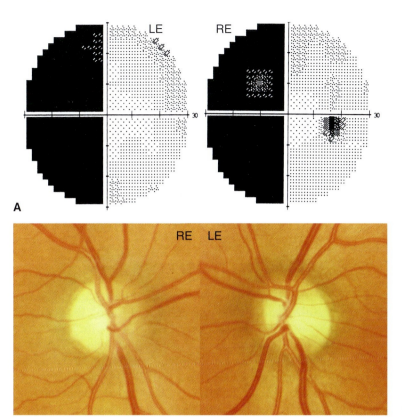

Figure 3–18. **Optic tract syndrome.**
A 43-year-old woman suffered a severe closed-head injury from an airplane crash. **(A)** A complete left homonymous hemianopia is present. This visual field result is said to be nonlocalizing, as it could represent injury anywhere from the right optic tract to occipital cortex. **(B)** The right optic disc has mild pallor, with loss of nerve fiber striations superiorly and inferiorly. The left optic disc (the eye with the temporal visual field defect) demonstrates "bow-tie" atrophy, with pallor that extends temporally and nasally. A 0.6 log unit (LU) relative afferent pupillary defect (RAPD) is also present in the left eye. The disc pallor and RAPD offer clinical evidence that the site of injury is the right optic tract. **(C)** The loss of axons originating in the nasal hemiretina (representing the temporal visual field) creates the distinctive bow-tie pattern of pallor.

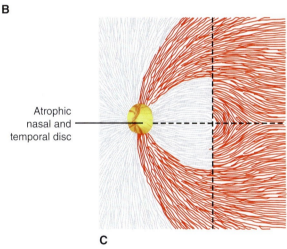

complete and absolute. Unilateral left hemispheric lesions may affect the ability of the patient to name the letters seen (alexia), but not the visual acuity. Patients with homonymous hemianopia often read only one-half of the visual acuity chart in their remaining field with each eye. A symmetric bilateral decrease in visual acuity *can* be caused by *bilateral* homonymous defects, resulting from bilateral lesions in the posterior visual pathway.

▶ OPTIC TRACT

Pupillary fibers exit the optic tract just before the lateral geniculate nucleus, travelling in the brachium of the superior colliculus to synapse in midbrain pretectal nuclei. Disruption of the right optic tract produces a small but *measurable afferent pupillary defect* in the left eye, because the temporal visual field lost in the left eye normally provides more pupillary input than the nasal visual field lost in the right eye. Thus, optic tract lesions produce homonymous, incongruous visual field defects (see Figure 3–17A), frequently with a small relative afferent pupillary defect (RAPD) in the eye contralateral to the lesion. Similar to all pregeniculate lesions, optic disc pallor eventually develops with axonal atrophy over time. The resultant pallor in the contralateral eye appears as a band or *bow-tie* of atrophy across the disc in some patients (see Figure 3–18).

▶ LATERAL GENICULATE NUCLEUS

ORGANIZATION

The LGN is the major destination of the axons that originated in the ganglion cell layer of the retina in each eye. Each optic tract terminates at its respective LGN, with individual axons synapsing in alternating layers depending on their eye of origin (see Chapter 5 for details).

VISUAL FIELD DEFECTS

Isolated lesions of the LGN are especially rare and are usually associated with vascular disease. Visual field defects are homonymous, somewhat incongruous, and may produce a unique sector-shaped pattern due to the neuronal architecture and a dual blood supply (see Figures 3–17C, D and 5–12; Figure 3–19).

▶ OPTIC RADIATIONS

ORGANIZATION

Neurons in the lateral geniculate nuclei project their axons to the occipital cortex, which is located at the most posterior extent of the brain. The primary visual cortex (Brodmann area 17) occupies the posterior tip of each hemisphere, extending onto the mesial surface of each hemisphere above, below, and into the calcarine fissure. Superior projections representing the inferior visual fields travel rather directly from the LGN through the parietal lobe to the cortical area above the calcarine fissure. The lower projections (representing the superior visual fields) cannot travel directly posterior, as the temporal horn of the ventricular system is in the most direct path. Instead, the lower projections are diverted somewhat anteriorly to curve laterally around the ventricular system, sweeping anteriorly through the temporal lobe (Meyer loop), then regaining an alignment parallel to the superior (parietal) fibers after this brief detour (see Figure 3–17). Fibers representing the peripheral fields sweep more anteriorly, about 5 cm from the anterior tip of the temporal lobe. Temporal lobectomy surgery for intractable seizures that extends beyond this point interrupts these fibers, producing superior homonymous visual field defects.

VISUAL FIELD DEFECTS

Lesions involving the optic radiations (geniculostriate pathway) are homonymous, with increasing congruity the more posterior the lesion. *Temporal lobe lesions* result in superior homonymous visual field defects, or at least defects that are denser above the horizontal meridian than below (see Figure 3–17E). The classic finding is homonymous, superior, wedge-shaped "pie in the sky" defects. *Parietal lobe lesions* create homonymous visual field defects that are denser below than above (see Figure 3–17F). Patients with visual field defects from parietal lobe lesions are rarely seen by ophthalmologists, as these hemispheric lesions usually cause serious associated neurological dysfunction that prevents the patient from being aware of the visual loss (or at least from complaining about it). These neurological deficits also preclude formal visual field testing in most patients.

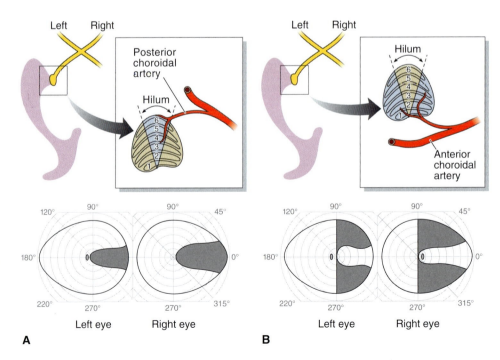

Figure 3-19. **Lateral geniculate nucleus sectoranopia.** Vascular lesions of the lateral geniculate nucleus (LGN) can affect the central hilum of the LGN if the branch from the posterior choroidal artery is involved, or the peripheral portions of the nucleus if the blood supply from the anterior choroidal artery is involved, resulting in two unique homonymous visual field defects. (Modified from Kline LB: *Neuro-ophthalmology Review Manual*, 7th ed. Thorofare, NJ: SLACK; 2013.)

▶ OCCIPITAL LOBE ORGANIZATION

The primary visual cortex stretches from the posterior pole of the brain along the mesial surface of the hemispheres, extending into the folds of the calcarine fissure. The central visual field is represented at the occipital tip, with the more peripheral visual field represented deeper in the interhemispheric fissure (Figure 3–20). The calcarine fissure separates the upper projections above (inferior visual fields) from the lower projections below (superior visual fields).

The posterior tip and 40% to 50% of the contiguous mesial surface of the occipital lobes are devoted to central vision (see Figure 3–20). The previous section on retinal anatomy pointed out the small size of the receptive fields in the macular area and the large concentration of ganglion cells and axons representing central vision. This retinal arrangement corresponds to the disproportionately large area of the visual cortex that is devoted to the central visual field.

VISUAL FIELD DEFECTS

Occipital lobe lesions produce visual field defects that are homonymous and highly congruous. Additional characteristics are discussed below.

Watershed Infarcts

The tip of the occipital cortex represents a watershed zone of anastomoses between the middle and posterior cerebral arteries. Hypotensive events can cause an infarct of this area due to the vulnerability of watershed zones in cerebral hypoperfusion, producing a central homonymous visual field defect (Figure 3–21B, C). Small, paracentral homonymous visual field defects can cause blurred vision and difficulty reading despite a

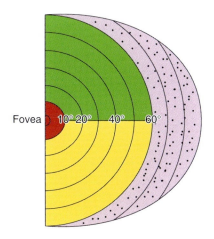

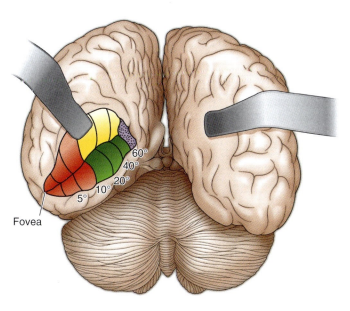

Figure 3-20. **Cortical map and corresponding visual field.**
The illustration shows the posterior aspect of the brain with the cerebral hemispheres spread apart (revealing the mesial surfaces) and the calcarine fissure exposed (in the left hemisphere). The shaded area represents the primary visual cortex. The center of the visual field (fovea) corresponds to the exposed tip of the occipital lobe, with the more peripheral visual field shown as degrees of the eccentricity from the center. Observe how the degree lines labeled on the left visual cortex (*bottom*) correspond to the right hemifield (*top*). The central visual field occupies far more cortex relative to the more peripheral field: Greater than 80% of the primary visual cortex is devoted to the central 30° of visual field. The area beyond 60° corresponds to the monocular temporal crescent (*stippled area*).

normal visual acuity and fundus examination, and can be very difficult to diagnose (Figure 3–22).

Macular Sparing

All unilateral retrochiasmal lesions spare central acuity, but *macular sparing* refers to the tendency of occipital lesions to produce homonymous visual fields that spare the central 5° of the visual field (see Figure 3–21A). This situation occurs with ischemic events involving the posterior cerebral artery, as the middle cerebral artery keeps the occipital tip perfused, sparing this area of cortex that serves central vision.

Respect of the Horizontal Meridian

Because the visual cortex is anatomically divided by the calcarine fissure (with separate vascular supplies),

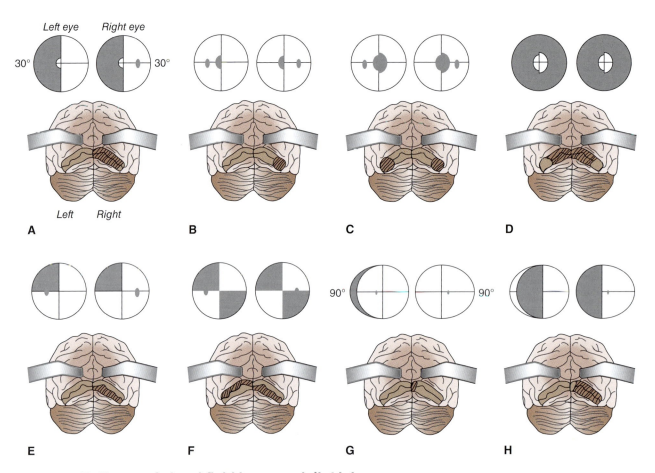

Figure 3–21. Patterns of visual field loss: occipital lobe.
The mesial surfaces of the occipital lobes are exposed to show lesions and their corresponding visual field defects. The visual fields in **(A)–(F)** are shown from the perspective of automated perimetry (with a 30° radius); the visual fields in **(G)** and **(H)** show the entire visual field, as produced by Goldmann perimetry. **(A)** Left homonymous hemianopia with central sparing from a right occipital lobe infarction. **(B)** Left central homonymous visual field loss from an infarct of the tip of the right occipital lobe, at the watershed zone between the middle and posterior cerebral arteries (see Figures 3–22 and 5–17). **(C)** Bilateral central homonymous visual field loss from bilateral infarctions of the occipital lobe tips. Such lesions can occur from profound hypotensive episodes with bilateral watershed infarcts. **(D)** Bilateral homonymous visual field defects with central sparing from bilateral occipital lobe infarction. This situation is most likely to occur from sequential, rather than simultaneous, strokes in the right and left posterior cerebral artery circulation. **(E)** Left homonymous superior quadrantanopia from a lesion involving the lower bank of the right occipital lobe, below the calcarine fissure (see Figure 3–23). **(F)** Bilateral homonymous visual field defects (checkerboard pattern) from an infarct above the calcarine fissure on one side and below it on the other side. **(G)** Loss of the temporal crescent in the visual field of the left eye, with no corresponding homonymous defect in the visual field of the right eye, caused by a lesion involving the mesial surface of the right occipital lobe at its anterior limit. **(H)** Sparing of the temporal crescent in the visual field of the left eye in the presence of a left homonymous hemianopia, due to a lesion involving the right occipital lobe that spares the most anterior extent of the primary visual cortex (see Figure 3–25).

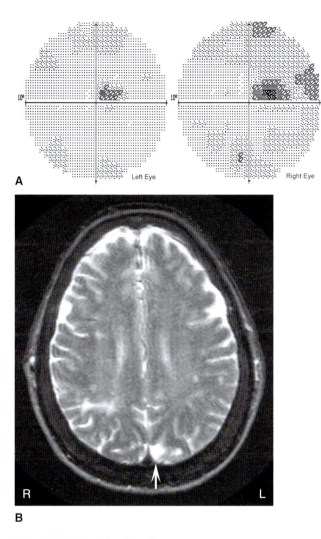

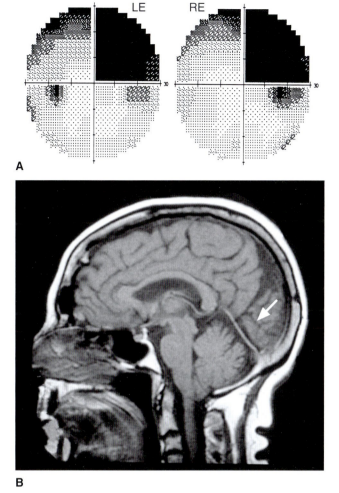

Figure 3-22. Elusive homonymous paracentral scotoma.
A 66-year-old woman presented with the sudden onset of blurred vision, especially noticed when reading. She complained bitterly of missing letters and words. However, her visual acuity was 20/20, Humphrey 30-2 perimetry was normal, and the eye examination was normal. **(A)** The cause of her complaint was not evident until Humphrey 10-2 perimetry was performed, showing a tiny paracentral right homonymous visual field defect (note that this test has a 10° rather than 30° radius). **(B)** Magnetic resonance imaging confirmed the suspected occipital lobe infarct at the tip of the left occipital lobe (*arrow*).

Figure 3-23. Quadrantanopia.
A 70-year-old woman was found to have a visual field defect during a routine examination. The patient was unaware of any visual loss and had no known history of stroke. **(A)** Humphrey 30-2 perimetry demonstrates a right superior homonymous quadrantanopia (respecting both the vertical and horizontal meridians). **(B)** Magnetic resonance imaging (T1-weighted sagittal view) demonstrates cortical atrophy of the left visual cortex confined to the area below the calcarine fissure (*arrow*), presumably from a remote infarct.

Bilateral Lesions of the Occipital Lobe

Bilateral lesions that involve the occipital tip may cause a symmetric decline in the visual acuity (unlike unilateral occipital lobe lesions), with bilateral central homonymous visual field defects. Careful perimetry may reveal mismatched bilateral homonymous defects along the vertical meridian (see Figure 3–21C). The opposite situation can also occur: Bilateral occipital infarcts with bilateral central sparing can result in peripheral field loss with remaining central islands of vision (see Figure 3–21D; Table 3–3). An unusual but striking visual field defect results from infarction of the occipital lobe below

lesions above or below the calcarine fissure can cause homonymous visual field defects that respect the horizontal meridian (see Table 3–1). The visual field defects are not likely to be confused with optic-nerve-related visual field loss, because they are always homonymous and always respect the vertical meridian as well (see Figure 3–21E; Figure 3–23).

TABLE 3-3. PERIPHERAL VISUAL FIELD LOSS WITH PRESERVATION OF THE CENTRAL VISUAL FIELD

Location	Disorders	Comments
Visual cortex	Bilateral occipital infarcts with macular sparing	Visual fields in both eyes are by necessity affected. Small steps that respect the vertical meridian may be identified by careful perimetry. The funduscopic examination is normal.
Optic disc	Advanced glaucoma	Optic disc will display severe glaucomatous atrophy (cupping). Perimetry of the remaining central island of vision may reveal nasal segments that respect the horizontal meridian.
	Optic disc drusen	Visible disc drusen, or buried in a "lumpy-bumpy" disc (see Figure 4–40).
	Chronic atrophic papilledema	Usually bilateral, but may be asymmetric (see Figure 4–25).
Retina	Central retinal artery occlusion with cilioretinal sparing	Acutely, retinal edema can be seen that spares distribution of a cilioretinal artery (see Figure 14–4).
	Retinitis pigmentosa	Bilateral (see Figure 3–6).
Other	Nonorganic visual loss or poor performance on automated perimetry	Patients with nonorganic visual loss often have poor visual acuity (implying a central scotoma) and paradoxically produce a markedly constricted visual field with intact central test points.

the calcarine fissure on one side, and above on the other side. The resultant bilateral homonymous (mixed) quadrantanopia produces a "checkerboard field" (see Figure 3–21F). Bilateral occipital lobe infarctions are often asymmetric, but are always homonymous and almost always highly congruous (Figure 3–24).

Temporal Crescent

All points in the primary visual cortex have binocular input except the deepest portion of the primary visual cortex, which corresponds to the 30° of temporal visual field (temporal crescent) in the contralateral eye, unmatched by the smaller nasal visual field of the ipsilateral eye (see Figure 3–1). Sometimes this area is spared in a posterior cerebral artery stroke (see Figure 3–21H; Figure 3–25). An isolated lesion in this area of visual cortex can cause a *monocular* temporal crescent field defect (defying the rule that occipital lesions are always homonymous and congruous), but is a very rare occurrence (see Figure 3–21G).

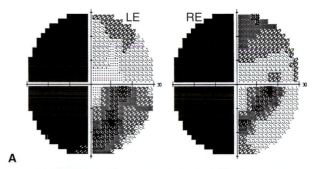

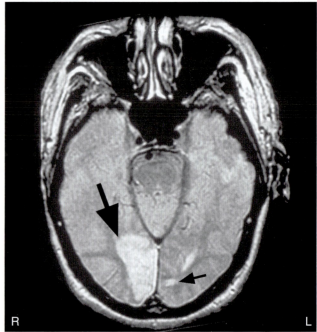

Figure 3-24. Bilateral occipital infarcts.
An 82-year-old man complained of sudden visual loss in his left eye. Visual acuity was 20/30 in both eyes. **(A)** Humphrey 30-2 perimetry demonstrates a complete left homonymous hemianopia, but also a congruous right inferior homonymous defect. **(B)** Corresponding infarcts are seen on magnetic resonance imaging (T1-weighted axial image with contrast): a large infarct of the right occipital cortex (*large arrow*), and a smaller, discreet infarct in the left occipital lobe (*small arrow*) that does not involve the occipital tip (sparing central vision).

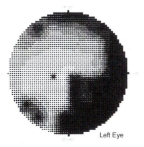 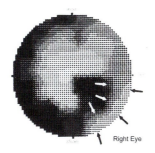

Figure 3–25. Sparing of the temporal crescent.
This is a full-field automated static visual field (Octopus perimeter) of a patient with a left posterior cerebral artery occlusion and occipital infarct. The radius of this perimetric plot is a full 90°, an expanse that is far more typical of Goldmann perimetry than automated tests (note the position of the blind spot in the visual field of the left eye). The arrows show a portion of the temporal crescent that has been spared. The occipital cortex that represents the temporal crescent is deep in the interhemispheric sulcus and was not involved in the ischemic event. The temporal crescent is peculiar because it is entirely monocular—it is the temporal extent of the visual field (60°–90°) that is unmatched by the limited nasal field of the opposite eye (which extends only to 60°).

▶ KEY POINTS

- The visual field extends 90° temporally, 60° nasally, and approximately 70° superiorly and inferiorly in each eye.
- Cataract and other anterior segment disorders cause a diffuse depression of the entire visual field.
- Diseases that affect the *deep (outer) retina* (such as retinitis pigmentosa) cause visual field defects that do not respect the horizontal or vertical meridians.
- Diseases affecting axons in the optic nerve, optic disc, or retinal nerve fiber layer demonstrate patterns of visual field loss that parallel the nerve fiber arrangement, such as nasal step, arcuate, altitudinal, temporal wedge, and cecocentral visual field defects.
- The status of the visual fields from both eyes in all patients with visual loss must be known, even when the patient's complaint is attributed to only one eye.
- Lesions that affect the central body of the chiasm cause bilateral temporal (bitemporal) visual field defects that are often asymmetric between the two eyes.
- Binasal visual field defects are almost always the result of bilateral optic neuropathies rather than lateral chiasmal compression.
- The combination of an optic-nerve-related visual field defect in one eye and a superior temporal visual field defect in the other suggests a lesion at the junction of the optic nerve and chiasm (junctional scotoma).
- Lesions in the optic tract and posterior visual pathway produce contralateral homonymous visual field defects.
- Between the chiasm and occipital lobe, lesions that are more posterior (closer to the occipital lobe) produce homonymous visual field defects that tend to be more congruous.
- Complete homonymous hemianopias are nonlocalizing, in that the degree of congruity cannot be assessed.
- Unilateral homonymous hemianopias do not affect visual acuity.
- Optic tract lesions produce homonymous, incongruous, visual field defects, frequently with a small RAPD and "bow-tie" atrophy of the optic disc, all contralateral to the lesion.
- Temporal lobe lesions result in homonymous visual field defects that are denser above than below (often superior wedge-shaped defects).
- Parietal lobe lesions create homonymous visual field defects that are denser below than above.
- The temporal visual field from 60° to 90° (temporal crescent) is seen only by the ipsilateral eye, with monocular input to the (contralateral) visual cortex at the anterior limit of the primary visual cortex.
- Occipital infarcts may occasionally cause a complete homonymous hemianopia that spares the temporal crescent in the eye contralateral to the lesion.
- Occipital lesions often produce homonymous visual field defects that spare the central 3° to 5° of the visual field.

SUGGESTED READING

Books

Anderson DR: *Testing the Field of Vision.* St. Louis, MO: CV Mosby Co; 1982.

Barton JJS, Benatar M: *Field of Vision: A Manual and Atlas of Perimetry.* Totowa, NJ: Humana Press; 2003.

Budenz, DL: *Atlas of Visual Fields.* Philadelphia, PA: Lippincott-Raven; 1997.

Hart WM Jr: Clinical perimetry and topographic diagnosis in diseases of the afferent visual system, in Slamovits TL, Burde R (eds): *Neuro-ophthalmology,* Vol. 6 of *Textbook of Ophthalmology.* Podos SM, Yanoff M (eds). London: Mosby Year Book; 1991:1.1–1.29.

Lee AG, Brazis PW: Visual field defects, in *Clinical Pathways in Neuro-ophthalmology: An Evidence-Based Approach.* New York, NY: Thieme; 1998:151–170.

Miller NR, Newman NJ: Topical diagnosis of lesions in the visual sensory pathway, in Miller NR, Newman NJ (eds): *Walsh and Hoyts' Clinical Neuro-ophthalmology*, Vol. 1, 5th ed. Baltimore, MD: Williams and Wilkins Co; 1998:237–386.

Walsh TJ (ed): *Visual Fields: Examination and Interpretation (Ophthalmology Monographs)*, Vol. 3, 2d ed. San Francisco, CA: American Academy of Ophthalmology; 1996.

Articles

Barton JJS, Hefter R, Chang B, et al: The field defects of anterior temporal lobectomy: a quantitative reassessment of Meyer's loop. *Brain* 2005;12:2123–2133.

Frisen L, Holmegaard L, Rosencrantz M: Sectorial optic atrophy and homonymous, horizontal sectoranopia: a lateral choroidal artery syndrome? *J Neurol Neurosurg Psychiatry* 1978;41:374–380.

Horton JC: Wilbrand's knee of the primate chiasm is an artifact of monocular enucleation. *Trans Am Ophthalmol Soc* 1997;95:579–609.

Horton JC, Hoyt WF: The representation of the visual field in human striate cortex. A revision of the classic Holmes map. *Arch Ophthalmol* 1991;109:816–824.

Jacobson DM: The localizing value of a quadrantanopia. *Arch Neurol* 1997;54(4):401–404.

Kedar S, Zhang X, Lynn MJ, Newman NJ, Biousse V: Congruency in homonymous hemianopia. Am J Ophthalmol 2007;143:772–780.

Keltner JL, Johnson CA: Automated and manual perimetry. A six-year overview. Special emphasis on neuro-ophthalmic problems. *Ophthalmol* 1983;91:68.

Manfre L, Vero S, Focarelli-Barone C, et al: Bitemporal pseudohemianopia related to the "tilted disk" syndrome: CT, MR, and fundoscopic findings. *Am J Neuroradiol* 1999;20:1750–1751.

Mills RP: Automated perimetry in neuro-ophthalmology. *Int Ophthalmol Clin* 1991;31(4):51.

CHAPTER 4

Optic Nerve Disorders

- ▶ ANATOMY OF THE OPTIC NERVE 85
  - Intraocular course 85
  - Intraorbital course 87
  - Intracanalicular course 88
  - Intracranial course 88
- ▶ CLINICAL EXPRESSION OF DISEASE 88
  - Pallor and cupping 88
  - Optic disc swelling (edema) 89
  - Accompanying signs 90
- ▶ ISCHEMIC OPTIC NEUROPATHIES 92
  - Nonarteritic anterior ischemic optic neuropathy 92
  - Arteritic anterior ischemic optic neuropathy 96
  - Diabetic papillopathy 99
  - Papillophlebitis 100
  - Radiation optic neuropathy 100
- ▶ OPTIC NEURITIS 100
- ▶ OPTIC PERINEURITIS 105
- ▶ PAPILLEDEMA 106
  - Mechanism of papilledema 106
  - Idiopathic intracranial hypertension (pseudotumor cerebri) 107
  - Other causes of papilledema 115
- ▶ COMPRESSIVE OPTIC NEUROPATHIES 115
  - Optic nerve sheath meningiomas 115
  - Other causes of optic nerve compression 117
- ▶ INTRINSIC NEOPLASMS 118
  - Optic nerve glioma 118
  - Lymphoproliferative disorders 119
  - Other intrinsic neoplasms 119
- ▶ INFLAMMATORY OPTIC NEUROPATHIES 119
- ▶ INFECTIOUS OPTIC NEUROPATHIES 120
  - Optic disc edema with a macular star 120
  - Cat-scratch neuroretinitis 121
  - Other infectious neuropathies 122
- ▶ TOXIC AND NUTRITIONAL OPTIC NEUROPATHIES 122
- ▶ HEREDITARY OPTIC NEUROPATHIES 124
  - Autosomal dominant (Kjer) optic atrophy 124
  - Leber hereditary optic neuropathy 125
- ▶ TRAUMATIC OPTIC NEUROPATHY 127
- ▶ GLAUCOMA 128
- ▶ OPTIC DISC DRUSEN 129
- ▶ ANOMALOUS OPTIC DISCS 132
  - Crowded optic discs 134
  - Elevated discs without drusen 134
  - Tilted optic discs 134
  - Myelinated retinal nerve fibers 134
  - Hypoplasia 134
  - Aplasia 134
  - Coloboma 134
- ▶ KEY POINTS 135

In Chapter 3, the organization of axons in the sensory visual system provided the basis for understanding the patterns of visual field defects. In this chapter, the neuroanatomy of the anterior sensory visual system forms the foundation for understanding optic nerve disorders and their clinical expression.

▶ ANATOMY OF THE OPTIC NERVE

The optic nerve originates at the confluence of retinal ganglion cell axons as they traverse the scleral canal to exit the globe, and ends anatomically as these axons merge with the axons of the fellow optic nerve at the chiasm. Anatomic divisions of the optic nerve include intraocular, intraorbital, intracanalicular, and intracranial portions (Figure 4–1).

INTRAOCULAR COURSE

The short intraocular course of the optic nerve is often referred to as the *optic nerve head*, and the portion that can be seen with the ophthalmoscope is called the *optic disc*. The optic disc is usually oval, measuring about

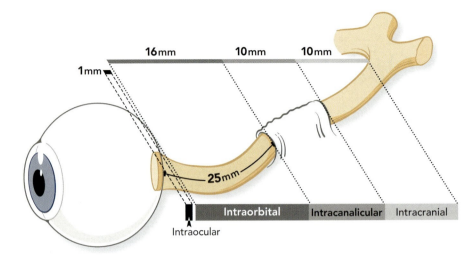

Figure 4-1. **Anatomic divisions of the optic nerve.**

1.5 by 1.75 mm, with its long axis typically oriented vertically. In most subjects, the *optic cup*, devoid of axons, is seen centrally, surrounded by the pink, doughnut-shaped neuroretinal rim (Figure 4–2A). The rim consists of axons seen end-on, as they pass from the nerve fiber layer and make a right-angled turn into the scleral canal. Although the number of axons in normal subjects is relatively constant, the diameter of the scleral canal varies among individuals. When the scleral opening is small, the axons are crowded into a small space (Figure 4–2B). These small, cupless discs are often referred to as "*discs at risk*," as they are frequently associated with optic disc infarction (anterior ischemic optic neuropathy [AION]). Individuals with large scleral openings may have large disks with large central cups, which may be mistaken for the pathological cupping characteristic of glaucoma.

Optic nerve axons congregate into bundles as they pass through the *lamina cribrosa*. This fibrous diaphragm is contiguous with the sclera and has approximately 200 openings. The lamina cribrosa further divides the intraocular optic nerve head into prelaminar, laminar, and postlaminar portions. Optic disc swelling occurs when the prelaminar axons swell due to failure of orthograde axoplasmic flow at the level of the lamina cribrosa. Axoplasmic stasis and disc swelling can be caused by compression, ischemia, toxins, or inflammatory processes, and is not disease specific.

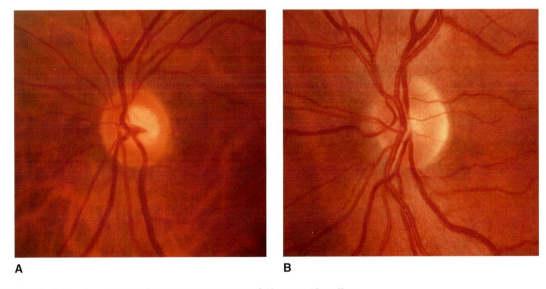

Figure 4-2. **Ophthalmoscopic appearance of the optic disc.**
(A) The normal left optic disc has a cup-to-disc ratio of 0.5. Note the pink color of the neuroretinal rim surrounding the cup, the central position of the retinal artery and vein, and the branching pattern of the retinal vasculature. **(B)** A normal left optic disc with a small cup-to-disc ratio, less than 0.1. This optic disc configuration is associated with an increased risk of developing anterior ischemic optic neuropathy.

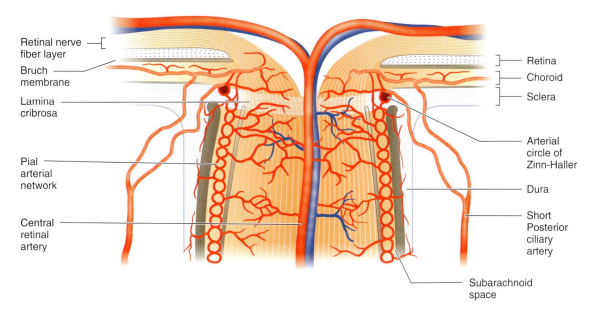

Figure 4-3. Anterior optic nerve anatomy and blood supply.
Observe the abundant blood supply to the retrobulbar optic nerve from the pial plexus on the surface of the nerve and some contribution from the central retinal artery. In contrast, the prelaminar and laminar portions of the optic nerve head do not receive any significant contribution from the central retinal artery, but rely almost entirely on the short posterior ciliary arteries, which also supply the high-flow choroid. (Reproduced with permission from Weinstein JM. The pupil. In Slamovits TL, Burde R, associate editors. Neuro-ophthalmology, vol 6. In Podos SM, Yanoff M, editors: Textbook of ophthalmology. St Louis, 1991, Mosby.)

Behind the globe, two to six short posterior ciliary arteries (branches of the ophthalmic artery) penetrate the sclera in a circumferential fashion around the exiting optic nerve. These vessels form an incomplete anastomotic ring at the level of the choroid (arterial circle of Zinn-Haller), supplying both the high-flow vasculature of the choroidal circulation and the optic nerve head. Although the central retinal vessels pass through the optic nerve head, their contribution to its vascular supply is negligible (Figure 4–3). Insufficient blood flow through the posterior ciliary arteries from thrombosis, hypotension, vasculitic occlusion, or other disease causes ischemic optic neuropathy.

There are high concentrations of mitochondria in the axons of the prelaminar and laminar regions of the optic nerve. This is thought to be due to the much higher energy requirements for conduction in this unmyelinated portion of the optic nerve. This may also explain the vulnerability of the prelaminar optic nerve to processes that affect mitochondria, including heritable, toxic, and nutritional disorders, but also possibly anterior ischemic optic neuropathy and glaucoma.

INTRAORBITAL COURSE

After passing through the lamina cribrosa, the retinal ganglion cell axons acquire myelin sheathing, doubling the diameter of the optic nerve to more than 3 millimeters. The myelin sheath is produced by *oligodendrocytes*, the same cell type found in the white matter tracts of the central nervous system. Peripheral nerves are myelinated by Schwann cells. Thus, the optic nerve is histologically a white matter tract of the brain, rather than a peripheral nerve. This is evident clinically in several ways: The optic nerve does not usually regenerate like other cranial nerves, and optic neuritis is a frequent occurrence in multiple sclerosis (MS), a disease affecting white matter in the brain and spinal cord.

The orbital portion of the optic nerve is approximately 25 mm in length from the posterior aspect of the globe to the orbital apex. Because the globe is only 15 mm anterior to the orbital apex, the optic nerve describes a gently curved path; the extra length allows full movement of the globe without being tethered by the optic nerve (see Figure 4–1). In the orbit, the optic nerve is surrounded by the optic nerve sheath, which is continuous with the intracranial dura through the optic canal posteriorly, and bounded by the sclera anteriorly. The sheath encloses an extension of the intracranial meninges, with pia, arachnoid, and cerebrospinal fluid continuous with the intracranial subarachnoid space. Elevated intracranial pressure can be transmitted through the optic canal directly to the optic nerve head, causing bilateral optic disc edema (papilledema). Meningiomas can arise within the orbit from the dural optic nerve sheath, just as they develop from the intracranial meninges.

At the orbital apex, the nerve sheath fuses with a fibrous ring (annulus of Zinn) that forms the insertion of the superior oblique and the four rectus muscles. This connection explains why eye movement can cause pain when the optic nerve is inflamed in retrobulbar optic neuritis.

The vascular supply of the intraorbital optic nerve is more robust and redundant than that of the optic nerve head. Branches of the ophthalmic artery provide numerous longitudinal pial vessels to the surface of the optic nerve, which in turn yield penetrating vessels that extend toward the center of the nerve. The central retinal artery enters the nerve approximately 10 mm behind the globe, also contributing to the vascular supply of this segment of the intraorbital optic nerve (see Figure 4–3). Given such a hardy blood supply, ischemic insults to the retrobulbar optic nerve are rare, in contrast to the relatively frequent occurrence of optic disc infarction (ie, AION).

INTRACANALICULAR COURSE

The intracanalicular portion of the optic nerve is approximately 10 mm long, beginning where the optic nerve enters the optic foramen in the lesser wing of the sphenoid, and ending where the optic nerve exits the optic canal and enters the intracranial cavity. From the orbit, the optic canal is directed medially and superiorly to enter the intracranial cavity. The optic canal is separated from the sphenoid sinus by very thin papyraceous bone, and the course of the optic nerve can be seen as a convexity in the lateral wall of the sinus. In addition to the optic nerve, the optic canal also contains the ophthalmic artery (and some accompanying sympathetic fibers).

Space-occupying lesions within the bony confines of the optic canal (such as an intracanalicular meningioma) do not have to be large to compress the intracanalicular optic nerve and cause visual loss, and may not be easily seen on neuroimaging. Blunt accelerating or decelerating trauma to the orbital rim can transmit forces to the optic canal, causing optic nerve tears, contusion, and shearing injury to the optic nerve, with or without canal fractures. Hemorrhage or edema within this confined space may produce additional ischemic injury.

INTRACRANIAL COURSE

The intracranial portion of the optic nerve extends from the nerve's entrance into the intracranial space to the chiasm. Its length is approximately 10 mm, but varies greatly between individuals (from 3 to 18 mm). The optic nerves angle superiorly at approximately 45° from the skull base and converge toward the midsagittal plane to form the chiasm. The anterior clinoid bone is superior and lateral to the optic nerve as the nerve emerges from the optic foramen. The inferior frontal lobes and olfactory tracts are located above the nerve. The vascular supply of the optic nerve in this location includes the carotid arteries, located laterally, as well as the anterior cerebral arteries and the anterior communicating arteries, located superiorly. As the carotid artery emerges from the cavernous sinus, the ophthalmic artery is its first intracranial branch, travelling on the inferior surface of the optic nerve to enter the optic foramen. Carotid-ophthalmic artery aneurysms (commonly large and bilateral) or dolichoectatic enlargement and displacement of the carotid artery can cause compression of the intracranial optic nerve.

▶ CLINICAL EXPRESSION OF DISEASE

Acquired optic nerve disorders commonly result in pallor, pathological cupping, or swelling of the optic disc. Congenital optic disc anomalies, discussed at the end of this chapter, produce a broad spectrum of optic disc appearances that can easily be confused with acquired disease.

PALLOR AND CUPPING

The axons that make up the optic nerve may be affected by disease anywhere along their course, from their origin in the inner retina to their synaptic endpoint in the lateral geniculate nucleus. Fatal injury to an axon results in retrograde and orthograde degeneration of the axon, and eventual death of the retinal ganglion cell of origin. Axonal injury remote from the optic disc may cause optic nerve dysfunction without any *acutely* observable optic disc abnormality, but over time optic disc atrophy and nerve fiber layer dropout in the inner retina becomes visible, revealing the extent of the damage. In the majority of neuro-ophthalmic disorders, axonal loss manifests as pallor of the normally pink neuroretinal rim, without apparent loss of neuroretinal rim mass. Diffuse disc pallor is a final common pathway for many optic neuropathies, and is nondiagnostic. However, the location of segmental pallor is often instructive, such as the sectoral or altitudinal pallor in AION, unilateral "bow-tie" atrophy with optic tract lesions (bilateral with chiasmal lesions), or temporal pallor characteristic of the toxic/nutritional or hereditary optic neuropathies (see Figures 4–10D; 4–34A, C; 5–4B; 5–9B). Loss of axons may also manifest as optic nerve cupping, as the central cup enlarges from axonal dropout. Optic disc cupping is characteristic of glaucoma, but can occur in other optic neuropathies. Cupping *with pallor* of the remaining neuroretinal rim suggests a cause other than glaucoma (see Figure 4–39B).

OPTIC DISC SWELLING (EDEMA)

The term "optic disc *edema*" implies that optic disc swelling is the result of extracellular fluid from vascular transudation, which is usually *not* the case. "Optic disc *swelling*" is a better term, but commonly the two terms are used interchangeably (and we succumb to the popular usage of "edema" in this book—but only occasionally).

Swelling of the prelaminar axons causes elevation and expansion of the optic nerve head. Axons swell when the normal process of anterograde axoplasmic flow is dammed up by mechanical, ischemic, or toxic-metabolic processes occurring in the mitochondria-rich region of the axons anterior to the lamina cribrosa (Figure 4–4). The normally distinct border of the optic disc and surrounding retina become blurred as swollen peripapillary axons become elevated and opaque. Transudation of fluids from injured axons and disc vessels also contribute a small amount to the disc's swollen appearance. A number of insults to the optic nerve can result in optic disc swelling (Table 4–1). Elevated intracranial pressure transmitted to the optic nerve head within the confines of the optic nerve sheath can cause stasis of axoplasmic flow at the level of the lamina because of regional pressure differentials. Anterior ischemic optic neuropathy produces optic disc swelling as a result of ischemia. Inflammation from infection, demyelination, or scleritis can also produce disc swelling. Because optic disc swelling can be caused by many disease processes, the history, examination,

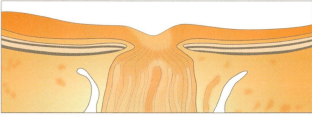

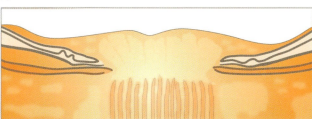

Figure 4-4. Prelaminar swelling in optic disc edema.
(A) Cross section of optic disc through normal optic nerve. **(B)** Optic disc with papilledema. Observe the swelling anterior to the lamina cribrosa from axoplasmic stasis in papilledema. (Reproduced with permission from Liu GT, Volpe NJ, Galetta SL: Neuro-ophthalmology: Diagnosis and Management, Book with DVD-ROM: 2nd edition. Saunders/Elsevier, 2010.)

▶ **TABLE 4–1. CAUSES OF OPTIC DISC ELEVATION**

Papilledema (elevated intracranial pressure)
Optic neuritis
Anterior ischemic optic neuropathy
  Nonarteritic
  Arteritic (GCA)
  Diabetic papillitis

Compression
  Graves orbitopathy
  Meningioma
  Orbital masses

Infiltration (inflammatory and neoplastic)
  Sarcoidosis
  Lymphoproliferative disorders
  Glioma

Infection
  Syphilis
  Lyme disease
  Cat-scratch disease
  Toxoplasmosis

Leber hereditary optic neuropathy (LHON)
Venous congestion
  Retinal vein occlusion
  Papillophlebitis
  Dural cavernous fistula

Other ocular disorders
  Uveitis
  Hypotony
  Cystoid macular edema

Systemic
  Hypertensive emergency (malignant hypertension)
  Severe anemia
  Hypoxemia
  Cyanotic heart disease
  Uremia

Optic disc tumors
  Hemangioma, hemangioblastoma
  Melanocytoma
  Metastasis

Trauma
Toxic
  Amiodarone
  Methanol

Pseudopapilledema
  Anomalous discs
  Optic disc drusen
  Gliosis
  Tilted discs

Abbreviation: GCA, giant cell arteritis.

ancillary testing (such as neuroimaging), and clinical course are the keys to determining the diagnosis. Important features in developing a differential diagnosis are listed in Figure 4–5, with individual disorders covered in detail in this chapter.

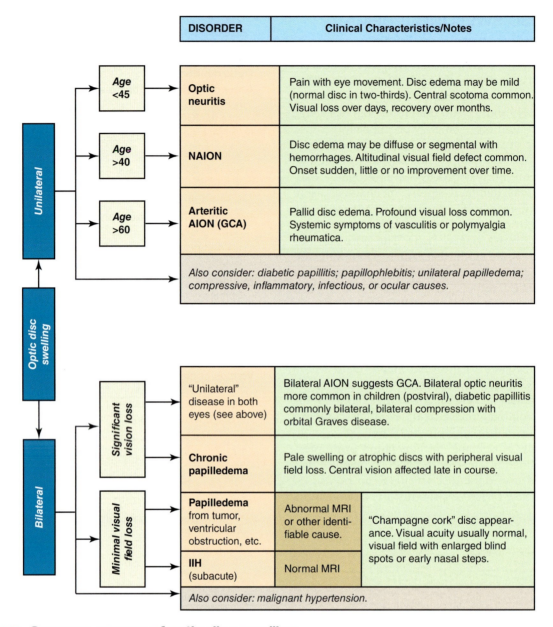

Figure 4-5. Common causes of optic disc swelling.
Although there are many causes of optic disc swelling, a thorough history and examination helps to narrow the possibilities. The more common diagnostic possibilities can often be distinguished by whether one or both optic discs are involved, the age of the patient, and the degree and time course of visual loss. Abbreviations: AION, anterior ischemic optic neuropathy; GCA, giant cell arteritis; MRI, magnetic resonance imaging; NAION, nonarteritic anterior ischemic optic neuropathy.

Infiltration of the optic nerve head by cancer cells, inflammatory cells, and/or infectious organisms is another mechanism of optic nerve head elevation. Generally, these processes also incite concomitant optic disc swelling.

Some anomalous, but otherwise normal optic discs may be elevated, giving the false appearance of optic disc edema (Table 4-2; see Figure 4-43B).

ACCOMPANYING SIGNS

Rapid expansion of the optic disc from axonal swelling can cause damage to the optic disc and peripapillary vasculature, resulting in hemorrhages at many levels: deep, dark peripapillary subretinal hemorrhages; dot/blot intraretinal hemorrhages; nerve fiber layer hemorrhages (usually flame shaped); and (rarely) preretinal or vitreous hemorrhage (Figures 4-6 and 4-7). Cotton-wool spots are areas of nerve fiber layer infarction and can be seen on the optic disc as well as in the nerve fiber layer of the retina (Figure 4-8). Vascular changes can include telangiectasia on the disc surface (increased capillarity) or venous stasis (increased venous caliber). Telangiectasia on the disc and within the peripapillary retina can accompany Leber hereditary optic neuropathy (LHON;

▶ **TABLE 4-2. DISTINGUISHING TRUE OPTIC DISC SWELLING FROM ANOMALOUS OPTIC DISCS (PSEUDOPAPILLEDEMA)**

Common Features of Anomalous Optic Discs
- Often cupless with small diameter
- Venous pulsations often present, but may be absent
- Increased number of central retinal vessels arising from the apex of the disc (increased branching on the disc)
- Scalloped or irregular disc margin, optic disc drusen may be visible
- Vessels cross disc margin without being obscured
- Usually do not leak but can stain with IVFA

Common Features of True Optic Disc Swelling
- Central cup usually relatively preserved unless swelling is extreme
- Increased "capillarity" on the optic disc
- Opacification of the peripapillary NFL, obscuring vessels as they cross the disc margin
- Concentric circumferential peripapillary chorioretinal folds (Paton lines) or radial choroidal folds may be present
- Glistening tiny "pseudodrusen": lipoproteinaceous residues on surface of optic discs in long-standing optic disc swelling
- Cotton-wool spots on or around the optic disc
- Retinal hemorrhages: splinter hemorrhages (most common), but may have dot and blot, subretinal, or even preretinal subhyaloid hemorrhages
- Absent venous pulsations (however, 20% of normal discs lack venous pulsations)
- Leakage and staining with IVFA

Abbreviations: IVFA, intravenous fluorescein angiography; NFL, nerve fiber layer.

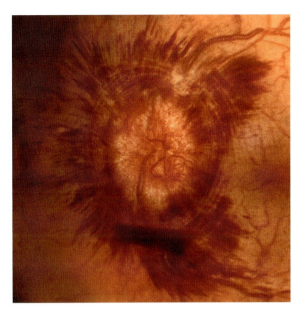

Figure 4-6. **Severe optic disc edema.** Massive optic disc edema is present in this patient with intracranial hypertension and systemic hypertension. The optic nerve is elevated and enlarged. Hemorrhage is present in the nerve fiber layer (flame-shaped hemorrhages) and within the retina (dot/blot hemorrhages). The swollen nerve elevates and laterally displaces the choroid and retina, creating concentric chorioretinal folds called *Paton lines*.

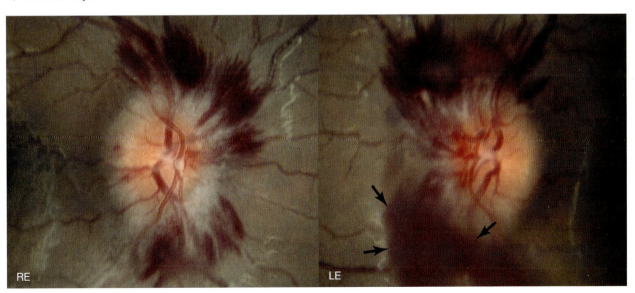

Figure 4-7. **Optic disc edema with retinal hemorrhages.**
This patient with papilledema has hemorrhages in the nerve fiber layer (NFL) of the retina, producing flame-shaped hemorrhages, as seen in the right eye. The shape of the hemorrhages reflects the anatomic arrangement of the nerve fiber layer in the inner retina. The left eye has preretinal hemorrhages (*arrows*) in addition to NFL hemorrhages. Preretinal blood can flow over the surface of the retina, constrained only by the vitreous (hyaloid). This type of hemorrhage is called *subhyaloid*. Preretinal blood can also break through into the vitreous and create a diffuse vitreous hemorrhage, obscuring the view of the retina.

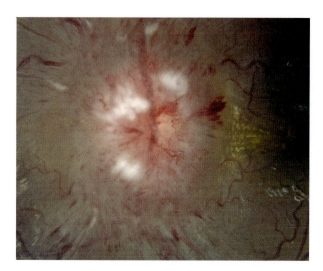

Figure 4–8. Optic disc edema with cotton-wool spots.
The white patches on the surface of this disc with grade 5 papilledema are infarcts of the nerve fiber layer, called cotton-wool spots. Their presence suggests ischemia. Though more common in ischemic conditions such as malignant hypertension, they can be present in severe optic disc edema from any cause. Also note the macular edema residues forming a partial macular star.

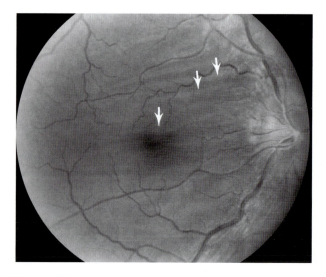

Figure 4–9. Choroidal folds and optic disc edema in idiopathic intracranial hypertension.
This clinical photograph shows linear macular striations (*arrows*) that can occur when the expanded optic nerve sheath indents the posterior globe, shortening the axial length of the eye (which induces a hyperopic refractive shift).

see Figure 4–35A). Collateral veno-venous vessels on the disc can be seen with optic nerve sheath meningioma, chronic papilledema, or compensated retinal vein occlusion. An increase in the diameter of the intraocular portion of the optic nerve from axonal swelling produces concentric peripapillary chorioretinal folds, called Paton lines (see Figure 4–6). Macular choroidal folds, oriented radially to the disc, frequently occur as a result of indentation of the posterior globe by an engorged optic nerve sheath expanded by high cerebrospinal fluid pressure, but can also occur in orbital Graves disease or from any intraorbital mass (Figure 4–9). Macular edema can occur with massive disc swelling of any cause (see Figure 4–8) but is most frequently seen accompanying optic disc edema in infectious or postinfectious autoimmune processes (neuroretinitis) (see Figure 4–32A).

▶ ISCHEMIC OPTIC NEUROPATHIES

Anterior *ischemic* optic neuropathy (AION), as its name implies, is the result of ischemia. The designation of *anterior* indicates that the ischemic insult causes damage to the optic nerve head and is visible with the ophthalmoscope. AION is thought to be caused by hypoperfusion of one or more of the short posterior ciliary arteries that supply the optic nerve head. *Nonarteritic* AION (NAION) is very common, and is most likely the result of vascular insufficiency from thrombosis and/or hypotension in patients with atherosclerotic disease. *Arteritic* AION occurs less often (5–10% of AION), and is caused by vasculitic occlusion of the arterial supply to the optic nerve head due to giant cell arteritis (GCA). This more devastating form of AION can cause bilateral blindness, as well as significant systemic vascular morbidity.

The term *posterior ischemic optic neuropathy (PION)* indicates an infarct of the optic nerve posterior to the optic disc, with a normal-appearing optic disc initially. PION is rare (due to the robust vascular supply of the retrobulbar optic nerve as discussed earlier), and occurs almost exclusively in two settings: vasculitis (mainly GCA), or profound blood loss and/or hypotension that occurs during surgery or as a result of trauma.

NONARTERITIC ANTERIOR ISCHEMIC OPTIC NEUROPATHY

NAION is a common cause of sudden, painless, monocular visual loss in adults typically 50 to 70 years old (Figure 4–10). Systemic hypertension (50%) and/or diabetes mellitus (25%) are commonly present. Frequently, patients have other systemic manifestations of atherosclerotic disease such as angina pectoris, previous myocardial infarctions, or history of stroke. Sleep apnea, migraine, renal dialysis, and smoking are other potential associated conditions.

Symptoms

Visual loss in this condition ranges from profound to mild, and is frequently first noted by patients when

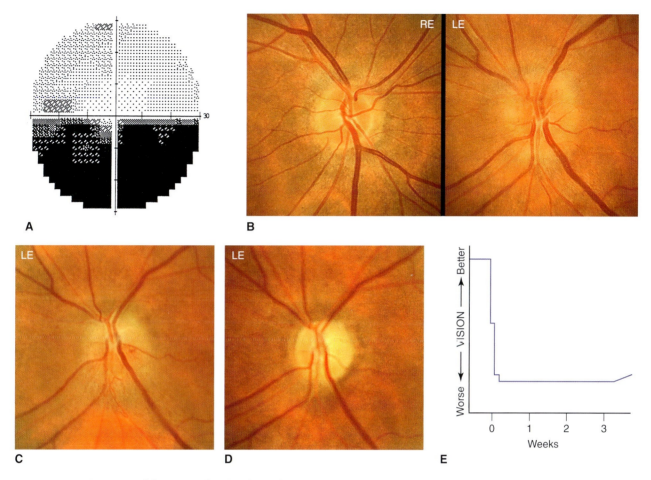

Figure 4–10. **Nonarteritic anterior ischemic optic neuropathy.**
A 62-year-old man awoke with painless visual loss in his left eye. **(A)** A dense inferior altitudinal visual field defect was present in the left eye (the visual field in the right eye was normal). **(B)** The right disc was normal, but note the absence of a central cup, showing that this patient has the typical cupless "disc at risk" for AION. The left optic disc was swollen. The optic disc edema primarily involved the upper half of the optic disc, corresponding to the inferior visual field defect. **(C)** After 6 weeks, the upper pole of the left optic disc was less swollen, but pale. Paradoxically, the lower pole appeared more swollen, with telangiectatic vessels that may represent "luxury perfusion" to the remaining normal nerve. **(D)** After 6 months, the upper portion of the left optic disc became pale, and the lower half remained pink. **(E)** Time course of visual loss. The visual loss in this disorder is sudden, but may decline stepwise over several days. Some patients may have slight improvement in their central vision with time, but the visual field defect is typically permanent.

they awaken from sleep. The visual loss is generally painless but can be associated with a mild ocular ache. The visual deficit is usually stable after onset, but some patients may have a stepwise decline in vision over several days. A subset of patients (5–10%) has a relentlessly progressive stepwise decline in vision for weeks following the initial event.

Signs

The visual field loss is commonly a mix of central and altitudinal visual field defects (Figure 4–10A), but any disc-related visual field defect can occur. Not uncommonly, patients are quite specific in their history, stating that they have lost the lower (or upper) half of their vision. Occasionally, central acuity is spared, but the vast majority of the time the visual field defect includes central vision.

The optic disc swelling is frequently ruddy or hyperemic and may be diffuse or segmental. For example, a dense inferior altitudinal visual field defect may be associated with segmental swelling of the superior pole of the optic disc, with relative preservation of the inferior pole (see Figure 4–10B). The discs are commonly small and cupless "disks at risk," a finding that may only be appreciated by viewing the contralateral (unaffected) optic disc (see Figure 4–10B). This finding is so widespread that patients thought to have NAION who have a moderate or large cup-to-disc ratio should be considered to have some other process (such as arteritic AION) until proven otherwise. Peripapillary nerve fiber hemorrhages frequently accompany the disc edema. The remainder of the fundus is generally unremarkable, although retinal arterioles may reflect evidence of systemic hypertension, diabetes, or atherosclerotic disease. The disc swelling generally resolves within 3 to 6 weeks, leaving optic disc pallor (see Figure 4–10C, D).

Causes

NAION is thought to be a stroke of the optic nerve head, resulting from insufficient blood flow through the posterior ciliary arteries. Atherosclerosis that accompanies aging, or that is accelerated by systemic vascular diseases such as hypertension and diabetes, narrows the lumen to a critical level where thrombosis or even mild hypotension results in ischemia. The crowded, cupless optic discs commonly identified in these patients may initiate and perpetuate a cascade: ischemia causing edema, edema in the narrow confines of the crowded disc causing further ischemia from increased tissue pressure, with a downward spiral of increasing edema and ischemia.

The timing of this ischemic event, characteristically occurring at night and in the early morning, may be explained by nocturnal hypotension, a concept first described by Hayreh et al (1994). Systemic blood pressure is normally lower at night when patients are sleeping. Hypertension (and other vascular disorders) can damage arterial compliance and local autoregulation, such that nocturnal hypotensive swings reach a critical level that precipitates NAION. Long-acting antihypertensive medications may further accentuate nocturnal hypotension. Not infrequently, patients who present with AION report having been changed to stronger or longer-acting antihypertensive medication in the weeks or months before the event. Obviously, withdrawal of the patient's antihypertensive medications is not the answer, but it is reasonable to suggest to the patient's physician that long-acting antihypertensives be taken in the morning, or that shorter-acting drugs be considered to avoid nocturnal hypotension.

Differential Diagnosis

The most important consideration in the differential diagnosis is distinguishing NAION from arteritic AION caused by GCA (see Figure 4–5). In every case of AION, the physician should ask specific questions regarding the systemic symptoms of vasculitis (discussed below). AION may be difficult to distinguish from optic neuritis in adults aged 35 to 45 years, and the patients may need both possibilities investigated (Table 4–3). Table 4–1 lists other causes of optic disc elevation.

Evaluation

A sedimentation rate, C-reactive protein, and complete blood count should be drawn in most cases to address the possibility of an arteritic cause. Patients without known diabetes or hypertension should be assessed for these two diseases, and it is reasonable to send patients to their medical physician for a thorough examination. Patients younger than 45 years without known risk factors should have a serological evaluation for hyperlipidemia, vasculitis (rheumatological studies), hypercoagulable states, and syphilis (Table 4–4). Patients with symptoms suggestive of sleep apnea may need a sleep study.

Neuroimaging is generally not indicated as long as the history is convincing for AION (sudden onset, stable course), and the examination is consistent (optic disc swelling). If optic neuritis is a consideration, magnetic resonance imaging (MRI) may be needed to assess the possibility of MS. Patients who present with recent visual loss and *optic nerve pallor* may require neuroimaging to evaluate for possible compressive neuropathy (such as a meningioma, parasellar or sellar tumor, or compressive orbital Graves disease).

Treatment

No proven, effective treatment is known for NAION. However, oral or intravenous corticosteroids in the acute phase are thought to be effective by some authorities, such as Hayreh and Zimmerman (2008). The use of optic nerve sheath fenestration in this condition was explored by the ischemic optic neuropathy decompression trial (IONDT). The study showed that this surgery was not beneficial and may even be harmful. The use of a daily aspirin may decrease the risk of an event in the contralateral eye, as discussed below. Obviously, underlying precipitating factors should be addressed, such as blood loss, anemia, sleep apnea, or factors inducing hypotension. As discussed above, a patient's medications for systemic hypertension should be reviewed. A potential association of NAION with drugs for erectile dysfunction (phosphodiesterase-5 inhibitors) has been proposed, but a causative link is not convincing. It is reasonable to caution patients who have had one eye affected regarding the potential risk of these drugs.

Clinical Course

Patients should have repeat visual fields after several weeks and after several months, to ensure that the visual field loss is not progressive. Once NAION has finished its course and optic pallor ensues, this process is unlikely to occur again in the same eye. One proposed rationale is that the death of axons from an ischemic event frees up space for the remaining

► **TABLE 4–3. OVERLAPPING PROFILES: COMPARISON OF ARTERITIC AND NONARTERITIC AION, AND NONARTERITIC AION AND OPTIC NEURITIS**

	Arteritic and nonarteritic AION may be difficult to distinguish in older patients	Nonarteritic AION and optic neuritis may be difficult to distinguish in younger patients	
	Arteritic AION (GCA) **5–10% of AION**	**Nonarteritic AION** **90–95% of AION**	**Optic Neuritis**
Age	>50 years (very rare <50 years)	45–70 years	<45 years
Sex	F > M	F = M	F > M
Optic disc appearance	Usually pale edema, occasionally disc may be normal (in PION). Any cup/disc configuration.	Sectoral or diffuse hyperemic optic disc edema with peripapillary hemorrhage and cotton-wool spots. Cup/disc ratio small.	Only 1/3 have optic disc edema (2/3 have a normal disc). Usually disc edema is mild, without hemorrhage or cotton-wool spots.
Eventual optic atrophy	Diffuse pallor, but can have cupping.	Sectoral or diffuse pallor (no cupping).	Diffuse pallor.
Vision loss	Acute, severe.	Acute, less severe.	Subacute (declines over days/week).
Other eye	75% involved acutely if untreated.	Rarely involved acutely; 30% lifelong risk, 15% 5-year risk.	Unusual for adults to present with bilateral symptoms (but subclinical involvement of opposite eye by visual field in 50%).
Pain	Scalp tenderness and headache.	Unusual.	Often have pain with eye movement that precedes vision loss.
Other eye symptoms	TVL preceding AION, diplopia.	None.	Phosphenes acutely, and Uhthoff phenomenon after recovery.
Systemic symptoms or findings	GCA symptoms: headache, scalp tenderness, jaw or tongue claudication, fever, night sweats, malaise, weight loss	Risk factors include hypercholesterolemia, hypertension, diabetes, other vascular disease.	MS symptoms: numbness, imbalance, diplopia, paraparesis, incontinence, others.
Vision prognosis	Some can improve initially with IV steroids.	Visual field rarely improves (but visual acuity can improve some).	Dramatic improvement is the rule: over weeks to months.
Immediate treatment considerations	Immediate institution of high-dose steroids to salvage vision and reduce risk to the other eye.	No proven treatment. Acute-phase corticosteroids may help Hayreh (2008).	Consider IV methylprednisolone as per ONTT; do not use low-dose oral corticosteroids alone.
Labs	Elevated ESR and CRP (but not always).	Normal ESR and CRP.	Normal ESR and CRP.
MRI	Only helpful to exclude other entities; optic nerve enhancement possible.	Only helpful to exclude other entities; optic nerve enhancement very rarely.	Helpful; may show optic nerve enhancement or white matter changes suggestive of MS.
IVFA	IVFA can show delayed filling of and staining of optic disc, and choroidal hypoperfusion.	Delay in filling and staining of optic disc, but usually no choroidal hyperperfusion.	No delay in filling. Disc will stain if swollen.

Abbreviations: CRP, C-reactive protein; ESR, erythrocyte sedimentation rate; GCA, giant cell arteritis; IV, intravenous; IVFA, intravenous fluorescein angiography; MRI, magnetic resonance imaging; MS, multiple sclerosis; ONTT, Optic Neuritis Treatment Trial; PION, posterior ischemic optic neuropathy; TVL, Transient visual loss.

▶ **TABLE 4-4. HEMATOLOGIC ABNORMALITIES THAT CAN CAUSE VASCULAR OCCLUSIONS**

Hypercoagulable States
　Protein C deficiency
　Protein S deficiency
　Antithrombin III deficiency
　Antiphospholipid antibodies
　　• Lupus anticoagulant
　　• Anticardiolipin antibodies
　Factor V Leiden mutation (activated protein C resistance)
　Hyperhomocysteinemia

Erythrocyte Disorders
　Polycythemia
　Sickle-cell disease and others

Leukemias

axons, effectively reversing the crowding of the optic disc. About one-half of patients with NAION may experience *minimal* improvement in visual function with time, usually manifest as slight improvement in visual acuity (see Figure 4–10E). The incidence of occurrence in the fellow eye is 20% to 40%, although it generally occurs years later. Simultaneous or sequential events in both eyes should raise strong suspicions of a vasculitic (eg, GCA) or other cause (eg, amiodarone toxic optic neuropathy). Unlike retinal vascular events, NAION has not been shown to be associated with an increased risk of cerebrovascular or cardiovascular events.

ARTERITIC ANTERIOR ISCHEMIC OPTIC NEUROPATHY

Arteritic anterior ischemic optic neuropathy is caused by vasculitic closure of the posterior ciliary arteries from GCA. The visual loss is usually more profound than nonarteritic AION, and may occur in both eyes at the same time or in rapid succession. Patients with GCA are usually older than 60 years, and the disease becomes more common with each decade of life. Arteritic AION is unusual before 60 years of age, and only a small number of patients with this diagnosis in their 40s have been documented. Among patients with GCA, women outnumber men 3 to 1, and it is much less common in African-Americans.

Causes

GCA is an idiopathic systemic vasculitis consisting of inflammation in the wall of small and medium-sized arteries, usually involving the extracranial arteries of the head. The inflammatory process can greatly expand the wall thickness, obliterating the lumen of the vessel and obstructing blood flow, with resultant ischemic consequences (Figure 4–11).

Symptoms

Patients with GCA may present with rapid and profound blindness from ischemic optic neuropathy in one or both eyes. Permanent visual loss is frequently preceded by transient visual loss lasting seconds to minutes, similar to amaurosis fugax (see Table 1–3). Although the visual loss itself is painless, patients commonly complain of a new (more or less continuous) headache, scalp tenderness, and jaw claudication. Scalp tenderness may be caused by inflamed arteries in the scalp, or be secondary to scalp ischemia. Scalp tenderness may be so intense that patients complain of pain when lying on a pillow, combing their hair, or wearing a hat. Jaw pain with chewing, pain on swallowing, and talking-induced tongue pain can result from claudication of the involved muscles. Additional manifestations of this systemic vasculitis include weight loss, poor appetite, generalized malaise, myalgia, arthralgia, and low-grade fever.

Polymyalgia rheumatica (PMR) is a chronic rheumatological disorder characterized by proximal shoulder and buttock pain without tenderness. PMR may be a precursor or concomitant accompaniment of GCA.

Signs

Visual field defects from arteritic AION may be similar to those found in nonarteritic AION, though the visual acuity and field are frequently much more severely affected. Not uncommonly, patients present with NLP (no light perception) vision. The optic disc appearance may be indistinguishable from nonarteritic AION, but more commonly it is diffusely edematous and chalky pallid (see Figure 4–11A). On occasion, arteritis can cause a posterior ischemic optic neuropathy (PION), in which the optic disc appears normal or is only minimally affected acutely. Acute, profound visual loss in a patient older than 55 with an unimpressive disc and retina, or in whom visual loss exceeds the observed optic disc edema, should be considered GCA until proven otherwise (Table 4–5). Bilateral or rapidly sequential AION also requires immediate consideration of GCA. In contrast to nonarteritic AION, glaucomatous-like optic disc cupping may develop following arteritic AION.

The occasional occurrence of a retinal infarct in the distribution of a cilioretinal artery in the setting of AION is highly suggestive of arteritis. This association is not surprising because the optic disc and peripapillary choroid share a common blood supply—the short posterior ciliary arteries. Ophthalmic artery involvement can cause simultaneous ischemic optic

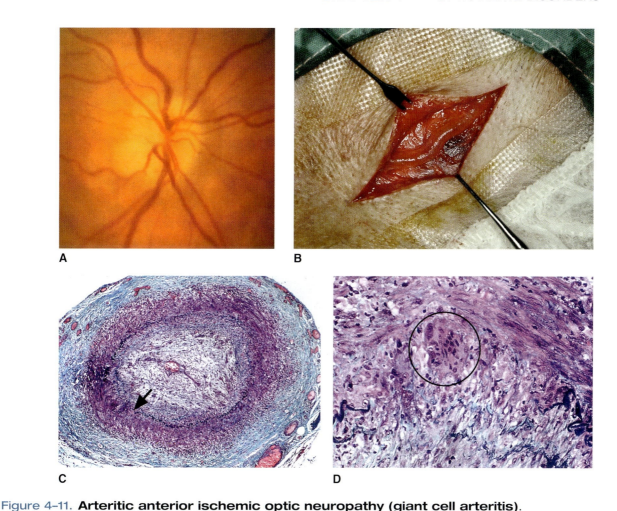

Figure 4–11. **Arteritic anterior ischemic optic neuropathy (giant cell arteritis).**
A 74-year-old woman described brief episodes of visual loss in her right eye for several days, followed by a "skim" over the right eye 2 days before her evaluation, and awoke the next day with "no vision" in the right eye. She reported general malaise and tenderness of her scalp over the temples for two weeks. The examination showed light perception vision only in the right eye, with pale optic disc swelling. Although the erythrocyte sedimentation rate (ESR) was relatively normal for her age (41 mm/hr), giant cell arteritis (GCA) was suspected on the basis of the history and examination. The patient was admitted for high-dose intravenous steroids, and a temporal artery biopsy confirmed the diagnosis of GCA. **(A)** Pale optic disc edema was present in the right eye. **(B)** Temporal artery exposed at biopsy. The artery appeared large and pale. **(C)** Temporal artery cross section. Hematoxylin and eosin (H&E) stain, x100. The lumen is obliterated by massive thickening of the arterial wall. Fracture of the internal elastic lamina is seen (*arrow*). **(D)** A multinucleated giant cell is seen at higher magnification (*circled*).

neuropathy and central retinal artery occlusion, a rare combination that can be caused by the profound ischemia possible from GCA.

Inflamed temporal arteries (or other scalp arteries) can frequently be palpated as a firm "cord" with a poor or absent pulse, explaining this disorder's alternate name: *temporal* arteritis. Fortunately, these frequently involved arteries are also easily surgically accessible for biopsy.

Visual loss occurs in 30% to 40% patients with GCA. If the disorder is unrecognized and untreated, visual loss in the second eye can occur in up to three-quarters of patients with arteritic AION, usually within several weeks. Early recognition of this process is vital to prevent bilateral blindness. Other vascular consequences of GCA are listed in Table 4–6.

Differential Diagnosis

The evaluation of patients presenting as AION is directed at determining whether the process is arteritic or nonarteritic, as discussed in previously (see Figure 4–5). Fluorescein angiography has been advocated by some experts as a potential way of distinguishing these two entities. Patients who have profound insufficiency of the posterior ciliary arteries resulting from GCA may demonstrate areas of choroidal hypoperfusion on the early sequences

▶ **TABLE 4-5. ACQUIRED CAUSES OF PROFOUND VISUAL LOSS WITH A RELATIVELY UNREMARKABLE FUNDUS EXAMINATION**

Retrobulbar Optic Neuritis
Young adults with monocular visual loss and RAPD.

Neuromyelitis Optica (Devic Disease)
Severe vision loss often bilaterally, usually associated with long longitudinal transverse myelitis.

Compressive Optic Neuropathy
Optic disc becomes pale eventually, but may look normal at first.

Posterior Ischemic Optic Neuropathy
GCA: Patients >55 years with acute visual loss and symptoms of systemic vasculitis.
Perioperative vision loss: usually associated with profound blood loss and/or hypotension.
Radiation optic neuropathy: usually occurs several years after radiation to head.

Acute Traumatic Optic Neuropathy
Pallor may take weeks to develop following injury.

Disorders of the chiasm
Often a mix of chiasm, optic nerve, and optic tract visual field patterns.

Retrochiasmal Lesions
Unilateral retrochiasmal lesions: contralateral homonymous hemianopia that does not affect visual acuity.
Bilateral occipital lobe disease: (see Table 5-3) Bilateral, symmetric congruous visual field loss and symmetric visual acuity loss.

Retrobulbar Inflammatory or Infiltrative Disorder
Neurosarcoidosis, idiopathic orbital inflammatory syndrome may not cause optic disc pallor or swelling initially.

Retinal Artery Occlusion
After the acute retinal edema has resolved, retinal findings may be subtle.

Paraneoplastic Optic Neuropathy and Retinopathy
Bilateral, symmetric, slowly progressive visual loss.

Toxic and Nutritional Optic Neuropathies (and Toxic Maculopathies)
Bilateral, progressive loss of central vision

▶ **TABLE 4-6. ISCHEMIC MANIFESTATIONS OF GIANT CELL ARTERITIS (GCA)**

Ophthalmic
  Anterior ischemic optic neuropathy
  Posterior ischemic optic neuropathy
  Central or branch retinal artery occlusion
  Choroidal infarction
  Ocular ischemic syndrome
  Ischemic cranial neuropathies
  Ischemia of extraocular muscles

Systemic
Common
- Jaw, tongue, and swallowing claudication, rarely tongue "sores"
- Headache and scalp tenderness, rarely scalp necrosis
- Malaise, anorexia, weight loss, fever, night sweats
- Polymyalgia rheumatica

Uncommon
- Cardiovascular (myocardial infarction, aortic involvement)
- Mesenteric vascular insufficiency
- Stroke

Evaluation

Although no pathognomonic blood test is available for identifying GCA, an elevated Westergren sedimentation rate (usually >50) and elevated C-reactive protein (CRP)

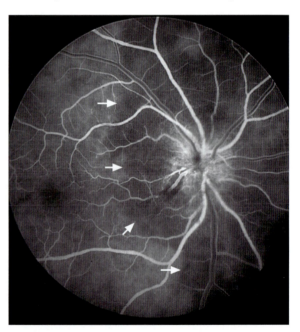

Figure 4-12. Intravenous fluorescein angiogram in arteritic anterior ischemic optic neuropathy.
The early phase of an intravenous fluorescein angiogram shows a typical large nonfilling segment of the choroid (*arrows*) in a patient with anterior ischemic optic neuropathy from giant cell arteritis.

of intravenous fluorescein angiography (IVFA), with a marked delay in choroidal filling (Figure 4-12).

Patients with prominent bilateral optic disc edema and minimal visual loss are more likely to have papilledema from elevated intracranial pressure than bilateral arteritic AION, as the visual loss is typically profound in arteritic AION.

Patients older than 55 with acute, profound visual loss but minimal optic disc or retinal findings may have posterior ischemic optic neuropathy (PION) from GCA; other entities in the differential diagnosis are listed in Table 4-5.

add weight to the clinical suspicion of this disorder. Thrombocytosis, anemia of chronic disease, and mild liver enzyme abnormalities may be present as well.

The erythrocyte sedimentation rate (ESR) is a nonspecific indicator of inflammation, and is also elevated in patients with infectious, collagen-vascular, renal, or neoplastic disorders, and in diabetic patients. The normal sedimentation rate increases with age. The upper limit of normal for a given age can be estimated by dividing the age by two in men, and adding 10 before dividing by 2 in women. Even with this criterion, some patients with an elevated ESR have no demonstrable disease. *On the other hand, the ESR may be normal in up to 20% of patients who have GCA.* Therefore, this important clinical test must be interpreted in the context of the patient's other signs and symptoms. An elevated CRP has proven to be more sensitive (100% in one study), and the combination of an elevated CRP *and* ESR yields a specificity of 97% for GCA.

A *definitive* diagnosis can be made only by identifying characteristic pathological features in a biopsy of an affected artery (see Figure 4–11C, D). A temporal artery biopsy should be performed on all patients suspected of having GCA, even those patients in whom the clinical diagnosis seems certain. A positive biopsy may not change the short-term treatment plan, but it is invaluable in managing the patient in the months and years following the diagnosis, particularly if patients develop significant systemic morbidity related to steroid therapy.

The vasculitis in GCA is not continuous, and may be found in patches along an artery with normal or healing intervening areas. Therefore, temporal artery biopsies should be at least 2 to 3 cm in length, because a short biopsy specimen, or one that is not completely serially sectioned, may miss the pathological area. A single arterial specimen is diagnostic in 80% to 90% of patients who have GCA. Most physicians advocate a biopsy of the contralateral temporal artery or other symptomatic scalp artery if the initial temporal artery biopsy is negative in a patient with compelling clinical findings. Biopsy of two sites increases the sensitivity to greater than 90%. Some physicians biopsy the temporal artery on both sides during the same surgery.

Thus, a patient suspected of having GCA should have a sedimentation rate and C-reactive protein drawn, and steroids should be immediately administered (described in more detail below). A temporal artery biopsy should be performed within 1 to 2 weeks of beginning steroids if possible, as the rate of a definitively positive biopsy (showing diagnostic giant cells) will decrease after several weeks of steroid therapy. However, even after months of treatment, discontinuities of internal elastic lamina may still be identified, suggesting "healed" arteritis.

The clinical presentation, ESR, CRP, and temporal artery biopsy are usually sufficient to establish a definitive diagnosis. In atypical cases, neuroimaging may be required, and the differential diagnoses outlined in Figure 4–5 and Table 4–5 will need to be addressed. GCA is by far the most common vasculitis causing ischemic optic neuropathy in patients older than 50 years, but occasionally laboratory studies may be needed to address other vasculitides such as systemic lupus erythematosus, polyarteritis nodosa, herpes zoster, or Churg-Strauss disease.

Treatment

Immediate administration of steroids may prevent bilateral blindness—an outcome that is not uncommon when the diagnosis or treatment is delayed. In patients with acute visual loss, high-dose intravenous steroids may actually recover some vision. A common regimen is 250 mg of intravenous methylprednisolone every six hours over several days. This treatment often requires hospitalization based on the age and potential for medical complications in these patients. Patients without acute visual loss but with clinical findings suggestive of GCA should be started immediately on 60 to 80 mg of oral prednisone daily, until a biopsy can be performed to determine further management.

Patients with GCA frequently require oral corticosteroids for 1 year or more. Most patients can be tapered to lower doses over a period of months by careful monitoring of the patient's sedimentation rate, C-reactive protein, and symptoms. Collaboration with the patient's medical physician is of paramount importance, given the potential systemic complications of corticosteroid therapy. Occasionally, immunosuppressive therapies such as methotrexate may be added as a steroid-sparing agent, to permit a more rapid taper of prednisone (particularly in diabetic patients).

DIABETIC PAPILLOPATHY

Diabetic patients with optic disc edema and visual loss may have diabetic papillopathy (also called diabetic papillitis). This condition has features that suggest it is clinically different from typical nonarteritic AION: (1) the patients are younger (aged 15–40 years), (2) visual field defects and visual acuity loss is much less severe, (3) the condition is often bilateral, and (4) the visual deficits are more likely to improve with time (Figure 4–13). Though more common in patients with type I diabetes, this condition can also occur in patients with type II diabetes. The optic disc edema is usually diffuse rather than focal, and the discs display a fine, diffuse telangiectasia that may be difficult to distinguish from neovascularization. When it is bilateral, diabetic papillitis may mimic papilledema (often referred to as "diabetic pseudopapilledema"). Diabetic papillitis and AION may be indistinguishable in some cases. The precise etiology of diabetic papillitis is uncertain, but likely represents a form of optic nerve head ischemia. There is

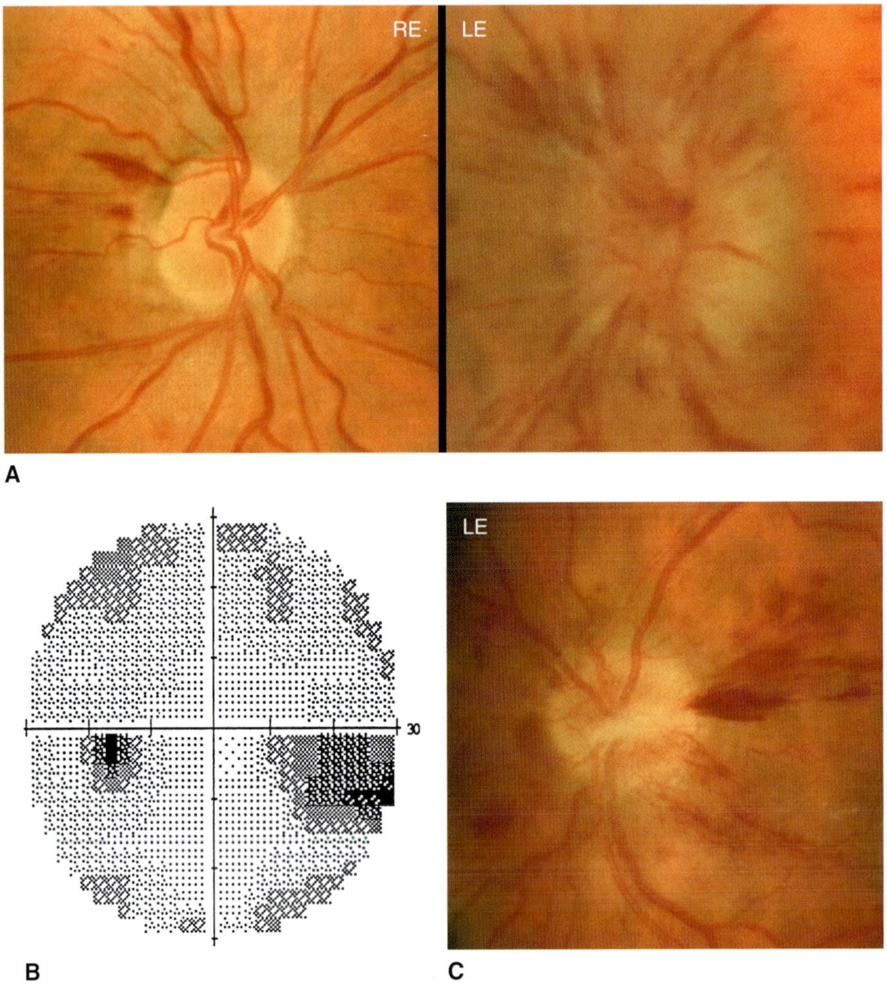

Figure 4-13. Diabetic papillopathy (papillitis). A 37-year-old insulin-dependent diabetic patient described a sudden change in the vision of his left eye. **(A)** The right optic disc is not swollen, but diabetic retinopathy is evident in both eyes. The left optic disc is diffusely swollen with disc and peripapillary hemorrhages. **(B)** Automated perimetry of left eye showed only a small inferior nasal step, far less than expected from the degree of optic disc swelling. The visual acuity was 20/80. The visual field in the right eye was normal. **(C)** Three months later, the optic disc swelling in the left eye was nearly resolved, with mild pallor remaining. The central acuity improved to 20/40, but the visual field defect remained unchanged.

no proven effective treatment, though oral, periocular, and intravitreal steroids have been advocated.

PAPILLOPHLEBITIS

Papillophlebitis is a poorly defined cause of unilateral optic disc swelling that occurs most commonly in healthy patients aged 20 to 30 years. Patients present with painless, minimal visual loss. The optic disc shows diffuse hyperemic disc swelling, with dilated veins and flame-shaped peripapillary hemorrhages. The optic disc appearance suggests a central retinal vein occlusion (CRVO), but the hemorrhages do not extend far from the disc, and are not found in the retinal periphery (Figure 4-14). This entity is most likely a variant of central retinal vein occlusion, and the clinical evaluation should be the same as a CRVO in a young person: assessment for hypercoagulable states (see Table 4-4).

RADIATION OPTIC NEUROPATHY

Radiation optic neuropathy (RON) is a cause of subacute, painless visual loss, typically occurring years after radiation therapy (external beam and gamma knife) for ocular or central nervous system (CNS) tumors. It can occur with optic disc edema, similar to AION, or as a retrobulbar or chiasmal process with normal-appearing optic discs initially. The vision loss is usually stepwise progressive and is severe. Patients may have evidence of concomitant radiation retinopathy or CNS radionecrosis.

The clinical scenario is unusual in that RON occurs as a sudden event 1 to 2 years (or more) after the radiation treatment. This acute event occurs as an ischemic process from an occlusive microvasculopathy, likely as a culminating event set in motion by initial damage to arteriolar and capillary endothelial cells.

Evaluation of patients with RON must address the possibility of recurrence of the original tumor or other processes. Corticosteroids, hyperbaric oxygen, and anticoagulation have been used with limited success.

▶ OPTIC NEURITIS

Optic neuritis typically causes acute monocular visual loss in young adults aged 15 to 45 years, associated with pain induced or worsened by eye movement (Figure 4-15). Three-quarters of patients with optic neuritis are women.

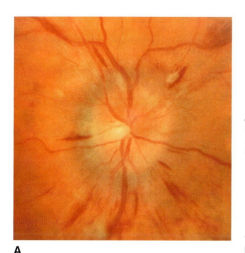
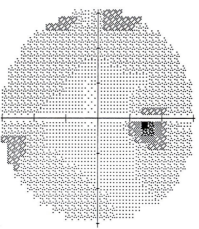

Figure 4-14. **Papillophlebitis.** A 35-year-old man described a "smudge" in the vision of his right eye. The best corrected visual acuity was 20/40 in the right eye and 20/20 in the left eye. **(A)** Optic disc edema with peripapillary hemorrhages, cotton-wool spots, and venous engorgement was present in the right eye. Unlike a central retinal vein occlusion, no hemorrhages were present in the retinal periphery. The fundus abnormalities and symptoms gradually cleared over 4 months. **(B)** Automated perimetry of the right eye shows minimal diffuse depression with a mean deviation of −4.43. The left eye had a normal visual field (mean deviation of −2 decibels).

The term *optic neuritis* means inflammation of the optic nerve, and therefore could be used to describe any condition that causes optic nerve inflammation. However, most physicians reserve this term for primary demyelinating events such as the optic neuropathy associated with MS or idiopathic conditions that have a similar clinical course.

Much of the clinical knowledge regarding optic neuritis comes from the Optic Neuritis Treatment Trial (ONTT), a National Institutes of Health (NIH)-funded, national, prospective, randomized study that evaluated the treatment of acute optic neuritis. This important study provides information regarding not only the treatment of optic neuritis, but also the presentation characteristics, visual outcome, and risk of MS in patients with optic neuritis.

Symptoms

Optic neuritis usually causes monocular visual loss, described by patients as a haze, cloud, or dimness with poor color vision. The visual loss may progress over 2 to 7 days, at which point the vision begins to slowly improve, with normal or near-normal visual function usually achieved over several weeks or months (see Figure 4-15F). Retrobulbar pain, made worse with eye movement, usually precedes visual symptoms and continues during the phase of visual decline. As discussed above, the pain likely originates from extraocular muscle traction on an inflamed optic nerve at the annulus of Zinn. Occasionally, patients report seeing brief spots of light (phosphenes, photopsias) induced by eye movements or loud sounds. A neurological history and review of symptoms may reveal previous or concomitant neurological events that suggest a diagnosis of MS, such as transient episodes of numbness, weakness, loss of bowel or bladder control, or imbalance.

Many patients with active or recovered optic neuritis may note dimming of vision in the affected eye when their body temperature is elevated, such as after exercise, after a shower or sauna, or with a fever. This transient visual loss is called *Uhthoff phenomenon* and results from temporary impairment of optic nerve fiber conduction, which may be caused by elevated body temperatures or changes in the pH or ion content of the blood.

Signs

Visual acuity is usually affected. Color vision and contrast sensitivity deficiencies may be more severe than would be predicted from visual acuity alone (see Figure 2-7C). Potential visual field defects include any optic disc-related visual field abnormality. Although a central scotoma is the classic finding, altitudinal visual field defects are also at least as common (and were more common in the ONTT than central scotomas), making the distinction between this disorder and AION difficult in some cases. It is not unusual to find slight visual field abnormalities in the asymptomatic eye. The RAPD is frequently measurably larger than expected from the visual field defect. However, patients who have had optic neuritis in the fellow eye may have a minimal or no RAPD. Even after a patient's visual acuity, visual field, and color vision have recovered, the RAPD tends to persist, as does the brightness sense disparity between an affected and unaffected eye.

The prolonged conduction velocity of an affected optic nerve can be demonstrated as a delay (increased latency) in the signal generated with visually evoked potential (VEP) testing. This test is not useful in the diagnosis of optic neuritis in a symptomatic eye, as common clinical tests of visual function present more compelling evidence of a previous or current optic neuritis. However, VEP testing is employed frequently by neurologists seeking evidence of demyelination in multiple sites in non-ocular, mono-symptomatic patients suspected of having MS. The *Pulfrich phenomenon* (see Box 2-4) may be observed by patients with unilateral optic neuritis, as a direct consequence of delayed signal conduction in an affected optic nerve.

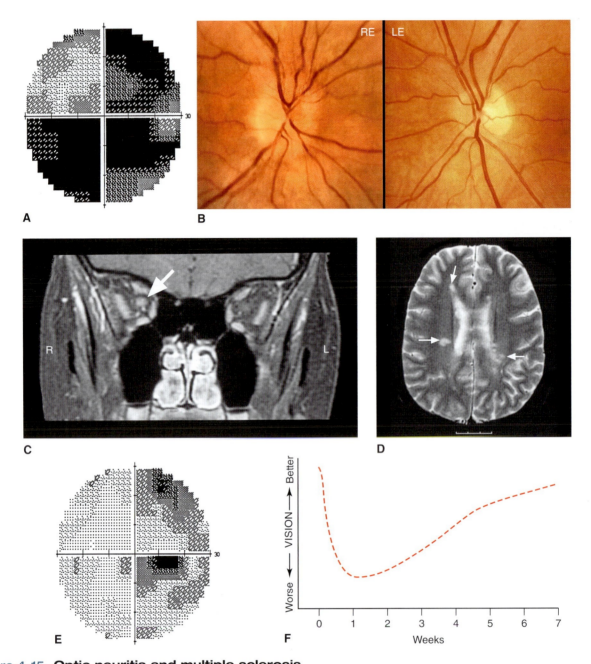

Figure 4–15. **Optic neuritis and multiple sclerosis.**
A 32-year-old woman had pain with eye movement and decreased vision in her right eye. **(A)** The initial visual field of the right eye showed dense visual field loss in three quadrants. The visual acuity was 20/80 and a 1.2 log unit relative afferent pupillary defect (RAPD) was present. The left eye was normal. **(B)** Mild diffuse disc edema was present in the right eye; the left optic disc was normal. **(C)** Magnetic resonance imaging (MRI) of the orbits (T1-weighted image with contrast, coronal view) revealed enhancement of the right optic nerve (*arrow*). **(D)** MRI of the brain (T2-weighted image, axial view) revealed periventricular white matter plaques characteristic of multiple sclerosis (MS) (*arrows*). Additional T2 signal abnormalities were seen in the right pons (*not shown*). As recommended by the Optic Neuritis Treatment Trial (ONTT), three days of high-dose intravenous methylprednisolone were administered. **(E)** Within 3 weeks of onset, the visual field demonstrated dramatic improvement. A shallow central scotoma remained, with a visual acuity of 20/40. Eventually the visual field and acuity normalized, but a small RAPD was still present 2 years later. **(F)** Time course of visual loss. Optic neuritis typically causes a decline in vision over several days to a week, followed by a slow but steady recovery over several months. Patients often achieve near-normal visual acuities and visual fields, but may indefinitely note a subjective difference in the brightness or quality of vision in the affected eye.

The optic disc initially appears normal in two-thirds of patients, consistent with a demyelinating event that is posterior to the optic nerve head. The remaining one-third of patients demonstrate optic disc swelling that is usually diffuse and mild, occasionally with a few associated disc and nerve fiber layer hemorrhages (see Figure 4–15B). The macula is unaffected, unlike the macular edema and edema residues seen in neuroretinitis. With time, optic disc pallor becomes evident in almost all patients, but may be subtle. Optic disc pallor can sometimes be seen in an asymptomatic eye, suggesting a previous subclinical optic neuritis. Uveitis and peripheral retinal venous sheathing are described in some patients with MS, but are usually found in the far periphery of the retina (requiring indirect ophthalmoscopy to be seen).

Causes

The presumed cause of optic neuritis is an autoimmune attack primarily on the myelin (oligodendroglial) coat of the optic nerve, rather than on the axons (although some axonal loss also occurs). The myelin internodes allow rapid signal conduction (saltatory conduction). Loss of myelin in the optic nerve dramatically affects vision because the conduction of visual information is slowed when saltatory conduction breaks down. With time, even with incomplete repair, saltatory conduction and sensory action potentials return to near normal. This is the same process of myelin damage that occurs in the myelinated white-matter tracts in the brain in MS. It is no surprise that many patients with optic neuritis either have, or will develop, MS.

Differential Diagnosis

The differential diagnosis in young patients with recent profound visual loss, a large RAPD, and a *normal* optic disc is a relatively short list consisting of optic neuritis and a number of other less likely disorders (see Table 4–5). Compressive optic neuropathy is possible in such patients, but the necessity of neuroimaging in patients with optic neuritis (see following section) addresses this potential diagnosis. A longer list of potential causes must be considered in those patients with disc swelling, including AION (Table 4–3), Leber hereditary optic neuropathy (LHON), and infiltrative or infectious neuropathies (see Figure 4–5).

Evaluation

In considering a multitude of clinical tests to assess young patients presenting with classic optic neuritis, the ONTT established that neuroimaging was the only test helpful in determining treatment. As will be discussed below, the presence of white matter plaques (see Figure 4–15D) suggests consideration of treatment with high-dose intravenous steroids. MRI of the brain and orbits with gadolinium should be obtained to address treatment considerations, evaluate for systemic MS, and look for any unexpected findings (such as an optic nerve sheath meningioma). MRI of the orbits with fat suppression often demonstrates variable enhancement of the involved optic nerve (see Figure 4–15C), but may be normal.

Treatment

The ONTT randomized 457 patients with optic neuritis into three treatment groups: no treatment (placebo tablets), moderate-dose oral prednisone, and high-dose intravenous methylprednisolone for three days (followed by oral prednisone for 11 days). A summary of the outcomes of the study and resultant treatment recommendations is presented in Table 4–7. Patients in the intravenous steroid group in the ONTT were admitted to the hospital, and were treated with 250 mg of intravenous methylprednisolone every 6 hours for 3 days, followed by an 11-day oral prednisone taper.

▶ **TABLE 4–7. FINDINGS AND RECOMMENDATIONS OF THE ONTT**

Findings	Recommendations
Patients who received moderate-dose oral steroids alone had a significantly higher rate of recurrence of optic neuritis than the other two groups.	*Do not treat patients with optic neuritis with oral prednisone alone.*
Patients with two or more white matter plaques on contrast-enhanced MRI were more likely to have neurological events suggestive of MS than patients with normal MRI. The risk of developing MS was reduced in those patients with MRI findings who received intravenous steroids, but only for about 2 years; by 3 years no lasting effect was evident.	MRI with contrast is helpful in predicting the probability of MS and should be done if the diagnosis is uncertain. Those patients with white matter plaques should be considered for intravenous methylprednisolone treatment to reduce the short-team risk of developing other neurological symptoms. Because there is no proven long-term advantage, prescribing no treatment is a reasonable approach.
Patients treated with intravenous steroids improved more quickly than untreated patients, but all patients improved to the same degree within 6 months to 1 year.	Although intravenous steroids offer no long-term advantage for visual recovery, a more rapid recovery may be beneficial in those patients whose only or better eye is affected.

Abbreviations: MRI, magnetic resonance imaging; MS, multiple sclerosis; ONTT, Optic Neuritis Treatment Trial.

Many physicians have modified this regimen to make it practical for home intravenous therapy, administering 500 mg of methylprednisolone twice a day, or even 1000 mg daily, for 3 to 5 days.

Another consideration in determining who to treat includes any underlying medical conditions that would present a significant risk to the patient if he or she were to receive corticosteroid treatment. Complications from intravenous steroid therapy in young, otherwise healthy subjects in the ONTT were rare but included single cases of transient psychosis, elevated blood sugar, and acute pancreatitis.

Clinical Course

The ONTT demonstrated that about 90% of patients improved within one year to a visual acuity better than 20/30, regardless of treatment. Subjective and objective improvement in the visual field should be evident 3 to 5 weeks after onset (see Figure 4–15E, F). Failure to improve is still compatible with a diagnosis of optic neuritis, but at that time, other items in the differential diagnosis should be considered. A continued, relentless decline in vision over months is very atypical for optic neuritis and requires reinvestigation with repeat MRI or computed tomography (CT) studies of the orbit and brain.

Steroid-dependent optic neuropathies improve while a patient is on steroids, but worsen when the steroids are tapered. This pattern is far more typical of inflammatory processes or neoplasia than optic neuritis, and additional investigation should be directed accordingly (Table 4–8).

Patients with white matter plaques on MRI, or other neurological symptoms in addition to visual loss should be evaluated by a neurologist for MS. The 15-year data from the longitudinal optic neuritis study (LONS) of the ONTT patients showed that 50% of patients (75% if lesions on MRI, 25% if MRI is normal) will develop clinically diagnosable MS in their lifetime (Box 4–1). Several studies support the use of interferon therapy in patients with a single demyelinating event and MRI lesions to reduce the probability of developing MS (Box 4–2). However, the following must be considered in treatment decisions: Treating all such patients subjects the group

▶ **TABLE 4–8. STEROID-DEPENDENT DISORDERS AFFECTING VISION**

Neoplastic
  Optic nerve glioma
  Optic nerve sheath meningioma
  Chromophobe adenoma
  Craniopharyngioma
  Medulloblastoma
  Lymphoproliferative optic nerve infiltration/ compression
  Meningeal carcinomatosis

Paraneoplastic
  Retinopathy
  Optic neuropathy

Inflammatory
  Sarcoidosis
  Idiopathic orbital inflammatory syndrome
  Vasculitis: granulomatosis with polyangiitis (Wegener granulomatosis), Behçet disease, GCA
  Tolosa Hunt syndrome
  IgG4-related systemic disease

Other
  Autoimmune optic neuropathy
  Neuromyelitis optica (Devic disease)

Abbreviation: GCA, giant cell arteritis.

▶ **BOX 4–1. MULTIPLE SCLEROSIS**

Multiple sclerosis (MS) is an autoimmune disorder with focal, patchy destruction of white matter in the brain, spinal cord, and optic nerves of unknown cause. The disease is more common in women (2:1 female:male ratio), and is most common in adults aged 25 to 40 years. The risk of developing MS increases 20-fold in first-degree relatives of patients with MS. The incidence of MS increases with increasing distance from the equator. Patients who move after 15 years of age carry with them the risk of developing MS of their original locale. Patients who move before 15 years of age seem to acquire MS with the risk of the new location.

MS occurs in four basic forms: remitting and exacerbating, primary progressive, secondary progressive, and large lesion form. Optic neuritis is a common feature of remitting and exacerbating and secondary progressive MS, but is rare in other forms.

Systemic findings in MS include extremity weakness, cerebellar dysfunction (causing vertigo and ataxia), paresthesias of the face and body, and urinary retention or incontinence. Many patients have episodes of reversible neurological dysfunction that may be separated by many months or years. Approximately one-third of patients with MS have no physical disability or decreased life expectancy, but 10% of patients may have a relentlessly progressive form. Patients who are older at the time of diagnosis have a poorer prognosis than do younger patients and are more likely to have the primary progressive form.

A diagnosis of MS is made by identifying neurological symptoms that are separated in time and space (affecting different areas of the central nervous system). Although magnetic resonance imaging abnormalities and cerebrospinal fluid findings of oligoclonal bands and elevated IgG levels are supportive, MS remains a clinical diagnosis.

> **BOX 4–2. TREATMENT OF PATIENTS WITH MONO-SYMPTOMATIC DEMYELINATING EVENTS**

Three prospective studies randomized patients with their first acute demyelinating event (not only optic neuritis) and magnetic resonance imaging (MRI) lesions to treatment with interferon or placebo. Each of the three studies showed that treatment significantly reduced the subsequent development of clinically definite multiple sclerosis (CDMS).

Controlled High-Risk Subjects Avonex Multiple Sclerosis Prevention Study (CHAMPS). Randomized 383 patients: intravenous (IV) steroids were followed by weekly intramuscular (IM) Avonex, or IV steroids and IM placebo. At 3 years the study was terminated because the development of MS was clearly lower in the Avonex-treated group.

Early Treatment of Multiple Sclerosis Study (ETOMS). Randomized 308 patients to weekly IM Rebif or IM placebo, showing that the Rebif-treated group was less likely than the placebo group to develop CDMS (34% vs 45%).

Betaseron in Newly Emerging Multiple Sclerosis for Initial Treatment (BENEFIT) study. Randomized 468 patients to alternate-day subcutaneous Betaseron or subcutaneous placebo, with the treated group less likely than the placebo group to develop CDMS (28% vs 45%).

---

that would not have developed MS to the side effects, risks, and cost of interferon therapy.

Variations

Optic neuritis can occur in systemic lupus erythematosus (SLE) and other autoimmune disorders. Optic neuritis can occur in response to a viral illness or immunization, or may be idiopathic, with a presentation and course identical to the optic neuritis associated with MS but without ever manifesting systemic symptoms. Optic nerve inflammation that is secondary to contiguous ocular, orbital, or sinus disease is discussed separately below.

Children may present with bilateral optic disc edema and visual loss, presumably from a postinfectious optic neuritis or meningoencephalitis (acute disseminated encephalomyelitis [ADEM]). These childhood cases are less likely than those of adults to be at risk of future development of MS. Symptomatic bilateral optic neuritis in adults is unusual, although the ONTT demonstrated minimal visual field defects in the asymptomatic eye of many patients with optic neuritis.

Neuromyelitis optica (NMO; Devic disease) is an inflammatory demyelinating disorder that is similar to MS in several ways, but is a distinct disease. It is important to distinguish NMO from MS because both treatment and prognosis are different. In NMO, the target of the autoimmune attack appears to be the astrocyte, rather than oligodendroglia as in MS. NMO is characterized by unilateral or bilateral optic neuritis, and lower extremity weakness or paralysis from spinal cord demyelination, usually occurring in children and young adults (Figure 4–16; see Figure 1–1). The spinal cord characteristically has three or more contiguous longitudinal segments involved on neuroimaging. Unlike MS, patients frequently present with bilateral optic neuritis, with eyes affected simultaneously or in quick succession. Vision is usually more severely affected and less likely to recover in NMO than in MS, and pain with eye movement is less common. About 70% of affected individuals have a positive serum NMO antibody, an antibody directed against aquaporin 4, which is a water channel expressed in astrocyte foot processes. Treatment considerations include immunosuppressive agents such as azathioprine and rituximab, with high-dose intravenous steroids and plasma exchange for acute episodes. Interferon beta medications used to treat MS can actually worsen NMO, so distinguishing NMO from MS is particularly important.

▶ OPTIC PERINEURITIS

Optic perineuritis (OPN) is an optic neuritis look-alike that is uncommon but needs to be recognized because the disease mechanism and treatment are different from demyelinating optic neuritis. OPN is an inflammatory disorder within the spectrum of idiopathic orbital inflammatory syndrome (IOIS; discussed in Chapter 8) that involves the optic nerve sheath and intraorbital tissues, but demyelination is not the primary pathological mechanism. OPN can be seen with scleritis, GCA, tuberculosis, syphilis, and granulomatosis with polyangiitis (Wegener granulomatosis), but most commonly is an isolated idiopathic disorder. It is more common in women than men and is typically, but not exclusively, unilateral. OPN is frequently abrupt in onset and painful, with variable visual involvement. Depending on the site of involvement, the disc may be swollen or normal in appearance. MRI characteristically shows a doughnut ring of inflamed optic nerve sheath on coronal sections, or a "tram track" sign on axial cuts (see Figure 8–4). Optic nerve sheath biopsies show nonspecific inflammatory lymphocytic infiltration and thickening of the nerve sheath, occasionally with granulomatous inflammation.

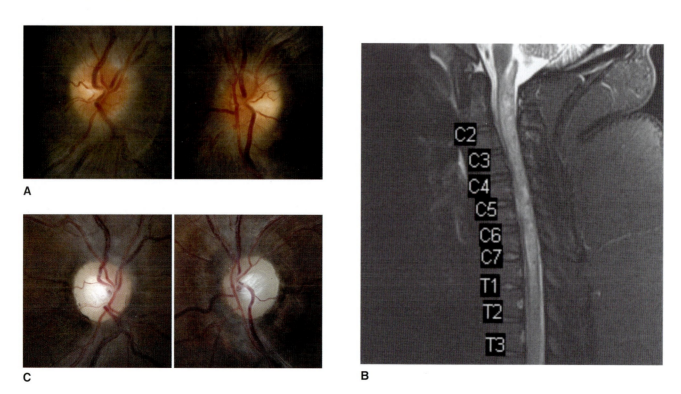

Figure 4–16. **Neuromyelitis optica.**
An 18-year-old African-American woman presented with bilateral vision loss with optic disc edema (**A**), lower extremity weakness, and urinary incontinence. Cervical-spine magnetic resonance imaging (MRI) showed C1 to T1 transverse long longitudinal myelopathy (**B**), in addition to bilateral optic nerve enhancement (*not shown*). Neuromyelitis optica (NMO) antibody was positive. Methotrexate and monthly intravenous methylprednisolone resulted in improvement in vision and other neurological symptoms. Optic disc edema resolved, with subsequent bilateral optic disc pallor (**C**).

▶ PAPILLEDEMA

Papilledema means swelling of the papilla (optic disc). However, the term is generally reserved to describe bilateral optic disc swelling that results from elevated intracranial pressure.

MECHANISM OF PAPILLEDEMA

Cerebrospinal fluid (CSF) is produced by the choroid plexus in the ventricles, flowing through the midline third ventricle and cerebral aqueduct to the fourth ventricle. From the fourth ventricle, CSF flows through the foramina of Magendie and Luschka into the subarachnoid space surrounding the brain and spinal column, as well as into the orbital extension of the subarachnoid space bounded by the optic nerve sheath. CSF is absorbed by the arachnoid granulations into the adjacent dural venous sinuses (Figure 4–17).

High CSF pressure in the brain is conveyed through the optic canal into the space bounded by the optic nerve sheath in the orbit, increasing the tissue pressure within the optic nerve head, causing stasis of orthograde axoplasmic flow. Axoplasmic stasis causes swelling of the prelaminar axons, resulting in optic disc swelling. Secondarily, elevation of the venous pressure within the nerve head leads to venous engorgement and tortuosity, capillary dilation, and hemorrhage. Trabeculations exist between the optic nerve sheath and pia of the optic nerve, and vary between individuals in their impedance to transmission of CSF between the brain and orbit. Variation in sheath anatomy may account for the marked asymmetry or unilaterality of optic disc edema seen occasionally, or (rarely) the absence of disc edema in patients with intracranial hypertension.

Elevation of the superior sagittal sinus venous pressure (from conditions such as venous sinus thrombus, dural arteriovenous malformations (AVMs), right heart failure, or radical neck dissection) reduces CSF absorption and may cause intracranial hypertension. Damage or malfunction of the arachnoid granulations (meningitis, subarachnoid hemorrhage, toxins, or drugs) or obstruction of ventricular outflow (aqueductal stenosis, tumor) can also cause a rise in CSF pressure (see Figure 4–17). Expanding brain tumors are obviously one of the more worrisome causes of papilledema.

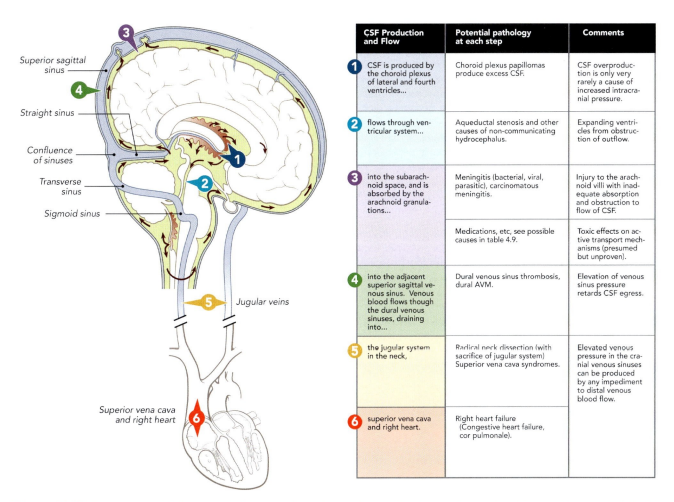

Figure 4–17. **Causes of intracranial hypertension related to impediments of cerebrospinal fluid flow and absorption.**

Although many of the causes of intracranial hypertension are evident on neuroimaging, a significant group of patients have normal neuroimaging. Idiopathic intracranial hypertension (pseudotumor cerebri) refers to a group of predominantly obese females with elevated intracranial pressure and papilledema, without obvious cause.

IDIOPATHIC INTRACRANIAL HYPERTENSION (PSEUDOTUMOR CEREBRI)

Idiopathic intracranial hypertension (IIH) is a condition of unknown cause that produces elevated intracranial pressure and papilledema, primarily in obese females between puberty and menopause. Neuroimaging is essentially normal, without tumor or identifiable obstruction of the ventricular system (Box 4–3). The female to male ratio is approximately 8 to 1. Obesity is present in more than 90% of women with this disorder, 60% of men, and 30% of children (Figure 4–18).

The terminology surrounding IIH is somewhat confusing and imprecise. This clinical disorder is often called *pseudotumor cerebri*, but this term technically includes any condition other than tumor that causes intracranial hypertension. Use of the term *benign intracranial hypertension* (BIH) raises objections, because the condition may have severe visual consequences. The designation *idiopathic intracranial hypertension* seems to clearly define the clinical group discussed here, but in some cases a potential cause can be implicated with reasonable certainty, and the disease may then not qualify as truly idiopathic (Table 4–9). The best suggestion is to use the term IIH for the idiopathic condition discussed in this section, unless an identifiable cause can be named to complete the designation, such as "intracranial hypertension secondary to vitamin A toxicity."

Symptoms

The most common symptom associated with IIH is headache, although in some cases it can be conspicuously absent. Patients often report that the headache is more painful when bending over or coughing. Another frequent finding is pulsatile tinnitus, often described as "hearing a swishing heartbeat" in one or both ears. Patients frequently describe brief (2–5 second) episodes

▶ BOX 4–3. DIAGNOSTIC CRITERIA FOR IDIOPATHIC INTRACRANIAL HYPERTENSION

Symptoms *All symptoms, when present, must be attributable to intracranial hypertension or papilledema only.* Common symptoms include headache, transient visual obscurations, peripheral visual field loss, pulsatile tinnitus, horizontal diplopia. Less commonly; neck, back, and shoulder pain; nausea, vomiting, or photophobia. Atypical symptoms should raise the suspicion that intracranial hypertension or papilledema is secondary, and the investigation should be directed to find an underlying primary disorder. Note that patients may have IIH and be entirely asymptomatic, with the diagnosis made after the incidental discovery of papilledema.

Signs *All signs, when present, must be attributable to intracranial hypertension or papilledema only.* No focal neurological signs should be present with the exception of unilateral or bilateral sixth cranial nerve palsies. Note that papilledema is not required to make the diagnosis; in rare cases the diagnosis is suspected by symptoms and confirmed by lumbar puncture in patients with normal optic discs. Patients with normal discs without papilledmea are not at risk for vision loss.

Neuroimaging *MRI or contrast-enhanced CT shows no evidence hydrocephalus, mass, structural lesion, or vascular abnromality.* MRI (with and without contrast) with MR venography is the best imaging protocol, and should be done in all atypical cases (men and non-obese women), as these studies will address the possibility of dural venous outflow obstruction, AVMs and other disorders masquerading as IIH.

Lumbar Puncture *Elevated intracranial pressure measured documented by LP, with normal CSF composition.* The opening pressure should be greater than 250 mm of water, with values between 200 and 250 mm suspicious but non-diagnostic. The diagnostic threshold is based on an LP performed in the lateral decubitus position, with legs extended in a relaxed patient. There are currently no diagnositic opening pressure criteria for LPs performed in other positions, such as the prone position when performed with radiologic guidance.

No other cause of intracranial hypertension identified This final disclaimer is necessary as there are some conditions and drugs that appear to be causative; so even though the other criteria have been met, the condition is not truly *idiopathic*, but secondary. This then would be called "intracranial hypertension caused by…".

Abbreviations: AVM, arteriovenous malformation; CSF, cerebrospinal fluid; CT, computed tomography; IIH, idiopathic intracranial hypertension; LP, lumbar puncture; MR, magnetic resonance; MRI, magnetic resonance imaging.

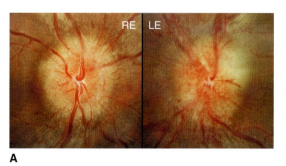

A

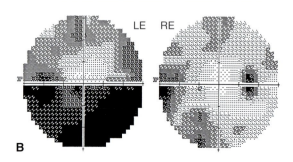

B

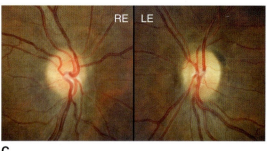

C

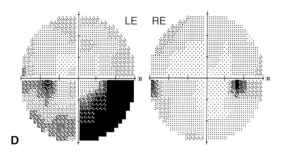

D

Figure 4–18. Idiopathic intracranial hypertension.
A 40-year-old woman presented with a history of headache and transient visual obscurations in her left eye for 8 months, and blurred vision in her left eye for 2 months. Magnetic resonance imaging (MRI) with contrast of the brain was normal, and a lumbar puncture revealed an opening pressure of 368 mm of water with normal cerebrospinal fluid studies. Acetazolamide 500 mg twice a day and an effective weight loss program was instituted with resolution of optic disc edema in about 6 months. **(A)** Bilateral optic disc edema at presentation. Paton lines can be seen at the temporal edge of the left disc. **(B)** Visual fields on presentation. The visual field in the left eye shows a dense inferior altitudinal visual field defect. In the right eye, an inferior nasal step is identified. **(C)** Optic disc photographs from 1 year after presentation show resolution of the optic disc edema, with mild pallor remaining. **(D)** The visual field defects also improved, but a dense inferior nasal step remains in the left eye.

▶ **TABLE 4–9. OTHER CAUSES OF INTRACRANIAL HYPERTENSION**

Some patients may meet all the criteria for IIH as described in Box 4–9, except for the last one: *no other cause identified*. The conditions and drugs associated with intracranial hypertension are listed by the degree of certainty with which they can be implicated as the primary cause of intracranial hypertension.

Highly Likely
Causes of increased intracranial venous pressure (see Figure 4–17)
- Dural venous sinus thrombosis
- Arteriovenous malformations
- Jugular venous insufficiency (bilateral radical neck dissections)
- Superior vena cava syndrome
- Right heart failure with pulmonary hypertension

Medical disorders
- Addison disease
- Hypoparathyroidism
- Sleep apnea
- Renal failure
- Iron-deficiency anemia

Drugs
- Tetracycline, doxycycline, and minocycline
- Vitamin A: dietary, vitamin pills, related retiniod medications
- Levonorgestral (contraceptive implants and intrauterine devices)
- Steroid withdrawal after prolonged administration

Probable Causes
Drugs
- Anabolic steroids (may cause venous sinus thrombosis), chlordecone (Kepone)
- Ketoprofen or indomethacin in Bartter syndrome
- Thyroid replacement therapy in hypothyroid children
- Growth hormone replacement in deficient patients

Possible Causes
Drugs
- Diphenylhydantoin
- Lithium carbonate
- Nalidixic acid
- Sulfa antibiotics

Causes Frequently Cited but Unproven
Drugs
- Corticosteroid intake
- Multivitamin intake
- Oral contraceptive use

Other
- Hypovitaminosis A
- Hyperthyroidism
- Pregnancy
- Menarche
- Menstrual irregularities

Abbreviation: IIH, idiopathic intracranial hypertension.

---

of unilateral or bilateral visual loss with postural changes called *transient visual obscurations* (TVOs). The phenomenon is most likely related to brief drops in perfusion of the swollen optic nerve head with even slight dips in systemic blood pressure. Permanent visual loss may occur if the optic disc swelling becomes chronic. Marked engorgement of the optic nerve sheath can also flatten the posterior aspect of the globe. This condition can produce blurred vision as the result of macular choroidal folds (see Figure 4–9), or can create a hyperopic shift in the patient's refraction by shortening the axial length of the eye. Transient or lasting horizontal diplopia may occur from associated sixth cranial nerve dysfunction.

Important concerns in the patient's history include medications over the previous year, weight gain or loss, head trauma, symptoms of sleep apnea, and any previous intracranial or head/neck surgery. Vitamin A consumption by tablet or diet (liver, fad diets) should be assessed. Menstrual irregularities and hormonal changes are common in women in this age group, so their reported association with IIH is tenuous at best.

Signs

The appearance of optic disc swelling may be variable (Figure 4–19). The classic appearance is a diffuse, uniform elevation of the optic disc that gives it a "champagne cork" appearance. Nerve fiber layer hemorrhages and deep peripapillary retinal hemorrhages are common (see Figure 4–18A). The severity of optic disc edema is often asymmetric between the two eyes, and occasionally swelling is unilateral. Not infrequently, it may be difficult to distinguish anomalous optic discs from true papilledema (see Table 4–2). Patients with CSF pressures of 200 mm or more reportedly lack normal pulsations of the central retinal vein at the optic disc. However, at least one-fifth of normal discs lack pulsations, so their absence is a "soft" sign at best.

Visual function testing reveals normal visual acuity and visual fields with early optic disc swelling. Expansion of the optic disc and the resulting lateral and upward displacement of the peripapillary retina can produce both relative and absolute enlargement of the blind spot on formal perimetry (Figure 4–20). Over time, chronic disc swelling and ischemic damage cause axonal death and optic atrophy, producing visual field defects. Nasal steps are the most common early defect (see Figure 4–18B, D), with concentric depression of the entire visual field in advanced stages. Central vision is rarely affected until late in the course (or with acute fulminant disc swelling), thus visual acuity alone is of little help in assessing the progress of the disease. Rarely central vision can be affected by an associated peripapillary choroidal neovascular membrane and

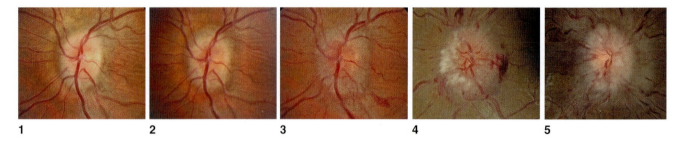

Figure 4-19. Modified Frisén grading of papilledema.
(1) *Grade 1 papilledema.* A C-shaped 270° halo of axonal swelling obscures the disc margin most of the way around the disc, but with a gap (sharp disc margin) at the temporal portion of the disc. **(2)** *Grade 2 papilledema.* The halo of swollen axons is 360° around the disc, including the temporal portion. **(3)** *Grade 3 papilledema.* In addition to obscuring the entire disc margin as in grade 2, the disc edema obscures some of the major vessels at the margin of the disc. **(4)** *Grade 4 papilledema.* The disc swelling is sufficient to obscure some of the major vessels on the surface of the disc itself. **(5)** *Grade 5 papilledema.* The optic disc swelling is severe, characterized by partial or total obscuration of all vessels over the surface of the disc.

subretinal hemorrhage (Figure 4–21), choroidal folds, and macular edema.

Elevated intracranial pressure in IIH does not seem to damage intracranial structures, and neurological deficits apart from visual loss should raise suspicion of some other disorder. The single exception to this rule is sixth cranial nerve paresis. Presumably, changes in intracranial pressure (and the brain's position in the cranium) may stretch and injure the sixth cranial nerves, given their firm attachment to the brainstem and to the skull base.

Causes

In IIH, there is no overt structural obstruction to the circulation of CSF. Studies have shown that the problem lies in defective reabsorption of CSF at the level of the arachnoid granulations. The association of this condition with certain medications is consistent with this idea, because toxins could potentially interfere with the transport mechanisms required for CSF absorption by the arachnoid granulations (see Table 4–9).

The role of obesity in this disorder is unclear, but it seems to be a causative factor, because IIH often resolves with weight loss alone. Many investigators have suspected a hormonal mechanism related to lipid metabolism. IIH may be associated with sleep apnea, a disorder that is also more common in obese patients.

Differential Diagnosis and Evaluation

The differential diagnosis of bilateral optic disc elevation is found in Figure 4–5. The most important entities to address in the differential diagnosis of papilledema include brain tumors, obstruction of the ventricular system, or dural-sinus thrombosis. For this reason neuroimaging should be performed immediately (Figure 4–22). Although a CT scan is usually sufficient for ruling out a space-occupying intracranial mass, MRI with contrast is superior to CT in imaging the brain for processes such as infiltrating tumors, and is particularly advantageous when magnetic resonance venography (MRV) is also performed to evaluate for venous sinus thrombosis (Figure 4–23), arteriovenous malformations, or vascular tumors.

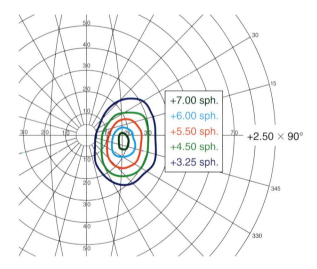

Figure 4-20. Enlarged blind spot with papilledema.
Patients with papilledema are frequently noted to have enlarged blind spots on perimetry. This is most likely a refractive effect from elevation of the peripapillary retina due to optic disc edema, rather than from optic nerve dysfunction. This Goldmann plot of the blind spot in a patient with papilledema shows that the blind spot becomes smaller as increasing plus lenses are used to bring the patient's focal point forward, providing sharper focus on the elevated peripapillary sensory retina.

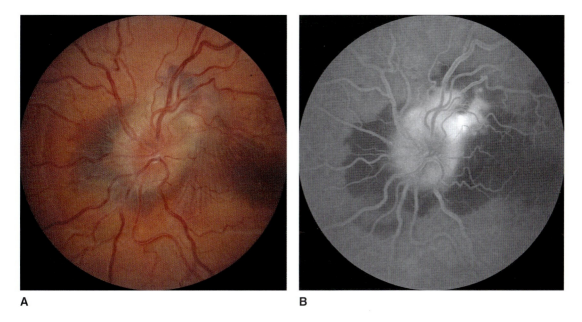

Figure 4-21. Papilledema with associated peripapillary choroidal neovascular membrane. Patients with optic disc edema can develop a peripapillary choroidal neovascular membrane (CNVM). This may precipitate a sudden change in vision, and is a reason for decreased central acuity (not typical with papilledema). It may be that the swollen optic nerve stretches or stresses the surrounding edge of Bruch membrane, allowing choroidal vessels access to the subretinal space. **(A)** Optic disc edema with subretinal blood. **(B)** Intravenous fluorescein angiography (IVFA; late sequence) shows staining of the swollen optic disc, hyperfluorescence of the CNVM at the superior pole of the disc, and blocking of the normal choroidal fluorescence by the subretinal blood.

Blood pressure should be measured (with appropriate-sized cuffs) on all patients, because severe hypertension may present with bilateral optic disc edema (Figure 4–24). Patients with intracranial hypertension *and* systemic hypertension may have a poorer visual prognosis. Abrupt lowering of blood pressure in either circumstance (IIH or severe hypertension) may precipitate acute, severe, and permanent visual loss. Malignant hypertension causes optic disc edema and retinal ischemia, as well as posterior reversible encephalopathy syndrome (PRES). Patients with PRES demonstrate CNS edema, typically of the occipital lobes, with headache, confusion, seizures, and visual loss.

Truly *idiopathic* intracranial hypertension is uncommon in males. Some men with this initial diagnosis have been discovered to have occult dural arteriovenous malformations, sleep apnea, or other identifiable underlying pathology.

Baseline automated threshold perimetry (eg, Humphrey 30-2 or 24-2) and optic disc photographs should be performed, because these parameters are the most reliable indicators of disease progression and treatment effectiveness.

A lumbar puncture must be performed to make the diagnosis of IIH, even when the clinical presentation is classic. In addition to documenting the opening pressure, the CSF must be examined for evidence of hemorrhage, infection, or neoplasm. The opening pressure is measured in the lateral decubitus position with legs and head in a neutral, relaxed position. Opening pressures greater than 250 mm H_2O confirm the presence of intracranial hypertension; pressures between 200 and 250 mm H_2O are suggestive but less certain. Only rarely are additional lumbar punctures of any utility once elevated intracranial pressure is established. This procedure is not an effective form of treatment, because the CSF volume is quickly regenerated. Lumbar puncture is also not a reliable way of monitoring the effectiveness of medical treatment, since CSF pressure has marked hour-to-hour fluctuations.

Diagnosis and treatment of this disorder is best performed when an ophthalmologist and neurologist work together. The ophthalmologist follows the important indicators of disease progression and the potential for lasting visual morbidity—the visual fields and disc appearance. The neurologist's role is to confirm the diagnosis with a neurological examination and lumbar puncture, and to aid in the medical management of headache.

Treatment

Treatment alternatives include observation, diet, medication, and surgery. Patients without significant visual field defects may require neither medical nor surgical treatment. This is especially true if a suspected precipitating cause has been eliminated, such as vitamin A or

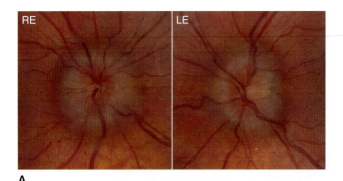

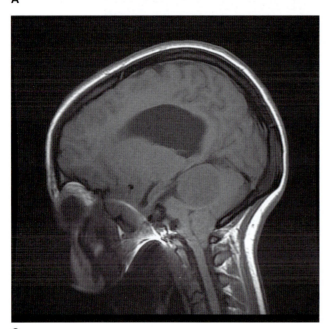

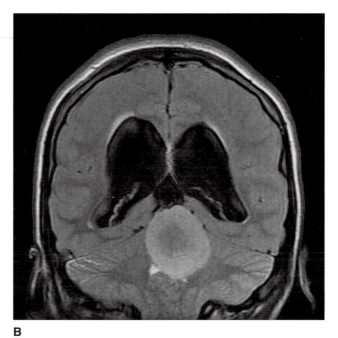

Figure 4–22. Papilledema from a posterior fossa mass.
A 14-year-old girl was evaluated for occasional headache by her optometrist and referred to the neuro-ophthalmologist with elevated optic discs. She described two episodes of near syncope within the previous month, one of which occurred after a ride at the fair, but otherwise had a negative neurological and general medical review of systems. On examination, the visual acuity was 20/20 in both eyes with normal visual fields. The fundus examination revealed bilateral optic disc edema **(A)**. Urgent neuroimaging was arranged, though understandably questioned by a relatively asymptomatic patient and her mother. Magnetic resonance imaging (MRI) revealed a posterior fossa mass with obstructive hydrocephalus, seen in a coronal T1 flair image **(B)**. A sagittal T1 image showed inferior cerebellar tonsil herniation of approximately 1.5 cm **(C)**. The patient was taken directly from the MRI scanner for admission to the neurosurgical intensive care unit, followed by a craniotomy and resection of the tumor. Pathology revealed a low-grade glioma. This case illustrates the importance of prompt neuroimaging for patients with papilledema, *particularly children*.

antibiotics, patients recovering from meningitis or head trauma, or obese patients in a successful weight loss program.

The effectiveness of weight loss cannot be overemphasized. Loss of even a few pounds can be more effective than any medication. Despite the potential discomfort of the physician talking to a young obese woman about her weight, weight loss is a very effective treatment modality and must be addressed clearly with the patient. The patient's family physician or internist, or a reputable, medically-based weight loss program should be sought to provide sound and safe weight loss advice and treatment. Bariatric surgery is a consideration in the morbidly obese, but the risks of this surgery must be carefully weighed. Although the rapid weight loss with bariatric surgery may be ultimately beneficial in IIH, there is the potential for worsening of papilledema and vision loss if patients become hypotensive or anemic.

Acetazolamide (Diamox) is a carbonic anhydrase inhibitor that reduces intracranial pressure by decreasing CSF production. This drug is generally effective when given in doses of at least 500 milligrams twice a day, often with convincing improvement in 3 to 4 weeks (see Figure 4–18). Side effects include paresthesias of extremities and face, dysgeusia (especially with carbonated beverages), and dyspepsia. Fortunately, serious side effects including anaphylaxis, aplastic anemia, and

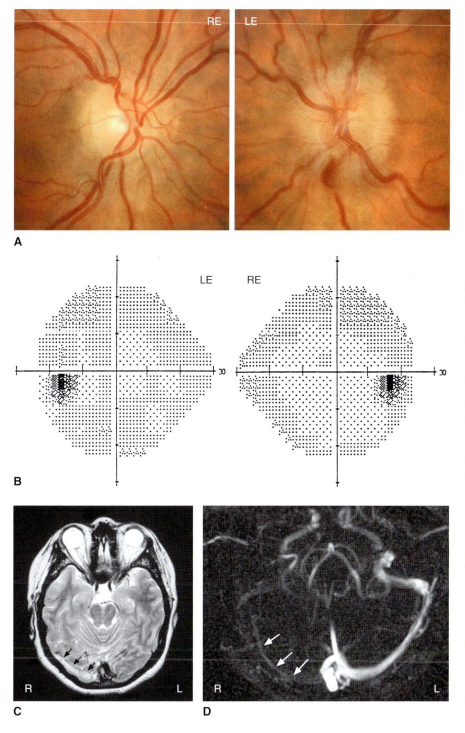

Figure 4-23. **Intracranial hypertension from dural sinus thrombosis.** A 32-year-old woman complained of severe headache, increasing in intensity over 3 weeks. **(A)** Optic disc edema was bilateral, more prominent in the left eye. **(B)** The visual fields were relatively normal, with only slight enlargement of the blind spots. **(C)** Magnetic resonance imaging (MRI) of the brain (T2-weighted image, axial view) revealed bright signal (rather than the normal flow void) in the right transverse sinus (*arrows*) and sigmoid dural sinuses, indicative of thrombosis. **(D)** Magnetic resonance angiography (MRA) demonstrated absence of flow in the right transverse (*arrows*) and sigmoid sinus. The patient was admitted to the neurology service and treated with both acetazolamide and anticoagulants. Although the optic disc edema resolved within 2 months, headache continued to be a chronic problem.

Stevens-Johnson syndrome are extremely rare. Topiramate (Topamax) may be helpful alone or in combination with acetazolamide. Topiramate is also a carbonic anhydrase inhibitor, and has the added advantage of also being a headache treatment and acting as an appetite suppressant. Furosemide (Lasix) is less effective in the treatment of this disorder. Although long-term oral corticosteroids are counterproductive, short-term high-dose intravenous steroids prior to surgical treatment may be useful in fulminant cases.

An optic nerve sheath fenestration or neurosurgical shunting procedure (ventriculoperitoneal or lumboperitoneal shunt) may be needed for patients with progressive visual field loss despite medical therapy (Figure 4–25). Optic nerve sheath fenestration effectively reduces the transmitted CSF pressure at the optic

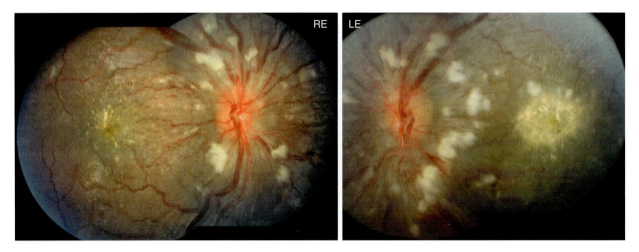

Figure 4-24. **Bilateral optic disc edema from severe (malignant) hypertension.**
A 9-year-old boy was referred for blurred vision and presumed papilledema. Bilateral hyperemic optic disc edema was present with retinal hemorrhages, cotton-wool spots, retinal arteriolar narrowing, and macular edema residues, as seen in this montage of retinal photographs. The blood pressure was 200/105. The patient was admitted to the pediatric intensive care unit for management of a hypertensive emergency. Neuroimaging was consistent with posterior reversible encephalopathy syndrome (PRES). Further evaluation confirmed renovascular hypertension.

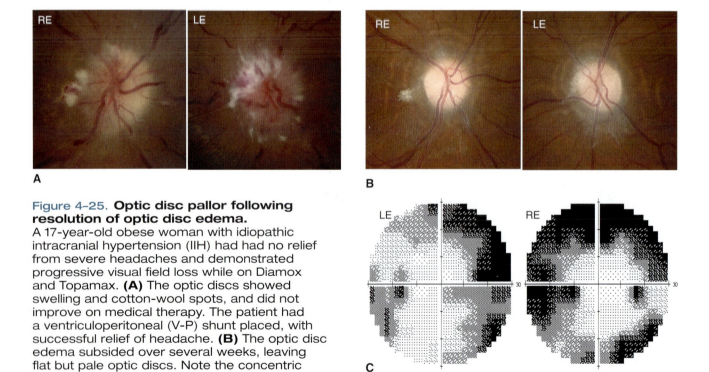

Figure 4-25. **Optic disc pallor following resolution of optic disc edema.**
A 17-year-old obese woman with idiopathic intracranial hypertension (IIH) had had no relief from severe headaches and demonstrated progressive visual field loss while on Diamox and Topamax. **(A)** The optic discs showed swelling and cotton-wool spots, and did not improve on medical therapy. The patient had a ventriculoperitoneal (V-P) shunt placed, with successful relief of headache. **(B)** The optic disc edema subsided over several weeks, leaving flat but pale optic discs. Note the concentric "bathtub rings" around the optic discs serving as high water marks as the edema resolved. Hard exudates are also seen in the papillomacular retina of the right eye as the edema cleared.
(C) The patient's initial visual fields improved following placement of the V-P shunt, but she was left with permanent visual field loss, consistent with the presence of optic disc pallor. Despite this initial success, the potential for V-P shunt failure requires that the patient's visual fields and optic disc appearance be monitored closely over time. When the optic disc is pale (atrophic), it may not be capable of swelling; in this circumstance, following the disc appearance is less helpful than following the visual fields to watch for progression of the disease.

disc by opening the sheath, thereby allowing CSF to be diverted into the intraconal orbital tissues for absorption. Optic disc edema is reliably reversed by this procedure, but its long-term effectiveness is uncertain. The CSF pressure (as measured by lumbar puncture or intracranial monitor) is not significantly affected by optic nerve sheath fenestration, but investigators have reported improvement in headache in 50% of patients and contralateral optic disc edema improvement in 70% of patients. However, a patient with severe headache that is unresponsive to vigorous medical treatment may benefit most from a neurosurgical shunt.

Focal narrowing of the transverse sinuses on MRV in patients with IIH may be seen. It is likely that this finding is the *result* of elevated intracranial pressure in most cases rather than the *cause*, but the significance of this finding in IIH is not entirely clear. This has led to consideration of interventional radiologic procedures such as endovascular dilation and stenting of narrowed dural venous sinuses, particularly if a significant pressure gradient is measured across the narrowed area. This approach remains very controversial, and the physician needs to be aware that the requirement for anticoagulation with stenting may complicate the possibility of urgent optic nerve sheath fenestration or neurosurgical shunting in these patients, should they be required.

Clinical Course

Frequent, formal visual field testing is required to follow the course of a patient with chronic papilledema, because visual acuity may remain 20/20 despite severe peripheral visual field loss. Obviously, serial observations of the optic disc appearance provides the most direct and objective information about the course of the disease. Formal grading of the optic disc edema is clinically helpful (see Figure 4–19), but should not replace serial fundus photography as the "gold standard" for following the appearance of the optic disc over time. Regular follow up visits (that include perimetry and optic disc assessment) are required regardless of the treatment, because treatment failure may occur at any time. Shunt failure may occur without causing headache, and may produce insidious peripheral visual loss that may go unnoticed until the visual loss is severe and damage to the optic disc is irreversible.

The majority of patients requiring medical treatment respond well to acetazolamide, with resolution of optic disc edema from 3 to 6 months. When the optic disc edema is gone, a trial period off of acetazolamide with careful observation is reasonable, especially if the patient has been successful with weight loss. Some patients never have a recurrence, while in others the condition is a chronic, life-long problem.

OTHER CAUSES OF PAPILLEDEMA

Because many of the signs and symptoms of elevated intracranial pressure involve the eyes, the ophthalmologist is often the first physician to encounter patients with intracranial tumors, dural sinus thrombosis, and other neurological or neurosurgical conditions. Many of these conditions are diagnosed when the ophthalmologist investigates papilledema with neuroimaging. Obviously, prompt referral to the appropriate specialist is the most important course of action. However, the ophthalmologist still has an important role in the multidisciplinary management of such patients, because his or her serial observations of optic disc appearance and visual fields often determine the therapeutic course.

▶ COMPRESSIVE OPTIC NEUROPATHIES

Mechanical compression of the optic nerve can cause axonal death, but also can cause demyelination without permanent axonal injury. Ischemia also plays a major role in the pathogenesis of compressive neuropathies, because tumors can disrupt local perfusion by mechanical pressure, or "steal" the blood supply. Unlike other cranial nerves, optic nerve axons do not regenerate after a lethal injury. However, successful reversal of optic nerve (or chiasmal) compression can result in significant improvement in visual field defects, presumably the result of remyelination and recovery of partially injured axons. Prompt diagnosis is therefore important, as early intervention may offer the best chance for visual recovery.

OPTIC NERVE SHEATH MENINGIOMAS

Optic nerve sheath meningiomas are a cause of unilateral progressive visual loss, most common in women (female:male ratio of 3:1) in their 40s (Figure 4–26). Meningiomas of the optic nerve sheath represent a third of primary optic nerve tumors, 5% of all orbital tumors, and 1% of all meningiomas (most are intracranial). Usually unilateral, they can be bilateral, particularity when associated with neurofibromatosis type 2 (NF-2).

Symptoms and Signs

Patients describe an insidious, painless, loss of vision in one eye. Any type of optic nerve–related visual field defect can occur. A classic pattern seen with Goldmann perimetry is a central scotoma that gradually connects (or breaks out) to the periphery. Proptosis may develop, depending on the bulk and location of the meningioma. Diplopia can occur if the tumor restricts free movement

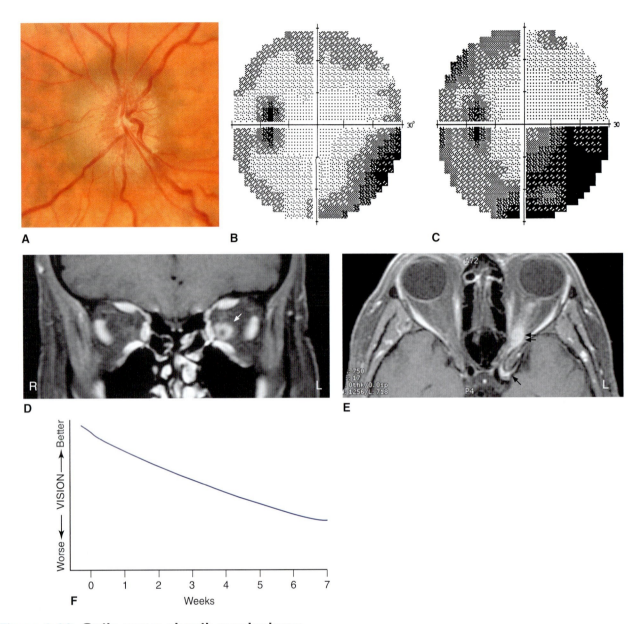

Figure 4–26. Optic nerve sheath meningioma.
A 51-year-old woman had left optic disc edema for 3 years, with normal computed tomography (CT) scans. A subjective decline in vision led to further investigation, with the diagnosis of an optic nerve sheath meningioma based on magnetic resonance imaging (MRI) studies. **(A)** Chronic, diffuse edema of the left optic disc was present. The appearance of the optic disc changed little in over 3 years since her diagnosis was made. **(B)** Automated perimetry of the left eye at the time of diagnosis shows an inferior nasal step. The visual acuity was 20/20. **(C)** Four years later, the nasal step has enlarged, and is nearly an altitudinal defect. The visual acuity at this time is 20/40. **(D)** MRI of the orbit (with contrast, coronal plane). The meningioma is seen as an enhancing mass surrounding the compressed, nonenhancing optic nerve (*arrow*). **(E)** MRI (axial plane) reveals that the meningioma is present in the orbit (*double arrows*) and extends through the optic canal intracranially (*single arrow*), but does not include the chiasm. **(F)** Time course of vision loss. A steady decline of vision is the general rule with compressive lesions.

of the globe. Rarely, gaze-evoked amaurosis can occur as compression of the optic nerve or its vascular supply is induced with eccentric gaze.

The classic triad of findings with optic nerve sheath meningiomas include (1) disc pallor, (2) optic disc veno-venous collateral vessels, and (3) progressive visual loss; however, not all of these elements are invariably present. The optic nerve may be pale and atrophic or swollen, depending on the location and duration of the lesion. Retino-choroidal venous collaterals (also called optociliary shunts) on the optic disc occur in response to obstruction of central retinal venous outflow. Neuroimaging may show thickening of the nerve/nerve sheath complex. CT imaging of the orbits often shows enhancement of the sheath, which spares the nerve itself, appearing as a "railroad track" on axial images and as a "bull's eye" on coronal views.

Causes

Optic nerve sheath meningiomas arise from the meningeal components of the optic nerve sheath in the orbits. Similar to intracranial meningiomas, the tumor rarely metastasizes, but causes local injury by compression of adjacent structures. In the orbit, the tumor tends to encircle the optic nerve, causing injury by myelin displacement, axonal disruption, or compromise of the optic nerve's blood supply. Some meningiomas have hormone receptors, with potentially massive growth when exposed to exogenous hormones (such as birth control pills) or the high levels of progesterone and estrogen produced during pregnancy.

Variations

Optic nerve sheath meningiomas may extend into the optic canal, or may originate from the dura within the optic canal. The confines of the canal may allow a small meningioma to cause marked compression of the optic nerve that may be difficult to visualize on neuroimaging. Meningiomas arising from the orbital sheath often extend through the optic canal and into the intracranial cavity. Meningiomas can also arise from the intracranial dura, compressing the intracranial optic nerve or the chiasm. Sphenoid wing meningiomas commonly have intraorbital and intracranial components. These tumors can also extend laterally, producing a characteristic filling in of the temporal fossa that can be palpated on examination.

Unlike in adults, meningiomas in children tend to be very aggressive, and often result in death.

Differential Diagnosis and Evaluation

The triad of pallor, optic disc collateral vessels, and progressive visual loss can also be present with sarcoidosis or optic nerve glioma. Optic nerve sheath meningiomas can also appear similar to retinal vein occlusions on ophthalmoscopy: Vein occlusions can produce collateral "shunt" vessels similar to those seen with optic nerve sheath meningiomas; meningiomas can secondarily produce an element of venous stasis; and both conditions may cause disc edema. The optic disc edema and visual field loss from optic nerve sheath meningioma may be mistaken for ischemic optic neuropathy or optic neuritis initially (particularly when the vision loss is "suddenly" discovered by the patient), but the slow, relentless decline in vision is highly suggestive of a compressive optic neuropathy (see Figure 4–26F).

Neuroimaging is required when a compressive optic neuropathy is suspected, either with MRI of the brain and orbits (with contrast and orbital fat suppression) or CT imaging of brain and orbits with contrast. Sometimes the enlarged appearance of the nerve may be difficult to distinguish from optic nerve glioma or inflammatory conditions such as sarcoidosis or optic perineuritis. Performing both MRI and CT may narrow the diagnosis and aid in assessing the intracranial extent of growth. Very rarely, biopsy of the mass is required to make a diagnosis and plan treatment.

Treatment

Observation is a reasonable approach in those patients who have good vision and stable clinical course. The natural history of optic nerve sheath meningiomas is highly variable: They may remain static for many years, or they can progress relatively rapidly. Radiation is the treatment of choice for patients with significant vision loss or progressing symptoms; it has proven to be very effective in reversing or at least stabilizing vision loss. Surgery is not an option in most patients, as excision of the optic nerve sheath meningioma invariably strips the vascular supply of the optic nerve, resulting in blindness. The decision to perform surgery for intracranial extension when present is complex and depends on whether there is a threat to the contralateral optic nerve or chiasm; the size, location, and growth of tumor; and remaining sight in the affected eye.

Optic nerve sheath meningiomas can be followed by neuroimaging. But careful monitoring of optic nerve function is perhaps even more important, because tumor progression may not always be evident on neuroimaging, and the status of the patient's vision is critical in treatment decisions. Therefore, visual acuity testing, perimetry, measuring the RAPD, or other tests of optic nerve function (eg, contrast sensitivity and color vision testing), as well as ocular motility and orbital examination (eg, monitoring proptosis) need to be followed over time.

OTHER CAUSES OF OPTIC NERVE COMPRESSION

Orbital Graves disease (thyroid eye disease) can cause compression of the optic nerve within the orbit by marked enlargement of the extraocular muscles. The manifestations of Graves disease are discussed in detail in Chapter 8. It is important to note that an optic neuropathy can occur even in the absence of the external signs of thyroid eye disease (see Figure 8–7). Other space-occupying lesions affecting the orbital portion of the optic nerve include capillary hemangiomas, orbital varices, mucoceles, metastatic tumors, fibrous dysplasia, or infectious cysts; all of which therefore can present as compressive optic neuropathies. Like optic nerve sheath meningiomas, any space-occupying lesion in the orbit can cause gaze-evoked amaurosis.

The intracanalicular portion of the optic nerve is vulnerable to compression from dural meningiomas or osseous disorders such as fibrous dysplasia. The intracranial optic nerve can be affected by the same processes that affect the chiasm (discussed in Chapter 5), notably intracranial meningiomas (parasellar and sphenoid wing meningiomas), and aneurysms of the anterior circle of Willis.

▶ INTRINSIC NEOPLASMS

OPTIC NERVE GLIOMA

Optic nerve gliomas occur primarily in children; 70% of patients present before 10 years of age (Figure 4–27). Decreased vision may be the presenting complaint, but often strabismus and nystagmus resulting from poor vision may be noted first by the child's family. Proptosis can occur, depending on the extent and bulk of orbital involvement. Patients can present with a normal-appearing optic disc, optic disc edema, or optic atrophy (pallor).

About one-half of optic nerve gliomas arise in the orbital portion of the optic nerve, with the remainder arising intracranially. Approximately 50% of patients with optic nerve gliomas have neurofibromatosis type I. Approximately 15% of patients with neurofibromatosis type I harbor an optic nerve glioma.

Pathologically, the tumor is a pilocytic astrocytoma (juvenile type), with benign cytological appearance. In children the tumor enlarges slowly or may appear inactive. Gliomas of the anterior visual pathway that arise in adulthood behave very differently, as they exhibit malignant behavior and rapidly lead to blindness and death (Figure 4–28).

Neuroimaging of childhood gliomas typically reveals a fusiform swelling of the optic nerve and/or chiasm. This condition may be associated with endocrine dysfunction and hypothalamic involvement, necessitating an endocrine evaluation in all children with optic nerve or chiasmal glioma. As previously discussed, a pediatric evaluation for systemic signs of neurofibromatosis is also required.

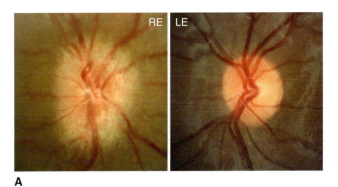

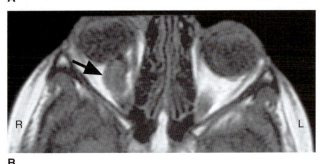

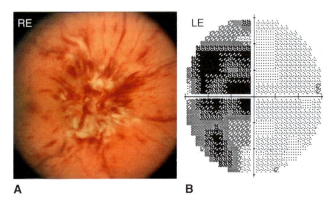

Figure 4–28. Glioma of the anterior visual pathway in an adult.
A 36-year-old man with a diagnosis of glioblastoma multiforme in the right parietal region had received both conventional and gamma-knife radiation therapy. A complete left homonymous hemianopic visual field defect was present. The patient then presented with visual loss in the right eye, decreasing to NLP (no light perception) over 2 weeks. Neuroimaging demonstrated anterior extension of the malignant glioma into the right optic nerve. **(A)** Marked optic disc elevation and retinal venous stasis was present in the right eye; the left optic disc was normal. **(B)** Automated perimetry shows that only the nasal hemifield of the left eye remained, as the right eye was NLP. The visual field loss was the result of involvement of the right optic tract and right optic nerve.

Figure 4–27. Optic nerve glioma and neurofibromatosis.
A 6-year-old girl was seen by her ophthalmologist with a "right eye turning in." A diagnosis of neurofibromatosis (NF-1) had recently been made on the basis of café-au-lait spots and a known family history of NF-1. The patient's visual acuity was 20/80 at the time of diagnosis, and had remained stable for more than 3 years without treatment. **(A)** Diffuse elevation and edema of the right optic disc is evident. The left optic disc is normal. **(B)** Magnetic resonance imaging (MRI) (T1 axial view) reveals massive enlargement of the optic nerve (*arrow*) with proptosis.

Treatment is controversial, but most physicians favor a conservative "watch and wait" approach given the usual static course in children. Surgical resection may be considered in patients with a blind eye and disfiguring proptosis or isolated orbital involvement. Indications for and effectiveness of radiation treatment and chemotherapy are uncertain.

LYMPHOPROLIFERATIVE DISORDERS

Neoplastic involvement of the optic nerve may present with grotesque infiltration and elevation of the optic nerve head, or as an initially normal-appearing disc that gradually turns pale from a retrobulbar process. Acute leukemic infiltrative optic neuropathy is a true oncologic emergency because prompt radiation treatment may be sight-saving (Figure 4–29). Infiltrative optic neuropathies should be considered in patients with visual loss and a known lymphoproliferative disorder or who are systemically ill, or those whose history and examination do not fit the patterns of common optic neuropathies. Infectious (such as tuberculosis) and inflammatory (sarcoidosis) entities may be infiltrative in nature, and should be considered in the differential diagnosis (Table 4–10). In addition, patients whose optic neuropathy improves on steroids, only to worsen when steroids are stopped (steroid-dependent neuropathy) may have an infiltrative optic neuropathy or fungal infection such as aspergillosis or mucormycosis) (see Table 4–8). MRI of brain and orbits with contrast may show optic nerve enhancement or other intracranial foci.

OTHER INTRINSIC NEOPLASMS

Melanocytomas are rare pigmented tumors of the optic disc, more common in dark-skinned patients

▶ **TABLE 4–10. INFILTRATIVE OPTIC NEUROPATHIES**

Lymphoproliferative Disorders
Leukemia
- Monocytic
- Acute myelocytic
- Acute lymphocytic
- Chronic lymphocytic

Lymphoma
Plasmacytoma
Multiple myeloma

Metastatic Carcinoma (esp. breast and lung)

Carcinomatous Meningitis (esp. breast and lung)

Inflammatory Disorders
Sarcoidosis
Systemic lupus erythematosus
Granulomatosis with polyangiitis
  (Wegener granulomatosis)

Infectious Processes
Tuberculosis
Syphilis
Cryptococcosis
Toxoplasmosis
Toxocariasis
Cytomegalovirus
Coccidiomycosis
Aspergillosis
Lyme disease

(Figure 4–30). Histologically they are composed of nevus cells. Generally, they are asymptomatic and benign, but rarely can become malignant.

▶ INFLAMMATORY OPTIC NEUROPATHIES

Inflammation of the optic nerve can be caused by many processes. Primary inflammatory optic neuropathies include sarcoidosis (Figure 4–31; Box 4–4), and idiopathic orbital inflammatory syndrome (discussed in Chapter 8). Inflammation accompanies infectious,

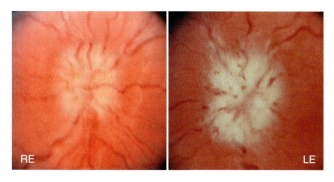

Figure 4-29. **Acute leukemic optic nerve infiltration.**
A 10-year-old boy with acute lymphocytic leukemia presented with bilateral blurred vision. Both optic nerves were enlarged and elevated, with hemorrhages and cotton-wool spots present, suggesting acute leukemic optic nerve infiltration (pictured). Urgent radiation of the optic nerves resulted in partial recovery of visual loss.

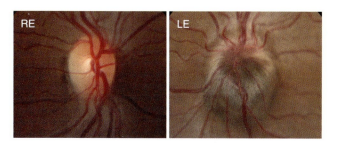

Figure 4-30. **Melanocytoma.**
A melanocytoma of the left optic disc was discovered incidentally. The normal right optic disc is shown for comparison.

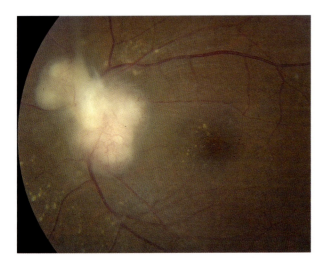

Figure 4-31. Sarcoid optic neuropathy. In addition to optic disc edema, this patient with neurosarcoidosis also demonstrates peripapillary granulomas.

neoplastic, autoimmune, and other optic neuropathies, making it difficult to categorize the primary disease process (see Table 4–10).

▶ INFECTIOUS OPTIC NEUROPATHIES

OPTIC DISC EDEMA WITH A MACULAR STAR

Optic disc edema with a macular star (ODEMS) is a descriptive term that includes a number of different disease processes, characterized by the presence of optic disc edema and macular edema. The term *neuroretinitis* is often used interchangeably with ODEMS, but neuroretinitis has come to specifically imply a infectious cause.

Noninfectious entities that can produce coexistent optic disc and macular edema include hypertensive retinopathy and postoperative cystoid macular edema (Irvine-Gass syndrome). Hypertensive retinopathy is invariably

---

▶ BOX 4-4. SARCOIDOSIS

Sarcoidosis is a multisystem idiopathic granulomatous inflammatory disorder, commonly with pulmonary and dermatologic manifestations, that can also affect the eye, orbit, and intracranial visual system. The disease is commonly diagnosed in patients in their 30s and 40s, but can occur at any age. In the United States, sarcoidosis is at least ten times more prevalent in African-Americans than Caucasians.

Pathologically, affected tissues are infiltrated with noncaseating granulomas. Although this disorder is clinically and pathologically similar to tuberculosis, no causative agent has been identified in sarcoidosis.

Although some patients with proven sarcoidosis are asymptomatic, others may exhibit severe systemic and neurological consequences. Most patients present with constitutional symptoms: malaise, weakness, fever, weight loss, and diaphoresis. Pulmonary involvement is common, and is manifest as hilar and mediastinal adenopathy often evident with a routine chest x-ray, but best seen with computed tomography (CT) imaging. Lung parenchymal involvement can cause coughing and shortness of breath, and wheezing. Cutaneous manifestations include erythema nodosum, nodular granulomas, lupus pernio, and mucous membrane (including conjunctival) lesions. Similar to hilar adenopathy, painless and symmetric peripheral lymphadenopathy is common. Other affected organs include liver, spleen, lacrimal and parotid glands, muscles, heart, and the central nervous system.

Potential ocular and orbital involvement includes granulomatous uveitis, as well as infiltration of the conjunctiva, extraocular muscles, lacrimal gland, and optic nerve.

Involvement of the central nervous system is designated as *neurosarcoidosis* and commonly affects the optic nerves, chiasm, and optic tracts. Other cranial neuropathies can occur. The facial nerve is the most common cranial nerve to be affected. Meningeal or ventricular disease can cause elevated intracranial pressure and papilledema. Meningeal neurosarcoidosis can also produce a mass effect with compression of adjacent structures, and may be difficult to distinguish from meningioma both clinically and neuroradiologically. Parenchymal disease can cause neuroendocrine disturbances (such as diabetes insipidus from hypothalamic involvement), seizures, encephalopathy, or white matter changes that mimic multiple sclerosis. The spinal cord, peripheral nerves, and muscles can also be affected by sarcoidosis.

The diagnosis of sarcoidosis is often made on the physical examination, imaging studies (hilar adenopathy on chest imaging, lesions on brain magnetic resonance imaging [MRI]), or serological tests (elevated angiotensin-converting enzyme [ACE], hypercalcemia, hypergammaglobulinemia). In some patients, a lumbar puncture and cerebrospinal fluid analysis may be needed to distinguish neurosarcoidosis from infectious and neoplastic processes. Pathological diagnosis can be made by identifying affected tissues (examination, gallium scan, positron emission tomography [PET] scan, and other imaging), that may be biopsied (by bronchoscopy or by brain, meningeal, skin, lymph node, lacrimal gland, or conjunctival biopsy). If the diagnosis is not established by biopsy, the diagnosis should be considered "suspicious but unproven."

Sarcoidosis almost always responds promptly to treatment with intravenous or oral steroids; therefore, failure to respond to treatment should lead to questioning this diagnosis. Steroid-sparing agents (eg, cyclophosphamide, methotrexate, and cellcept) and surgical therapy for the complications of sarcoidosis may be required to augment therapeutic effects and mitigate corticosteroid side effects.

bilateral with other retinal signs (see Figure 4–24), and cystoid macular edema does not usually develop a "star." Exudative lesions in the retinal periphery (Coats disease, capillary hemangiomas) can cause macular stars, but the disc is usually unaffected. Diabetic maculopathy, occasionally accompanied by diabetic papillopathy or optic disc neovascularization, tends to produce circinate edema residues, and is not likely to be confused with this entity. Macroaneurysms of retinal vessels near the disc can cause macular exudates and optic disc edema. Optic disc edema from any cause, when extreme, may be associated with macular edema and a star. This observation suggests that all causes of disc edema may need to be considered in the differential diagnosis of ODEMS when the degree of optic disc swelling is extreme.

The precise pathophysiology of neuroretinitis is not known, but likely involves an exudative process in the vessels of the disc and macula triggered by the infectious organism or the subsequent immune response to the infection (postinfectious autoimmune mechanism). The availability of sensitive serological tests for the etiologic agent in cat-scratch disease (*Bartonella henselae*) demonstrates that this organism a common cause of neuroretinitis. Other infectious processes that can cause neuroretinitis include *toxoplasmosis*, toxocariasis, syphilis, Lyme disease, and viral entities. A bilateral, recurrent, idiopathic neuroretinitis with a poor visual outcome was been described by Purvin and Chioran (1994).

CAT-SCRATCH NEURORETINITIS

Patients with neuroretinitis caused by cat-scratch disease (CSD) are typically young adults or children who develop a febrile illness several weeks after exposure to a cat (Figure 4–32). The disease is transmitted by a scratch from an infected cat, or may be transmitted by fleas from the cat to the human.

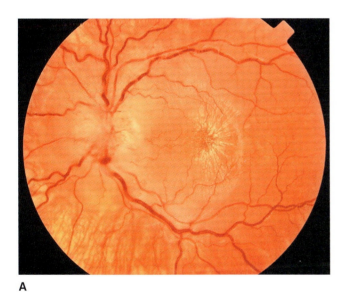

A

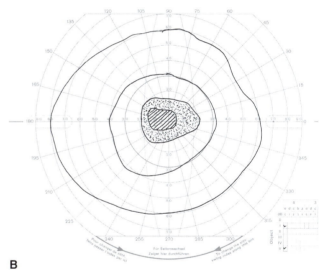

B

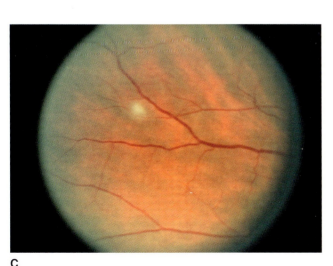

C

Figure 4–32. Neuroretinitis from cat-scratch disease.
A 10-year-old girl complained of blurred vision in her left eye that began 2 weeks after a self-limited, 4-day febrile illness. She frequently played with the family's kitten. Enzyme immunoassay for *Bartonella henselae* was positive. **(A)** The left fundus shows optic disc edema and edema residues forming a macular star. Focal disc elevation suggesting a granuloma can be seen on the temporal disc.
(B) Goldmann perimetry shows a dense cecocentral scotoma. Visual acuity was CF 2'. The patient was treated with oral doxycycline hyclate, 100 mg daily for 10 days. In one month, the acuity improved to 20/100, and was 20/20 within four months, with normalization of the visual field defect. **(C)** Peripheral fundus. Deep chorioretinal white spots are often present in both eyes even when the neuroretinitis is confined to one eye, as demonstrated in another patient with cat-scratch disease neuroretinitis.

Symptoms

The systemic symptoms include fever, malaise, and general lymphadenopathy that usually resolve after 1 or 2 weeks. Only a small percentage of patients with CSD develop neuroretinitis and visual loss. Visual symptoms usually begin 2 to 3 weeks after the systemic symptoms have subsided. Many patients do not recall an antecedent systemic illness. The examiner should question the patient specifically about fever, malaise, cough, adenopathy, exposure to cats and kittens, as well as known or potential sexually transmitted diseases when appropriate.

The time course of visual loss is similar to optic neuritis, as it may progress over several days or weeks and then slowly improve over several months. Pain with eye movement can occur, but is not nearly as frequent as with optic neuritis.

Signs

Central and cecocentral scotomas are the most common visual field defect. The visual deficit generally cannot be accounted for by the maculopathy alone, suggesting optic nerve dysfunction as well. As with optic neuritis, there are usually color vision defects and an RAPD.

The optic disc shows mild to moderate diffuse edema, frequently with a focal elevation of the optic disc that has the appearance of an optic disc granuloma. The optic disc edema is accompanied by white edema residues in the inner macula that line up radially in Henle layer, forming a star (see Figure 4–32A). Acutely the macular edema may be subtle, and the patient may be thought to have optic neuritis. Usually within a week or so of the onset of visual symptoms, the characteristic edema residues in the macula appear. The radial star pattern may completely encircle the fovea, or be limited to only one sector. A few vitreous cells may be present. Deep, white choroidal patches are occasionally seen in the retinal periphery, even in the fellow asymptomatic eye (see Figure 4–32C).

Evaluation

Patients with a classic history and examination may not require an extensive evaluation. All patients should have blood pressure measured, as macular stars can occur in hypertensive retinopathy. Laboratory studies that may be helpful include complete blood count with differential, toxoplasmosis titer, and syphilis and Lyme disease serologies. A positive serologic titer (indirect fluorescence assay) for *Bartonella henselae* is specific, and thus may be helpful in confirming the suspected cause. However, a negative titer does not exclude CSD.

Treatment

The visual prognosis for CSD neuroretinitis is good, with most patients experiencing a significant recovery regardless of treatment. This natural history of recovery makes it difficult to assess the efficacy of treatment. Many physicians treat CSD neuroretinitis with a course of ciprofloxacin, doxycycline, or other antibiotics if the clinical course is protracted.

OTHER INFECTIOUS NEUROPATHIES

Infectious agents can affect the optic nerve by (1) direct infiltration of the optic nerve by the organism, (2) by inciting a local inflammatory response or autoimmune attack on the optic nerve, (3) by local mass effect from an infectious focus, or (4) by compromise of the vascular supply by vasospasm or vascular occlusion from the products of an inflammatory response. Many agents have been implicated (see Table 4–10), but syphilis can affect the visual pathway in so many varied ways, it should be included in the differential diagnosis in most forms of optic neuropathy.

▶ TOXIC AND NUTRITIONAL OPTIC NEUROPATHIES

Slow, bilateral, and symmetrical loss of central vision is characteristic of toxic and nutritional optic neuropathies. Toxins and nutritional deficiencies are usually grouped together for two reasons: In many cases they are both present as co-conspirators causing an optic neuropathy, and toxins and nutritional deficiencies produce clinical findings that are bilateral and essentially identical. In addition, there is increasing evidence that both toxic and nutritional optic neuropathies injure the optic nerve by affecting the mitochondria (Box 4–5).

Visual fields reveal bilateral cecocentral scotomas (Figure 4–33). The optic discs may appear normal initially, but inevitably develop temporal pallor. Careful observation may reveal nerve-fiber layer dropout in the papillomacular bundle. Causes discussed in the following paragraphs include alcoholism and vitamin deficiencies, and ethambutol and other drug toxicities. Additional causes are listed in Table 4–11.

Alcoholism is a common cause of toxic/nutritional optic neuropathy. The nutritional deficiencies that inevitably accompany alcoholism may be the most damaging factor, but a toxic effect of alcohol and its by-products may also play a role. Most patients demonstrate remarkable improvement with vitamin supplementation, particularly with folate and B complex vitamins. Referral to a substance abuse specialist is needed to prevent the recurrent cycle of alcohol abuse and nutritional deprivation. The combination of alcoholism and cigarette smoking may have synergistic optic nerve toxicity (tobacco-alcohol amblyopia).

Deficiency of B vitamins, folic acid, and niacin may cause a nutritional optic neuropathy. Vitamin-deficiency

▶ BOX 4-5. MITOCHONDRIAL OPTIC NEUROPATHIES

Retinal ganglion cells are particularly sensitive to mitochondrial dysfunction—mitochondrial insults typically are first manifest as vision loss from an optic neuropathy. Mitochondrial disorders affecting the optic nerve can be congenital or acquired. Congenital/hereditary abnormalities can be the result of mutations in the mitochondrial DNA (such as Leber hereditary optic neuropathy [LHON]), and will therefore display the pattern of exclusive maternal transmission. However, it is also possible to have mitochondrial disorders from nuclear DNA mutations at chromosomal sites that code for products destined to function in the mitochondria (such as dominant optic atrophy and the OPA1 gene), which will display a classic Mendelian genetic pattern as autosomal dominant or recessive. Each of these hereditary mitochondrial disorders can have variable penetrance and other systemic manifestations. This list of known heritable mitochondrial disorders is growing. Understanding the mechanism of mitochondrial dysfunction may allow a more directed approach to therapy, including gene therapy.

Acquired mitochondrial optic neuropathies are usually the result of toxic/nutritional factors that affect mitochondrial function and result in axonal damage and cell death. Ethambutol is the most common example, as well as other antibiotics whose mechanism of action against bacteria/viruses can directly damage mitochondria and result in optic neuropathy and vision loss.

Some patients can have both a genetic defect and susceptibility, and an acquired trigger in the form of an antibiotic or nutritional deficiency that can precipitate an optic neuropathy, such as vision loss in patients with LHON triggered by antibiotics or alcohol. This may be the mechanism of an epidemic of optic neuropathy in Cuba in 1991–1993 and so-called "tropical amblyopia."

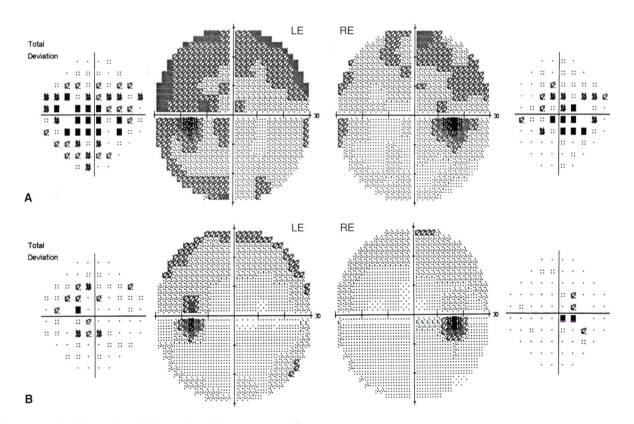

Figure 4-33. Toxic/nutritional optic neuropathy.
A 59-year-old man reported the gradual onset of poor vision in both eyes. He admitted drinking too much alcohol but believed he ate a well-balanced diet. Visual acuity was 20/80 in each eye, with a normal slitlamp and ophthalmoscopic examination. **(A)** The visual field on presentation showed bilateral cecocentral scotomas, best appreciated by looking at the total deviation plots. A nutritional optic neuropathy was suspected, and the patient was started on a multivitamin, as well as folate 1 mg daily, and was referred to his general medical physician to address his diet and probable alcoholism. **(B)** Four weeks later, the automated visual field had improved significantly, with improvement of visual acuity to 20/30 in each eye. The patient's visual acuity and visual fields were normal when tested after an additional 6 weeks. The patient said he was compliant with his vitamin therapy, but admitted his alcohol was only minimally reduced.

TABLE 4–11. COMMON TOXIC/NUTRITIONAL OPTIC NEUROPATHIES

Drugs
  Antibiotics
- Ethambutol (Myambutol, antimycobacterial)
- Isoniazid (INH, antimycobacterial)
- Linezolid (Zyvox, antibiotic)
- Chloramphenicol (inexpensive antibiotic commonly used in impoverished nations)
- Streptomycin (generic aminoglycoside antibiotic)

  Halogenated hydroxyquinolines (Clioquinol is an antifungal drug and antiprotozoal drug)
  5-Fluorouracil (chemotherapeutic)
  Disulfiram (Antabuse, used to treat chronic alcoholism)
  Amiodarone (Cordarone, Pacerone, used to treat cardiac dysrhythmias)

Toxins
  Methanol
  Ethylene glycol
  Heavy metals (lead, arsenic)
  Carbon monoxide
  Cyanide

Nutritional Deficiencies
  Thiamine (B_1)
  Vitamin B_{12} (pernicious anemia)
  Folate

Mixed Toxic/Metabolic and Nutritional
  Tobacco-alcohol amblyopia
  Cuban epidemic of optic neuropathy (CEON)
  Other "tropical amblyopias"

Abbreviation: INH, isonicotinylhydrazine.

Data from Sadun AA: Mitochondrial optic neuropathies: toxic/metabolic. Meeting syllabus of the North American Neuro-ophthalmology Society, 2012: 71–76; Miller NR, Hoyt WF: *Walsh and Hoyt's Clinical Neuro-ophthalmology*: New York: Lippincott Williams & Wilkins; 2005: 447–463.

optic neuropathies are uncommon in the modern era, but can occur rarely in circumstances such as anorexia or after Roux-en-Y bariatric surgery. Optic neuropathy from malabsorption of vitamin B_{12} (pernicious anemia) may be difficult to diagnose, because the optic neuropathy may appear before a significant anemia and macrocytosis develop.

Ethambutol, a cyanonitrile, is commonly used to treat tuberculosis and atypical mycobacterial infections. Like other antibiotics, its effect on the optic nerve may be related to optic nerve mitochondrial toxicity (see Box 4–5). Toxicity to the optic nerve may occur at a previously tolerated dose when other toxic agents are added to a patient's regimen, or when weight loss from the chronic infection increases the dose per kilogram of body weight. Cessation of the medication usually allows slow improvement of the patient's vision, often taking several months.

Amiodarone has been associated with a bilateral optic neuropathy very similar to anterior ischemic optic neuropathy. This common antiarrhythmic drug is most likely to be used in the very population at risk for AION, so a causative link is difficult to prove. However, patients with presumed amiodarone optic neuropathy differ from AION in that both optic nerves are affected simultaneously, the vision loss is gradual over weeks and months rather than sudden, the vision loss is less severe, and the optic disc edema persists longer, and vision can improve with cessation of the drug. Note that amiodarone (and methanol) are exceptions to the rule that most toxic optic neuropathies do not manifest optic disc edema.

▶ HEREDITARY OPTIC NEUROPATHIES

The designation of *hereditary optic neuropathy* describes many different genetic abnormalities that are transmitted in a variety of inheritance patterns. Autosomal recessive inheritance is associated with severe visual loss from infancy. Dominant inheritance patterns characteristically have milder disease with delayed onset, which may be difficult to distinguish from toxic/nutritional optic neuropathy. Leber hereditary optic neuropathy (LHON) is transmitted as a mitochondrial mutation, with a unique non-Mendelian inheritance pattern. Optic atrophy may also occur with heritable neurodegenerative disorders associated with spinocerebellar disorders, deafness, ataxia, and motor and sensory neuropathies. Although a great number of genetic defects can lead to an optic neuropathy, there is increasing evidence that most of these genetic defects impair energy production in the mitochondria. It may be that the highly metabolic optic nerve is particularly vulnerable to mitochondrial energy compromise (see Box 4–5).

AUTOSOMAL DOMINANT (KJER) OPTIC ATROPHY

This dominantly inherited disorder causes a bilateral, symmetric, slowly progressive central or cecocentral visual field loss (Figure 4–34). Visual abnormalities usually begin in childhood, between 4 and 10 years of age, and may progress into the early teens. By the mid-teens the vision stabilizes, typically with a visual acuity around 20/100. Classically, the Farnsworth-Munsell 100 Hue test demonstrates a tritanopic (blue-yellow) axis. The inheritance pattern may not be obvious in the family history, as incomplete penetrance is common. Although many patients are aware that their vision has been subnormal their entire life, some patients are not symptomatic until adulthood. The family history should be explored

CHAPTER 4   OPTIC NERVE DISORDERS   125

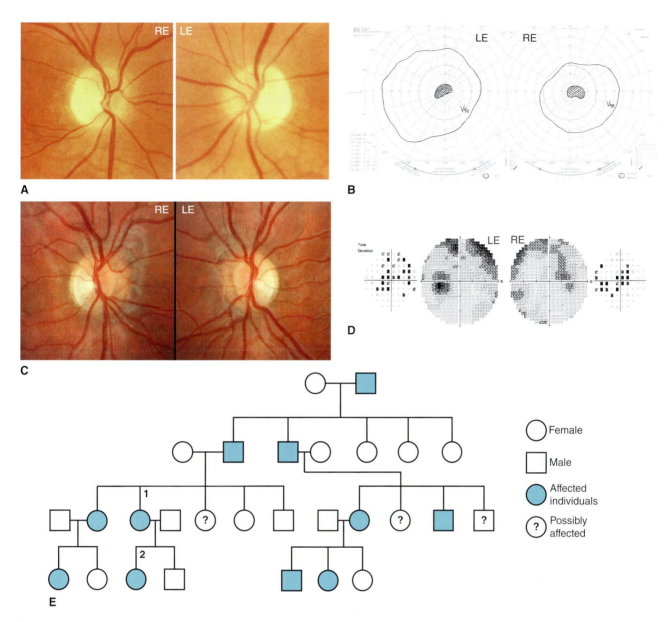

Figure 4–34. **Dominant optic atrophy.**
A 43-year-old woman has had subnormal vision her entire life. With a known family history of visual loss, she also brought her 18-year-old asymptomatic daughter for evaluation. (**A**) The mother's optic discs show diffuse pallor, with more striking pallor temporally. (**B**) Bilateral cecocentral scotomas were present with Goldmann perimetry. The visual acuity was 20/200 in both eyes. (**C**) The daughter's optic discs showed bilateral temporal pallor. (**D**) The daughter's automated perimetry showed bilateral shallow central scotomas. The visual acuity was 20/50 in each eye. (**E**) Four generations of this family are known or suspected to be affected by this autosomally dominant hereditary neuropathy (Kjer). (1, *the mother*; 2, *the daughter*.)

in detail by constructing a family tree if possible, identifying all known or potentially affected individuals. The optic discs typically display temporal pallor, but may appear relatively normal. Nerve fiber layer defects in the papillomacular bundle may be evident. About two-thirds of patients have a genetic defect linked to a region of chromosome 3q, called the OPA1 gene, which codes for products important in mitochondrial function.

LEBER HEREDITARY OPTIC NEUROPATHY

LHON is a heritable disorder causing painless visual loss predominantly in men (90%) over a broad range of ages, but typically between 20 and 30 years (Figure 4–35). LHON is but one form of mitochondrial optic neuropathy (see Box 4–5).

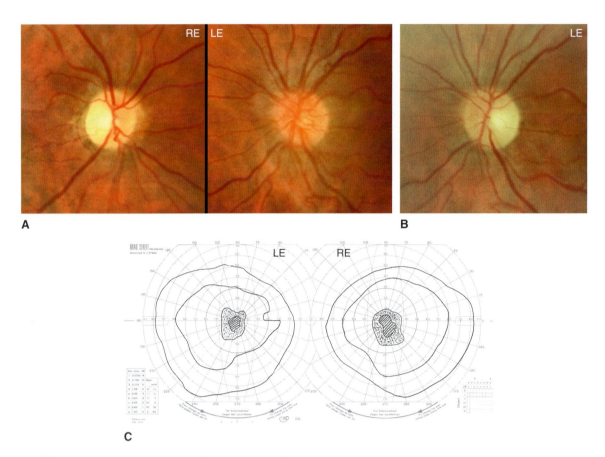

Figure 4–35. **Leber hereditary optic neuropathy.**
A 19-year-old man described the sudden onset of blurred vision in his right eye, which continued to progressively worsen. Two months after the onset of visual loss in his right eye, the vision in the left eye declined rapidly. Leber hereditary optic neuropathy (LHON) was confirmed with the identification of a mitochondrial DNA mutation at position 3460. **(A)** Optic discs, 2 months after onset of visual loss in the right eye, just before symptoms began in the left eye. Minimal temporal pallor of the right optic disc is present. The left optic disc is hyperemic, with subtle peripapillary telangiectatic vessels present. **(B)** Left optic disc, 3 months after presentation, after both eyes are affected. The disc hyperemia and telangiectasia have resolved, with mild temporal pallor now present. **(C)** Goldmann visual fields demonstrate bilateral cecocentral scotomas.

This hereditary defect is peculiar because patients have normal vision at birth and for 2 to 3 decades of life until *acute* visual loss occurs in one eye, followed by a similar event in the fellow eye within weeks or months. The precipitating factors are unknown, but alcohol or tobacco abuse or a nutritional deficiency is suspected to play a role. The visual field defect is usually a central or cecocentral scotoma that may continue to worsen over several months. The effect on the visual acuity ranges from mild to profound.

The optic disc may be mildly hyperemic with swelling of the peripapillary nerve fiber layer, or may appear normal. Dilation of small retinal capillaries is the classic finding, but it is difficult to identify unless specifically sought. Unlike neovascularization of the optic disc, these vessels do not leak on IVFA. Disc pallor develops shortly after visual loss, with loss of the peripapillary vascular changes; therefore, these characteristic peripapillary telangiectatic vessels may be best identified in the unaffected eye.

The genetic abnormality responsible for LHON is in the *mitochondrial* DNA. Although most genetic information is contained in the nuclear DNA (chromosomes), small strands of circular DNA in the mitochondria code for certain crucial components involved in energy-producing mitochondrial oxidative phosphorylation. Three genetic defects in mitochondrial DNA have been conclusively linked to LHON. These disorders are designated by the position of the point mutations in well-conserved regions of the mitochondrial DNA sequence: 11778 (70% of patients, also called the Wallace mutation), 14484, and 3460.

The inheritance pattern of mitochondrial genetic disorders is unique. At conception, the mitochondrial DNA in the sperm is excluded from the fertilized egg. The offspring receives mitochondrial DNA virtually exclusively from the mother. Thus, the genetic defect in LHON is passed from a female carrier to both male and female offspring. All daughters are carriers, and can occasionally manifest the disease. It is not clear why women with this genetic defect are so unlikely to manifest the disease, but Giordano et al (2010) present the idea that estrogens may have a protective effect. All sons have the genetic defect and frequently, but not invariably, manifest the disease, but they do not pass the defect to their children. The disorder is therefore exclusively maternally inherited, but manifests mostly in male offspring.

Many patients with LHON are initially thought to have optic neuritis, because the clinical presentation may be similar. However, pain with eye movement (a common finding in optic neuritis) is absent in LHON. When the clinical presentation is suggestive of LHON, genetic testing can provide confirmation and spare the patient an otherwise extensive evaluation. Once the mutation has been identified, genetic counseling for the patient and family is indicated. Because of a potential association with cardiac conduction abnormalities, an electro cardiogram should be obtained in patients with LHON. Also, patients at risk for LHON should be advised not to use tobacco and to limit alcohol intake, as these and other environmental factors may play a role in triggering visual loss. Treatment with oral supplements directed at mitochondrial function, such as coenzyme Q_{10} have been disappointing. Effective treatment is likely just on the horizon—drugs such as idebenone, a coenzyme Q_{10} analogue, are showing some promise. Approximately 10% of patients have an inexplicable spontaneous recovery, often years after vision loss (more likely with 14484 than 3460 or 11778 mutations).

▶ TRAUMATIC OPTIC NEUROPATHY

Traumatic optic neuropathy (TON) can occur through direct or indirect mechanisms. Examples of *direct* traumatic optic neuropathies include the impact of a BB shot on the intraorbital nerve, injury from a needle during retrobulbar injection, or impaling of the optic nerve by a bone fragment from a fracture of the optic canal (Figure 4–36). *Indirect trauma* is more common, occurring with blunt trauma (deceleration or acceleration) involving the orbital rim or forehead, such as a child going headfirst over the handlebars of a bicycle or tricycle. Indirect traumatic optic neuropathy can occur in the absence of fractures involving the optic canal or orbit and with few external signs of injury.

Symptoms

Visual loss is usually immediate at the time of trauma, and often severe (about half of patients are NLP). An important subgroup of patients may have a lucid interval, followed hours or days later by a precipitous drop

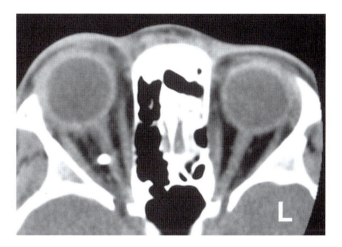

Figure 4-36. **Direct optic nerve trauma.** A 12-year-old boy was injured when a BB struck his right orbit. The entry wound was in the temporal conjunctiva, just missing the globe. Computed tomography (CT) scan (axial image) shows the BB adjacent to the right optic nerve. Acutely, the right optic disc appeared normal but turned pale over 4 weeks.

in vision, presumably caused by expanding optic nerve edema or hemorrhage within the confines of the optic canal.

Signs

TON may initially present with a normal-appearing optic disc and retina. Optic disc pallor, and occasionally cupping (especially in children and young adults), becomes evident over 1 or 2 months. Rarely optic disc edema may be present acutely, which suggests a trauma-associated AION. Optic nerve trauma is usually not an isolated finding. The potential for coincident trauma involving the adnexa, orbit, and globe, as well as head and body trauma must be actively addressed.

Causes

The mechanism of direct trauma is no mystery—axons and their support tissue are damaged by shearing, compression, contusion, and/or interruption of their vascular supply. The mechanisms of indirect-traumatic optic neuropathy include the transmission of forces to the orbital apex and optic canal by the conical shape of the bones forming the orbit (Figure 4–37), and shearing forces generated by violent movement of the intraorbital optic nerve relative to its fixed position posteriorly where it enters the optic canal (or anteriorly where it connects to the globe). Additional damage to the optic nerve may be caused by optic nerve edema or hemorrhage within the confines of the bony optic canal. A compartment syndrome may develop with ischemia to the

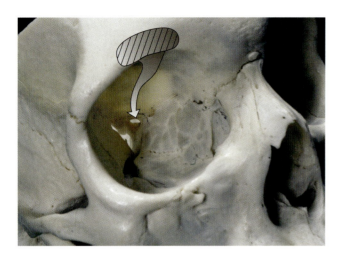

Figure 4–37. Indirect traumatic optic neuropathy.
Forces generated from a blow to the orbital rim can be transmitted to the optic canal, contusing the optic nerve even in the absence of fracture.

optic nerve, causing even further edema and compression. This cycle of edema and ischemia is most likely the mechanism in patients whose visual loss is delayed for hours or days following trauma.

Differential Diagnosis

In most patients, the presentation of traumatic optic neuropathy is self-evident, with history, examination, and other manifestations of trauma leaving little doubt. Occasionally patients may present with a pale optic nerve and an uncertain history; these patients require neuroimaging. Progressive visual loss with optic nerve pallor is not consistent with traumatic optic neuropathy and suggest a compressive optic neuropathy.

Evaluation

Because a search for skull and orbital fractures is indicated in most cases, a CT scan of the brain and orbits may be more appropriate than MRI as an initial study. Coronal slices provide the most information (and advances in CT technology no longer require extension of the neck in these patients with potential cervical spine injury). As discussed above, the high likelihood coincident trauma to the globe, adnexa, orbit, and head must be explored. Evaluation of patients with optic nerve injury may be complicated by the fact that these patients may have life-threatening higher-priority traumatic injuries that must be addressed first.

Treatment

Debate regarding the treatment of traumatic optic neuropathy is ongoing. Theoretically, the use of high-dose intravenous corticosteroids in the acute setting seems reasonable, but to date there is no convincing evidence that this treatment is effective. In fact, the Corticosteroid Randomization After Significant Head Injury (CRASH) study reported an *increase in mortality* in head injury patients given high-dose steroids. There may still be a role for high-dose steroids in patients without demonstrable concomitant head injury, but such treatment would need to be individualized and the patients made aware of the potential risk and lack of proven efficacy. Surgical decompression of the optic canal, either transcranially or with an ethmoid sinus approach, has also been offered as a treatment of traumatic optic neuropathy. The rationale for this procedure seems reasonable given our understanding of the mechanisms of injury, but efficacy is unproven, and the potential for surgical morbidity must be considered. Surgery to relieve fracture fragments compressing or impinging on the optic nerve is controversial. Stable, metallic foreign bodies in the orbit may not require removal.

In summary, there is no proven effective treatment for traumatic optic neuropathy. The visual acuity in TON has been shown to improve without any treatment in at least 25% of patients. Therefore, observation may be the most reasonable course of action in most cases.

▶ GLAUCOMA

The most common disorder affecting the optic nerve—glaucoma—is so prevalent and complex that an entire subspecialty of ophthalmology is devoted to the study and treatment of this optic neuropathy. Glaucoma is not a single entity, but rather a collection of disorders related by the presumed mechanism of elevated intraocular pressure causing injury to the optic nerve. However, the role of intraocular pressure is poorly understood, the site of injury (optic nerve vs ganglion cells) is unclear, and the mechanism of glaucomatous optic atrophy (with cupping rather than pallor) is unknown. In many patients, the cause of elevated intraocular pressure is evident—such as blockage of aqueous outflow by hemorrhage, inflammatory products, or mechanical apposition of the iris (examples of *secondary* glaucoma). Secondary forms of glaucoma are often acute or subacute and accompanied by other ocular signs and symptoms, such as eye pain and redness. The most common form of glaucoma is *primary* open angle glaucoma (POAG), an idiopathic disorder of elevated intraocular pressure characterized by slow atrophy of the optic nerve manifested as an enlarging central cup and progression of peripheral visual field defects. Patients with POAG usually do not have pain or redness and can remain asymptomatic until progression to profound vision loss (Figure 4–38). A thorough discussion of glaucoma is beyond the scope of this book, but it is important to recognize this very common optic neuropathy as its evaluation and treatment is quite different from the other optic neuropathies discussed in this chapter.

Most forms of glaucoma are characterized by elevated intraocular pressure. However, the intraocular pressure does not always correlate with the progression of visual field loss, and visual loss may occur even in patients with apparently normal pressures. Patients with *low tension* (also called *normal tension*) glaucoma may require consideration of other diagnostic possibilities, such as a compressive optic neuropathy.

Atrophy of axons causes enlargement of the optic cup, predominantly with loss of neuroretinal tissue at the superior and inferior aspects of the cup, resulting in vertical elongation of the cup that "notches" the neuroretinal rim. Glaucoma does not typically cause pallor of the neuroretinal rim. Patients with cupping and rim pallor likely have another underlying diagnosis and require further investigation (eg, neuroimaging).

Visual field loss from glaucoma usually correlates relatively well with the degree and location of optic disc cupping. The pattern of visual field loss is remarkably similar to chronic optic disc edema, with preservation of central vision until late in its course. New visual field changes may be heralded by characteristic flame-shaped hemorrhages at the disc margin.

Occasionally, other optic neuropathies are misdiagnosed as glaucoma. Visual field defects that do not correlate with optic disc cupping, the presence of pallor of the neuroretinal rim, and early loss of central vision suggest a diagnosis other than glaucoma (Figure 4–39).

▶ OPTIC DISC DRUSEN

Optic disc *drusen* [Ger. pl. of *Druse*, stony nodule, geode] are mineralized hyaline-like crystals of unknown origin embedded in the substance of the prelaminar optic nerve head (Figure 4–40). Optic disc drusen are present in approximately 1% of whites, and are frequently bilateral (75%). Optic disc drusen can be inherited as an autosomal dominant trait with incomplete penetrance.

Microscopically, drusen appear as concentric layers of hyalinoid material, with positive staining for amino acids, acid mucopolysaccharide, calcium, and hemosiderin, but not amyloid.

Symptoms

Optic disc drusen are frequently an incidental discovery in a routine eye examination. Occasionally, patients present complaining of peripheral visual loss. Rarely, patients may experience a relentless, progressive, stepwise decline in peripheral vision. Transient visual obscurations, similar to those seen in papilledema, may occur with optic disc drusen.

Signs

In children and young adults, optic disc drusen may be buried within the disc and not visible with ophthalmoscopy (Figure 4–41). The discs are elevated, often with a "lumpy-bumpy" contour, and may simulate optic disc edema (pseudopapilledema) (see Table 4–2). Over time, the drusen emerge, perhaps because of atrophy of the overlying nerve fibers. Optic disc drusen in adults are usually evident with the ophthalmoscope, appearing as glistening, yellowish, "rock candy" crystals poking up through the nerve fibers of the disc. Subretinal and splinter hemorrhages may be present. Peripapillary choroidal neovascular membranes can occur in association with

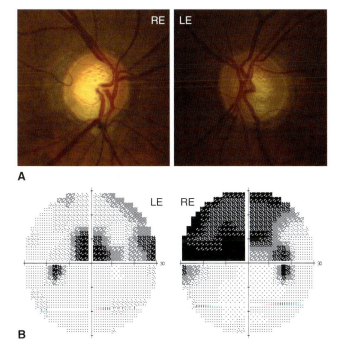

Figure 4-38. Primary open angle glaucoma. A 54-year-old man has primary open angle glaucoma. **(A)** Both discs show a large cup-to-disc ratio, about 0.9. The thin remaining neuroretinal rim is still pink, not pale. The rim is especially thin at the inferior poles, where it is "notched" to the rim. **(B)** Automated Humphrey 30-2 perimetry shows superior altitudinal visual field defects, corresponding to the notching of the inferior neuroretinal rims. Despite the severe visual field loss, the patient remains 20/30 in both eyes. This is the same patient depicted in Figure 3–9, where progression of visual field loss over time is shown.

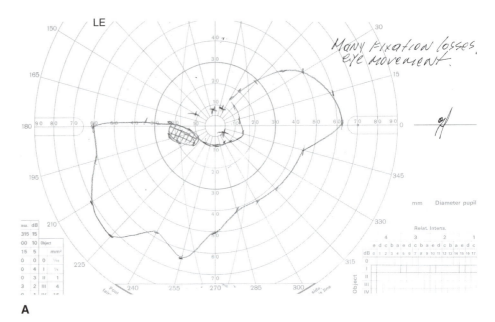

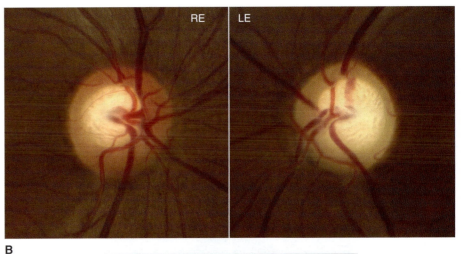

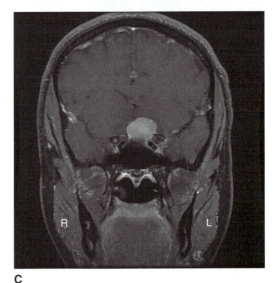

Figure 4-39. **Cupping and pallor of the optic disc.** A 45-year-old woman described gradual vision loss in her left eye. The patient was previously diagnosed with glaucoma in the left eye, but did not have elevated intraocular pressures. Visual acuity was 20/20 in the right eye, and CF 4' in the left eye. **(A)** Goldmann perimetry from the left eye shows a dense central scotoma with superior visual field loss that respects the horizontal meridian, consistent with an optic nerve–related visual field defect. However, a central scotoma would be most unusual for glaucoma. The visual field in the right eye was normal (not pictured). **(B)** The right optic disc is normal, with a cup-to-disc ratio of 0.6. The left eye has a cup-to-disc ratio of 0.8, which seems compatible with the diagnosis of glaucoma. However, not only is the optic disc cupped, but the neuroretinal rim is pale, raising further suspicions that glaucoma may not be the correct diagnosis. **(C)** The presence of a central scotoma and optic disc pallor with cupping raised concerns for a compressive optic neuropathy and led to neuroimaging. Magnetic resonance imaging (MRI; coronal T1 with contrast is pictured) was consistent with a planum sphenoidale meningioma compressing the prechiasmatic left optic nerve.

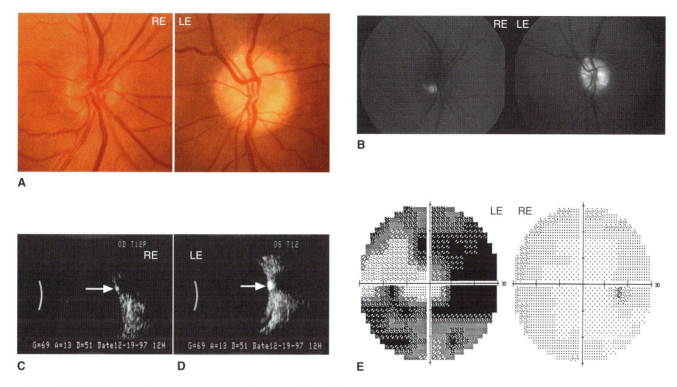

Figure 4–40. **Optic disc drusen and visual field loss.**
A 62-year-old man reported that the vision in his right eye has been better than in his left eye for many years. **(A)** The right optic disc appears normal; optic disc drusen are evident on the left. **(B)** By using the barrier filters for fluorescein angiography without fluorescein dye injection, auto-fluorescence can be detected. Faint auto-fluorescence can be seen in the inferior portion of the right disc, suggesting buried optic disc drusen. Diffuse auto-fluorescence of the left optic disc is evident. **(C)** B-mode ultrasound of the right eye shows the highly echoic buried disc drusen (*arrow*), even though drusen were not evident with the ophthalmoscope. **(D)** B-mode ultrasound of the left eye shows the bright echo signals from florid optic disc drusen (*arrow*). **(E)** In the left eye, dense peripheral visual field loss is evident, with preservation of the central acuity (20/25). The right eye has a normal visual field and visual acuity.

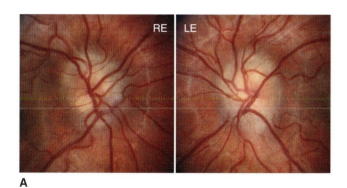

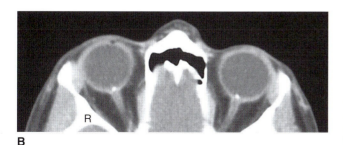

Figure 4–41. **Pseudopapilledema from buried optic disc drusen.**
A 16-year-old woman was noted to have elevated optic discs and headaches. Visual acuity and visual fields were normal. A computed tomography (CT) scan of the brain was reportedly normal. B-mode ultrasound of the optic discs revealed buried optic disc drusen (as in Figure 4–40). **(A)** The optic discs are elevated with a "lumpy-bumpy" contour. **(B)** Review of the patient's CT scan (axial view, bone windows) revealed the radiodense drusen.

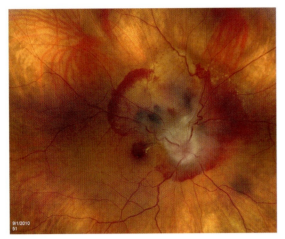

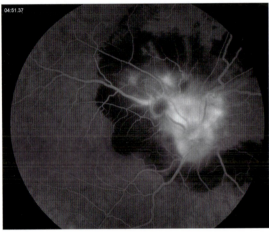

Figure 4-42. **Drusen of the optic disc with peripapillary choroidal neovascular membrane.**
(A) Extensive peripapillary subretinal hemorrhage is evident in this retinal montage photograph. **(B)** Intravenous fluorescein angiography (late phase) shows hyperfluorescence of a peripapillary choroidal neovascular membrane superiorly, and blockage of choroidal hyperfluorescence from extensive subretinal blood.

disc drusen (Figure 4-42). Optic disc drusen may be associated with retinitis pigmentosa and angioid streaks.

Optic disc–related visual field defects, with corresponding loss of the retinal nerve fiber layer, may be present. Curiously, central visual acuity is almost never affected. Optic disc drusen are a potential cause of peripheral constriction with preservation of central vision (see Table 3-3).

Causes

The precise mechanism of visual loss in patients with optic disc drusen is unknown, but it likely relates to the typical crowded configuration of the optic discs. Axonal atrophy may occur secondary to compression of optic nerve axons, but the position and extent of disc drusen does not correlate well with the visual field defects. Some patients present with an acute event, demonstrating true optic disc swelling in addition to the presence of disc drusen, implicating a drusen-related AION.

Differential Diagnosis and Evaluation

Buried disc drusen may give the appearance of optic disc edema (pseudopapilledema). On the other hand, tiny, glistening edema residues often accompany chronic optic disc edema and should not be mistaken for drusen (see Table 4-2). Disc drusen not evident with the ophthalmoscope are best identified with orbital ultrasound, appearing as focal, highly echoic densities (see Figure 4-40C, D). The calcific component of the drusen also makes them highly visible on CT images that include the optic nerve head (see Figure 4-41B). Drusen exhibit autofluorescence, demonstrated with the standard barrier and exciter filters of the fluorescein angiogram camera (without fluorescein) (see Figure 4-40B). Optical coherence tomography (OCT) can also be used to visualize optic disc drusen.

The discovery of optic disc drusen in a patient with elevated optic discs may save the patient an extensive evaluation for optic disc edema. However, the presence of optic disc drusen does not preclude other diseases—patients with optic disc drusen can also have true papilledema. The physician should actively seek evidence of other potential disorders and investigate any findings not consistent with disc drusen. For example, progressive visual loss would not be typical for optic disc drusen, and such patients require further evaluation including neuroimaging to look for possible optic nerve compression.

Treatment

As discussed above, the mechanisms of visual loss from optic disc drusen are not entirely understood. Some physicians suggest topical agents (eg, Alphagan [brimonidine tartrate]) to lower the intraocular pressure in an effort to improve the ocular perfusion gradient.

▶ ANOMALOUS OPTIC DISCS

The term *anomalous optic disc* implies a congenital rather than an acquired abnormal optic disc appearance. Disc anomalies may be minor and not affect optic nerve function (crowded, elevated, or tilted discs), or may represent significant maldevelopment of the visual pathway (hypoplasia, aplasia, or coloboma) (Figure 4-43).

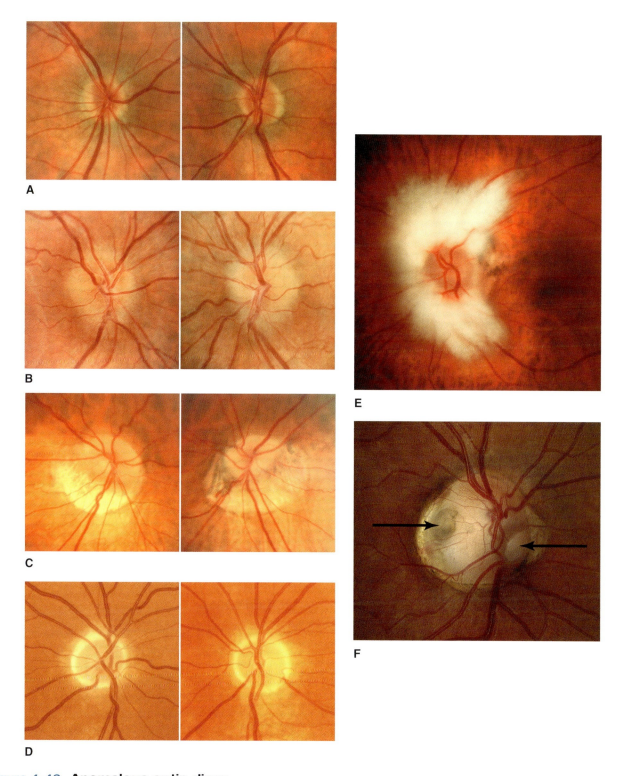

Figure 4-43. **Anomalous optic discs.**
(A) Small, cupless optic discs. (B) Anomalously elevated optic discs without identifiable drusen. (C) Tilted optic discs with an inferior temporal conus in a patient with high myopia. (D) Optic disc hypoplasia with a double-ring sign. (E) Myelinated nerve fiber layer simulating optic disc edema. (F) Optic nerve head pits (*arrows*).

CROWDED OPTIC DISCS

Small optic discs that are "cupless" may be at risk for AION (see discussion of AION; Figure 4–43A).

ELEVATED DISCS WITHOUT DRUSEN

Some anomalous optic discs that appear elevated may not harbor disc drusen (see Figure 4–43B). This optic disc appearance typically occurs in young patients and is usually bilateral, mimicking papilledema. Concern is heightened when drusen are not clinically identified. Some of these optic discs may eventually develop drusen. Table 4–2 lists some characteristics to help distinguish true papilledema from pseudopapilledema.

TILTED OPTIC DISCS

This anomaly results from an oblique insertion of the optic nerve on the globe, and is a frequent finding in axial myopia (see Figure 4–43C). The nasal edge of the disc is elevated, and the temporal edge and adjacent retina are depressed relative to the normal plane of the peripapillary retina. These discs appear vertically elongated, with a white crescent temporally where the retinal pigment epithelium stops short of the disc edge. The depression of retina temporal to the disc may cause a refractive scotoma, occasionally simulating the bitemporal visual field defects of chiasmal disorders (see Figure 3–14, Table 3–2). Inferior, superior, and temporal tilted discs also occur.

MYELINATED RETINAL NERVE FIBERS

Myelination of the anterior visual pathway begins at the lateral geniculate nucleus during gestation, proceeding anteriorly and reaching the lamina cribrosa of the optic nerve at about term. In less than 1% of the population, myelination abnormally proceeds into the eye and retinal nerve fiber layer for a variable extent. This creates white, opaque patches with feathered edges in the nerve fiber layer of the retina, usually adjacent to the optic disc, which may be confused with optic disc swelling or retinal ischemia (see Figure 4–43E). Occasionally, myelinated nerve fiber patches can occur in the peripheral retina, not adjacent to the optic disc. Myelinated retinal nerve fibers are not associated with disease, and generally do not cause symptomatic visual loss.

HYPOPLASIA

Optic disc hypoplasia represents incomplete development of the optic disc, characterized by a small optic disc with a larger concentric, variably pigmented ring (double-ring sign; see Figure 4–43D). Visual function may be poor or relatively good. Disc hypoplasia may occur in one or both eyes, and has been reported in children born to diabetic mothers, or mothers who have been exposed to alcohol, LSD (lysergic acid diethylamide), quinine, or antiepileptic drugs during pregnancy. Disc hypoplasia can be associated with other congenital neurological and systemic abnormalities, and should prompt a thorough neurological investigation when discovered in children. The older clinical term septo-optic dysplasia (de Morsier syndrome) correctly implies that optic disc hypoplasia can accompany other congenital CNS abnormalities such as neuroendocrine axis dysfunction, but the absence of the septum pellucidum is neither significant nor prognostic. A hypoplastic appearance of the optic disc can also be caused by arrested development resulting from craniopharyngiomas or gliomas. Neuroimaging and determination of endocrine function may be required in the evaluation of optic disc hypoplasia in children.

APLASIA

A complete failure of optic nerve development is rare and usually associated with lethal congenital neural abnormalities.

COLOBOMA

Incomplete closure of the fetal fissure in ocular development can initiate a broad spectrum of optic disc and chorioretinal development abnormalities, termed *colobomas*. One extreme coloboma is the morning glory syndrome, consisting of marked excavation of an enlarged disc with embryonic glial remnants extending from the disc in the form of a flower. *Optic nerve pits* represent a mild abnormality in the spectrum of developmental disc anomalies, but associated macular subretinal fluid can cause a profound effect on vision (see Figure 4–43F). Optic disc and chorioretinal colobomas are typically located inferior and temporal to the disc, along the site of the fetal fissure (Figure 4–44). Visual dysfunction generally parallels the degree of optic disc malformation. Developmental optic disc abnormalities may be associated with forebrain abnormalities, particularly basal encephaloceles.

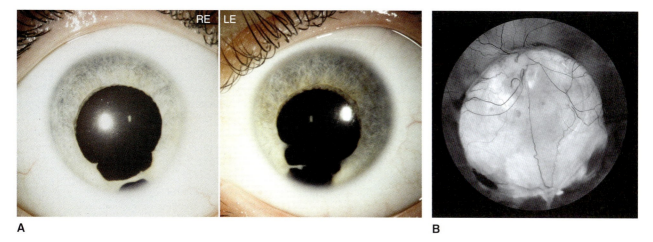

Figure 4-44. Ocular coloboma.
(A) Bilateral inferonasal iris defects suggest that this patient had incomplete closure of the fetal fissure during embryonic development. **(B)** Fundus map of the patient's right eye was digitally created from many individual 30° photographs. A large coloboma involves the retina and optic disc (seen at the superior edge). The left eye was nearly identical.

▶ KEY POINTS

- Anterior ischemic optic neuropathy is a common cause of unilateral optic disc edema and sudden visual loss in patients older than 45 years.
- AION may be nonarteritic, or secondary to GCA.
- A prompt diagnosis and immediate corticosteroid treatment of GCA can prevent bilateral blindness.
- When GCA is suspected, an ESR and CRP should be sent and corticosteroid therapy should be instituted immediately, with a temporal artery biopsy arranged following these steps.
- Optic neuritis is a cause of visual loss in young patients characterized by pain with eye movement and an optic disc that may be swollen or normal in appearance.
- High-dose intravenous corticosteroids should be considered when patients with optic neuritis have white matter changes visible on MRI.
- Papilledema may be caused by intracranial tumors and ventricular obstruction, or may be an idiopathic disorder in young, obese females (eight times more common in women than in men).
- Papilledema should be initially investigated by a blood pressure measurement, neuroimaging, and lumbar puncture (if imaging reveals no mass or obstruction).
- Chronic papilledema can cause slowly progressive profound visual field loss despite normal visual acuity; patients must be followed with serial perimetry.
- A gradual, insidious decline in vision with optic nerve pallor suggests a compressive optic neuropathy such as a meningioma, orbital mass, or orbital Graves disease.
- Optic nerve gliomas in children are frequently associated with neurofibromatosis (type I), and commonly behave in a benign fashion.
- Acute leukemic infiltrative optic neuropathy is an ophthalmic emergency; radiation therapy may be sight-saving.
- The term *neuroretinitis* designates optic disc edema associated with macular edema (with edema residues that typically form a macular star), which is often the result of an infectious process or subsequent immune response.
- Toxic and nutritional deficiencies cause progressive, bilateral, cecocentral scotomas.
- Leber hereditary optic neuropathy (LHON) is associated with specific point mutations in mitochondrial DNA, and typically causes acute visual loss in one eye, followed within weeks by a similar event in the other eye, usually in young men between 15 and 30 years old.
- Trauma to the optic nerve can occur without fractures, because the forces from blunt trauma to the brow or cheek are mechanically funneled to the orbital apex and optic canal.
- Optic disc drusen can be associated with peripheral (not central) visual field defects.

SUGGESTED READING

Books

Burde RM, Savino PJ, Trobe JD: Prechiasmal visual loss, in *Clinical Decisions in Neuro-ophthalmology*. 2d ed. St. Louis, MO: Mosby Year Book; 1992:41–73.

Corbett JJ, Martin TJ: Pseudotumor cerebri, in Youmans JR (ed): *Neurological Surgery*, 4th ed. Vol. 4. Philadelphia, PA: Saunders; 1995:2980–2997.

Corbett J, Wall M: The optic nerve head: elevated discs, in Rosen ES, Thompson HS, Cumming WJK, et al (eds): *Neuro-ophthalmology*. London: Mosby International Limited; 1998.

Digre KB, Corbett JJ: *Practical Viewing of the Optic Disc*. New York, NY: Heinemann; 2000.

Feldon SE: Tumors of the anterior visual pathways, in Jakobiec FA, Albert DM (eds): *Principles and Practice of Ophthalmology*. Philadelphia, PA: WB Saunders Co. 1994.

Fraunfelder FT, Fraunfelder FW, Chambers WA: *Clinical Ocular Toxicology: Drugs, Chemicals, and Herbs*. Philadelphia, PA: Saunders/Elsevier; 2008.

Hayreh, Sohan. *Ischemic Optic Neuropathies*. Berlin, New York: Springer; 2011.

Katz B, Wall M: The optic neuropathies, in Slamovits TL, Burde R (assoc eds): *Neuro-ophthalmology*: in Podos SM, Yanoff M (eds): *Textbook of Ophthalmology*, Vol 6. London: Mosby; 1991:3.1–3.40.

Kline LB, Foroozan R (eds): Optic nerve disorders, *Ophthalmology Monographs*, Vol. 10. San Francisco, CA: American Academy of Ophthalmology; 2007.

Lee AG, Brazis PW: *Clinical Pathways in Neuro-ophthalmology: An Evidence-Based Approach*, 2d ed. New York, NY: Thieme; 2003.

Liu GT, Volpe NJ, Galetta SL, Galetta SL: Visual loss: optic neuropathies (Chap 5), Optic disc swelling (Chap. 6), Papilledema and Other Causes, in *Neuro-ophthalmology: Diagnosis and Management*, 2d ed. Philadelphia: Saunders Elsevier; 2010.

Miller NR, Newman NJ, Biousse V, et al. (eds): The visual sensory system, in *Walsh and Hoyts' Clinical Neuro-ophthalmology*: 6th ed, Vol. 1. Baltimore, MD: Williams and Wilkins; 2005.

Sadun AA, Glaser JS: Anatomy of the visual sensory system, in *Neuro-ophthalmology*: Philadelphia, PA: Lippincott; 1991:61–82.

Spoor TC: *Atlas of Optic Nerve Disorders*. New York, NY: Raven Press; 1992.

Articles

Optic Nerve Anatomy

Barron MJ, Griffiths P, Turnbull DM, et al: The distributions of mitochondria and sodium channels reflect the specific energy requirements and conduction properties of the human optic nerve head. *Br J Ophthalmol* 2004;88:286–290.

Hayreh SS: Anatomy and physiology of the optic nerve head. *Trans Am Acad Ophthalmol Otolaryngol* 1974;78:240–254.

Clinical Expression of Disease

Quigley HA, Anderson DR: The histological basis of optic disc pallor. *Am J Ophthalmol* 1977;83:709–717.

Sadun AA, Rismondo V: Evaluation of the swollen disc, in Schachat A (ed): *Current Practice in Ophthalmology*. Boston, MA: Mosby Year Book; 1992:177–186.

Nonarteritic Anterior Ischemic Optic Neuropathy

Beck RW, Servais G, Hayreh SS: Anterior ischemic optic neuropathy. IX. Cup-to-disc ratio and its role in pathogenesis. *Ophthalmology* 1987;94:1503–1508.

Hayreh SS, Zimmerman MB: Nonarteritic anterior ischemic optic neuropathy: role of systemic corticosteroid therapy. *Graefes Arch Clin Exp Ophthalmol* 2008;246:1029–1046.

Hayreh SS, Zimmerman BM, Podhajski P, et al: Nocturnal arterial hypotension and its role in optic nerve head and ocular ischemic disorders. *Am J Ophthalmol* 1994;117:603–624.

Ischemic Optic Neuropathy Decompression Trial Research Group: Ischemic optic neuropathy decompression trial: twenty-four month update. *Arch Ophthalmol* 2000;118(6):793–798.

Ischemic Optic Neuropathy Decompression Trial Research Group: Optic nerve decompression surgery for nonarteritic anterior ischemic optic neuropathy is not effective and may be harmful. *JAMA* 1995;273(8):625–632.

Rizzo JF, Lessell S: Optic neuritis and ischemic optic neuropathy: overlapping clinical profiles. *Arch Ophthalmol* 1991;109:1668–1672.

Arteritic Anterior Ischemic Optic Neuropathy (Giant Cell Arteritis)

Hayreh SS, Podhajsky PA, Raman R, et al: Giant cell arteritis: validity and reliability of various diagnostic criteria. *Am J Ophthalmol* 1997;123:285.

Keltner JL: Giant-cell arteritis: signs and symptoms. *Ophthalmol* 1982;89:1101–1110.

Parika M, Miller NR, Lee AG, et al: Prevalence of a normal C-reactive protein with an elevated erythrocyte sedimentation rate in biopsy proven giant cell arteritis. *Ophthalmol* 2006;113:1842–1845.

Weyand CM, Bartley GB: Giant cell arteritis: new concepts in pathogenesis and implications for management. *Am J Ophthalmol* 1997;123:392.

Radiation Optic Neuropathy

Kline LB, Kim JY, Ceballos R: Radiation optic neuropathy. *Ophthalmol* 1985;92:1118–1126.

Lessell S. Friendly fire: neurogenic visual loss form radiation therapy. *J Neuroophthalmol* 2004;24:23–250.

Optic Neuritis

Beck RW, Cleary PA, Anderson MM, et al: A randomized, controlled trial of corticosteroids in the treatment of acute optic neuritis. *N Engl J Med* 1992;326:581–588.

Beck RW, Cleary PA, Trobe JD, et al: The effect of corticosteroids for acute optic neuritis on the subsequent development of multiple sclerosis. *N Engl J Med* 1993;29:1764–1769.

Comi G, Fillipi M, Barkhof F, et al: Effect of early interferon treatment on conversion to definite multiple sclerosis: a randomized study. *Lancet* 2001;357:1576–1582.

Flippi M, Rovaris M, Ingles M, et al: Interferon beta-1a for brain tissue loss in patients at presentation with syndrome suggestive of multiple sclerosis: a randomized, double-blind, placebo-controlled trail. *Lancet* 2004;364:1489–1496.

Jacobs LD, Beck RW, Simon JH, et al: Intramuscular interferon beta-1a therapy initiated during a first demyelinating event in multiple sclerosis. CHAMPS study group. *N Engl J Med* 2000;343:898–904.

Kappos L, Polman CH, Freedman MS: Treatment with interferon beta-1b delays conversion to clinically definite and McDonald MS in patient with clinically isolated syndromes. *Neurology* 2006;67:1–8.

Optic Neuritis Study Group: Multiple sclerosis risk after optic neuritis: final optic neuritis treatment trial follow-up. *Arch Neurol* 2008;65(6):727–732.

Optic Neuritis Study Group: High- and low-risk profiles for the development of multiple sclerosis within 10 years after optic neuritis. *Arch Ophthalmol* 2003;121:944–949.

Optic Neuritis Study Group: The clinical profile of optic neuritis: experience of the optic neuritis treatment trial. *Arch Ophthalmol* 1991;109:1673–1678.

Optic Neuritis Study Group: Visual function 15 years after optic neuritis: a final follow-up report from the optic neuritis treatment trial. *Ophthalmology* 2008;115(6):1079–1082.

Neuromyelitis Optica

Lennon VA, Wingerchuk DM, Kryzen TJ, et al: A serum autoantibody marker of neuromyelitis optica: distinction from multiple sclerosis. *Lancet* 2004;364:2106–2112.

Morrow MJ, Wingerchuk D: Neuromyelitis optica. *J Neuroophthalmol* 2012;32(2)154–166.

Wingerchuk DM, Lennon VA, Pittock SJ, et al: Revised diagnostic criteria for neuromyelitis optica. *Neurology* 2006;66(10):1485–1489.

Optic Perineuritis

Purvin V, Kawasaki A, Jacobson DM: Optic perineuritis: clinical and radiographic features. *Arch Ophthalmol* 2001;119:1299–1306.

Idiopathic Intracranial Hypertension (Pseudotumor cerebri)

Burgett RA, Purvin VA, Kawaski A: Lumboperitoneal shunting for pseudotumor cerebri. *Neurology* 1997;49:734.

Corbett JJ, Savino PJ, Thompson HS, et al: Visual loss in pseudotumor cerebri. *Arch Neurol* 1982;39:461–474.

Corbett JJ, Thompson HS: The rational management of idiopathic intracranial hypertension. *Arch Neurol* 1989;46:1049–1051.

Friedman DI, Jacobson DM: Diagnostic criteria for idiopathic intracranial hypertension. *Neurology* 2002;59:1492–1495.

Friedman DI, Jacobson DM: Idiopathic intracranial hypertension. *J Neuroophthalmol* 2004;24:138–145.

Frisén L: Swelling of the optic nerve head: a staging scheme. *J Neurol Neurosurg Psychiatry* 1982;45:13–18.

Wall M: Idiopathic intracranial hypertension: mechanisms of visual loss and disease management. *Semin Neurol* 2000;20(1):89–95.

Wall M, George D: Idiopathic intracranial hypertension. A prospective study of 50 patients. *Brain* 1991;114:155–180.

Neoplasms

Haik BG, Saint Louis L, Bierly J, et al: Magnetic resonance imaging in the evaluation of optic nerve gliomas. *Ophthalmology* 1997;94:709–717.

Hoyt WF, Baghdasssarian SA: Optic glioma of childhood. Natural history and rationale for conservative management. *Br J Ophthalmol* 1969; 53(12):793–798.

Hoyt WF, Meshel LG, Lessell S, et al: Malignant optic glioma of adulthood. *Brain* 1973;96:121–132.

Lee AG: Neuro-ophthalmology: management of optic pathway gliomas. *Neurosurg Focus* 2007;23(5):E1.

Lindblom B, Truwit CL, Hoyt WF: Optic nerve sheath meningioma: definition of intraorbital, intracanalicular, and intracranial components with magnetic resonance imaging. *Ophthalmology* 1992;99:560–566.

Listernick R, Louis DN, Packer RJ, et al: Optic pathway gliomas in neurofibromatosis-1: controversies and recommendations. *Ann Neurol* 2007;61(3):189–198.

Miller NR: New concepts in the diagnosis and management of optic nerve sheath meningioma. *J Neuroophthalmol* 2006;26(3):200–208.

Sibony P, Krauss H, Kennerdal J, et al: Optic nerve sheath meningiomas. Clinical manifestations. *Ophthalmology* 1984;91:1313–1326.

Wilson WB: Meningiomas of the anterior visual system. *Surv Ophthalmol* 1981;26:109–127.

Zimmerman CF, Schatz NJ, Glaser JG: Magnetic resonance imaging of optic nerve meningiomas. *Ophthalmology* 1990;97:585–591.

ODEMS and Neuroretinitis

Brazis PW, Lee AG: Optic disc edema with a macular star. *Mayo Clin Proc* 1996;71:1162–1166.

Golnik KC, Marotto ME, Fanous MM, et al: Ophthalmic manifestations of *Rochalimaea* species. *Am J Ophthalmol* 1994;118:145–151.

Purvin VA, Chioran G: Recurrent neuroretinitis. *Arch Ophthalmol* 1994;112:365–371.

Toxic/Nutritional

Sadun AA: Mitochondrial optic neuropathies. *J Neurol Neurosurg Psychiatry* 2002;72:423–425. doi:10.1136/jnnp.72.4.423

Sadun AA: Mitochondrial optic neuropathies: toxic/metabolic. Meeting syllabus of the North American Neuro-ophthalmology: Society, 2012: 71–76.

Dominant Optic Atrophy

Cohn AC, Toomes C, Potter C, et al: Autosomal dominant optic atrophy: penetrance and expressivity in patients with OPA1 mutations. *Am J Ophthalmol* 2007;143:656–662.

Hoyt CS: Autosomal dominant optic atrophy: a spectrum of disability. *Ophthalmology* 1980;87:245–251.

Leber Hereditary Optic Neuropathy

Giordano C, Montopoli M, Perli E, et al: Oestrogens ameliorate mitochondrial dysfunction in Leber's hereditary optic neuropathy. *Brain* first published online October 13, 2010 doi:10.1093/brain/awq276.

Klopstock T, Yu-Wai-Man P, Dimitriadis K, et al: A randomized placebo-controlled trial of idebenone in Leber's hereditary optic neuropathy. *Brain* 2011;134:2677–2686.

Newman NJ, Biousse V, Newman SA, et al: Progression of visual field defects in Leber hereditary optic neuropathy: experience of the LHON treatment trial. *Amer J Ophthalmol* 2006;141(6):1061–1067.

Newman NJ: Leber's hereditary optic neuropathy—new genetic considerations. *Arch Neurol* 1993;50:540.

Newman NJ, Wallace DC: Mitochondria and Leber's hereditary optic neuropathy. *Am J Ophthalmol* 1990;109:726–730.

Traumatic Optic Neuropathy

Anderson RL, Panje WR, Gross CE: Optic nerve blindness following blunt forehead trauma. *Ophthalmology* 1982;89:445–455.

Edwards P, Arango M, Balica L, et al: CRASH trial collaborators. Final results of MRC CRASH, a randomized placebo-controlled trial of intravenous corticosteroid in adults with head injury—outcomes at 6 months. *Lancet* 2005;365:1957–1959.

Purvin V: Evidence of orbital deformation in indirect optic nerve injury. *J Clin Neuroophthalmol* 1988;8(1):9–11.

Spoor TC, Hartel WC, Lensink DB, et el: Treatment of traumatic optic neuropathy with corticosteroids. *Am J Ophthalmol* 1990;110:665–669.

Steinsapir KD: Treatment of traumatic optic neuropathy with high-dose corticosteroid. *J Neuroophthalmol* 2006;26:65–67.

Steinsapir KD, Goldberg RA: Traumatic optic neuropathy. *Surv Ophthalmol* 1994;38:487–518.

Wu N, Yin ZQ, Wang Y: Traumatic optic neuropathy therapy: an update of clinical and experimental studies. *J Int Med Res* 2008;36:883–889.

Anomalous Optic Discs

Borchert M: Reappraisal of the optic nerve hypoplasia syndrome. *J Neuroophthalmol* 2012;32(1):58–67.

Lambert SR, Hoyt CS, Narahara MH: Optic nerve hypoplasia. *Surv Ophthalmol* 1987;32:1–9.

Rosenberg MA, Savino PJ, Glaser JS: A clinical analysis of pseudopapilledema. I. Population, laterality, acuity, refractive error, ophthalmoscopic characteristics, and coincident disease. *Arch Ophthalmol* 1979;97:71–75.

Savino PJ, Glaser JS, Rosenberg MA: A clinical analysis of pseudopapilledema. II. Visual field defects. *Arch Ophthalmol* 1979;97:71–75.

Witmer MT, Margo CE, Drucker M: Tilted optic disks. *Surv Ophthalmol* 2010;55(5):403–428.

Paraneoplastic and Inflammatory Optic Neuropathies

Chan JW: Paraneoplastic retinopathies and optic neuropathies. *Surv Ophthalmol* 2003;48:12–38.

Scott TF: Neurosarcoidosis: progress and clinical aspects. *Neurology* 1993;43:8–12.

Stern B, Corbett JJ: Neuro-ophthalmologic manifestations of sarcoidosis. *Curr Treatment Options Neurol* 2003;9:63–71.

CHAPTER 5

Disorders of the Chiasm and Retrochiasmal Visual Pathways

- ► CHIASM AND PARASELLAR REGION 139
  - Signs and symptoms: neuroanatomic correlation 139
  - Disorders of the chiasm 143
  - Evaluation and management 147
- ► OPTIC TRACT 147
  - Anatomy 147
  - Signs and symptoms 147
  - Disorders of the optic tract 147
- ► LATERAL GENICULATE NUCLEUS 148
- ► OPTIC RADIATIONS 150
  - Parietal lobe signs and symptoms 151
  - Temporal lobe signs and symptoms 154
- ► OCCIPITAL LOBE 155
  - Anatomy and pathophysiology 155
  - Signs and symptoms 155
- ► EVALUATION AND MANAGEMENT OF PATIENTS WITH HOMONYMOUS VISUAL FIELD LOSS 156
- ► KEY POINTS 157

This chapter explores the chiasm and parasellar region. As in the previous chapter addressing the optic nerve, the clinical expression of disease is discussed in the context of neuroanatomy. Visual field defects resulting from disorders of the chiasm and parasellar region were addressed in the discussion of the organization of the visual system in Chapter 3.

► CHIASM AND PARASELLAR REGION

The chiasm is formed by the confluence of the right and left optic nerves. Axons from the optic nerves are re-routed in the chiasm to form the right and left optic tracts (Box 5–1). The intracranial optic nerves and chiasm ascend at an angle of 45° from the skull base (Figure 5–1A). From a superior perspective, the chiasm is shaped like the Greek letter chi (χ), the origin of its name. The chiasm is approximately 4-mm thick, 12-mm wide, and 8-mm long.

Lesions affecting the chiasm, and their accompanying signs and symptoms, are readily understood when one considers the structures around the chiasm. The chiasm is located about one centimeter above the pituitary gland, which rests in the sella turcica of the sphenoid. The hypothalamus is directly above, and the pituitary stalk (infundibulum), connecting the hypothalamus and pituitary, is posterior. The cavernous sinuses form the lateral walls of the sella turcica. The third ventricle extends to the posterior notch of the chiasm.

The chiasm is positioned within the circle of Willis and receives its blood supply from multiple sources so infarction is uncommon. Mass lesions arising from sellar and parasellar regions (pituitary adenomas, craniopharyngiomas, meningiomas, and aneurysms) are the most common disease processes affecting the chiasm. Mass lesions cause injury to chiasmal axons or their myelin sheath from compression, vascular compromise, or both.

SIGNS AND SYMPTOMS: NEUROANATOMIC CORRELATION

The Chiasm

The patterns of visual field loss that arise from disorders of the chiasm are a logical consequence of the axonal decussation, and are discussed in Chapter 3 (see Figures 3–11 and 3–12). The classic pattern consists of bitemporal visual field defects that respect the vertical meridian. Since disorders that affect the chiasm are usually mass lesions, they rarely attack with pinpoint accuracy. Therefore, complex visual field defects resulting from insults to various combinations of optic nerve, the body of the chiasm, and optic tract are not uncommon. Curiously,

▶ BOX 5-1. DESTINATION OF AXONS PASSING THROUGH THE CHIASM

1. The overwhelming majority of axons passing through the chiasm enter the right or left optic tract (depending on which half of visual space they represent) and synapse in the *lateral geniculate nucleus* (retino-geniculate pathway).

2. Several small bundles of axons exit from the dorsal and posterior surface of the body of the chiasm and ascend bilaterally to synapse in the *suprachiasmatic, supraoptic,* and *paraventricular nuclei* of the hypothalamus. These fibers are likely involved in controlling diurnal rhythms and circadian neuroendocrine systems, but have no clinically testable visual function.

3. Some axons passing through the chiasm and into the optic tract exit in the brachium of the superior colliculus just before reaching the lateral geniculate nucleus. The major destination of axons in this pathway is the *pretectal brainstem nuclei* that participate in the afferent limb of the pupillary light reflex; other axons in this pathway (of uncertain function) synapse in the *superior colliculus* and the *accessory optic nucleus* of the midbrain, and the *pulvinar*.

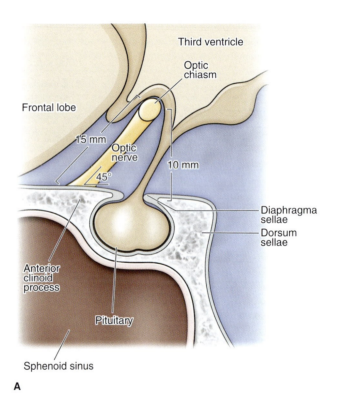

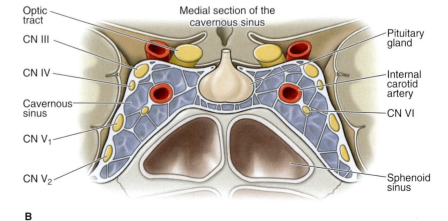

Figure 5-1. **Anatomy of the chiasm and parasellar region.** (A) Midsagittal view showing relationship of the chiasm to the pituitary gland and third ventricle. (B) Coronal perspective shows the location of the pituitary gland relative to the cavernous sinus.

trauma to the chiasm from head injury can occasionally produce "perfect" bitemporal visual field defects.

Patients who have dense bitemporal visual field defects may have no overlapping visual field to allow their eyes to obtain fusion and lock together. This situation can cause the *hemifield slide* phenomenon, in which each half of the binocular visual field slips and slides with respect to the other. Horizontal objects (eg, lines of print) may overlap or separate, or appear broken, dynamically slipping up and down, or even moving horizontally with respect to each other (Figure 5–2A). Related visual complaints include double vision and difficulty with tasks that require alignment, such as adding up a column of numbers. Reading can be particularly difficult because of misalignment of text and words that appear to fall off the line (see Figure 5–2B).

Another feature of bitemporal visual field loss is a *postfixation scotoma*. Objects located just beyond a near fixation point fall into the blind temporal hemifields of both eyes, and are therefore not seen (Figure 5–3). This condition creates difficulty with tasks such as cutting fingernails or toenails or threading a needle, and can cause individual words or letters to disappear with reading.

Lesions affecting the chiasm can cause *retrograde axonal atrophy*, which results in visible optic disc pallor and nerve fiber layer loss over time. Disorders affecting the body of the chiasm injure the crossing axons from each eye; axons that originate from each nasal hemiretina (representing the temporal hemifields in each eye). Retrograde axonal degeneration causes optic nerve pallor primarily at the midnasal and midtemporal portions of the optic disc; the nasal part of the disc receives axons from all ganglion cells located nasal to the optic disc, and the temporal portion of the disc receives maculopapillary axons from ganglion cells between the foveola and the disc. The axons at the superior and inferior poles, which sweep around from the unaffected temporal hemiretina, are preserved. This selective atrophy results in a horizontal band of optic disc pallor (bow-tie atrophy) in each eye, a pattern that can be seen in the eye(s) with temporal hemifield loss from chiasmal or optic tract lesions (Figure 5–4).

A relative afferent pupillary defect (RAPD) is often present with chiasmal disease, depending on the density and asymmetry of the visual field loss between the two eyes. *The RAPD is present in the eye with the greatest visual field loss, not necessarily the eye with the worst visual acuity.*

The Sellar and Parasellar Region

The *pituitary gland* is inferior to the chiasm within the sella turcica. In approximately 80% of individuals the body of the chiasm is directly above the pituitary gland. In approximately 10% the body of the chiasm

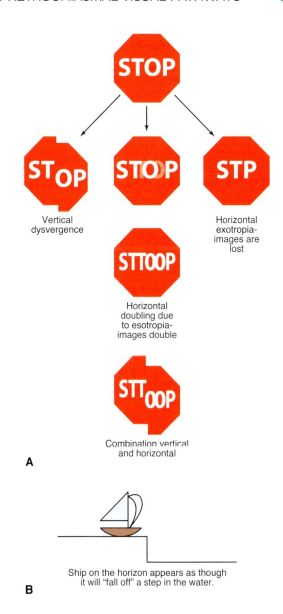

Figure 5–2. Hemifield slide with bitemporal hemianopia.
Dense bitemporal visual field defects have no overlapping visual field to allow the two eyes to obtain fusion and lock together; therefore, the two halves of the binocular visual field slip and slide with respect to one another. Horizontal objects (eg, lines of printed text) may appear broken, dynamically slipping up or down, or even moving horizontally with respect to each other **(A)**. Patients have complaints of double vision and difficulty with tasks that require alignment, such as adding up a column of numbers. Text may appear misaligned with words that appear to fall off the line. A boat may appear to be in danger of falling off the edge of the water **(B)**!

is located more anteriorly, over the tuberculum sella (*prefixed chiasm*), and in the remaining 10% the chiasm is more posterior than the sella (the *postfixed chiasm*), lying directly above the posterior wall or the dorsum sellae. The position of the chiasm determines whether

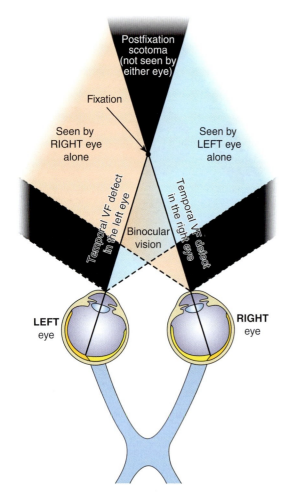

Figure 5-3. **Postfixation scotoma with bitemporal hemianopia.**
Objects located just beyond a near fixation point will fall in the blind temporal hemifields of both eyes and are therefore not seen. This creates difficulty with tasks such as cutting one's nails or threading a needle, and patients may complain of disappearing words and letters while reading. Abbreviation: VF, visual field.

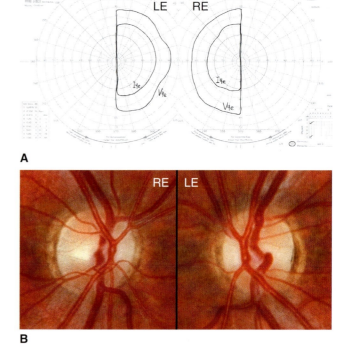

Figure 5-4. **Bilateral bow-tie atrophy from trauma to the chiasm.**
An 11-year-old boy with head trauma from an automobile accident had bitemporal visual field defects. **(A)** Goldmann visual fields show a complete bitemporal hemianopia, suggesting midline trauma to the body of the chiasm. **(B)** Bilateral bow-tie atrophy of the optic discs is evident (see Figure 3-18).

the optic nerves, body of the chiasm, or optic tracts will be primarily affected by masses that grow upward from the sellar region. On average, there is at least 1 cm between the dorsum sellae and the body of the chiasm. This space is the *inferior chiasmatic cistern*. Thus, tumors arising from the region of the sella may extend unimpeded superiorly toward the chiasm, but must be at least 1 cm in vertical height to begin to compress the chiasm and have any effect on vision (see Figure 5-1A). In addition to visual loss, chronic headache is common but not invariable among all types of sellar tumors.

The paired *cavernous sinuses* form the lateral walls of the sella turcica. This dural venous sinus contains the cavernous segment of the internal carotid artery; cranial nerves (CNs) III, IV, VI, V_1, and V_2; and sympathetic nerves (see Figure 5-1B). Sellar masses (eg, pituitary tumors) can extend laterally into the cavernous sinuses, causing diplopia (affecting CN III, IV, VI), ptosis or anisocoria (affecting CN III or the sympathetic nerves), and pain or facial numbness (affecting CN V).

Other Neighboring Structures

The posterior notch of the chiasm is immediately adjacent to the anterior extent of *the third ventricle*. Noncommunicating hydrocephalus due to aqueductal stenosis can cause expansion of the third ventricle, stretching the posterior aspect of the chiasm and impinging on the posterior decussating axons and causing central bitemporal visual field loss. Signs and symptoms associated with hydrocephalus may also be present including papilledema, CN VI palsies, headache, gait disturbances, and somnolence. Additionally, lesions that cause cerebral aqueductal stenosis may also produce symptoms of dorsal midbrain syndrome (discussed in Chapter 10).

The *hypothalamus* is directly contiguous with the chiasm superiorly, and diseases may seamlessly involve both structures (eg, chiasmal glioma or neurosarcoidosis). Disorders that affect the hypothalamus may be life threatening. Early symptoms of hypothalamic involvement include diabetes insipidus, marked behavior changes, and lethargy.

The ascending *intracranial internal carotid arteries* are lateral to the body of the chiasm. Arterial ectasia and aneurysm of the carotid arteries are rarely a source of chiasmal compression.

Chiasmal lesions are occasionally associated with acquired *seesaw nystagmus*; the reason is unclear, but it may be due to simultaneous involvement of adjacent brainstem structures.

DISORDERS OF THE CHIASM

As discussed above, extrinsic mass lesions are the most common cause of chiasmal visual field loss, and include pituitary tumors, meningiomas, craniopharyngiomas, other tumors (Figure 5–5), and occasionally giant aneurysms. In addition, processes that commonly affect the intracranial optic nerve, such as demyelination, gliomas, and inflammatory disorders, can also affect the chiasm. Table 5–1 lists disorders that can affect the chiasm.

Pituitary Adenomas

Pituitary macroadenomas are the most common extrinsic masses that cause chiasmal compression (and the most common lesion overall affecting the chiasm). Pituitary *macroadenomas* extend beyond the sella; *microadenomas* are contained within the sella, and therefore do not cause visual dysfunction. Pituitary tumors may be associated with hypersecretion (secreting pituitary adenomas), hyposecretion (compression of otherwise normal portions of the gland), or normal pituitary function. Most patients with visual loss from pituitary masses have nonsecreting adenomas, because patients with secreting adenomas generally seek medical help because of symptoms of endocrine dysfunction before the tumor is large enough to compress the chiasm and cause visual loss (Figures 5–6 and 5–7).

Many pituitary macroadenomas are surgically accessible by transsphenoidal microsurgery. This approach minimizes surgical morbidity and recovery time by approaching the pituitary fossa extracranially through the nose and sphenoid sinus. Successful decompression often results in improved vision, but patients who have developed optic atrophy prior to surgery have a less favorable prognosis, and typically have some degree of permanent visual field loss. Thus, early diagnosis and treatment are important to maximize visual recovery. Bromocriptine (eg, Parlodel) and cabergoline (eg, Dostinex) are dopamine agonists that reduce the size of prolactin-secreting pituitary tumors, but regrowth is the rule when the medication is discontinued. Radiation therapy may be a treatment alternative or adjunct in some cases.

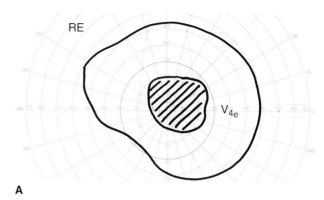

A

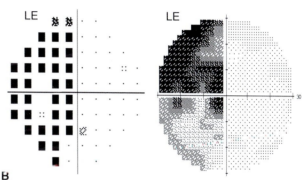

B

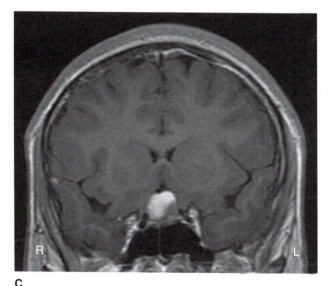

C

Figure 5–5. Junctional scotoma from pilocystic astrocytoma.
A 15-year-old boy presented with left monocular oscillopsia and vision loss. Visual acuity was 20/400 in the right eye and 20/20 in the left eye. Neuroimaging revealed a mass at the right anterior chiasm, and subsequent pathology from surgical resection revealed a pilocystic astrocytoma. Visual field testing on presentation was consistent with a right junctional scotoma. **(A)** Goldmann perimetry of the right eye showed a dense central scotoma. **(B)** Humphrey perimetry demonstrated a temporal visual field defect (total deviation and grayscale plots shown) in the asymptomatic left eye. **(C)** Magnetic resonance imaging of the brain (coronal view, T1 with contrast) shows the mass, which involves the right anterior chiasm.

▶ TABLE 5-1. DIFFERENTIAL DIAGNOSIS OF CHIASMAL DISORDERS

Etiology	Comments
Pituitary tumors/apoplexy	Discussed in detail in this chapter.
Meningiomas	
Craniopharyngiomas	
Chiasmal gliomas	Often involve the optic nerve(s) as well. See discussion in Chapter 4.
Other tumors/masses	Metastases, nasopharyngeal carcinomas, chordomas, dysgerminomas, hemangiomas, arachnoid cysts, sphenoid sinus mucoceles.
Sarcoidosis and other granulomatous diseases	See Box 4-4. Hypothalamic involvement can cause death.
Radiation neuropathy	Acute visual loss months to years after radiation.
Vascular causes	Suprasellar aneurysms, dolichoectatic vessels, arteriovenous malformations, cavernomas, and (rarely) infarction from arteritis.
Infection	Abscesses, neurosyphilis.
Optochiasmatic arachnoiditis	Foreign body (postsurgical), infectious, idiopathic.
Trauma	May have associated diabetes insipidus and basal skull fractures.
Demyelination	MS can cause chiasmal demyelination.
Posthypophysectomy empty sella	Herniation of the chiasm into an empty sella following surgical evacuation of a sellar mass can compress the intracranial optic nerves. Adhesions and inflammation can cause downward traction.
Posterior compression by an enlarging third ventricle	Acute noncommunicating hydrocephalus can cause expansion of the third ventricle into the posterior notch of the chiasm resulting in a central bitemporal visual field defect. Papilledema is usually present.

Abbreviation: MS, multiple sclerosis.

Pituitary Apoplexy

Acute enlargement of a pituitary adenoma can occur from spontaneous infarction and hemorrhage. The rapid expansion of the tumor within the sella can extend outward into the cavernous sinuses causing cranial neuropathies and motility disturbances, or upward into the optic nerves/chiasm/optic tracts, resulting in visual loss. Anterior extension may cause epistaxis or cerebrospinal fluid (CSF) rhinorrhea; posterior rupture can cause

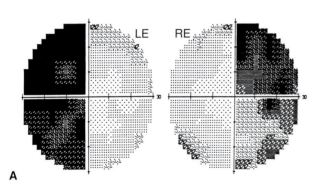

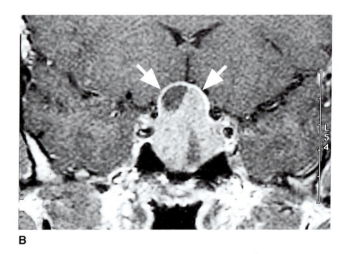

Figure 5-6. **Bitemporal visual field loss from a pituitary adenoma.**
A 34-year-old man described blurred vision, predominantly in his left eye. Visual acuity was 20/20 in the right eye and 20/50 in the left eye. The optic discs were normal. **(A)** Automated perimetry shows bilateral temporal visual field defects, denser in the left eye. **(B)** Magnetic resonance imaging (coronal view, T1-weighted image with contrast) reveals a mass arising from the sella and extending superiorly (*arrows*) compressing the chiasm. The cystic areas seen within the mass are regions of tumor necrosis.

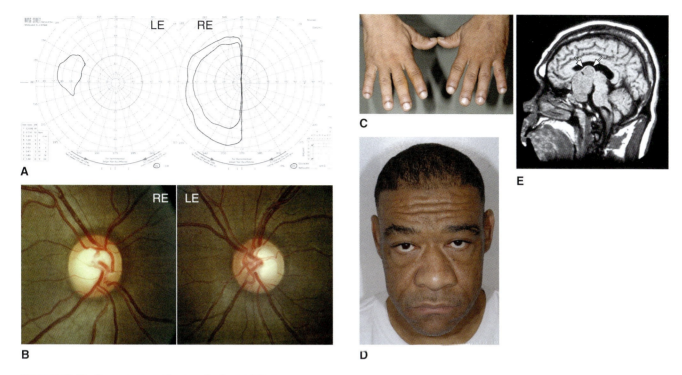

Figure 5-7. Acromegaly and visual loss.
A 34-year-old man described gradual loss of vision in his left eye over 9 months. Acromegalic features were noted. **(A)** Goldmann perimetry shows temporal hemifield loss in the right eye and profound visual field loss in the left eye with only a temporal island of vision remaining. Visual acuity was 20/20 in the right eye and 1/200 in the left eye. **(B)** The optic discs were relatively unremarkable, with only a hint of temporal pallor of the left optic disc. **(C)** The patient's hands showed disproportionate thickening of his fingers. **(D)** Coarse facial features including enlarged brow, nose, and jaw are demonstrated in this clinical photo (from a different patient with acromegaly). **(E)** Magnetic resonance imaging (T1 weighted, sagittal view) revealed a large sellar mass extending superiorly and elevating the floor of the third ventricle (*arrows*). A prominent brow and thickened skull are also evident on this scan. Subsequent evaluation confirmed the diagnosis of a growth-hormone-secreting pituitary adenoma.

inflammatory meningitis from blood and debris. The acute compromise of pituitary function (especially corticotropins) may be life threatening, and thus requires prompt diagnosis and medical treatment.

During pregnancy the pituitary gland enlarges, and it defervesces postpartum. The vascular changes associated with the pituitary gland's response to pregnancy can predispose patients to pituitary apoplexy, particularly after delivery (Sheehan syndrome).

Craniopharyngioma

Craniopharyngiomas are mixed solid and cystic midline tumors that arise from embryonic remnants of Rathke pouch, and are located in the region of the pituitary gland and stalk. These tumors can occur at any age, but the incidence is bimodal: more common in young patients (<20 years), with a second peak in the fifth and sixth decades of life (Figure 5–8). Tumor cysts contain desquamation products, necrotic tissue, and blood, often with punctate dystrophic calcification (a helpful sign on computed tomography (CT)). These large suprasellar tumors frequently cause pituitary and hypothalamic dysfunction, as well as hydrocephalus. Surgical treatments include shunting procedures for hydrocephalus, cyst aspiration, cyst shunting to a subcutaneous reservoir, and tumor debulking. Radiation (stereotactic radiotherapy) may be an alternative or adjunctive treatment.

Intracranial Meningiomas

Meningiomas that arise intracranially near the optic foramen (medial sphenoid ridge, tuberculum sellae) can cause optic nerve compression with monocular symptoms. Tumors that arise or extend posteriorly cause compression of the chiasm and result in bilateral visual field defects that are usually asymmetric between eyes. Visual loss is typically progressive, but may wax and wane. Growth may be accelerated during pregnancy because of progesterone and estrogen receptors that may be present in these tumors.

Treatment options include surgery and radiation. Intracranial meningiomas can encase arteries and nerves, often preventing complete surgical removal. Surgical debulking of the tumor is often combined with adjunctive radiation therapy.

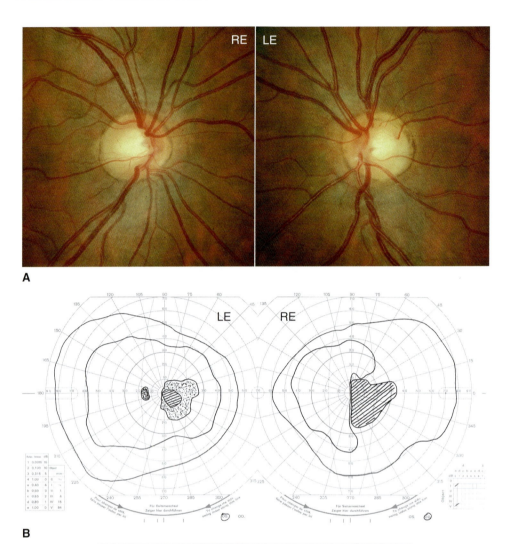

Figure 5-8. Craniopharyngioma. A 14-year-old boy complained of headache and blurred vision in his right eye. **(A)** The left optic disc showed temporal pallor; the right disc was relatively normal. **(B)** Goldmann perimetry showed a right homonymous, incongruous visual field defect. Visual acuity was 20/30 in the right eye and 20/100 in the left eye. **(C)** Magnetic resonance imaging (T1-weighted image, sagittal view) revealed a large inhomogeneous sellar mass (*large arrows*). The fluid material within the cystic mass has settled out into two layers (remember the patient is supine) (*small arrow*). Additional studies showed panhypopituitarism, and subsequent pathology showed the mass to be a craniopharyngioma. The visual function improved dramatically after resection, but the patient required repeated resections of solid tumor and drainage of cysts.

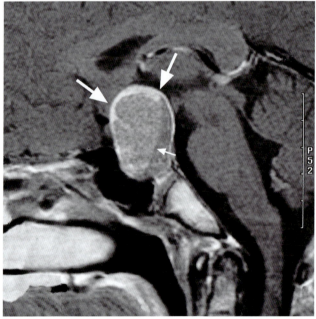

EVALUATION AND MANAGEMENT

Patients with signs and symptoms that suggest sellar/parasellar disease require neuroimaging. Magnetic resonance imaging (MRI) with contrast provides excellent anatomical and pathological detail of structures in this region. Orbital studies should also be included because the optic nerves may be primarily or secondary affected. CT may be helpful in identifying calcification and bone destruction (craniopharyngiomas and meningioma), and hyperostosis (meningioma).

A multidisciplinary approach is usually required for evaluation and management of sellar/parasellar disorders, often including neurosurgeons, neurologists, pediatricians, endocrinologists, medical oncologists, radiation oncologists, and otolaryngologists. The ophthalmologist plays an important role in making the initial diagnosis and in subsequent evaluation of the patient's visual function. Although neuroimaging is important in following patients regardless of treatment, post operative changes to the region may make the interpretation of these studies difficult. Sequential visual fields provide another perspective by which to judge the progress of the disease and efficacy of treatment.

▶ OPTIC TRACT

ANATOMY

The optic tracts extend posteriorly and superiorly from the chiasm, curving around the brainstem just lateral to the cerebral peduncles, and terminate in the lateral geniculate nuclei (LGNs). Pupillomotor axons leave the optic tract before it terminates in the LGN. The exiting pupillomotor axons travel through the brachium of the superior colliculus and synapse in the pretectal nuclei of the rostral midbrain. These in turn provide input to the Edinger-Westfal subnuclei of the oculomotor (CN III) nucleus (see Figure 11–4). This pathway constitutes the afferent limb of the pupillary light reflex, and is discussed in greater detail in Chapter 11. The major vascular supply of the optic tract is the anterior choroidal artery, a branch of the middle cerebral artery, but branches of the posterior cerebral arteries also participate; isolated ischemic events of the optic tract are rare.

SIGNS AND SYMPTOMS

In addition to visual field defects, optic tract lesions can cause optic atrophy and an RAPD.

Visual Fields

Disorders that affect the optic tract produce contralateral homonymous visual field defects that are often (but not always) incongruous, as described in Chapter 3 (see Figure 3–17).

Optic Atrophy

The optic tract carries axons that originate in the ganglion cells of the retina to their termination point in the LGN. Thus, similar to chiasmal lesions, optic tract lesions also can cause retrograde axonal death that produces optic atrophy within months of an insult. *Bow-tie* (or band) atrophy occurs (as described for chiasmal lesions) in the eye contralateral to the optic tract lesion—the eye with the temporal visual field defect. Although the reciprocal pattern (a vertical band or bow-tie) might be expected in the *ipsilateral eye* with nasal visual field loss, a loss of the nerve fiber layer striations above and below the disc, or a more diffuse mild pallor, is the rule (Figure 5–9). Lesions of the visual pathway beyond the LGN (postsynaptic) do not produce optic atrophy. Congenital lesions of the occipital cortex or geniculocalcarine fibers are an exception, because transsynaptic degeneration can occur from retro-geniculate lesions when acquired early in development.

Relative Afferent Pupillary Defect

The optic tract contains pupillomotor axons from the temporal hemiretina (nasal hemifield) of the ipsilateral eye, and axons from the nasal hemiretina (temporal hemifield) of the contralateral eye. The pupillomotor input from the contralateral eye is greatest, corresponding to the larger extent of the temporal hemifield and greater number of axons crossing in the chiasm. Therefore, a tract lesion has a greater impact on the afferent contribution of the contralateral eye, producing a small, but identifiable RAPD in the contralateral eye.

Neighboring Structures

Potential symptoms from involvement of nearby structures is generally the same as for the chiasm. A contralateral hemiparesis can occur from involvement of the adjacent cerebral peduncles.

DISORDERS OF THE OPTIC TRACT

Isolated lesions of the optic tract are infrequent. More commonly, both the optic tract and chiasm are involved by a mass lesion. Rarely, trauma, infarction, or demyelination can cause an optic tract lesion. The types of disorders that affect the optic tract, as well as their evaluation and management, are essentially the same as for the chiasm.

▶ LATERAL GENICULATE NUCLEUS

The LGN (also called the lateral geniculate body) is a thalamic nucleus positioned bilaterally along the lateral aspect of the midbrain. The nucleus is the destination of the axons that arose in the ganglion cell layer of the retinas, and is the origin of the geniculate-calcarine radiations. Each optic tract terminates at the ipsilateral LGN, with individual axons synapsing in alternating layers depending on the eye of origin (Figure 5–10). The arrangement of axons in the optic nerve (retinotopic organization) is preserved in the LGN but rotated 90°. As the optic tract approaches the LGN, an inward rotation occurs such that axons from the superior retinas synapse medially, with inferior projections rotated laterally. Exiting axons in the geniculo-striate pathway rotate outward to resume the original orientation.

The cell types in the lateral geniculate layers also differ. Large neurons occupy layers 1 and 2 (magnocellular layers), with smaller neurons in layers 3 through 6 (parvocellular layers). These two types of neurons have corresponding input from specific ganglion cells in the retina (M and P ganglion cells) and have distinct and separate axonal projections to the visual cortex. These parallel retino-cortical pathways are thought to subserve different components of visual perception (see Box 2–2).

The LGN has a dual blood supply. One portion of the nucleus is supplied by the anterior choroidal artery

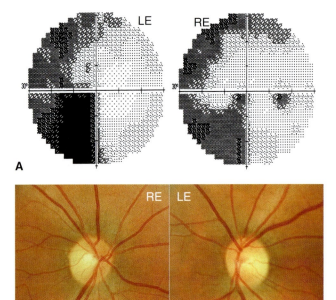
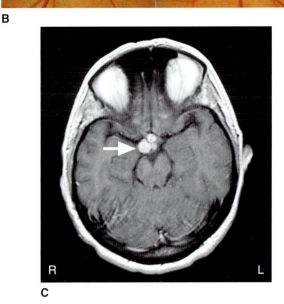

Figure 5-9. Optic tract.
A 40-year-old woman complained of decreased vision in her left eye. Examination revealed a visual acuity of 20/20 in each eye, but a relative afferent pupillary defect (RAPD) of 0.6 log units was identified in the left eye. **(A)** Automated perimetry showed a left incongruous homonymous visual field defect.
(B) Subtle bow-tie atrophy of the left optic disc was suspected. This finding, along with the visual field pattern and RAPD suggested a right optic tract lesion. **(C)** Magnetic resonance imaging (T1-weighted image with contrast, axial view) revealed a hemorrhagic lesion in the suprasellar cistern, just posterior to the chiasm, at the right optic tract (*arrow*). The lesion was excised, and the pathological diagnosis was a cavernous angioma.

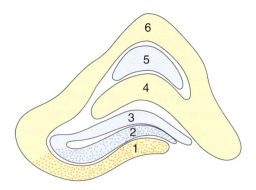

Ipsilateral eye: Layers 2, 3, and 5 (blue)
Contralateral eye: Layers 1, 4, and 6 (yellow)
Magnocellular ("M-cell") division: Layers 1 and 2 (stippled)
Parvocellular ("P-cell") division: Layers 3–6 (solid)

Figure 5-10. Layered structure of the lateral geniculate nucleus.
Axons from the ipsilateral eye (uncrossed axons from the temporal hemiretina) terminate in layers 2, 3, 5. Axons from the contralateral eye (crossed axons from the nasal hemiretina) synapse in layers 1, 4, 6. Layers 1, 2 are magnocellular regions, and layers 3, 4, 5, 6 are parvocellular.

(a branch of the middle cerebral artery); the lateral choroidal artery (a branch of the posterior cerebral artery) supplies the remaining area (Figure 5–11). Infarction in the distribution of one or the other of these two supply arteries produces the opposing "sectoranopia" visual field defects discussed in Chapter 3 (see Figure 3–19).

Isolated lesions of the LGN are rare. Pathological processes include ischemic infarction, hemorrhage

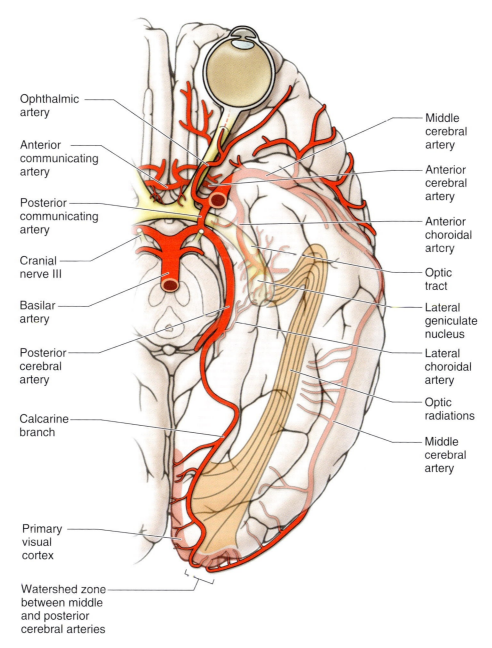

Figure 5–11. Vascular supply of the afferent visual system.
The intraorbital optic nerve and eye are supplied by branches of the *ophthalmic artery*. The intracranial optic nerve is supplied by the *internal carotid artery*, located laterally, as well as the *anterior cerebral artery* and the *anterior communicating artery*, located superiorly. The chiasm is positioned within the circle of Willis and receives its blood supply from multiple sources. The major vascular supply of the optic tract is the *anterior choroidal artery*—a branch of the middle cerebral artery—but branches of the posterior cerebral artery also participate. The lateral geniculate nucleus has a dual vascular supply: the *anterior choroidal artery* branching from the middle cerebral artery, and the *lateral choroidal artery*, a branch of the *posterior cerebral artery*. The *middle cerebral artery* travels over the lateral surface of the brain, yielding branches that penetrate into the parietal and temporal lobes to supply the optic radiations. Most of the primary visual cortex is supplied by the *posterior cerebral artery*, however, the tip of the occipital cortex is a watershed zone between the middle and posterior cerebral arteries.

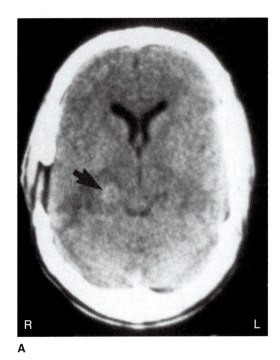

Figure 5-12. **Sectoranopia from lateral geniculate nucleus hemorrhage.** (A) Computed tomography of the brain shows a hemorrhage in right lateral geniculate nucleus (LGN). (B) Goldmann perimetry demonstrates an homonymous sectoranopia, a peculiar visual field defect unique to LGN lesions (see Figure 3-19).

(usually associated with arteriovenous malformations), trauma, and mass lesions (Figure 5-12).

▶ OPTIC RADIATIONS

From the lateral geniculate nucleus, the optic radiations carry visual information posteriorly, with superior fibers passing through the inferior parietal lobe and inferior fibers through the temporal lobe, to synapse in the primary visual cortex in the occipital lobe. Visual information is then relayed from the primary visual cortex *anteriorly* to other cortical areas of higher visual processing located in the occipital, temporal, and parietal lobes (Figure 5-13). Lesions involving the temporal, parietal, or occipital lobes can therefore affect vision in two ways: (1) lesions affecting the optic radiations or primary visual cortex will cause visual field defects, and (2) interruption of higher visual processes causes more complex symptoms of visual integration. A variety of curious symptoms can arise from lesions affecting these cortical areas of visual processing either directly or by interrupting connecting pathways from the primary visual cortex (*disconnection syndromes*). Disruption of other nonvisual cortical functions of the parietal and temporal lobes contribute additional neurological signs and symptoms that may be localizing.

The right and left hemispheres have different functions, and symptoms from lesions in these areas depend on which hemisphere is involved. The dominant hemisphere contains regions involved in language understanding and expression, whereas

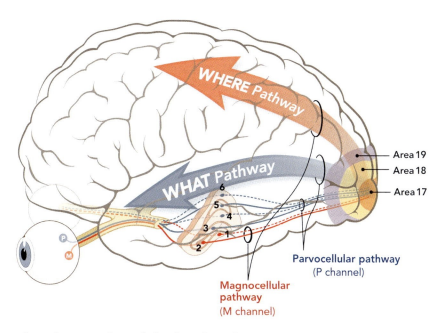

Figure 5–13. Dorsal and ventral occipitofugal pathways.
Visual information is conveyed from the retina to the lateral geniculate nuclei (LGNs) in parallel pathways: The P-system axons (*shown in blue*) synapse in the parvocellular layers of the LGN, and the M-system axons (*shown in red*) in the magnocellular layers of the LGN. The optic radiations continue this parallel arrangement, carrying visual information posteriorly to the primary visual cortex in the occipital lobe (Broadmann area 17). Visual information is then relayed from the primary visual cortex *anteriorly* through areas 18 and 19 to other cortical areas of higher visual processing: The P-system visual information forms a ventral pathway to the angular gyrus and regions in the temporal lobe; this is the "what" pathway, involved in language processing, naming objects, and identifying faces. The M-system forms the dorsal pathway to the parietal lobe and beyond; this is the "where" pathway for visuospatial processing. A lesion in the parietal or temporal lobes will often affect these pathways and produce corresponding disorders of higher cortical function, in addition to homonymous visual field defects from interruption of the optic radiations.

the nondominant hemisphere serves spatial senses and relationships. The left hemisphere is dominant in right-handed individuals (and most left-handed persons), with some left-handed persons having right hemisphere dominance. Only rarely are right-handers right-hemispheric dominant.

A broad spectrum of disease processes can affect the retrogeniculate visual pathways, as outlined in Table 5–2. Vascular events, especially embolic strokes, are common, as contrasted with the intracranial optic nerve, chiasm, and optic tracts, where mass lesions predominate.

The middle cerebral artery travels over the lateral surface of the brain, providing branches that penetrate the parietal and temporal lobes. The optic radiations are beneath the cortex; therefore, middle cerebral artery stroke resulting in visual field loss is also very likely to also affect the more superficial cortex, resulting in associated (cortical) neurological dysfunction (see Figure 5–11). The anterior choroidal artery supplies the optic tract, the anterior visual radiations in the temporal lobe, and the posterior limb of internal capsule. Infarctions in this territory commonly cause contralateral hemiparesis in addition to visual field loss.

PARIETAL LOBE SIGNS AND SYMPTOMS

The ophthalmologist rarely makes the initial diagnosis of a parietal lobe lesion because the neurological defects from parietal lobe dysfunction supersede the visual symptoms. Defects in verbal communication and intellect interfere with the patient's ability to recognize or complain about a visual deficit, and also make it difficult for the physician to test visual function.

Visual Fields

Visual field defects from parietal lobe lesions are homonymous with moderate congruity and are denser inferiorly (Figure 5–14). The patterns of visual field loss with parietal lobe disorders are discussed in Chapter 3 (see Figure 3–17).

Optokinetic Nystagmus

White matter tracts that connect the parietal and frontal cortex to the brainstem, located deep in the parietal lobe, are involved in the production of ipsilateral horizontal smooth pursuit eye movements. Damage to

TABLE 5-2. DISORDERS AFFECTING VISUAL PATHWAYS IN PARIETAL, TEMPORAL, AND OCCIPITAL LOBES

Process	Disorders	Comments
Congenital	Intrauterine ischemia, hemorrhage, maldevelopment, and trauma	Trans-synaptic degeneration with optic nerve pallor possible.
Vascular	Embolic stroke: emboli from heart, aortic arch, or from thrombosis or dissection of vertebral arteries	Commmon.
	Thrombotic stroke	Uncommon.
	Systemic hypotension	Watershed infarct of occipital lobe tip.
	Arteriovenous malformation	Can cause mass effect, ischemia, or hemorrhage.
Intracerebral hemorrhage	Hypertension, coagulopathies, infarcts, tumors	Acute symptoms and signs. Visual field defects may improve as hemorrhage clears.
Mass lesions	Glioma, meningioma, and metastatic tumors	Associated intracranial hypertension may cause headache, nausea and vomiting, or diplopia
	Lymphoma	Often associated with AIDS.
	Abscesses	Bacterial, fungal, and parasitic.
	Sarcoidosis	Can be an infiltrative or mass lesion.
Trauma	Penetrating or closed head injury, subdural or epidural hematomas	Closed head injury can cause transient cortical blindness.
Demyelination	Schilder disease, adrenoleukodystrophy, Pelizaeus-Merzbacher, metachromatic leukodystrophy, progressive multifocal leukoencephalopathy	Progressive dementia and spasticity.
	MS (unusual)	Patients are more likely to present with optic neuritis.
Degenerative	Alzheimer disease	Primarily affects visual-spatial organization.
Toxins	Carbon monoxide, nitrous oxide, ethanol, mercury, lead, cis-platin, cyclosporine, and methotrexate	Can cause cerebral blindness.
Others	Meningitis, encephalitis, subacute sclerosing panencephalitis, Creutzfeldt-Jakob (Heidenhain variety), acute ICP changes, and hyperglycemia	

Abbreviations: AIDS, acquired immune deficiency syndrome; ICP, intracranial pressure; MS, multiple sclerosis.

this pathway is clinically evident as an asymmetry in horizontal optokinetic nystagmus (OKN). Pursuit movements toward the side of the lesion are deficient, so decreased amplitude and frequency of OKN are noted when the optokinetic stimulus is moved toward the side of the lesion. This abnormality is independent of homonymous visual field defects that may be present.

Nondominant Parietal Lobe

Parietal lobe lesions in the nondominant hemisphere (usually the right hemisphere) affect *visual-spatial processing*. This defect may manifest itself as spatial disorientation in previously familiar places, difficulty copying simple figures (Figure 5–15), or difficulty constructing simple shapes from matchsticks. Patients may have left-right confusion, and often cannot accurately localize tactile stimuli or discern the position of their body in space (patients my lay at an oblique angle in bed).

Patients with *hemineglect* completely ignore the left side of space (from right parietal lesions), with or without an associated left homonymous hemianopia. In unilateral *visual hemi-inattention*, patients ignore one side if targets are presented simultaneously in both hemifields (*visual extinction*), even without a homonymous visual field defect. Nondominant parieto-occipital lobe lesions (and some drugs) can produce palinopsia. *Palinopsia* is the persistent or recurrent perception of an image after it is no longer in view. This can occur as multiple strobe-like freeze frames or a smeared "comet tail" image of an object

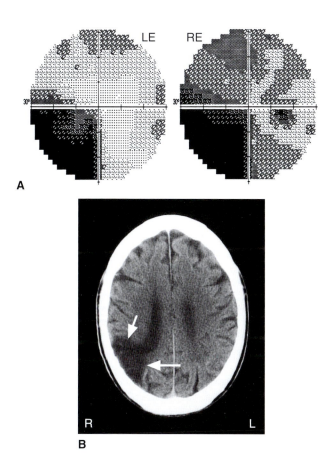

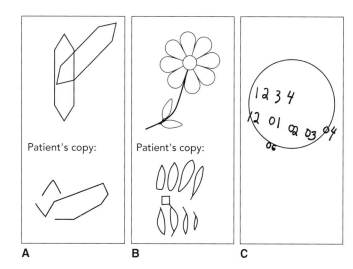

Figure 5–15. **Spatial disorientation with a right parietal lobe infarct.**
A patient with a right parietal stroke was asked to do the following tasks (with the patient's response as noted). **(A)** Copy the geometric shapes. **(B)** Copy the drawing of a flower. **(C)** Write the numbers on the face of a clock.

Figure 5–14. **Right parietal infarct.**
A 72-year-old man was evaluated for a left homonymous visual field defect. Optokinetic nystagmus was diminished when the stimulus was moving toward the right, and was normal in the opposite direction. **(A)** Automated perimetry showed a left homonymous visual field defect that was denser inferiorly, with intermediate congruity. **(B)** Computed tomography of the brain (axial image) shows a wedge-shaped area of low attenuation in the right parietal lobe (*between arrows*), most consistent with a subacute infarct.

in motion, or as the superimposition of a previously seen visual image over the current image. Parietal or parieto-occipital lesions can cause *polyopia*: seeing multiple copies of an image at one time. This phenomenon is a very rare cause of bilateral monocular diplopia and can occur with stroke, migraine, or in postictal states.

Dominant Parietal-Occipital Area

Alexia is the inability to read written language, assuming that the patient can see the words and is nonaphasic. *Agraphia* is the inability to write words. The interpretation and expression of written language depend on the angular gyrus in the dominant hemisphere, which is located at the confluence of the parietal, occipital, and temporal lobes. Lesions that affect the (left) angular gyrus can cause a constellation of signs and symptoms known as *Gerstmann syndrome*: alexia, agraphia, acalculia (inability to do simple math), light-left confusion, and finger agnosia (inability to name fingers).

Reading requires visual information from the primary visual cortex to be transferred to the angular gyrus in the (dominant) left hemisphere. Information from the left occipital cortex, representing the right hemifield, has a direct route to the left angular gyrus. However, information from the right occipital cortex (left hemifield) must be routed through the splenium of the corpus callosum to get to the left angular gyrus. A left parietal-occipital lesion can eliminate all visual input to the left angular gyrus: the left occipital lesion eliminates the right hemifield, and the left hemifield input from the right occipital cortex may be eliminated by inclusion of the fibers crossing at the splenium into the left parietal region (Figure 5–16). If the angular gyrus remained unharmed, then the patient would not be able to read (alexia) with the remaining left hemifield, but writing would be unimpaired. Thus, the peculiar clinical situation of *alexia without agraphia* is diagnostic of a left parietal-occipital lesion.

Balint Syndrome

Bilateral parietal-occipital lesions can produce a peculiar constellation of signs and symptoms known as *Balint syndrome*, consisting of ocular apraxia (inability to

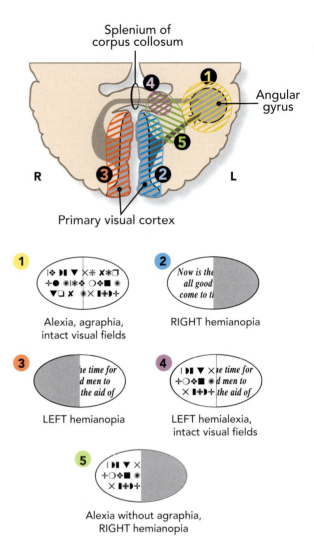

Figure 5-16. Potential lesions involving the angular gyrus and its interconnections.
The angular gyrus (located in the left hemisphere) receives information from the visual cortex and allows the interpretations of written language. It is also the coordinator for writing (motor) language. The brain depicted in this figure is oriented as would be seen on magnetic resonance imaging, axial view (note *R*, right and *L*, left). Several interesting potential lesions and their consequences are illustrated: **(1)** Lesions involving the angular gyrus itself would cause an inability to write (*agraphia*) and an inability to interpret written language even though it can be seen (*alexia*, illustrated as nonsense symbols). **(2)** Lesions of the left primary visual cortex produces a right hemianopia only. **(3)** Likewise, a lesion of the right primary visual cortex produces a left hemianopia, with normal reading comprehension in the remaining visual field. **(4)** Very rarely, a lesion involving the splenium of the callosum, interrupting the pathway from the right visual cortex to the angular gyrus, could produce hemialexia with normal visual fields.
(5) A more common situation seen clinically is a lesion that involves the left visual cortex and the crossing fibers in the corpus callosum, leaving the angular gyrus otherwise intact. Such patients can write without difficulty but are unable to read (even their own writing) with their remaining hemifield: *alexia without agraphia*.

voluntarily move the eyes on command to fix on an object in the visual field), optic ataxia (inability to accurately reach out and grasp or touch an object guided by vision), and simultanagnosia (inability to appreciate the totality of a visual scene). Balint syndrome is usually caused by bilateral watershed vascular infarcts or bilateral metastasis. Unilateral optic ataxia can occur with unilateral lesions in the contralateral parietal-occipital region.

TEMPORAL LOBE SIGNS AND SYMPTOMS

Visual Fields

Temporal lobe damage causes homonymous visual field loss with some degree of incongruity, and most dense superiorly (see Figure 3–17). The optic tract lies just below the anterior optic radiations, and marked incongruity seen in some temporal lobe lesions may be the result of concomitant optic tract involvement.

Sensory Hallucinations and Disturbances

The role of the temporal lobe in integrating sensory input is evident when tumors or seizures disrupt its function. Olfactory and gustatory hallucinations (uncinate fits), as well as formed visual hallucinations, partial complex seizures, deja vú, jamais vú, and presque vú sensations may occur.

Occipitotemporal Region

Lesions in the occipitotemporal region can produce visual agnosia and central achromatopsia. *Visual object agnosia* is the inability to visually recognize objects that are seen, despite functioning vision, speech, and intellect (classically described as "a percept stripped of its meaning"). Patients retain the ability to name objects by touch, or through other nonvisual sensory modalities. Visual agnosia is usually due to bilateral occipitotemporal stroke, and is an example of a disconnection process: Information from intact primary visual cortex (visual fields may be normal) is cut off from areas of higher cortical function. *Prosopagnosia* is visual agnosia confined to the inability to recognize faces or individual items within a class of items (eg, kinds of plants, animals, automobiles). *Central achromatopsia* is the loss of color discrimination in otherwise intact visual fields as a result of ventromedial occipitotemporal lesions (affecting area V4). This rare entity can be unilateral (hemiachromatopsia) or bilateral. Central achromatopsia is unlikely to occur in isolation, and is usually associated with homonymous superior visual field defects or prosopagnosia. Lesions affecting the lateral occipitoparietal (V5) area can cause *akinetopsia*. This condition is an exceedingly rare abnormality of motion perception, perceived as a series of frozen staccato images with missing frames between images.

▶ OCCIPITAL LOBE

ANATOMY AND PATHOPHYSIOLOGY

The primary visual cortex, designated as area 17 of Brodmann, lies primarily on the medial surface of the occipital lobe, within the central hemispheric sulcus. Area 17 occupies a strip of cortex above and below the calcarine fissure, and extends into the fissure and variably out onto the occipital tip (see Figure 3–20).

Brodmann areas 18 and 19 are immediately adjacent and receive projections from the primary visual cortex for further processing. The vascular supply is discussed in Chapter 3, within the context of visual field defects (see Figure 5–11). Unlike parietal and temporal lobe lesions, occipital lobe infarcts commonly cause visual field defects without any other accompanying neurological symptoms (so-called "silent strokes"). Thromboembolism from the heart and vertebrobasilar system is the most common cause of occipital lobe disease.

SIGNS AND SYMPTOMS

Visual Fields

Occipital lobe lesions produce highly congruous homonymous visual field defects (Figure 5–17). Other visual field characteristics of localizing value are summarized in Figure 3–21. The *Riddoch phenomenon* describes the ability of individuals to detect motion in an otherwise blind hemifield. Although reportedly a characteristic of occipital hemianopias, it can occur with any retrochiasmal visual field defect. This statokinetic dissociation is most likely the result of increased sensitivity caused by retinal summation of a moving object, but may represent visual processing via an alternative visual pathway.

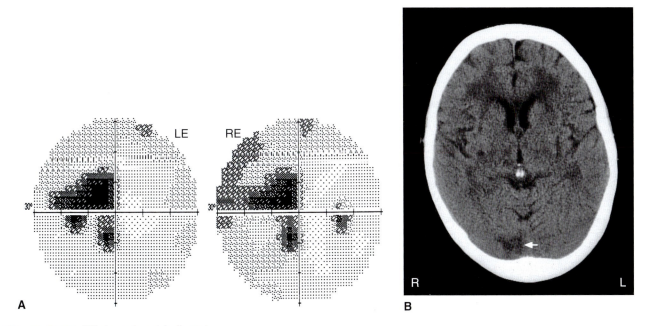

Figure 5–17. Watershed infarct.
A 53-year-old man described visual loss after a syncopal episode. **(A)** Automated perimetry shows a left homonymous paracentral scotoma that is highly congruous. **(B)** Magnetic resonance imaging (T2-weighted image, axial plane) reveals an infarct at the tip of the right occipital cortex, in the watershed zone between the middle and posterior cerebral circulations.

Vertebrobasilar Insufficiency

Vertebrobasilar insufficiency can cause reversible ischemia to the occipital lobes resulting in bilateral transient visual loss. Emboli, thrombosis, arterial dissection, and hypotension are the potential vascular mechanisms. In addition, positional compression of the vertebral arteries (eg, from head turn or chiropractic manipulation) can occur as a result of the course of the vertebral arteries within the bony foramina of the upper cervical spine. Because the vertebrobasilar system also supplies the brainstem, transient motility disturbances, nystagmus, vertigo, tinnitus, dysarthria, dysphagia, drop attacks, crossed hemiparesis, facial paresthesias, and headache (discussed in Chapter 14) may also occur.

Cortical Blindness

Bilateral infarctions of the retrogeniculate visual pathways can cause bilateral blindness, with normal pupillary responses and a normal ocular examination. Absolute, total visual loss is rare. As previously discussed, occipital events can occur with no other neurological signs or symptoms. The right and left occipital events do not have to be simultaneous: Patients may not recognize a unilateral homonymous visual field defect (especially if it is associated with hemi-neglect), and may become symptomatic only when the contralateral side is affected. *Anton syndrome* consists of denial of blindness with elaborate confabulation in patients with cortical blindness. Closed head injury, especially in children, can cause cortical blindness that is usually transient. These and other important causes of cortical blindness are outlined in Table 5–3. Cortical blindness may be difficult to distinguish from functional visual loss.

Hallucinations

Occipital lobe disturbances with an irritative focus can produce positive visual phenomenon, usually as unformed hallucinations (Box 5–2). By far, the most common example is the scintillating scotoma from migraine. *Formed* visual hallucinations are more likely to occur from pathology in other higher areas of visual processing, (especially the temporal lobe and occasionally the parietal lobe), or as the result of release phenomenon from visual loss anywhere in the afferent visual system (see Table 1–2).

▶ EVALUATION AND MANAGEMENT OF PATIENTS WITH HOMONYMOUS VISUAL FIELD LOSS

Perimetry provides the most compelling clinical evidence of an intracranial process affecting the afferent visual system, and often can help the physician localize the lesion. All patients who complain of blurred or poor vision need to have visual field testing in both eyes, even when the patient's complaints are confined to one eye. Patients with a homonymous visual field defect frequently attribute their problem to the eye on the side of the homonymous field loss.

Obviously, patients with homonymous visual field loss will need neuroimaging. However, the physician can provide more appropriate acute care and can guide diagnostic neuroimaging by using the history, visual fields, and accompanying symptoms to localize intracranial lesions.

An MRI of the brain with and without contrast provides the best study for disorders affecting the posterior visual pathways (especially with tailored MRI sequences and techniques such as fluid attenuated inversion recovery (FLAIR) and diffusion-weighted imaging). Computed tomography (CT) is excellent for assessing acute hemorrhagic stroke, but does not clearly reveal acute nonhemorrhagic infarction until 3 to 4 days have elapsed. Similar to disorders of the chiasm, a multidisciplinary approach to the evaluation and management of patients with homonymous visual field defects is the rule. Magnetic resonance angiography (MRA), cerebral angiography, and occasionally biopsy of an intracranial

▶ TABLE 5–3. CAUSES OF CORTICAL BLINDNESS (BILATERAL HEMISPHERIC DISORDERS)

Acquired
Vascular
- Bilateral posterior cerebral artery infarction
- Post-cardiac surgery
- Cerebral angiography complication

Hypoxia
Posterior reversible encephalopathy syndrome (PRES)
- Hypertensive encephalopathy
- Peripartum state (eclampsia)
- Tacrolimus (FK-506)
- Cyclosporine

Carbon monoxide poisoning
Creutzfeldt-Jacob disease (Heidenhain variant)
Trauma
Progressive multifocal leukoencephalopathy
Alzheimer disease

Congenital
Hypoxemic-ischemic encephalopathy
Periventricular leukomalacia
Cortical dysplasia

Reproduced, with permission, from Liu G, Volpe NJ, Galetta SL: *Neuro-ophthalmology: diagnosis and management*, 2d ed. Philadelphia: Saunders Elsevier; 2010: 312.

▶ BOX 5-2. HALLUCINATIONS AND ILLUSIONS FROM CENTRAL NERVOUS SYSTEM DISEASE

Migraine	Migraine aura is classically a scintillating scotoma. Involvement of areas of higher visual processing can produce many effects: formed hallucinations and Alice in Wonderland syndrome.
Release phenomenon (Charles Bonnet syndrome)	Interruption of visual input anywhere in the visual system can cause fill-in or release hallucinations in the area of blindness (Charles Bonnet syndrome). Patients are not cognitively impaired, and are often reluctant to discuss these vivid, detailed, but nonthreatening hallucinations.
Alcohol withdrawal	Auditory and visual hallucinations (often animals, bugs, lilliputian illusions) followed by delirium tremens and seizures.
Hallucinogens and cocaine	Psychedelic drugs such as LSD cause colorful hallucinations and distortions. Can persist or recur years later, so history of drug use is relevant with positive visual phenomenon.
Prescription drugs	Including many antidepressants, anticonvulsants, antiparkinsonian agents; digitalis and other cardiovascular medications, steroids, thyroxine, NSAIDs are also potential sources.
Neurodegenerative disorders	*Parkinson disease* patients can have complex hallucinations (usually of people) from the disease itself, or as a side effect of treatment medications. *Alzheimer disease* can cause complex hallucinations with delusional and paranoid ideations.
Midbrain disease	Peduncular hallucinosis is episodic vivid, colorful visual hallucinations of animals or people (colorful clothes, dancing and moving) in the setting of midbrain disease, usually with accompanying CN III palsy and ataxia (but occasionally without obvious neurologic dysfunction).
Seizure	Occipital lobe: usually unformed, may be indistinguishable from migraine aura.
	Temporal lobe: more complex visual hallucinations also with bad smells or tastes and motor activity (eye and head turning, automatisms).
	Parietal lobe (rare): distortions similar to Alice in Wonderland syndrome.
Parieto-occipital lobe disease	Palinopsia.
Vestibular	Posterior fossa lesions can produce the sensation that the visual environment is upside down or tilted—ocular tilt phenomenon.
Psychiatric	Hallucinations and delusions with lack of insight are characteristic of psychosis.
Narcolepsy	Hallucinations on wakening (hypnopompic) or going to sleep (hypnagogic) can be normal. However, thirty percent of patients with narcolepsy have vivid (sometimes unpleasant and threatening) hypnagogic hallucinations.

Abbreviations: LSD, lysergic acid diethylamide; NSAIDs, nonsteroidal anti-inflammatory drugs.
Data from Norton JW, Corbett JJ: Visual perceptual abnormalities: hallucinations and illusions. *Semin Neurol* 2000;20(1):111–121.

---

mass may be required to make a definitive diagnosis of an intracranial process.

Acute or progressive neurological symptoms (including homonymous visual field loss) require urgent neurological consultation. Patients with new symptoms (<24 hours) suggestive of stroke may require hospitalization for evaluation and possible anticoagulation. Patients with symptoms of acute nonhemorrhagic stroke may benefit from clot lysis with intravenous tissue plasminogen activator (t-PA), but only if administered within 3 to 4 hours of symptom onset. The rapid assessment of such patients includes a CT of the brain to be sure there is no hemorrhagic component to the stroke. The t-PA can be administered intravenously or specifically to the site of blockage by angiographic catheter.

Embolic stroke requires investigation for a potential embolic source. The carotid arteries are not a likely source of emboli to the posterior visual system, but carotid duplex studies, in conjunction with transcranial Doppler of the vertebrobasilar system, may reveal the extent of systemic atherosclerosis or abnormal flow patterns. Standard (transthoracic) echocardiograms may not reveal intracardiac embolic sources—a transesophageal echographic study is required for a serious look at the heart and aorta as potential embolic sources.

Although the management of most patients with intracranial disease is beyond the scope of ophthalmology, the ophthalmologist has several important roles: to recognize the patterns of visual field loss and symptoms that suggest intracranial disease, to pursue the diagnosis with appropriate imaging and other studies, and to help patients understand and cope with the visual deficits (Box 5–3).

> **BOX 5-3. WHAT CAN THE PHYSICIAN DO FOR PATIENTS WITH HOMONYMOUS VISUAL FIELD DEFECTS?**

1. *Help the patient (and the family) understand the nature of the visual deficit.* When patients understand that the eyes are not the problem, they realize that the visual loss cannot be fixed with glasses. Also, the concept of homonymous loss is not easy for most patients to understand. For example, there is great benefit in explaining why the patient with a right homonymous visual field defect is not likely to see items to the right of the dinner plate, and why it is best to sit to the patient's left when engaging the patient in conversation.

2. *Help the patient with reading difficulties.* Patients with right homonymous defects have difficulty reading because they cannot see the next word of a sentence, and those with left homonymous defects cannot find their way back to the next line. A straight edge, such as a ruler or card, can help them keep track of the lines of print. Occasionally, patients find that rotating the reading material counterclockwise and reading up (for left homonymous defects) or clockwise and reading down (for right homonymous defects) allows them to read into the seeing hemifield. Note that stroke and other lesions may also affect the patient's ability to understand written language even when they see it clearly (alexia).

3. *Discuss safety issues.* In most cases (depending on the extent of the homonymous defect and local regulations), driving will be contraindicated. This information can be terribly distressing to patients, but must be discussed. It is helpful to explain why it is unsafe to them and others ("You could run over a whole troop of Girl Scouts hiking on the right side of the road, because you can't see to the right"). Patients are more willing to accept this news if they know they will be returning for future visual field testing to look for any improvement.

4. *Address the limitations of treatment.* Optical devices purported to help in this situation are usually disappointing. Placing a hemianopic prism (a base-out Fresnel prism over the temporal half of the spectacle lens on the side of the homonymous loss) is a way for patients to be more aware of movement and objects in the blind hemifield. This method, as well as small mirrors on the glasses or prism insets, are warning systems at best, allowing the patient to then turn the head to see more clearly with the seeing hemifield. Only a minority of patients find these methods useful, and they do not allow patients to qualify for driving.

5. *Discuss release hallucinations (Charles Bonnet syndrome) when present.* As discussed in Box 1–2, patients are often reluctant to mention this, so patients should be specifically asked about hallucinations. The physician can relieve much anxiety (the patient's and the family's) by explaining the nature of this common phenomenon.

6. *Visual training?* While practical suggestions provided by occupational therapists are very helpful, there is no convincing evidence that visual rehabilitation therapy (computerized side-vision exercises and other methods) restores vision lost in a stroke.

▶ KEY POINTS

- The body of the chiasm is 1 cm above the dorsum sellae—tumors arising from the sella must be sizable to affect vision.
- Most patients with visual loss from pituitary masses have nonsecreting adenomas, because secreting adenomas will cause other symptoms before they are large enough to cause chiasmal compression.
- Pituitary tumors can extend superiorly and involve the chiasm, resulting in visual loss, or laterally into the cavernous sinus, causing motility disturbances, pain, and facial numbness.
- Sellar/parasellar masses can compress the optic nerves, the body of the chiasm, or optic tracts individually or in any combination.
- Bow-tie optic atrophy is characteristic of pregeniculate (chiasm, optic tract) lesions that cause temporal hemifield loss.
- Chiasmal lesions are one cause of acquired seesaw nystagmus.
- CT may complement MRI in imaging lesions in the region of the sella, by defining tumor-associated calcification, bone destruction, and hyperostosis.
- Sequential visual fields are helpful in monitoring sellar/parasellar tumors, especially when post-surgical changes make neuroimaging difficult to interpret.
- The optic tract syndrome consists of an incongruous homonymous visual field defect, RAPD, and optic bow-tie atrophy—all contralateral to the lesion.
- Ischemic events are the most common cause of retrogeniculate visual field loss, whereas compression (mass lesions) is the most common disorder affecting the chiasm and optic tracts.
- The visual field loss in parietal lobe lesions may be accompanied by diminished OKN when the stimulus is moved toward the side of the lesion.
- Alexia, with or without agraphia, can occur in parietal-occipital lesions in the dominant hemisphere.
- Nondominant parietal lesions are associated with visual-spatial abnormalities: left-right confusion, hemi-neglect, and construction apraxia.

- Retrogeniculate lesions may be further localized by asking patients with right homonymous visual field defects to read and write, and patients with left homonymous visual field defects to draw a clock.
- Olfactory, gustatory, or formed visual hallucinations may be caused by temporal lobe disease.
- Bilateral occipital-temporal lesions can cause various forms of visual agnosia, central achromatopsia, and superior homonymous visual field defects.
- Vertebrobasilar insufficiency causes transient visual loss, usually associated with transient brainstem neurological signs and symptoms.
- MRI of the brain with and without contrast, provides the best overall view of disorders affecting the posterior visual pathways.

SUGGESTED READING

Books

Barton JS, Girkin CA: Disorders of higher visual function, in Kline LB, *Neuro-ophthalmology Review Manual*. 7th ed. Thorofare, NJ: SLACK; 2013.

Liu GT, Volpe NJ, Galetta SL: Disorders of higher cortical visual function, in *Neuro-ophthalmology, Diagnosis and Management*, 2d ed. Philadelphia, PA: Saunders Elsevier; 2010.

Liu GT, Volpe NJ, Galetta SL: Retrochiasmal disorders, in *Neuro-ophthalmology, Diagnosis and Management*, 2d ed. Philadelphia, PA: Saunders Elsevier; 2010.

Miller NR, Newman NJ (eds): Topical diagnosis of lesions in the visual sensory pathway, in *Walsh and Hoyts' Clinical Neuro-ophthalmology*, Vol 1, 5th ed. Baltimore, MD: Williams & Wilkins; 1998:237–386.

Rizzo M, Barton JJS: Central disorders of visual function, in *Walsh and Hoyts' Clinical Neuro-ophthalmology*, Vol 1, 5th ed. Baltimore, MD: Williams & Wilkins; 1998:387–486.

Articles

Bell RA, Thompson HS: Relative afferent pupillary defect in optic tract hemianopias. *Am J Ophthalmol* 1978;85:538–540.

Girkin CA, Miller NR: Central disorders of vision in humans. *Surv Ophthalmol* 2001;45:379–405.

Kedar S, Zhang X, Lynn MJ, et al: Homonymous hemianopias: clinical-anatomic correlations in 904 cases. *Neurology* 2006;66:906–910.

Newman SA, Miller NR: Optic tract syndrome: neuro-ophthalmologic considerations. *Arch Ophthalmol* 1983;101:1241–1250.

Norton JW, Corbett JJ: Visual perceptual abnormalities: hallucinations and illusions. *Semin Neurol* 2000;20(1):111–121.

Savino PJ, Glaser JS, Schatz NJ: Traumatic chiasmal syndrome. *Neurology* 1980;30:963–970.

Savino PJ, Paris M, Schatz NJ, et al: Optic tract syndrome. A review of 21 patients. *Arch Ophthalmol* 1978;96(4):656.

CHAPTER 6

Unexplained Visual Loss: Anterior Segment, Retinal, and Nonorganic Disorders

- ▶ OCULAR DISEASES 161
  Anterior segment disorders 161
  Retinal disorders 164
- ▶ ELUSIVE NEURO-OPHTHALMIC DISORDERS 173
  Amblyopia 173
  Retrobulbar and intracranial disorders 173
- ▶ NONORGANIC (FUNCTIONAL) DISORDERS OF VISION 173
  History 174
  Examining patients with functional visual loss 175
  Treatment 180
- ▶ KEY POINTS 181

Not uncommonly, patients present with complaints of visual loss in which the neuro-ophthalmic history and examination fail to provide a ready diagnosis. In fact, the final common pathway for unexplained visual loss and suspected nonorganic disorders is typically the neuro-ophthalmologist. Such patients may have no evident structural abnormalities of the eye, and the patient's complaints and history may not suggest any of the afferent visual disorders discussed in the previous chapters. This chapter discusses a variety of disorders that should be considered in patients who have unexplained visual loss.

▶ OCULAR DISEASES

Patients with unexplained visual loss may have subtle, undiagnosed ocular disease as the cause of their visual complaint. The neuro-ophthalmologist must therefore maintain an open mind during the entire examination, devoting as much attention to the slitlamp and retinal examinations as is given to testing the visual fields. The neurologist may need the help of an ophthalmology colleague, especially in patients with unexplained afferent visual complaints. This chapter discusses anterior segment and retinal disorders that mimic neuro-ophthalmic disorders.

ANTERIOR SEGMENT DISORDERS

Ocular Surface Disease

Tear film disorders, such as *dry eye syndrome*, commonly cause transient visual blurring that may range in duration from seconds to hours in one or both eyes (see Table 1–3). Dry eye syndrome is very common in women older than 40 years, but is also associated with collagen vascular disease (Sjögren syndrome and many others), medications, systemic disorders (such as sarcoidosis), and neurological conditions (eg, progressive supranuclear palsy [PSP], Parkinson disease, facial nerve palsies). Patients frequently describe blurring that begins 2 to 3 minutes into a task requiring concentration, such as reading or driving. Sometimes the blurred vision clears momentarily with a blink. The patient's visual acuity may vary widely between examinations. A foreign body sensation and conjunctival injection are often present, but may not be prominent. Tear film disorders resulting in inadequate tear coverage can actually cause excessive tearing, but this reflex tearing consists of watery tears that fail to adhere to the ocular surface. *Meibomian gland dysfunction* and *blepharitis* can cause destabilization of the tear film and further exacerbate dry eye syndrome (Box 6–1).

> **BOX 6-1. TEAR FILM**

The importance of the tear film in maintaining clear vision is not always appreciated by physicians. In addition to providing nutrients to the cornea, the tear film provides a smooth surface over the corneal curvature to optimize the optics of the eye. Tear film dysfunction is a very frequent cause of blurred vision, eye pain, red eyes, and tearing.

The tear film is complex, consisting of three distinct layers: (1) an inner mucous layer that adheres to the ocular surface, (2) an aqueous layer in the middle that is the thickest layer, (3) an outer lipid layer that retards evaporation. This arrangement allows the tear film to distribute evenly over the ocular surface, pulled up as a sheet with each blink. Deficiencies in any of the three layers can cause the tear film to break up too soon or evaporate too quickly. Tear film dysfunction can result in overproduction of the aqueous component, which fails to adhere to the eye and simply accumulates until it falls over the lower eyelid. (Patients often question why artificial tears are recommended when their complaint is "too much tearing"). Tear film stability is also weakened by debris in the tear film, such as the products of chronic blepharitis.

Evidence of ocular surface disease at the slitlamp includes punctuate staining (with topical fluorescein or rose bengal) of the exposed area of the cornea, rapid tear breakup time (observing the fluorescein-stained tear film fall apart prematurely after a blink), deficient tear meniscus (normal adherence of tears along the lower lid margin is minimal or absent), and injection of the conjunctiva in the exposed area between the lids.

Patients with intermittent, variable blur and ocular pain/foreign body sensation or other signs of ocular surface disease may benefit from a trial of artificial tears (at least four times a day for several weeks) before (or concurrent with) further neuro-ophthalmic investigation. Ointment at night, punctal plugs, Restasis, and other measures may be helpful if indicated.

Irregularities of the corneal epithelium can cause intermittent blurring of vision, similar to tear film disorders. *Epithelial defects and punctate keratopathies* are usually obvious with the slitlamp examination, especially when the cornea is stained with topical fluorescein. *Corneal epithelial dystrophies* such as map-dot-fingerprint dystrophy may be subtle, and can escape notice if the slitlamp examination is cursory (Figure 6–1).

The slitlamp examination, augmented with fluorescein or rose bengal staining, is the primary means of diagnosing ocular surface disorders. Schirmer testing is a helpful adjunct to measure basal tear secretion.

For tear-film disorders, the use of artificial tears, punctal plugs, or cyclosporine ophthalmic emulsion (Restasis) can be curative in many patients. Artificial tears can also be helpful to some extent in patients with corneal surface abnormalities. Therefore, in patients in whom an ocular surface disorder is suspected, a trial of artificial tears may be indicated prior to initiation of an extensive neuro-ophthalmic evaluation.

Corneal Curvature

Irregular corneal astigmatism may be a cause of unexplained decreased visual acuity or monocular diplopia. This condition may result from contact lens wear, ocular surgery, or intrinsic disease of the cornea such as keratoconus (Figure 6–2). Patients with this diagnosis typically complain of blurred rather than dim vision. Visual field testing tends to be normal or show an overall slight depression. Often patients have seen many eye doctors, and have been given a variety of contact lens or eyeglasses prescriptions. Irregular corneal astigmatism is often first identified as an irregular reflex during retinoscopy. This is one case in which the pinhole acuity may exceed the best-corrected visual acuity. Keratometry and corneal topography are useful diagnostic tools for characterizing irregular corneal astigmatism. Placement of a diagnostic rigid contact lens will ameliorate corneal surface or contour abnormalities, and contact lens over-refraction will establish the true visual potential of the eye.

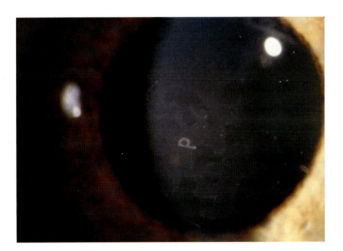

Figure 6-1. Corneal epithelial basement membrane dystrophy.
This common disorder disrupts the normally smooth optical surface of the cornea/tear film with ridges of epithelial irregularity. This may have a geographic appearance like a map, appear as dots on the surface of the cornea, or have irregular parallel ridges that resemble a fingerprint (hence, the alternative descriptive name: map, dot, fingerprint dystrophy). The map-like appearance and dots are evident on this clinical photograph of the cornea of a patient who presented with unexplained intermittent blurred vision.

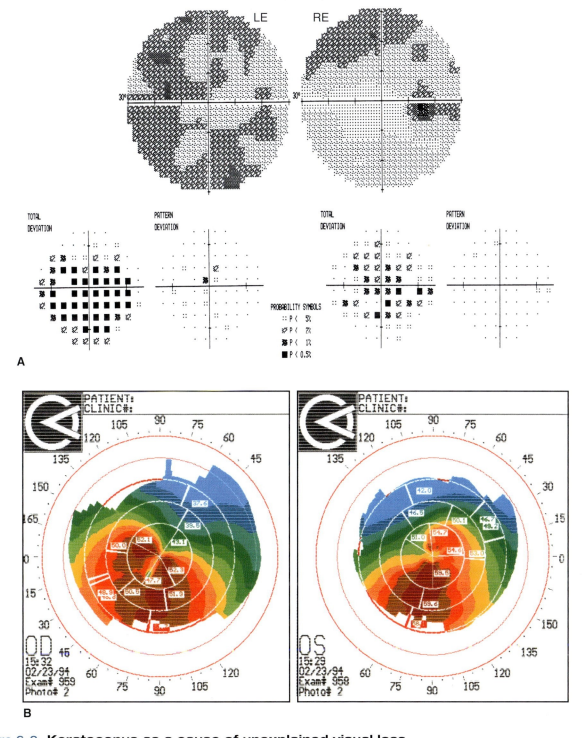

Figure 6–2. **Keratoconus as a cause of unexplained visual loss.**
A 37-year-old woman with a complaint of gradual visual loss in her left eye had a best-corrected visual acuity of 20/60 in the right eye and 20/400 in the left eye. The patient was referred for a neuro-ophthalmic evaluation for suspected optic neuritis. The examination revealed an irregular reflex on retinoscopy, no relative afferent pupillary defect, and a normal fundus examination. **(A)** Automated perimetry revealed diffuse depression of the visual field in both eyes, but with a normal pattern deviation. **(B)** Corneal topography showed marked irregular astigmatism consistent with the suspected diagnosis of keratoconus. The irregular astigmatism was confirmed as the cause of her visual loss by a diagnostic trial of rigid contact lenses, with an over-refraction yielding visual acuities of 20/25 in each eye.

Cataract

Another frequent masquerader of neuro-ophthalmic disease is cataract. Patients complain of the gradual onset of blurred (rather than dim) vision. Lens opacities do not cause focal visual field defects. The visual field is usually normal, or demonstrates a diffuse depression. Cataract may also cause monocular diplopia.

The *opalescent* nuclear sclerotic cataract is frequently unrecognized at the slitlamp, because it lacks the brunescent (yellow-brown) color of a typical nuclear sclerotic cataract, and often occurs in relatively young patients (aged 40–60 years). This type of cataract is also more frequent in myopic individuals (see Figure 1–3).

Posterior subcapsular cataract can cause variable visual blurring from glare, depending on lighting conditions. Subcapsular cataract may be more evident in the red reflex with the ophthalmoscope, retinoscope, or slitlamp (retro-illumination) than with direct illumination. *Cortical water clefts* that are located at the posterior pole of the lens can also cause significant visual problems. Both subcapsular and cortical water cleft cataracts can cause a disproportionate amount of visual loss when compared to their appearance with the slitlamp, due to their location near the optical nodal point of the eye.

The slitlamp and the potential acuity meter (PAM) are important diagnostic tools when cataract is suspected to be the cause of a visual complaint. The PAM is a device that projects an acuity chart onto the retina as a narrow beam, which can be maneuvered around any anterior segment opacities. Additional findings consistent with cataract as the cause of visual loss include the lack of a relative afferent pupillary defect (RAPD), a myopic shift in refraction, and a normal (or slightly depressed) visual field.

Refractive States

Every patient with subnormal visual acuity should have a refraction to determine the *best corrected visual acuity*. A surprising number of patients with simple refractive errors are referred with suspected neuro-ophthalmic diagnoses. As discussed in Chapter 2, performing retinoscopy in the course of a manifest refraction has other benefits, as it may reveal irregular corneal astigmatism or cataract.

Latent hyperopia should be suspected in patients in their 30s or 40s who complain of variable blurred vision, "eye strain" headaches, or difficulty reading. Such patients may have undercorrected hyperopia, which remains asymptomatic until their accommodative potential is reduced to a critical level in the early stages of presbyopia. Latent hyperopes must maintain constant accommodation to see clearly, and transient blurring of vision occurs with momentary lapses in this ocular marathon. Diplopia can occur when excessive focusing effort (accommodation) results in convergence spasm. A cycloplegic refraction may be required for confirmation of suspected latent hyperopia. A hyperopic change in the patient's corrective lenses is curative. Overcorrected myopic patients can present with symptoms similar to undercorrected hyperopes, because both require excessive accommodative effort to see clearly.

RETINAL DISORDERS

Retinal diseases can cause visual loss that may mimic optic nerve disorders. Most of the time retinal disorders are visible with the ophthalmoscope, but occasionally the retinal findings are scant. Usually, the RAPD in monocular retinal disorders is less than the RAPD that would be present from an optic neuropathy causing similar visual field loss. The pattern of visual field loss is helpful in some patients, but retinal vascular occlusions can produce visual field defects that are similar to optic nerve disease (Figure 6–3).

Central vision loss, and hence loss of visual acuity, occurs with macular disease. The Amsler grid is helpful in detecting metamorphopsia, a symptom that suggests macular rather than optic nerve disease. Photo-stress testing can also help distinguish between macular and optic nerve disorders, as discussed in Chapter 2. The introduction of optical coherence tomography (OCT), as discussed in detail in Chapter 1, has greatly improved our ability to diagnosis otherwise subtle macular disease that can mimic optic neuropathies. Intravenous fluorescein angiography (IVFA) and electroretinography (full-field or multifocal ERG) are needed in some cases of unexplained visual loss to look further for occult retinopathies. A few selected retinal disorders that often escape detection on examination or that may be confused with optic neuropathies are discussed in this section.

Retinal Vasculopathies

Branch retinal artery occlusions (BRAO) cause acute visual loss and focal visual field defects that can be similar to optic nerve disorders. Acutely, ophthalmoscopy reveals a whitish area of edematous ischemic retina, and often emboli can be seen in the retinal arterioles (see Figure 6–3). However, the retinal edema typically clears in days to weeks, leaving only subtle changes in the caliber of the affected retinal arterioles. Similarly, the retinal edema and "cherry red spot" from a *central retinal artery occlusion (CRAO)* (Figure 6–4A) soon resolve, leaving retinal arteriolar narrowing and mild diffuse optic nerve pallor. Distinguishing a long-standing CRAO from a primary optic neuropathy is often difficult, and

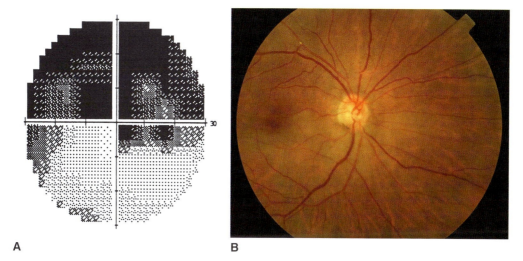

Figure 6-3. Retinal artery occlusion.
A 71-year-old man described the sudden loss of the superior visual field in his right eye. **(A)** The visual field was somewhat altitudinal, raising the possibility of anterior ischemic optic neuropathy. **(B)** However, the fundus examination showed no evidence of optic disc edema. Instead, retinal edema can be seen in the distribution of the inferior arcade vessels, diagnostic of a hemiretinal arterial occlusion. Note also the nonocclusive embolus (Hollenhorst plaque) lodged at the bifurcation in the superior temporal artery.

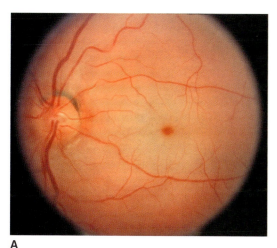
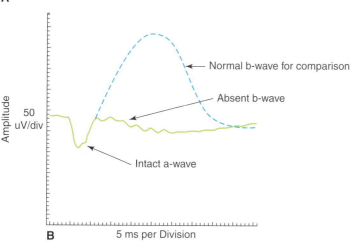

Figure 6-4. Central retinal artery occlusion.
(A) A 62-year-old woman with a history of a previous stroke had sudden visual loss in her left eye. Her evaluation led to a diagnosis of embolic central retinal artery occlusion (CRAO). The funduscopic examination in the affected eye (*pictured*) shows narrowing of the retinal arterioles; pale retina, especially in the macular area; and the cherry-red spot centrally. The cream-colored edematous nerve fiber layer is most evident where the nerve fiber layer is thickest, in the macula between the vascular arcades. Because of the anatomic peculiarities of the foveola, there are no axons to obscure the normal red color of the uninvolved choroidal circulation, which stands out against the pale surrounding macula, giving rise to the infamous cherry-red spot. When the retinal edema subsides (in days to weeks), the diagnosis will not be as obvious. **(B)** Electroretinogram (ERG) in a patient with a CRAO. A CRAO affects the inner retina, but the photoreceptors in the outer retina are supplied by the choroid, and so their function is preserved. This is evident in the ERG pictured, with preservation of the a-wave generated by the intact outer retina, but loss of the b-wave from ischemia of the inner retina. (Normal b-wave is shown for comparison; see Figure 2-28B).

CRAO should be considered in the differential diagnosis of visual loss and optic disc pallor. Intravenous fluorescein angiography is helpful in diagnosing both BRAO and CRAO, especially acutely. The electroretinogram (ERG) is diagnostic in central retinal artery occlusion, demonstrating preservation of the a-wave and loss of the b-wave from infarction of the inner retinal layers (see Figure 6–4B). Embolic retinal vascular occlusions are discussed in more detail in Chapter 14.

Central retinal vein occlusions (CRVO) and *branch retinal vein occlusions (BRVO)* cause marked retinal hemorrhages that are impressive and difficult to miss initially. Disc edema may also occur acutely, but the presence of peripheral retinal hemorrhages distinguishes a retinal vein occlusion from a primary optic neuropathy. After several months the retinal hemorrhages clear, leaving only a few markers of the event. Sometimes venous collateral vessels on the optic disc and slight disc pallor remain, mimicking the findings in optic nerve sheath meningioma.

Vasculitis can affect the retinal arteries or veins. In many patients, the consequences are catastrophic and obvious on examination. However, mild or focal disease can produce loss of visual acuity and visual field defects without profound visible changes in the retina (Figure 6–5). Retinal vasculitis is associated with a variety of systemic conditions, many of which can also cause central nervous system (CNS) disease. In addition to vasculitis, a number of other CNS and systemic diseases may present with vision loss and prominent retinal findings. *Acute posterior multifocal placoid pigment epitheliopathy (AMPPE)* is characterized by large extramacular lesions, and can be associated with cerebral vasculitis and stoke in some patients. *Microangiopathy of the brain, retina, and inner ear (Susac syndrome)* presents with branch retinal artery occlusions and CNS microinfarction. *Cerebral autosomal dominant arteriopathy with subcortical infarcts and leukoencephalopathy (CADASIL)* is a cause of stroke in young adults, with retinal findings including retinal

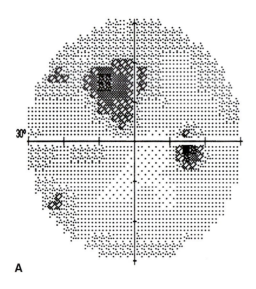

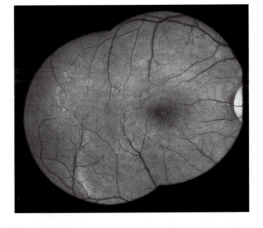

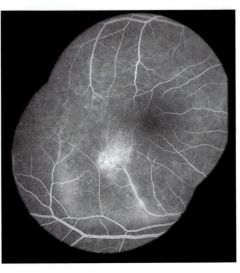

Figure 6–5. Syphilitic macular vasculitis. A 45-year-old man presented with decreased vision in his right eye. Serologic evaluation revealed active syphilis. **(A)** The initial automated visual field showed a superior paracentral visual field defect in the right eye; the left eye was normal. **(B)** The fundus examination demonstrated a normal optic disc and only very subtle changes in the macular vasculature. **(C)** Intravenous fluorescein angiography was performed because the visual field did not implicate an optic nerve disorder, demonstrating focal retinal vasculitis. The visual field defect cleared after treatment for neurosyphilis.

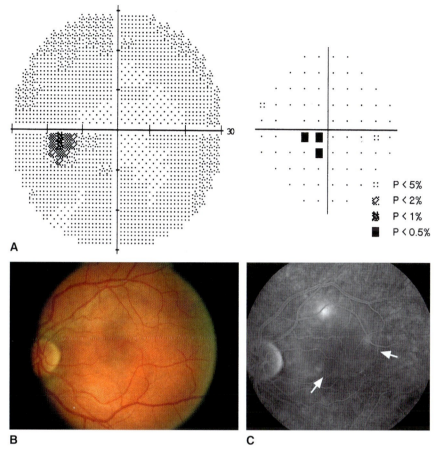

Figure 6-6. **Central serous chorioretinopathy.**
A 35-year-old woman complained of a painless decline in the vision of her left eye over 3 days. The visual acuity was 20/80. The relative afferent pupillary defect was only 0.3 log units—the first hint that this was not an optic neuritis. **(A)** Automated perimetry revealed a central scotoma. The shallow central depression is not evident in the grayscale, but can be seen in the total deviation probability plot. **(B)** The fundus examination suggested submacular fluid. The subtle retinal findings could easily be missed if the examiner (prematurely convinced of a diagnosis of optic neuritis) neglected a careful macular examination. **(C)** The diagnosis is confirmed by intravenous fluorescein angiography. Note the extent of the submacular fluid (*arrows*), and the punctate window defect in the retinal pigment epithelium, which is the source of the fluid.

arteriolar narrowing and sheathing, cotton-wool spots, and ischemic optic neuropathy.

Maculopathies

Age-related macular degeneration (ARMD) is common and often coexists with optic nerve disease such as anterior ischemic optic neuropathy in the older population. Visual field loss that can be attributed to ARMD should precisely match the shape and severity of the visible macular lesion (see Figure 3–7). Similar to optic neuritis, *central serous chorioretinopathy* causes central scotomas in young patients. Often an RAPD is small or absent. The fundus findings may be subtle, but OCT (or IVFA) is diagnostic (Figure 6–6). *Epiretinal membranes* tend to cause metamorphopsia rather than discreet scotomas, and are usually evident on careful ophthalmoscopy (Figure 6–7). *Vitreomacular traction (VMT)* and *macular holes* can cause decreased visual acuity and tiny central visual field defects—so small that the foveal threshold may be the only abnormal point with automated perimetry. Even with biomicroscopy using the 90-diopter lens or retinal contact lens, macular changes in the various stages of macular holes may be subtle, but fortunately OCT is diagnostic (Figure 6–8). *Cystoid macular edema (CME)* can occur as a consequence of many retinal and ocular disorders, and is not always evident with ophthalmoscopy. OCT is diagnostic of CME (Figure 6–9), and IVFA (showing late petaloid staining of the macular region) is needed only in atypical cases. CME can occur with diabetes, uveitis, and retinitis pigmentosa. CME can be associated with mild optic disc edema following intraocular surgery (known as Irvine-Gass syndrome).

Similar to toxic optic neuropathies, *toxic retinopathies* can present as mysterious, insidious bilateral, symmetrical visual loss. Chloroquine and hydroxychloroquine (Plaquenil) affect the macula primarily and cause retinal pigment epithelial changes early, and bull's-eye maculopathy late in their course. Hydroxychloroquine is a common medication used in treating connective tissue disorders, but toxicity is rare with the commonly used doses. Nicotinic acid (niacin), used in the treatment of hypercholesterolemia, can also cause a bilateral maculopathy (Figure 6–10). Thioridazine (Mellaril) toxicity causes decreased vision and nyctalopia, with retina pigment epithelial changes posterior to the equator. Agents causing toxic retinopathies are listed in Table 6–1.

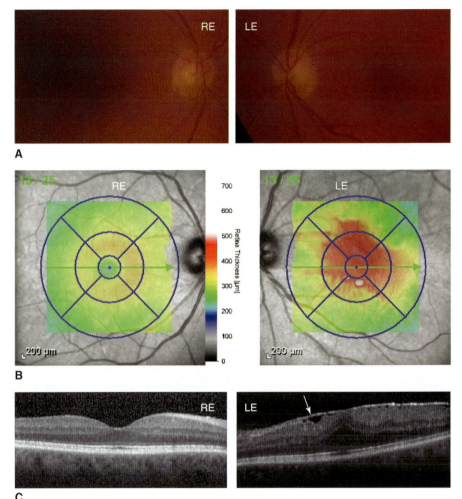

Figure 6–7. **Epiretinal membrane.**
A 54-year-old man was referred to the neuroophthalmology service for a complaint of progressive blurred vision in his left eye over 6 months, with a visual acuity of 20/30. Further history revealed that the vision in the eye was not just blurred but distorted—straight edges (his venetian blinds) were crooked in the middle. An Amsler grid showed central metamorphopsia (the patient's Amsler grid is shown in Figure 2–9C). **(A)** Fundus photographs. The right eye is normal. In the left eye, the foveal reflex is blunted, but pathologic changes are not obvious. **(B)** Optical coherence tomography (OCT) retinal thickness map. The color-coded retinal thickness map shows elevation of the left macula, with a normal right macula. **(C)** OCT cross section through fovea demonstrates an epiretinal membrane (*arrow*), pulling and distorting the macula—which is the cause of the patient's metamorphopsia.

Vitamin A deficiency can cause marked rod photoreceptor dysfunction and nyctalopia. Other manifestations include xerosis and conjunctival Bitot spots.

Retinal trauma is usually obvious from the history and fundus examination, but permanent subtle changes from trauma can occur. Berlin edema is a traumatic disorganization of macular photoreceptor orientation that appears acutely as a central sheen on ophthalmoscopy. This condition is generally reversible, but can result in permanent central visual loss.

Selected Retinopathies

Retinitis pigmentosa is a group of disorders with a variety of heritable patterns, typically associated with pigmented "bone spicules" along vessels in the retinal periphery, optic disc pallor, arteriolar narrowing, and vitreous cells. Some forms (so-called *sine pigmento*) may have rather unremarkable-looking fundi. When the rods (rather than cones) are primarily affected, patients may have prominent nyctalopia, with perimetry revealing a classic ring scotoma (corresponding to the region of the retina with the greatest rod concentration). The ERG is usually abnormal long before retinal changes are evident (see Figure 3–6).

Cone dystrophy (a subset of retinitis pigmentosa) is a group of heterogeneous heritable disorders characterized by predominantly cone dysfunction, usually presenting in middle-aged patients. Patients present with bilateral, symmetric declining visual acuity, central scotomas, and color vision abnormalities. Hemeralopia (rather than nyctalopia) is likely to be present (as the cones contribute most in photopic conditions). The fundus is unremarkable initially, only later showing retinal pigment epithelium (RPE) atrophy in the macula. This condition is often confused with a bilateral optic neuropathy. A multifocal ERG will reveal macular dysfunction in this condition, usually before macular signs are evident.

Stargardt disease is a hereditary macular degeneration that causes progressive bilateral central vision loss in young patients, usually presenting before 20 years of age. This disorder is the most common hereditary macular dystrophy. RPE changes in the fovea may be

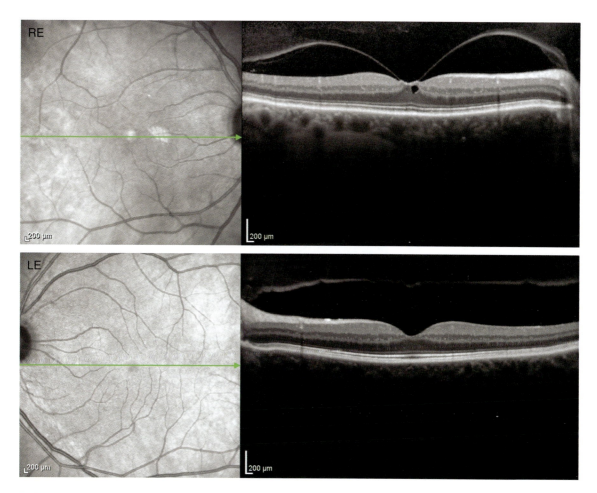

Figure 6-8. Vitreomacular traction.
A 73-year-old woman had successful cataract surgery in the right eye, but was disappointed as the best corrected visual acuity was 20/40. Automated perimetry was normal, with the exception of a decreased foveal threshold in the right eye. The fundus examination did not reveal the diagnosis, but optical coherence tomography (OCT) clearly shows vitreomacular traction (VMT) in the right eye, with distortion of the foveola (*top*). Note the normal OCT contour of the unaffected left eye (with unattached vitreous surface seen in the OCT cross section, *bottom*). VMT is often not evident on the funduscopic examination, and even intravenous fluorescein angiography is usually unrevealing. This diagnosis was often missed before the era of OCT imaging. Many patients at this stage of traction will progress to develop a macular hole, though some can have spontaneous release of the vitreous with restoration of normal foveolar architecture and improvement in visual acuity.

seen early, before the macula eventually develops the classic "beaten bronze" appearance. However, macular findings can be subtle early in this condition, and Stargardt disease can be confused with hereditary/toxic or other optic neuropathies. IVFA is diagnostic, with loss of the normal choroidal fluorescence (blocked by accumulation of lipofuscin in the RPE) (Figure 6–11). Genetic testing is available to look for associated mutations in the *ABCR* gene. There is no known treatment.

Cancer-associated retinopathy (CAR; also called paraneoplastic retinopathy) is a paraneoplastic syndrome in which autoantibodies are directed against the retina. CAR is classically associated with small-cell carcinoma of the lung or other visceral malignancies, but at least half of the time patients present with visual symptoms before a malignancy is discovered. Progressive bilateral visual loss may occur in the presence of a relatively unremarkable fundus, with perimetry typically showing a ring scotoma. Continuous photopsias, nyctalopia, and photosensitivity are common symptoms. The ERG demonstrates markedly reduced amplitudes early in the course. The diagnosis can be made by detecting the presence of antibodies (to the retinal protein *recoverin*) in the serum. However, many other retinal antigens (and corresponding antibodies) are known to produce CAR, so patients with suspected CAR should have an oncologic evaluation even if recoverin antibodies are negative. Treatment with corticosteroids, plasmapheresis, and intravenous immunoglobulin has been advocated but is generally disappointing. A CAR-like syndrome can also

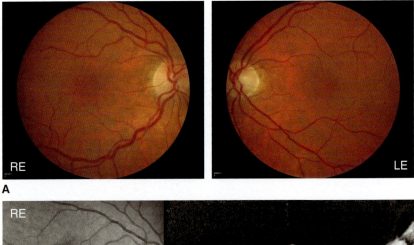
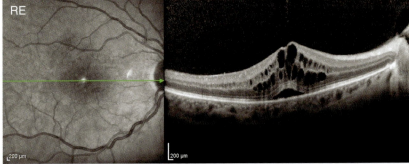
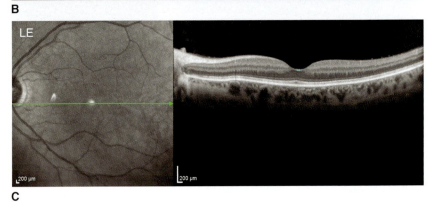

Figure 6-9. **Cystoid macular edema.**
(A) Fundus photographs show subtle abnormalities in the right macula, best seen by comparing to the normal left macula. **(B)** Optical coherence tomography (OCT) of the right eye, with cross section through the fovea. Unlike the fundus photograph, there is nothing subtle in this OCT, with marked elevation of the fovea and intraretinal cysts at multiple levels. **(C)** OCT of the left eye shows a normal foveal contour.

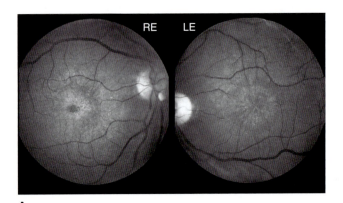
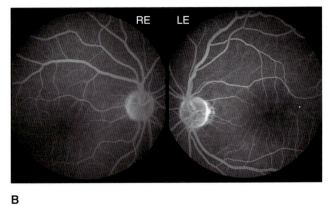

Figure 6-10. **Niacin toxicity.**
A 62-year-old man complained of gradual bilateral visual loss. Visual acuity was 20/50 in the right eye and 20/80 in the left eye. Bilateral central scotomas were identified on confrontation perimetry. The patient was taking 1 gram of niacin 3 times daily for hypercholesterolemia. **(A)** The ophthalmoscopic examination reveals a bilateral maculopathy, similar in appearance to cystoid macular edema (CME). **(B)** Intravenous fluorescein angiography demonstrates that the maculopathy does not stain like true CME. Niacin toxicity is one cause of this appearance of pseudo-CME.

TABLE 6-1. DRUGS KNOWN TO CAUSE TOXIC RETINOPATHIES

Drug	Description	Adverse Effects
Hydroxychloroquine (Plaquenil), Chloroquine (Aralen)	Antimalarial used in rheumatoid arthritis and lupus	Bull's eye maculopathy, corneal verticillata (whirl)
Quinine (Qualaquin)	*Rarely used* antimalarial, previously prescribed for nocturnal leg cramps	Retinal photoreceptor and ganglion cell toxicity
Thioridazine (Mellaril)	Antipsychotic drug rarely used (for patients unresponsive to standard regimens)	Pigmentary deposits on cornea and anterior lens capsule, pigmentary retinopathy
Tamoxifen (Nolvadex)	Anti-estrogen agent for breast cancer in premenopausal women	Crystalline deposits in the macula
Nicotinic acid (niacin, vitamin B_3)	Treatment for hypercholesterolemia: reduces high triglyceride levels, elevates low HDL levels	Atypical cystoid macular edema (see Figure 6–10)
Digoxin (Lanoxin)	Cardiac glycoside used to treat congestive heart failure and to slow the heart rate in patients with atrial fibrillation/flutter	Yellow vision (xanthopsia), color vision loss, positive visual phenomenon
Canthaxanthin	Carotenoid pigment used in "tanning pills"	Crystalline deposits in the macula
Vigabatrin (Sabril)	Antiepileptic drug used for infantile spasms and as adjunctive therapy for adult patients with refractory complex partial seizures	Peripheral visual field loss
Sildenafil (Viagra)	Used to treat erectile dysfunction	Halos and blue vision
Fingolimod (Gilenya)	Oral medication for treatment of relapsing forms of MS	CME, uveitis
Isotretinoin (Roaccutane, Accutane)	Retinoid used to treat cystic acne	Decreased night vision, papilledema from intracranial hypertension

Abbreviations: CME, cystoid macular edema; HDL, high density lipoprotein; MS, multiple sclerosis.

occur in the setting of systemic (non-oncologic) autoimmune disorders.

Melanoma-associated retinopathy (MAR) is another paraneoplastic retinopathy that may present in a similar fashion to CAR. In this condition, the ERG shows predominantly rod dysfunction. Patients with MAR usually have a known diagnosis of melanoma at the time of visual symptoms. The onset of MAR may correlate with metastatic disease. Other paraneoplastic retinopathy syndromes are being identified, characterized by the retinal antigenic site (the target of the paraneoplastic antibodies) including paraneoplastic ganglion cell neuropathy (PGCN), cancer-associated cone dysfunction (CACD), and diffuse uveal melanocytic proliferation (DUMP).

Acute zonal occult outer retinopathy (AZOOR) is a group of retinal disorders that present in a similar fashion, and likely have a common pathophysiology. This group includes multiple evanescent white dot syndrome (MEWDS), acute macular neuroretinopathy (AMN), acute idiopathic blind spot enlargement (AIBSE), and multifocal choroiditis. Visual loss in these disorders is sometimes preceded by a nonspecific flu-like illness, suggesting a possible post-viral, autoimmune origin. They occur predominantly in young women, presenting with vision loss and photopsias. Often, retinal findings are scant or absent. Intravenous fluorescein angiography or an ERG may be needed to define these elusive disorders. MEWDS is characterized by transient unilateral grayish-white dots at the level of the retinal pigment epithelium in the macula and peripapillary regions. Visual field abnormalities include enlargement of the blind spot, cecocentral scotomas, or generalized depression of the visual field. Patients usually have full recovery of vision within several months, although a few have persistent blind spot enlargement. AIBSE presents with photopsias and enlargement of the blind spot. AIBSE can occur with normal acuity and an unremarkable fundus examination, though often evidence of retinal and optic disc inflammation is present. This disorder is usually self-limited; the photopsias resolve, but the visual field defects may persist.

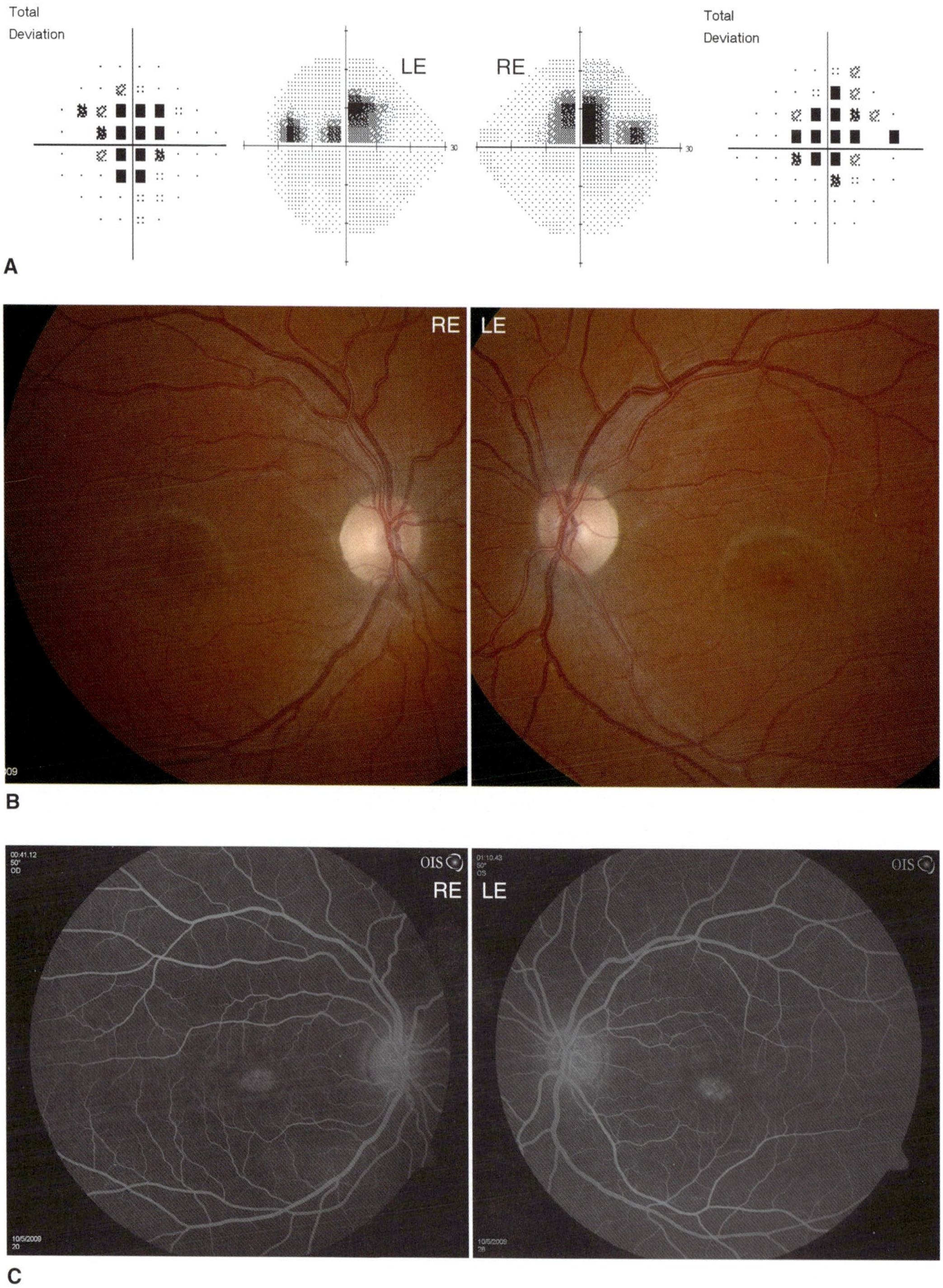

Figure 6-11. Stargardt disease.

A 16-year-old patient was noted to have poor visual acuity when she went to be tested for her driver's license. She reported that her vision may have been "a little blurry" for the last few years. Best corrected visual acuity was 20/80 in both eyes with bilateral central scotomas. The fundus examination was said to be unremarkable. A thorough work-up for a presumed bilateral optic neuropathy, including neuroimaging and genetic testing for Leber hereditary optic neuropathy, was negative. **(A)** Humphrey visual field testing (24-2) revealed bilateral cecocentral scotomas. **(B)** The funduscopic examination revealed subtle abnormalities prompting intravenous fluorescein angiography (IVFA). **(C)** IVFA (late venous phase at 1 minute) shows punctuate hyperfluorescence in the macula, but the most striking finding is the absence of normal choroidal background hyperfluorescence in all phases of the study (contrast the "silent choroid" in this IVFA with normal choroidal hyperfluorescence in Figure 1-5), characteristic of Stargardt disease. Genetic testing identified a mutation of the *ABCR* gene, confirming the diagnosis of Stargardt disease.

▶ ELUSIVE NEURO-OPHTHALMIC DISORDERS

AMBLYOPIA

Most patients with a monocular developmental amblyopia are aware that the vision in the affected eye has been poor lifelong. Occasionally, decreased vision from amblyopia is first discovered on a routine examination or vision screening in adulthood. Patients with amblyopic visual loss are unlikely to complain of a recent subjective change in their vision. An RAPD may be present, but is usually less than 0.6 log units. The visual field is usually normal, but may be modestly diffusely depressed. Color vision is usually normal. Focal visual field defects should not be present. Even with poor visual acuity, finding a discreet central scotoma with perimetry is unusual. There should also be an identifiable reason for amblyopia to exist, such as a congenital strabismus or anisometropia.

RETROBULBAR AND INTRACRANIAL DISORDERS

Retrobulbar and intracranial disorders that can cause visual loss in the presence of a normal fundus examination have been discussed in detail (see Table 4–5). A few guidelines are worth repeating:

1. It is essential to perform perimetry on both eyes to evaluate all patients who complain of monocular or binocular decreased vision. Patients with homonymous visual field loss may only complain of visual loss in one eye.
2. Unilateral stroke involving the retrochiasmal pathways does not cause visual acuity loss, even when the homonymous visual field loss is dense. However, bilateral lesions can cause decreased visual acuity in both eyes.
3. Optic neuritis may cause a subjective decline in the quality of vision, despite relatively normal visual acuity and perimetry. Additional vision tests, such as color vision or contrast sensitivity testing, may also be needed to characterize the defect.
4. Toxic and nutritional optic neuropathies often present a diagnostic challenge, because the optic nerves are often normal in appearance initially. Table 4–11 lists the agents and conditions commonly implicated.

▶ NONORGANIC (FUNCTIONAL) DISORDERS OF VISION

Visual complaints that have no physiological or organic basis are frequently referred to as *functional visual loss*. This section will concentrate on complaints of (afferent) visual loss, but nonorganic disorders can present in a variety of ways (Box 6–2). Patients with functional visual loss constitute a spectrum, ranging from the innocent "hysteric" to the deliberately deceptive "malingerer" (Box 6–3).

▶ BOX 6–2. NONORGANIC EYE DISORDERS

Visual loss. Discussed extensively in this chapter.

Pain, photophobia, asthenopia, and other discomfort. Dysesthesias are the most difficult nonorganic symptoms to deal with, because sensation is subjective. The physician needs to be cautious because many organic disorders do not have physical findings (as discussed in Chapter 13).

Diplopia. Diplopia that is nonorganic is often monocular, and the patient may describe more than two images (polyopia). However, most patients with monocular diplopia have disease (Table 1–5). Diplopia that clears when one or the other eye is covered is usually pathophysiological (an ocular motility disorder).

Convergence spasm. Convergence spasm produces an esotropia that can simulate an abduction deficit. Miotic pupils accompanying the esotropia is evidence that the esotropia is the result of an accommodative effort. Normal ductions can often be demonstrated by covering the opposite eye when testing. Horizontal versions should be normal, but testing versions may induce convergence spasm.

Normal versions can be more reliably demonstrated by having the patient fix on a distant object while moving the head (doll's head maneuver; see Figure 9–4).

Eyelid spasms. Voluntary blepharospasm may be difficult to distinguish from true blepharospasm, but may be noted to be absent when the patient is distracted or perceives that they are not being observed (see Figure 6–12). Voluntary blepharospasm cannot be maintained in upgaze.

Voluntary nystagmus. Voluntary nystagmus is a very high-frequency, low-amplitude, binocular, conjugate pseudo-nystagmus (not true nystagmus, back-to-back saccades). Requires obvious effort and cannot be sustained for more than 30 seconds.

Self-induced eye trauma. The trauma to the eye is certainly real, but the source of the lesion is self-induced. Sometimes seen when patients are seeking pain medications, or in psychiatric disorders (*Munchausen syndrome*).

Anisocoria. Anisocoria can present as a nonorganic disorder if a patient covertly instills a topical mydriatic agent.

Data from Fish RH, Foroozan R: Nonorganic visual disorders, in Kline LB. *Neuro-ophthalmology Review Manual*, 7th ed. Thorofare, NJ: SLACK; 2013:231–244.

▶ BOX 6–3. THE SPECTRUM OF PATIENTS WITH FUNCTIONAL VISION LOSS

HS Thompson wrote a classic treatise on functional vision loss in 1985. His characterizations of the spectrum of patients presenting with nonorganic vision loss is timeless and continues to provide insight for physicians dealing with the complexity of these patient encounters. Thompson discusses the continuum between the "malicious" and the "innocent" by discussing four overlapping profiles of patients with functional vision loss:

The deliberate malingerer willfully, knowingly, and maliciously feigns visual loss for personal gain. Such patients see the examination as a contest and appear stressed, "grumpy, and agitated." They may try too hard to act blind, stumbling over obstacles and never quite looking toward the examiner's voice. They are not at all happy with the conclusion of "good news" about their eye examination.

The worried impostor is aware that he is exaggerating his visual symptoms (for some sort of gain), but also is worried he might really have something bad. Like the deliberate malingerer, he is consciously falling short in each test—but differs as he starts to believe some of his own lies, worrying that he may really be sick. Such patients are less likely to argue with a good report, as they may be genuinely relieved.

The impressionable exaggerator is convinced that something is wrong, and is determined to be sure the physician does not miss it. Such patients tend to have a positive review of systems as they are happy to endorse any symptoms that will make the physician more concerned. These patients are suggestible, and seem to be responsive to the reassurance of normal examination.

The suggestible innocent has concluded that something is going terribly wrong, often after a minor injury or incident. Anxiety leads to further suggestibility and more dramatic symptoms (totally blind, tunnel vision), but the patient is far less concerned about the dire situation than would be expected. This type of patient embraces the physician's good news, and is quick to respond to a confident proclamation from the physician that he or she will get better.

Data from Thompson HS: Functional visual loss. *Am J Ophthalmol* 1985;100:209–213.

In children, functional visual loss may be a reaction to stress at home or school, or may be a form of attention-getting behavior. In contrast, adults may develop functional visual loss for financial gain following injury, or to support a claim for disability. These patients present an enormous challenge to the examining physician, exacting a disproportionate amount of time and worry, and requiring many (and lengthy) communications with other physicians, lawyers, and insurance personnel. In the remainder of this chapter, we will explore the variety of ways that functional patients can present to the ophthalmologist and present examination techniques that will help the examiner perform the most objective examination possible. Guiding principles for evaluating patients suspected of having functional visual loss are presented in Box 6–4.

HISTORY

The physician's suspicion of possible functional visual loss is often raised during the history. The pattern of visual loss may not fit the common sequence of known diseases. For example, trivial external trauma to the eye would not be expected to cause long-term disabling visual loss. In addition, potential secondary gain factors may become evident during the history. Some patients may be more focused on impending litigation or disability determination than on the diagnosis or treatment of their complaint. Patients who are naïve, worried, and eager to convince the physician of their visual deficit tend to have a positive review of ophthalmic symptoms, and often are suggestible in the history-taking process (Figure 6–12).

▶ BOX 6–4. GENERAL GUIDELINES FOR EVALUATING PATIENTS WITH FUNCTIONAL VISUAL LOSS

1. The ophthalmologist does not need to know every clinical "trick" for evaluating functional visual loss, but should develop a comfortable routine that can be performed efficiently and confidently when needed.
2. Remember that some patients with truly organic disease are also highly suggestible and may exhibit superimposed functional behavior, presumably to help the physician understand how bad their visual problem really is.
3. The physician should not make a diagnosis of functional visual loss until a thorough evaluation has been completed.
4. The physician is not obligated to, nor should he or she attempt to, confront suspected functional patients or convince them that their symptoms are "all in their head." The physician should stick to what he or she knows best—reporting the facts of a thorough examination to the patient and his or her physicians, without editorializing.
5. The ophthalmologist can do a tremendous amount of good for those patients who are on the innocent end of the spectrum by offering well-grounded reassurance after a thorough neuro-ophthalmic evaluation.

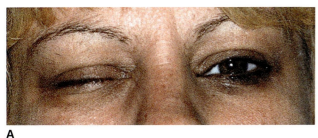
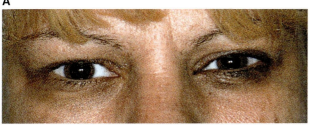
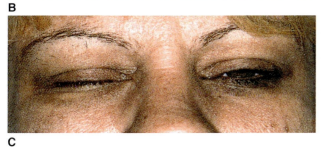

Figure 6–12. **Nonorganic ptosis.**
A 32-year-old woman said that she had a splash injury at work 2 months prior to her consultation, and since that time her "right eye won't open." **(A)** The patient had narrowed palpebral fissures in both eyes, more severe in the right eye. It was observed during the history that the eyelid appearance reverted to normal at times, but resumed the spastic appearance when attention was turned to her plight. **(B)** The patient was told that the spasm would be temporarily relieved with the dilating eyedrops used during the examination. After administration of cyclomydril into both eyes, the spasm was instantly and completely relieved, and the patient had a relatively normal appearance. After 30 minutes, the examiner commented that the effect of the eyedrops may be wearing off soon. **(C)** Within seconds, the patient's blepharospasm returned. The patient was instructed that the problem would resolve with treatment with eyedrops. Artificial tears were dispensed to the patient with a tapering schedule, with complete resolution of her symptoms.

Throughout the encounter with the patient, the physician should continually observe the patient's general behavior and visual capabilities. Does the patient's behavior suggest that the vision is better than stated: Can the patient successfully ambulate into the room and into the chair? Can the patient find and shake the physician's silently outstretched hand on meeting? Or, does the patient seem to exaggerate his or her plight with a messy, erratic signature, walking into walls, or never looking toward your voice?

EXAMINING PATIENTS WITH FUNCTIONAL VISUAL LOSS

Table 6–2 lists several practical methods for examining patients with suspected functional visual loss. Tests

▶ **TABLE 6–2. METHODS FOR EVALUATING SUSPECTED FUNCTIONAL VISUAL LOSS**

Visual acuity and central vision	One or both eyes affected	Exhaustive refraction beginning with smallest letters
		PAM
	Monocular functional visual loss	Fogging with phoropter
		Tests that separate the two eyes: duochrome, polarized, or liquid crystal glasses
		Tests of stereoacuity
	Very poor vision	OKN drum, mirror
		Threat, shocking visual material (not recommended)
Visual fields	Central scotomas or peripheral constriction	Tangent screen testing at 1 and 2 meters (tubular fields)
		Confrontation techniques
	Monocular visual loss	Binocular visual fields, repeat visual field testing

Abbreviations: OKN, optokinetic nystagmus; PAM, potential acuity meter.

generally fall into two categories: The first type of test demonstrates clearly that the patient's visual function is much better than they claim. For example, patients who say they are blind but who are tricked into reading the 20/30 line have *at least* a visual acuity of 20/30 in the eye in question. In contrast, other visual tests may demonstrate that the patient's responses to visual testing are nonphysiological, but do not prove a given level of visual function. For example, the production of tubular fields on tangent screen testing says nothing about whether the patient's visual fields are truly normal, but simply demonstrates that the patient is performing in a suggestible, nonphysiological fashion.

Visual Acuity

Although it is normally more efficient to start with the largest letters and work down when testing visual acuity, it is better to start with the smallest line of letters and work up when testing patients with suspected functional visual loss. Patients who are able to see the entire visual acuity chart at the beginning of the test may choose to read only the largest letters. Systems capable of presenting one line at a time are ideal, because they eliminate the frame of reference for the patient. For example, a patient with functional visual loss may happily read the 20/30 or 20/40 letters after having been presented with much smaller lines first. Conversely, the same patient is unlikely to attempt anything smaller than the 20/400 line if the examination had been carried out starting with the largest letters.

Patients should be encouraged to attempt to read lines that they say they cannot see. In the case of functional visual loss, the examiner can insist that the patient offer a guess, describe whether the letter is circular or square, or at least count the number of letters on the line in question. When the patient realizes that the examiner is going to methodically work on every single line in an exhaustive fashion, the patient is more likely to succumb and attempt to read smaller visual acuity lines than otherwise. Isolating letters or using the pinhole can offer further encouragement, as the examiner can describe these devices as "vision enhancers" for patients with poor vision.

The use of the phoropter to test visual acuity can also encourage patients with functional visual loss to reveal their true acuity. The examiner can tell the patient (honestly) that the phoropter is like a pair of binoculars, that it can magnify the letters, and that the patient will be surprised how well he or she can see with this magnifier. One effective phoropter technique starts with extra plus lens power added to the patient's refraction. As the plus is removed, the patient is encouraged to read now that more "magnification" has been added. In patients with bilateral visual loss, the examiner can announce that with both eyes open through the phoropter the patient should be able to see letters that are "twice as small." Following dilation, the examiner can offer further encouragement by suggesting that the patient's performance (with visual acuity or perimetry) should improve since "three or four times as much light" can now enter the eye.

An effective method of demonstrating normal visual acuity in patients with functional visual loss uses the *PAM*. As described earlier in this chapter, this device is usually used to predict postoperative visual acuity prior to cataract extraction by projecting a visual acuity chart on the macula with a thin beam of light that can be directed around media opacities. The same device can be used in patients with functional visual loss to extract a better assessment of true visual function. The examiner can state honestly that with this device even "legally blind patients" can see the smallest letters (which is true for many patients with cataract!). The test can be prefaced by noting that the machine will shine letters "directly on the brain" (technically true). The examiner should be cautioned that in some diseases that may be confused with functional visual loss (such as keratoconus), the measured acuity with the PAM may indeed be better than the best corrected visual acuity.

If the patient complains of visual loss in one eye only, tests performed with both eyes open can be particularly revealing when the patient is unsure which eye is actually being tested. Using the phoropter with both eyes open, the examiner can gradually add more plus to "fog" the better-seeing eye as the patient reads each line of the chart. Good acuity achieved in this manner can be accurately ascribed to the eye of complaint if the visual acuity in the normal but fogged eye alone is poor.

Specially designed charts and corresponding glasses allow each eye to be tested separately even though both eyes are open. In these tests, some of the test letters can only be seen by the right eye or the left eye alone. Examples include red-green lenses used with a duochrome vision chart, polarized glasses with selectively polarized optotypes, or liquid crystal shutter glasses and special video displays. These tests are not helpful if patients insist on closing one eye during the test.

Stereo acuity tests require excellent visual acuity in both eyes to be performed successfully (see Figure 2–13). Patients who are not aware of this physiological principle may be willing to perform this test, especially if the examiner suggests that it is a test of how well their "good eye" compensates for the "bad eye." A stereoacuity of 40 arc seconds requires a visual acuity of at least 20/25 in *both* eyes. This test may be of limited usefulness in patients who complain of bilateral visual loss.

The use of a handheld prism can help in patients with monocular visual loss. One method introduces a 4 prism-diopter base-out prism in the visual axis, which should induce a compensatory shift in fixation in a seeing eye. Another method uses a 4 to 8 prism-diopter base-up prism over the better eye to induce vertical diplopia while viewing the visual acuity chart: Patients who report seeing two lines or, even better, who can read the upper line (seen only with the "bad" eye) have revealed the true visual acuity of their affected eye.

The *optokinetic drum* (or tape) is helpful when patients declare complete blindness in one or both eyes. The optokinetic nystagmus that results from viewing this stimulus (see Figure 7–2) is proof of at least crude visual function. The moving stripes must be placed in an unavoidable position in front of the patient's affected eye. It is often helpful to ask patients if they "see anything" during the test. The presence of a brisk optokinetic response, despite a patient's insistence that he or she sees nothing at all, demonstrates that the visual acuity is at least in the 20/400 range, and that the patient is not fully cooperating. An even more compelling test is the use of a mirror tilted back and forth and side to side in front of the patients' face. This test provokes an orienting eye movement in response to the perceived environmental movement that is unavoidable in a seeing patient. Some physicians advocate presenting a visual threat to patients who feign total blindness to see if they react. An extension of this test is to present emotionally charged or embarrassing visual material to judge the patient's reaction. However, such testing indicates to the patient that the physician does not believe his or her complaints, generating defensiveness or even hostility that will mar the remainder of the examination.

Visual Fields

Demonstrating that patients with monocular functional visual loss have normal *visual acuity* is easier than proving that the *visual field* is normal. This is because performing perimetry without the patient being aware of which eye is being tested is not possible with standard formal perimetry. Patients can be encouraged to perform more accurate perimetry by suggesting that dilation can expand their side vision. Patients with functional visual loss may also be more cooperative when perimetry is called a "light sensitivity test" (especially those patients who complain of photosensitivity), rather than a peripheral vision test (see Figure 6–16C).

Some patients who insist on monocular visual loss will produce a homonymous hemianopic visual field defect when tested with both eyes open. However, a full visual field is obtained when the unaffected eye is tested alone. Clearly, these perimetry results are nonphysiological and suggest a nonorganic component (Figure 6–13).

Nonphysiological constriction of the visual fields can be evaluated with the use of the tangent screen (see Figure 2–25). A standard tangent visual field is carried

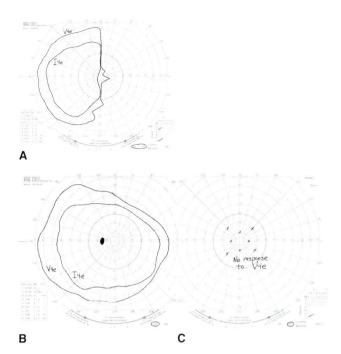

Figure 6–13. **Nonphysiological hemianopia.** A 45-year-old woman complained of visual loss in her right eye. There was no relative afferent pupillary defect, and the eye examination was normal. Goldmann perimetry was first performed with both eyes open, because nonorganic visual loss was suspected. The patient produced a hemifield defect, respecting the vertical meridian **(A)**. Perimetry was then performed on each eye in turn. The visual field in the left eye was normal, extending to both sides of fixation **(B)**. The patient did not respond to any stimuli with the right eye alone **(C)**. This result clearly demonstrates that the patient's performance is nonphysiological. This sequence of visual field testing can also be performed with confrontation perimetry.

out at 1 meter. If the same test is carried out at 2 meters (with the stimulus twice the size as the original) then the diameter of the projected visual field abnormality on the tangent screen should double in size. Patients with nonphysiological visual loss usually approximate the original boundaries of the field when tested at 2 meters, producing so-called "tubular or tunnel visual fields" (Figure 6–14).

With Goldmann perimetry, concentric constriction is the most common type of visual field produced with functional visual loss. Other commonly seen patterns are clearly nonphysiological, including crossing or inversion of isopters, stacking of isopters, and inconsistencies during testing (Figure 6–15). Spiraling of an isopter occurs when each meridian is tested in sequence several times, as the patient waits longer and longer to admit to seeing the kinetic stimulus (see Figure 6–15A). Star-shaped visual fields occur when random meridians are chosen in this same circumstance (see Figure 6–15B).

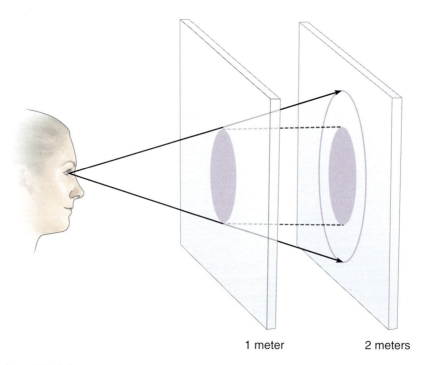

Figure 6–14. **Tunnel visual fields.**
The size of the visual field (and a true scotoma) should increase in area when the testing distance is increased, describing a funnel or *cone* shape. Thus, the projection of the visual field should be twice the diameter on the tangent screen when the testing distance is doubled (*solid lines*). Patients with nonphysiological visual field loss will often produce perimetric results (scotomas or peripheral constriction) that project to the same size, despite the increasing testing distance. From the illustration, it is evident why this nonphysiological perimetric pattern is called a *cylindrical* or *tunnel* field (*dashed lines*).

Automated perimetry in patients with nonorganic visual loss commonly shows a profound peripheral depression, with marked variability between tests (Figure 6–16A). Sometimes such patients will respond at the beginning of the test, when the cardinal points in a quadrant are tested, and respond less as the test progress, producing a "cloverleaf" pattern (see Figure 6–16B). Sequential visual fields over time may reveal marked variability—sometimes the patient forgets which part of his or her vision is supposed to be affected (Figure 6–17).

Figure 6–15. **Nonorganic visual field patterns with Goldmann perimetry.**
(A) *Spiraling isopters.* Patients who wait longer and longer to respond to the stimulus when it is tested along sequential radii (*as numbered*) produce a spiraling isopter. **(B)** *Star-shaped isopters.* If the perimetrist does not proceed sequentially (as in **A**), but chooses random radii (*as numbered*) to test, a jagged star-shaped pattern is produced when the patient is increasingly reluctant to respond. **(C)** *Crossing isopters.* Inconsistent responses produce the isopters that cross. This result is nonphysiological, as it suggests that the patient can see dim/small stimuli in areas where they cannot see bright/large stimuli. **(D)** *Tiny central island of vision.* Nonorganic visual fields that are only a few degrees in diameter are common.

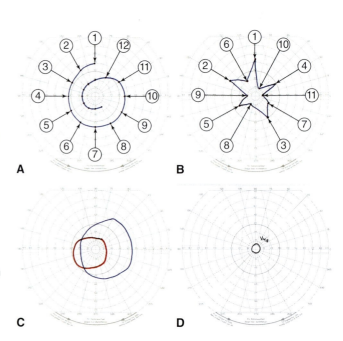

Several confrontation perimetry techniques may be useful when testing patients with functional peripheral visual loss. One technique is to begin with a peripheral finger-counting test at 4 meters or greater from the patient. The testing distance is then shortened to 1 meter, while explaining to the patient that he or she should be able to do much better now that you are so much closer. Some patients may be willing to cooperate at this closer distance, not realizing that although the fingers are nearer, they are actually far more peripheral. Another method disguises a confrontation visual field as a "rapid eye movement test." The patient is asked to rapidly look from the examiner's nose to the examiner's outstretched finger. The examiner places both (closed) hands at opposite points in the patient's peripheral visual field, randomly alternating a raised finger between hands. Consistent accuracy suggests intact peripheral visual fields; consistent inability to ever look correctly at the raised finger endorses suspicions of functional behavior.

Relative Afferent Pupillary Defect Test

As discussed in Chapter 2, most tests of visual function are subjective in the sense that the patient must cooperate and respond. One of the few objective tests available to the examiner is the RAPD test. For this reason, the RAPD test is one of the most important tests in the examination of all patients, particularly those in whom functional

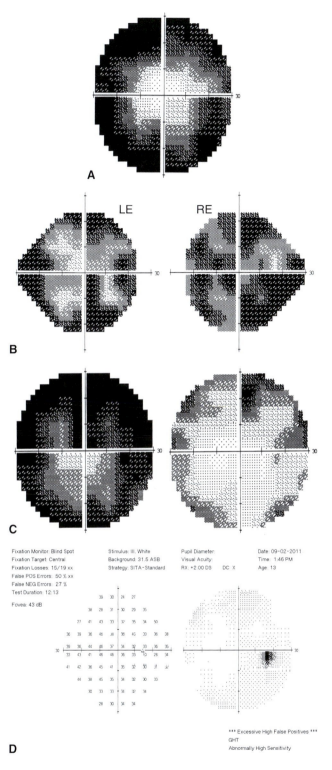

Figure 6-16. **Nonorganic visual field patterns with Humphrey perimetry.**
(A) *Peripheral depression (constricted visual field).* This pattern is often produced by patients with nonorganic visual loss who decide that they will only respond to the brightest central stimuli, or anxious patients who want to be "absolutely sure they really did see the stimulus." However, peripheral depression of the visual field can occur in many diseases (eg, glaucoma, chronic papilledema, retinitis pigmentosa). **(B)** *Cloverleaf visual field.* This pattern is produced when patients do well at the start of the test—when the four cardinal points in each quadrant are determined—but then do not respond well (produce many false negatives) to the rest of the test (due to fatigue, inattention, purposeful neglect). This is analogous to spiraling or star-shaped isopters with Goldmann perimetry. **(C)** *Variable and suggestible perimetry performance.* The visual field on the left is severely depressed. The physician was not convinced that this was a reliable visual field, so the patient returned a few days later for a repeat test on the same eye. This time the patient was told that the machine was set up for a "light sensitivity test" (true statement). The patient was more motivated to respond to the stimuli, and produced a dramatically improved visual field in the same eye, shown on the right. **(D)** *"Buckshot" visual field.* The bare areas in the grayscale are impossibly high thresholds (the computer has no shading for these out-of-range values) produced by patients who push the response button too often—even when they don't see the stimulus (many false positives). Patient who produce this pattern are not trying to convince the physician that they have a problem—it is the opposite: They want to convince the physician that they are normal (eg, to get driver's license, avoid treatment).

visual loss is suspected. However, it is important to note that patients with poor visual acuity from focal macular disease or patients who have a bilateral process may not have a clinically detectable RAPD despite true organic disease. On the other hand, a complaint of complete blindness in one eye with a normal visual field in the other eye is incompatible with a lack of an RAPD.

Electrophysiological Testing

The standard *electroretinogram (ERG)* tests only retinal function, and optic nerve or posterior visual pathway disease can certainly exist in the presence of a normal ERG. The examiner might be tempted to use the *visual evoked potential (VEP)* as the final authority in functional visual loss. The problem with this method is that the VEP can be abnormal despite a normal visual system if the patient does not appropriately accommodate, concentrate, and fixate on the alternating checkerboard pattern. Thus, an abnormal VEP does not offer final proof that an organic disorder exists. Even a normal VEP does not prove the visual system is normal, as retinal disorders and other diseases may have a normal VEP. Therefore, VEP is of limited help in proving or disproving functional visual loss.

TREATMENT

When the examination leads to the conclusion that functional visual loss is the cause of the patient's complaint, the patient (and patient's family if present) is presented with the "good news." The good news is that the examination showed the eyes and brain to be capable of normal vision and a full recovery, and that a full report supporting this conclusion will be provided. Patients who are on the "hysterical" end of the spectrum will benefit from this confident reassurance. Those who are truly "malingering" may by angry and argumentative, but will find it hard to argue with good news. A common response from such patients is, "If everything is OK, why can't I see?" The answer is that you do not know, but that in your experience the visual function will improve. Unless patients demonstrate abnormal behavior beyond their functional visual complaints, psychiatric referral is generally not helpful.

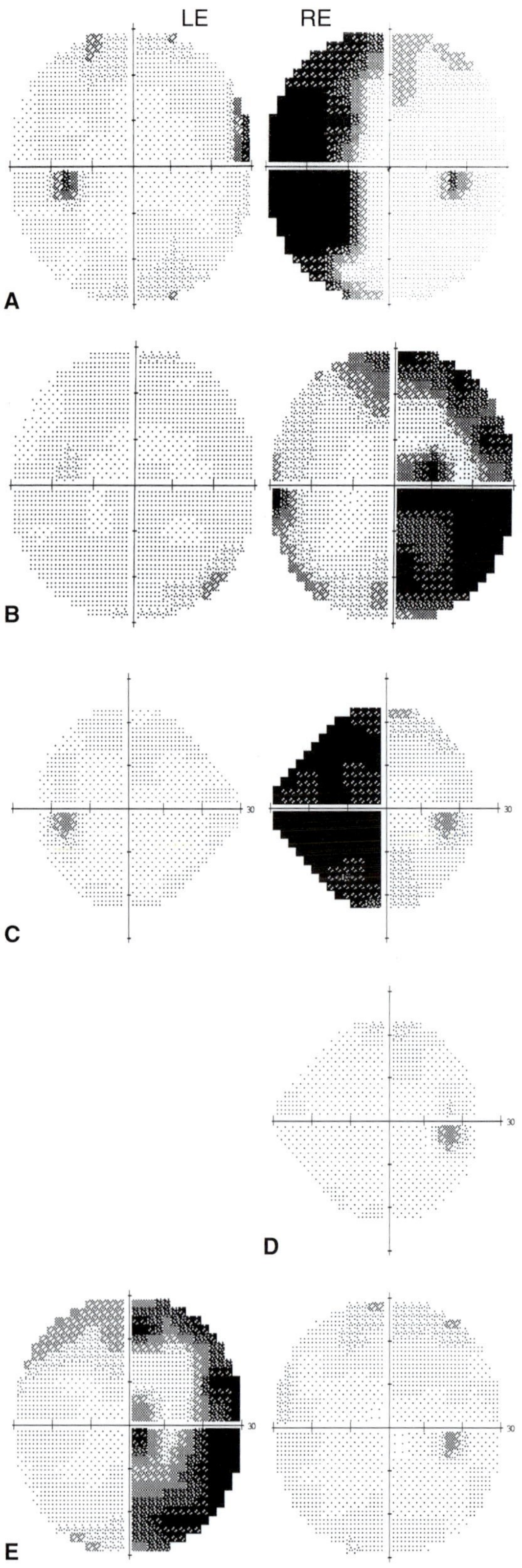

Figure 6–17. **Nonorganic visual field sequence.** A 14-year-old girl was evaluated for visual loss, ultimately determined to be nonorganic. **(A)** The initial Humphrey visual field (HVF) 30-2 showed *nasal* hemifield loss in the right eye, with a normal visual field in the left eye. **(B)** On a return visit 2 months later with no subjective change in her vision, the patient produced a visual field with *temporal* hemifield loss in the right eye. **(C)** After 6 months the visual field was repeated, now with *nasal* hemifield loss and perfect respect of the vertical meridian, seen in this 24-2 HVF. **(D)** The patient reported that she saw better when she looked to the right, so the patient was tested (same day as in **C**) with a slight face turn to the left, now producing a normal 24-2 HVF in the right eye. **(E)** Three year later, the patient's HVF 30-2 showed nasal hemifield loss in the *left* eye, with a normal visual field in the right eye!

▶ **KEY POINTS**

- Dry eye syndrome can cause transient visual blurring for periods ranging from seconds to hours.
- Ocular surface disease (eg, map-dot-fingerprint dystrophy) can cause variable visual blurring and may be subtle on slitlamp examination.
- Patients with a suspected ocular surface disorder may benefit from a trial of topical ocular lubricants prior to initiating an extensive neuro-ophthalmic work-up.
- Refraction and retinoscopy can make the diagnosis of irregular corneal astigmatism, cataract, and undiscovered refractive errors early in the evaluation, before an extensive search for unexplained visual loss is initiated.
- Findings that suggest a retinal rather than optic nerve disorder include an abnormal retina on fundus examination, a smaller RAPD than expected for visual loss, a positive photo-stress test, metamorphopsia with Amsler grid testing, and central as opposed to cecocentral visual field loss.
- OCT, IVFA, and ERG testing are important tools in evaluating patients with unexplained visual loss, as they may lead to the discovery of an undiagnosed retinal disorder.
- The fundus findings in retinal arterial occlusions may be minimal after resolution of retinal edema.
- Central serous chorioretinopathy, similar to optic neuritis, can cause a central scotoma in young patients.
- Cancer-associated retinopathy (CAR) can cause progressive bilateral visual loss in the presence of a relatively unremarkable fundus, and is usually associated with small cell lung cancer or other visceral malignancies.
- MEWDS (and other similar retinal inflammatory disorders) causes visual loss associated with photopsias, often with only subtle and transient retinal findings.
- Unilateral developmental amblyopia may be discovered incidentally, and is characterized by the lack of an acute visual complaint, absent (or small) RAPD, a normal fundus examination, and the presence of congenital strabismus or anisometropia.
- Functional visual loss in children may be a reaction to stress or an attention-getting behavior; in adults financial gain may be an unconscious or conscious factor.
- When a patient with functional visual loss has complaints in one eye only, tests performed with both eyes open can be particularly revealing, especially if the patient is unsure which eye is actually being tested.
- The physician does not need to confront the patient with functional visual loss, but should simply report the facts of a thorough examination to the patient and the patient's physicians.
- The ophthalmologist can do a tremendous amount of good in patients with nonorganic visual loss (especially in children) by offering well-grounded reassurance after a thorough neuro-ophthalmic evaluation.

SUGGESTED READING

Books

Liu GT, Volpe NJ, Galetta SL: Functional vision loss, in *Neuro-ophthalmology: Diagnosis and Management*, 2d ed. Philadelphia: Saunders Elsevier; 2010.

Miller NR: Neuro-ophthalmologic manifestations of nonorganic disease, in Miller NR, Newman NJ, Biousse V, et al. (eds): *Walsh and Hoyts' Clinical Neuro-ophthalmology*, Vol. 1, 6th ed. Baltimore, MD: Williams & Wilkins; 2005:1315–1334.

Sadun AA: Distinguishing optic nerve disease from retinal/macular disease, in Slamovits TL, Burde R (assoc eds): *Neuro-ophthalmology*, Vol. 6. in Podos SM, Yanoff M (eds): *Textbook of Ophthalmology*. London: Mosby; 1991:2.1–2.9.

Yannuzzi LA: *The Retinal Atlas*. Philadelphia, PA: Saunders/Elsevier; 2010.

Articles

Unexplained Visual Loss: Ocular Disorders

Chan JW: Paraneoplastic retinopathies and optic neuropathies. *Surv Ophthalmol* 2003;48(1):2–38.

Jacobson DM, Thirkill CE, Tipping SJ: A clinical triad to diagnose paraneoplastic retinopathy. *Ann Neurol* 1990;28:162–167.

Krachmer JH, Feder TS, Belin MW: Keratoconus and related noninflammatory corneal thinning disorders. *Surv Ophthalmol* 1984;28:293–322.

Quillen DA, Davis JB, Gottlieb JL, et al: The white dot syndromes. *Am J Ophthalmol* 2004;137(3):538–550.

Thirkill CE, Roth AM, Keltner JL: Cancer-associated retinopathy. *Arch Ophthalmol* 1987;105:372–375.

Waring GO III, Rodrigues MM, Laibson PR: Corneal dystrophies. I. Dystrophies of the epithelium, Bowman's layer and stroma. *Surv Ophthalmol* 1978;23:71–122.

Wilson CA, Choromokos EA, Sheppard R: Acute posterior multifocal placoid pigment epitheliopathy and cerebral vasculitis. *Arch Ophthalmol* 1988;106:796–800.

Functional Visual Loss

Acosta PC, Trobe JD, Shuster JJ, et al: Diagnostic strategies in the management of unexplained visual loss: a cost-benefit analysis. *Med Decis Making* 1981;1:125–144.

Gittinger JW: Functional hemianopia: a historical perspective. *Surv Ophthalmol* 1988;32:427–432.

Kathol RG, Cox TA, Corbett JJ, et al: Functional visual loss: 1. A true psychiatric disorder? *Psychol Med* 1983;13:307–314.

Kathol RG, Cox TA, Corbett JJ, et al: Functional visual loss. Follow-up of 42 cases. *Arch Ophthalmol* 1983;101:315–324.

Keane JR: Hysterical hemianopia. The "missing half" field defect. *Arch Ophthalmol* 1979;97:865–866.

Keane JR: Neuro-ophthalmic signs and symptoms of hysteria. *Neurology* 1982;32:757–762.

Keltner JL, May WN, Johnson CA, et al: The California syndrome. Functional visual complaints with potential economic impact. *Ophthalmology* 1985;92:427–435.

Scott JA, Egan RA: Prevalence of organic neuro-ophthalmologic disease in patients with functional visual loss. *Am J Ophthalmol* 2003;135:670–675.

Thompson HS: Functional visual loss. *Am J Ophthalmol* 1985;100:209–213.

Vaphiades MS, Kline LB: Functional visual disorders. Focal Points 2005: clinical modules for ophthalmologists, San Francisco: American Academy of Ophthalmology; 2005:23–33.

SECTION III

The Visual Motor System

The visual motor (efferent) system can be functionally divided into supranuclear/internuclear, nuclear/infranuclear, and orbit/extraocular muscle components. *Supranuclear* pathways originate in the cerebral cortex and are modulated by the cerebellum and vestibular apparatus to coordinate movement of both eyes with respect to the position and movement of the head and body. These areas and the functions they perform are *supranuclear* because they are higher up in the chain of command than the cranial nerve motor *nuclei* (for cranial nerves III, IV, and VI) that drive the extraocular muscles. *Internuclear* pathways provide direct connections between specific motor nuclei to coordinate binocular movement. *Infranuclear* pathways begin with the fascicles of cranial nerves III, IV, and VI and include the course of these cranial nerves to the extraocular muscles, delivering coordinated impulses to the muscles that move the eyes, eyelids, and pupil.

Disorders anywhere in the visual motor system can result in ocular misalignment (strabismus). The pattern of misalignment frequently suggests the site of the lesion, similar to the manner in which visual field defects identify the neuroanatomic location of afferent visual pathway lesions. Discussion of the ocular motor system begins with the techniques and tools used to examine the visual motor system (Chapter 7). The next three chapters work through the motor system in reverse order: extraocular muscles in the orbit and the neuromuscular junction (Chapter 8), cranial nerves III, IV, and VI (Chapter 9), and supranuclear control systems (Chapter 10). The pupil and facial nerve are also part of the efferent visual system and are discussed in Chapters 11 and 12, respectively. In each chapter, disorders and their signs and symptoms are discussed in the context of neuroanatomy.

CHAPTER 7

Examination of the Visual Motor System

- ▶ OVERVIEW AND TERMINOLOGY 185
- ▶ GENERAL OBSERVATIONS 186
- ▶ OCULAR MOTILITY 186
  - Fixation 186
  - Ocular versions and ductions 187
  - Vergence 187
  - Pursuit 188
  - Saccades 188
  - Ancillary methods 189
  - Assessing ocular alignment 190
  - Forced duction testing 192
  - Nystagmus 194
  - Eye movement recording 194
- ▶ PUPILS 194
- ▶ EYELIDS 195
  - Examination techniques 195
  - Ptosis 196
  - Eyelid retraction 197
  - Facial nerve disorders 197
- ▶ ORBIT AND ADNEXA 197
  - Inspection 197
  - Palpation 198
  - Auscultation 198
- ▶ ADDITIONAL ASSESSMENTS 199
  - Cranial nerve V 199
  - Cranial nerve VII 199
- ▶ KEY POINTS 200

This chapter expands the discussion of examination techniques summarized in Chapter 1 and is a companion to Chapter 2, which discusses examination of the afferent visual system. In this chapter, methods for examining the pupil and cranial nerves (CNs) III, IV, V, VI, and VII are presented, with greater detail provided in other chapters regarding examination of the pupil (chapter 11), CN VII (chapter 12), and CN V (chapter 13).

▶ OVERVIEW AND TERMINOLOGY

The purpose of the ocular motor system is to aim the visual axis of each eye at an object of interest. This function places an image of the object on the area of greatest retinal sensitivity: the foveola. Ideally, the motor system keeps the eyes steady and aligned with the fixation object even when the object is moving in three-dimensional space. The smooth tracking of a moving object is called *pursuit*. When a new object of interest is encountered, the motor system can quickly redirect gaze with a rapid movement to fixate on a new object of interest. This rapid refixation movement is called a *saccade*. Generally, when following or finding objects, both eyes move in the same direction (*conjugate gaze*). However, objects that move toward or away from the observer require a *disconjugate* eye movement (*vergence*). For example, an object approaching the observer's nose from a distance requires the eyes to *converge*, or turn in (right eye turns to the left, left eye turns to the right) to maintain fixation. *Divergence* occurs in the opposite setting: When the fixation object moves from near to far the eyes move outward—from a converged state to a more parallel alignment. Additional complexity is introduced when the *observer* is moving or when both the *observer and the object* are moving in space. Even in this complex situation, eye movement systems can provide stability of fixation, compensating for movement of the observer as an object is tracked.

When binocular fixation occurs, the brain can synthesize depth information from the slightly disparate views of the object (stereopsis). If the motor system fails to provide alignment, the brain cannot reconcile the two images, potentially resulting in *confusion* and *diplopia* (Box 7–1).

Six extraocular muscles insert on the globe and act in concert to rotate the eye horizontally and vertically. In addition, the globe can be rotated to a limited extent around the visual axis (*torsion*) to provide limited compensation for head or environmental tilt.

> ▶ **BOX 7-1. COMMONLY CONFUSED OCULAR MOTILITY TERMS**

Abduction/adduction Abduction is horizontal movement of an eye laterally, away from the nose. (A person who is *abducted* is taken away.) Adduction is horizontal movement of an eye medially, toward the nose.

Comitance/incomitance Ocular misalignments (strabismus) that maintain the same deviation in all gaze positions are said to be *comitant* (or concomitant). Comitance is a common feature of congenital strabismus. When the angle of deviation changes with the direction of gaze, the strabismus is said to be *incomitant*. Incomitance is the hallmark of cranial mononeuropathies, with increasing ocular misalignment in the direction of the palsied muscle.

Confusion/diplopia *Diplopia* refers to seeing the same image twice in a given field of view. However, patients are most often symptomatic with diplopia because it is accompanied by *confusion*. In confusion, two superimposed images occupy the central vision, causing confusion as to which is the real "straight ahead" image.

Ductions/versions *Ductions* describe the movement of a single eye, usually with the nontested eye covered. Common prefixes include Ab, away from the nose; Ad, toward the nose; supra, up; infra, down. *Versions* refer to the movement of both eyes together in the same direction (conjugate gaze). *Vergence* is movement of the two eyes in opposite directions (convergence and divergence).

Ocular motor nerves/oculomotor nerve The term *ocular motor nerves* refers to all three motor nerves, involved in ocular movement: cranial nerves (CNs) III, IV, and VI. The *oculomotor nerve* is CN III alone.

Palsy/paralysis/paresis These terms refer to impairment of function of a motor nerve. *Palsy* and *paralysis* suggest that the nerve is not working at all, whereas *paresis* denotes any level of weakness short of absolute. In practice the terms are often used interchangeably. These terms are also often applied to the *nerve* or the *muscle* it innervates: A CN IV palsy and a superior oblique palsy are the same thing.

Pursuit/saccades *Pursuit* ocular movements are slow, smooth, binocular ocular rotations that allow precise tracking of slow-moving objects (or movement of the observer). Pursuit is tested by having the patient track the examiner's slowly moving finger in the horizontal and vertical planes. *Saccades* are fast eye movements that redirect the eyes to a new object in the visual field. Saccades are tested by having the patient look from one of the examiner's fingers to the other in the horizontal and vertical plane. Optokinetic nystagmus (OKN) testing evaluates both pursuit and saccades. Pursuit and saccades are discussed in detail in Chapter 10.

Tropia/phoria A *phoria* (heterophoria) is an ocular deviation that occurs only when binocular fixation is disturbed, such as when one eye is covered. When viewing an object with both eyes, a subject with a phoria is capable of aligning the eyes to achieve fusion (single binocular vision). A *tropia* (heterotropia) is an ocular misalignment that is present even when both eyes are viewing, and may result in diplopia. Descriptive prefixes include *eso*, inward deviation (toward the nose); *exo*, outward; *hyper*, upward; *hypo*, downward—as in *esophoria* or *hypertropia*.

Right and left designations of tropias and phorias When a horizontal strabismus is incomitant *and* one eye is obviously the culprit, then it makes sense to say right esotropia or left exophoria. In *comitant* horizontal deviations, both eyes contribute equally to the problem and left or right is not designated. However, with vertical deviations, an eye *must* be designated and called *hypo* or *hyper*. Usually, the eye suspected of being the weakest is designated, but *left hypertropia* and *right hypotropia* say the same thing: The left eye is higher than the right.

The extraocular muscles are controlled by CNs III, IV, and VI, which originate in the brainstem. CN III also innervates the levator muscle (for elevating the upper eyelid) and carries parasympathetic input to the pupillary sphincter. The CNs are in turn coordinated by supranuclear regions in the brain. Other components of the efferent visual system include CN VII (the facial nerve), which innervates the orbicularis muscle that closes the eye and the sympathetic system that controls pupillary dilation. A brief discussion of the examination of CN V (trigeminal nerve) is included in this chapter, although it is primarily a sensory (afferent) cranial nerve.

▶ GENERAL OBSERVATIONS

The fine art of observation cannot be detailed in a textbook. The examiner should realize that the examination actually begins when the physician first encounters the patient—observing how the patient ambulates to the examination room, sits in the chair, and shakes the examiner's hand. Initial observations of the patient's facial movements, eyelids, and eye movements should be made during the history. Such observations are important because they may be more objective than when the patient is aware that his or her eyes and face are being scrutinized (see Figure 6–12).

▶ OCULAR MOTILITY

A general guide for evaluating ocular motility is presented in Table 7–1.

FIXATION

Fixation describes how the eyes remain trained on a single, stationary distant or near object. Fixation is

▶ **TABLE 7–1. EXAMINING OCULAR MOTILITY**

1. *Observe fixation*
   Observe throughout the examination, especially during visual acuity testing.
2. *Observe how the eyes move*
   Ocular versions and ductions
   Convergence
   Pursuit
   Saccades
3. *Measure eye alignment*
   Alternate cover testing and other tests
4. *Observe associated functions*
   Eyelid position
   Pupil size

---

normally *central*, with the eye pointed directly at the target object. Patients with central scotomas or anomalous retinal correspondence may display eccentric fixation. Fixation cannot occur if the patient's poor vision precludes seeing the fixation object. Patients with ocular misalignment may adopt a head turn or tilt, or may close one eye to avoid diplopia when both eyes are attempting to fixate.

Fixation is normally *steady*, without interruption. Abnormalities include square-wave jerks (brief, back-and-forth, horizontal saccadic diversions) from brainstem or cerebellar disease, or nystagmus.

Normal fixation is also *maintained*, that is, both eyes remain trained on the target, even if fixation is momentarily broken by a blink or brief occlusion of one eye. In young children, the determination of *central, steady, and maintained* fixation may be the only clues of central visual function that the examiner can determine. In adults, observations about fixation are usually made during visual acuity testing and throughout the motility examination.

OCULAR VERSIONS AND DUCTIONS

Ocular version testing looks for defects in the full range of conjugate gaze. The test is performed with both eyes open, observing each eye and comparing the two eyes at the extremes of gaze in the cardinal positions (Figure 7–1). The test is performed in a manner that allows observation of the action of each of the extraocular muscles. The actions of the vertically acting muscles are best tested when the eye is in adduction (superior and inferior oblique muscles) or abduction (superior and inferior rectus muscles). Ocular version testing also includes testing straight up and down to look for vertical gaze palsies.

In horizontal gaze, the normal eye can be abducted and adducted such that little or no sclera is visible in extreme gaze. This ability varies somewhat among individuals (especially with age) but normally should be symmetric between eyes. Vertical gaze is more difficult to judge because the eyelids move with vertical eye movements. Upgaze is particularly dependent on age, with increasing deficiency in normal patients with age. The upper eyelids need to be held up by the examiner to fully observe the eyes in the lower gaze positions. (However, it is important at some point to observe the position of the eyelids in downgaze.) The results of the motility examination can be recorded as shown in Figure 7–1.

Ocular duction testing is a monocular test, usually performed with the fellow eye covered, that examines the range of motion of a single eye. Ocular versions are performed first, followed by duction testing when necessary.

VERGENCE

Vergence testing examines the ability of the eyes to track an object from distant to near. It can be measured (in centimeters from the bridge of the nose) as the point at which an approaching accommodative target breaks down and is seen as double, and the point at which fusion is regained when the path of the target is reversed. However, these measurements are entirely dependent on the effort exerted by the patient, making interpretation difficult. Convergence effort can be maximized by having the patient focus on a near-card letter, rather than the examiner's finger. Another method is to use the patient's own finger as the convergence object, guided by the examiner from distant to near. Even blind patients can be tested in this manner because proprioceptive clues help the patient achieve convergence.

Convergence occurs by activation of both medial rectus muscles through a different supranuclear pathway than conjugate gaze. Disparities in medial rectus function between convergence and ocular versions may help to localize the lesion as supranuclear. For example, in an internuclear ophthalmoplegia (INO), an adduction deficit is present on attempted lateral gaze, but adduction is usually normal with convergence. This finding usually helps to distinguish the INO from an orbital restrictive process or partial CN III palsy.

Testing convergence is also important when *convergence insufficiency* is suspected. These patients have an exophoria or intermittent exotropia at near only and complain of vague discomfort (and occasionally diplopia) after extended near tasks. Usually a benign idiopathic condition, convergence insufficiency can also be associated with head trauma.

Convergence testing is also performed to observe the pupillary response to near (see Table 11–2) and

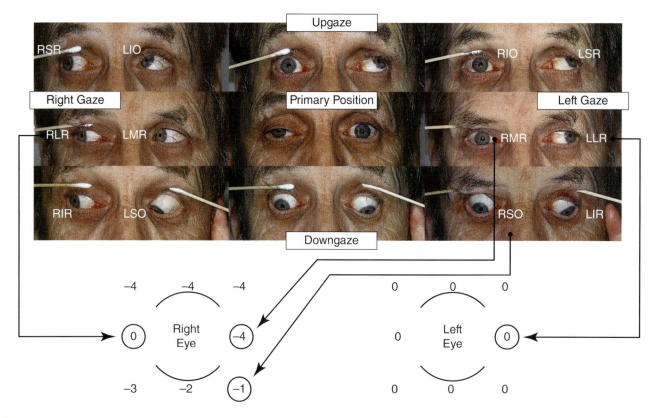

Figure 7-1. Observing and recording ocular versions. The cardinal positions of gaze are demonstrated. Note that six of the locations (outer columns) allow relative isolation of the action of individual extraocular muscles. Straight up and down assess vertical gaze. One method of recording observations of ocular versions is shown in the lower half of the illustration: 0 is normal motility and −4 means that the eye cannot get past primary position, with intermediate underaction graded −1, −2, or −3. A −5 designates that the eye cannot even achieve midposition, suggesting contracture of the opposing muscle. A "+" denotes an overaction (not shown in this example). The patient presented in this example has a right oculomotor nerve palsy. Observe how the numbers correspond to the action of individual muscles in each eye (*arrows*).

should be performed whenever the pupillary light reaction is poor.

PURSUIT

Pursuit testing checks the brain's supranuclear smooth-tracking mechanisms (discussed in Chapter 10). Pursuit is tested by asking the patient to follow the examiner's finger or other target as it slowly and smoothly moves between the extremes in the horizontal plane and then in the vertical plane. The pursuit target should be at least an arm's length from the patient to minimize confounding factors from convergence and accommodation. Abnormal pursuit may be *saccadic* (choppy) rather than smooth in one or both directions. Pursuit testing can be performed as an integral part of testing ocular versions—observations of how smoothly the patient can track the examiner's moving finger evaluates pursuit, and the ability of each eye to reach the endpoint at extreme gaze evaluates ocular versions.

SACCADES

Saccades are tested by asking patients to look rapidly from primary position (looking at the examiner's nose) to a target (the examiner's finger positioned in right and left gaze in the horizontal plane or straight up and down in the vertical plane). Supranuclear abnormalities may cause *hypometric* saccades, in which the eyes do not line up on the new fixation target in one quick movement, but require additional smaller saccades to finally arrive on target. *Hypermetric* saccades, in which the eyes overshoot the target, also occur. Unilateral slow saccades are identified by comparing the two eyes: The slow eye is still moving toward the target after the normal eye has completed its saccade. Unilateral slow saccades are seen in an eye with a neurogenic palsy, in contrast to saccades that are abruptly halted in restrictive disorders such as thyroid eye disease. Slow movement of the adducting eye alone suggests an internuclear ophthalmoplegia (INO). Attempted upward saccades produce convergence-retraction nystagmus in patients with dorsal midbrain syndrome (see Chapter 10).

ANCILLARY METHODS

Optokinetic Nystagmus Testing

Optokinetic nystagmus (OKN) testing was discussed briefly in the context of *afferent* visual system testing as an objective physiological response to test gross vision (see Table 6–2). The afferent limb of this physiological response begins with a moving visual stimulus, usually alternating black and white stripes on a rotating drum, but any interesting stimuli that are equally spaced at appropriate intervals moving across the visual field will work (Figure 7–2). The *efferent* limb consists of pursuit of the moving target in one direction and a refixation saccade in the opposite direction to acquire the next target. This test has value as a physiological stimulus that allows observation of saccade and pursuit movements, even in patients who may be incapable of cooperating with other examination techniques. In addition, the rapidly repeating saccades and pursuit greatly increase the clinical sensitivity of detecting abnormalities.

When performing an optokinetic test, the amplitude and frequency of the induced nystagmus should be observed, particularly when compared to the response from stimulus movement in the opposite direction. Box 7–2 lists the important clinical uses of the optokinetic response.

Oculocephalic (Doll's Head) Maneuver

The oculocephalic maneuver helps determine the level of a lesion in a gaze palsy because it uses the vestibular system to move the eyes. The test is performed by rotating the patient's head in the plane of the gaze palsy while the patient fixates on a stationary object. Patients who are unable to produce a gaze movement with this maneuver have a lesion at or below the level of vestibular input to the efferent visual motor system. Patients with a gaze palsy who can achieve full horizontal gaze with this maneuver but cannot do it volitionally have a supranuclaear palsy. The test can be performed for both horizontal and vertical gaze palsies.

Oculovestibular (Caloric) Testing

Similar to the oculocephalic maneuver, oculovestibular testing uses vestibular input to drive gaze movement and is especially useful in patients with altered consciousness who cannot cooperate with other examination methods.

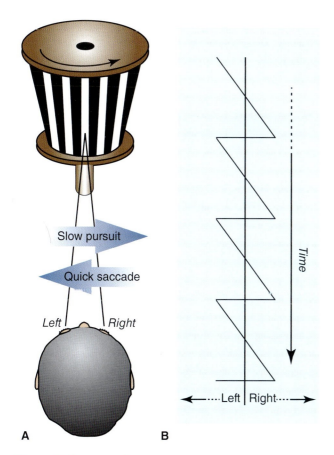

Figure 7–2. **Optokinetic nystagmus test.** (A) As the drum is rotated from left to right across the patient's field, pursuit movements are generated to follow the stimulus to the right, with rapid refixation saccades to the left. (B) A plot of the eye movements in response to the optokinetic stimulus is shown.

▶ **BOX 7–2. UTILITY OF OPTOKINETIC TESTING**

AFFERENT VISUAL SYSTEM
Objective determination of vision in patients with nonorganic vision loss

EFFERENT VISUAL SYSTEM
Dorsal midbrain syndrome. Upward saccades (downward moving optokinetic nystagmus [OKN] stimulus) generate convergence retraction nystagmus.
Internuclear ophthalmoplegia. The slowed adducting saccades (and abducting nystagmus of the opposite eye) are accentuated when the OKN stimulus is rotated toward the affected eye.
Progressive supranuclear palsy (early). The patient's eyes follow the stimulus but cannot generate a return saccade (the "drift" sign).
Congenital nystagmus. When an OKN stimulus is presented at the null point, the nystagmus induced is opposite in direction from the normal response in about two-thirds of patients.
Parietal lobe lesions may affect the pursuit response when the target is moved toward the side of the lesion, diminishing the amplitude of the nystagmus (when compared to rotation to the opposite side).

▶ BOX 7-3. PERFORMING CALORIC TESTING

The patient is positioned with the head elevated 30° so that the horizontal semicircular canals become vertical. Irrigation of *cold* water in one ear causes nystagmus with the fast phase to the *opposite* side; *warm* water results in the fast phase to the *same* side. The mnemonic is COWS, for Cold-Opposite and Warm-Same. Cold water in both ears simultaneously causes vertical nystagmus with the fast phase down, and bilateral warm water simultaneously results in the fast phase up. The mnemonic for bilateral simultaneous irrigation is CUWD, for Cold Up, Warm Down. These bovine mnemonics can be combined: "COWS chew their CU(W)D."

The test works by cooling or warming and thus inducing movement of the endolymphatic fluid within the semicircular canals. The induced flow simulates head rotation and results in a horizontal jerk nystagmus, as if the patient were rotating in a chair, without any actual movement of the patient's head. The saccade and pursuit components of the nystagmus can then be evaluated (Box 7-3).

ASSESSING OCULAR ALIGNMENT
Quantitative Tests

Alternate cover testing is a practical method for estimating and quantifying an ocular deviation. The patient is required to have sufficient vision in each eye to permit fixation. As the patient is fixating on a distant target, the examiner alternates a cover over each eye. As the cover is moved, the examiner observes how the uncovered eye moves to take up fixation. For example, an esotropic patient is made to fixate with his or her right eye by covering the left eye. When the cover is moved quickly from the left to the right eye, the left eye is observed to rotate laterally (abduct) in order to fixate on the target. A similar abducting movement is observed in the right eye as the cover is moved back to the left. This movement tells the examiner that the patient has an esodeviation whose magnitude is reflected by the distance the eye has to travel to refixate. This technique will reveal both heterophorias and heterotopias (see Box 7-1).

The deviation can be measured by using prisms that redirect the line of sight and correct the deviation (Figure 7-3). Vertical ocular deviations can be measured in the same manner (with base up or down prism).

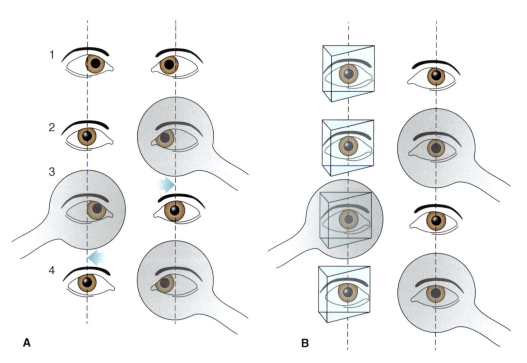

Figure 7-3. Alternate cover test.
(A) An esotropic patient (1) fixates on a distant target with the right eye when the left eye is covered (2). The left eye turns in while under the cover, which becomes evident as it moves out to take up fixation when the cover is moved to the right eye (3). Similarly the right eye is seen to move outward to fixate when the cover moves back to the left eye (4). **(B)** A base-out prism can "fix" the esodeviation (the prism apex points in the direction of the deviation). The examiner estimates the prism power, changing the value appropriately if movement still occurs with alternate cover testing. When all movement is neutralized (*as shown*), the power of the prism is a measure of the esodeviation in *prism diopters*. Exodeviations and vertical deviations can also be measured with alternate cover testing.

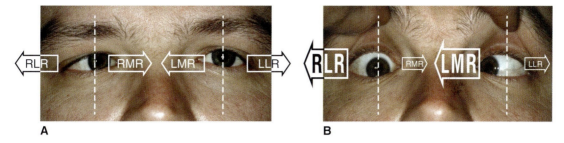

Figure 7–4. Primary and secondary deviation.
Secondary deviation is greater than primary deviation, as seen in this example of right lateral rectus palsy. **(A)** Primary deviation. When the normal left eye is fixating, the right eye deviates inward, reflecting the unopposed baseline tone of the right medial rectus. **(B)** Secondary deviation. When the palsied right eye is fixating, an enormous outflow to the weak right lateral rectus is required to maintain fixation. This outflow also goes to its yoke muscle—the left medial rectus—causing it to strongly deviate inwardly.

Combined vertical and horizontal deviation can be measured by neutralizing the horizontal and vertical components separately. The alternate cover test can be performed in any of the cardinal positions of gaze by having the patient maintain fixation and turning the patient's head. One method of documentation is to place the alternate cover test results on the same diagram on which ocular versions are recorded (see Figure 7–1).

The Hirschberg test can be used when the patient is not capable of fixating with one eye, such as in a patient with a sensory exotropia. With this method, the patient is instructed to look at the examiner's penlight; this action centers the light reflex on the fixating eye. Decentration of the light reflex in the deviating eye provides an estimate of the ocular misalignment: Each millimeter of decentration equals approximately 7° of ocular deviation when the light is 33 cm from the patient. This method can be further refined by placing prisms over the fixating eye until the light reflex is centered on the nonfixating eye (the Krimsky test). Other methods that measure ocular misalignment include the Maddox wing, amblyoscope, Lancaster red/green test, and Hess screen. *Diplopic visual fields* are performed using the Goldmann perimeter with both eyes open. The patient responds when the target light moves from an area of single vision to the point at which it doubles. A curvilinear isopter defines the area of single vision.

Primary and Secondary Deviation

Hering law of motor correspondence states that equal innervation is provided to *yoke muscles*. Yoke muscles are the corresponding muscles from each eye that move the eye in the same direction of gaze. For example, the right lateral rectus and the left medial rectus are activated together with equal innervation to perform right gaze and are therefore yoke muscles. If the right lateral rectus muscle is paretic but the left eye is fixating, then the esodeviation of the right eye reflects only the greater baseline tone of the right medial rectus over the paretic right lateral rectus. The observed deviation of the right eye is called the *primary* deviation. However, to fixate with the paretic right eye, enormous effort is required by the weak right lateral rectus to pull the eye straight. An equally strong innervation to the yoked left medial rectus results in a large esodeviation of the left eye, called the *secondary* deviation (Figure 7–4). *The secondary deviation is always greater than the primary deviation.* This principle may be helpful in determining which eye in an incomitant strabismus has a paretic muscle. It also has relevance because the *amount of deviation observed or measured in any test of ocular alignment depends on which eye is fixating*. Ambiguity can be avoided by using a consistent routine, such as always holding prisms over the right eye in the alternate cover test, and by recording how a given test was performed.

Red Glass Test

This test is performed by placing a red lens before the right eye (by convention) while the patient looks with both eyes at a point of light (penlight). Patients with ocular misalignment see a separate red and white light. The orientation and distance separating the red and white lights is a measure of the ocular misalignment. If the right eye is esotropic, the red light appears to be to the right of the white light (uncrossed diplopia). The red light is seen to the left of the white light in an exotropia (crossed diplopia). If the right eye is hypertrophic, the red light appears below the white light, and above it if the right eye is hypotrophic. As the light is moved to each of the cardinal positions of gaze, the subjective separation reported by the patient can help determine the degree and type of incomitance.

Single Maddox Rod

Similar to the red glass test, a red Maddox rod lens over the right eye can be used to dissociate the two eyes and measure ocular misalignment. The lens transforms the white light into a red *line*, oriented perpendicular to the Maddox rod striations (Figure 7–5). The advantage of this device is that the examiner can isolate the vertical component of a deviation (how far the white light is above or below the red horizontal line). The single Maddox rod is particularly useful in exploring vertical deviations with the three-step test (described in the following section). The lens can be rotated with the striations horizontal (producing a *vertical* line) to isolate the horizontal deviation (how far the white light is to the left or right of the red vertical line).

Bielschowsky Three-Step Test

The three-step test is a sequence of measurements of vertical ocular misalignment that logically isolates a weak vertically acting muscle. This test assumes that only one vertically acting muscle is paretic, which is not always the case. The amount of hypertrophia (by alternate cover testing or single Maddox rod) is compared in right and left gaze and in right and left head tilt. Figure 7–6 explains the logic behind these comparisons and how the weak muscle is determined. In practice, the vast majority of isolated, weak vertically acting muscles are superior oblique palsies. It is instructive to understand how the three-step test works because on rare occasions the sequence is needed to diagnose a muscle palsy other than a superior oblique palsy. Memorizing the sequence for superior oblique palsies is of great utility, even if the details of the test are soon forgotten. Right superior oblique palsies produce a *right* hypertrophia, which is greater in *left* gaze and with a *right* head tilt (mnemonic: right superior oblique palsy is right-left-right; left superior oblique palsy is left-right-left). Long-standing palsies do not always obey the rules of the three-step test, so this test may be less useful with chronic motility disorders.

Double Maddox Rod

A double Maddox rod test consists of a red Maddox rod lens over the right eye and a white Maddox rod lens over the left eye (in a trial lens frame), oriented so that the patient perceives two horizontal lines when viewing a penlight. The examiner helps the patient adjust the lenses so that both lines appear to the patient to be level and parallel. The degree of ocular torsion can be measured directly by the axis of the Maddox rods (using the astigmatism axis scale on the trial frame). This test is useful in measuring torsion from superior oblique palsies (see Figure 9–6B).

FORCED DUCTION TESTING

Abnormal ocular motility may occur because free movement of the eye is restricted. If the eye has a nonrestrictive

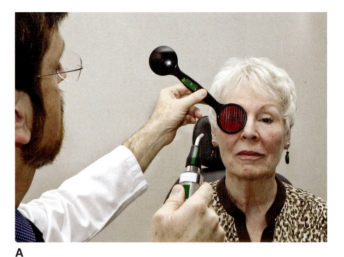

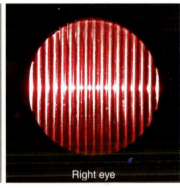

Figure 7–5. **Single Maddox rod.** **(A)** The patient is being tested for a vertical deviation. The Maddox rod is held over the right eye (with the ridges oriented vertically). **(B)** The patient looks at the light source and sees the light with the left eye but a red horizontal line with the right eye. Observe how the line perceived by the patient is perpendicular to the striations of the Maddox lens. **(C)** With both eyes, the horizontal line and the point of light are superimposed and serve as a measure of vertical misalignment. The patient's observations of the images from the right and left eyes are opposite the actual relative positions of the eyes. In this patient, the line (seen by the right eye) is *below* the light, consistent with a right *hypertropia*.

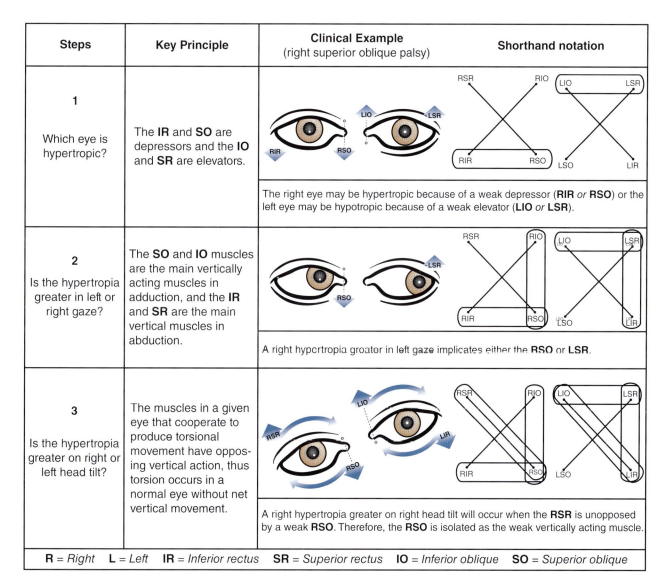

Figure 7–6. **Bielschowsky three-step test.**
The three-step test is a logical sequence of observations designed to find which muscle is the cause of vertical misalignment. The test is valid only if a single muscle is at fault, and may not work for long-standing deviations. The first column asks the key clinical question at each stage, and the second column states the principles involved. The remaining columns refer to this specific example of a right superior oblique palsy. The final column shows the classic shorthand notation often used to follow the logic of the three-step test. Potentially paretic muscles are circled at each step of the test, finally isolating a single muscle that is included in each step's circle. Note that the muscles are labeled *in their field of action*, not their anatomic location. For example, the right superior oblique (RSO) is labeled "down and in." Observe that in the clinical example pictured the corneal light reflex and position of the limbus relative to the eyelid margin offer clues that this patient has a right hypertropia.

strabismus (neurogenic, myasthenia), the examiner should be able to complete an attempted eye movement by the patient by physically moving a topically anesthetized eye to complete the duction. In a few cases (especially patients with profound horizontal motility deficits), a cotton-tipped applicator at the limbus can be used to push the eye (Figure 7–7A). However, the most rigorous method is to use toothed forceps to hold and move the eye at the muscle insertion. Using forceps to perform forced ductions is a routine part of strabismus surgery (when the patient is under anesthesia). It can be performed in the clinic by using topical anesthetic drops/ointment followed by 10% cocaine-soaked cotton-tipped applicators held at the site to allow grasping of a muscle insertion with a toothed forceps. The test is performed by grasping the insertion of the *opposing* muscle. The patient is instructed to look into the field of action of the weak muscle (the palsied direction) while

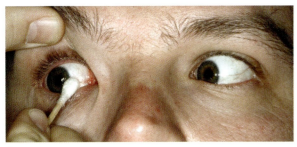

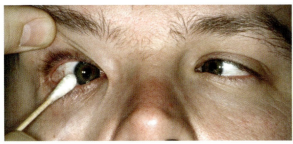

Figure 7-7. Forced duction testing. Although toothed forceps are preferred to perform forced ductions, this patient with a large abduction deficit could be adequately assessed with topical anesthetic and a cotton-tipped applicator. This patient is shown in Figure 7-4. **(A)** With the patient looking in right gaze, the examiner can easily push the globe into abduction without encountering resistance. This action suggests that no restrictive disorder is present, and that the abduction deficit is most likely neurogenic. **(B)** The force generation portion of the test is performed by holding the right eye in adduction as the patient attempts right gaze. Very little pressure is required to hold the eye, suggesting that the lateral rectus is generating little or no power.

the examiner moves the eye in the same direction. (A similar method that may be less traumatic to the eye is to grasp the junction of the conjunctiva and Tenon capsule at the limbus with the forceps). In restrictive strabismus, the examiner will feel resistance or be unable to complete the duction.

The amount of force generated by a muscle can be judged by grasping the insertion of the *palsied* muscle when the eye is out of the field of action of the muscle. The examiner then judges the force generated while the patent is asked to look into the field of action of the weak muscle (see Figure 7-7B).

Forced duction and force generation testing are needed only infrequently in neuroophthalmology. These tests are helpful when a restrictive component is suspected but not evident by other clinical tests, such as in orbital trauma with suspected medial or inferior rectus muscle entrapment and orbital Graves disease. Disorders that are initially nonrestrictive (such as CN palsies) can develop a restrictive component with time because the antagonist muscle may develop contractures. The forced duction test must therefore be interpreted with caution in patients with long-standing ocular misalignment.

Another method for evaluating the possibility of a restrictive motility disorder is to measure the change in intraocular pressure from primary position to eccentric gaze. For example, attempted upgaze in orbital Graves disease may rotate the globe against a large, noncompliant, inferior rectus muscle, raising the intraocular pressure. A restrictive process is suspected when there is an elevation of 5 mm Hg or more in the intraocular pressure when measured in extreme upgaze (with a Perkins or other handheld tonometer), compared to the pressure in primary position.

NYSTAGMUS

The presence of nystagmus can be observed during ocular version testing. Important characteristics include the type (jerk or pendular), direction (if jerk), amplitude, and frequency at each cardinal position of gaze, as well as at near. Latent nystagmus is present only when one eye is covered. By consciously examining for nystagmus on all patients, the physician gains confidence in distinguishing physiological (normal) endpoint nystagmus from pathological findings. Nystagmus is discussed in detail in Chapter 10.

EYE MOVEMENT RECORDING

Several methods exist to quantitatively measure and record eye movements and nystagmus. Placement of a coil-embedded contact lens on the eye, within the framework of a magnetic field, allows precise measurement of ocular rotations. Noncontact methods include infrared photodiodes and video-based methods.

Dynamic recording of motility disorders helps in the clinical determination of a diagnosis, but perhaps more importantly, it increases understanding of the complex mechanisms involved in ocular movement. Much of our current understanding of the neurophysiology of eye movements comes from the study of eye movement recordings in patients with motility disturbances.

▶ PUPILS

The pupil size in light and in darkness should be recorded, with particular attention to differences in pupil size (anisocoria). Patients who do not have a brisk pupillary response to light should have the pupillary response to near observed. Further details of the pupillary examination are discussed in Chapter 11. The relative afferent pupillary defect (RAPD) test is discussed in Chapter 2.

► EYELIDS

Evaluation of the eyelids is an important part of the neuro-ophthalmic examination. Abnormal eyelid position and function can be caused by disorders involving CN III, the oculosympathetic pathway, and CN VII, as well as supranuclear pathways, or as a result of neuromuscular diseases. To avoid unwarranted neurological investigations, it is also important for the physician to recognize non-neurological eyelid abnormalities (such as ptosis from levator dehiscence or eyelid edema).

EXAMINATION TECHNIQUES

The size of the ocular fissure is the net result of forces opening the eye (eyelid retractors) and those closing the eye (eyelid protractors). Thus, an ocular fissure that is abnormally narrow may be the result of a retractor weakness (ptosis) or protractor hyperactivity (orbicularis spasm). A palpebral fissure that is abnormally wide can result from retractor hyperactivity (such as eyelid retraction in orbital Graves disease) or protractor weakness (as in acute facial palsy). It is not always obvious which eye is abnormal when there is an asymmetry of the palpebral fissures. Does the eye with the smaller fissure have eyelid ptosis, or does the opposite eye have eyelid retraction? Furthermore, ptosis on one side may cause contralateral eyelid retraction, because the effort generated to lift the ptotic eyelid is shared bilaterally. This form of eyelid retraction promptly reverses when the examiner gently lifts the ptotic eyelid. Important elements of the eyelid examination are summarized in Table 7–2 and Figure 7–8.

► TABLE 7–2. EXAMINATION OF EYELID POSITION AND FUNCTION

Examination Component	Method of Measurement or Observation	Examples of Abnormalities
Observe eyelid position	Record as millimeters of ptosis, the MRD, or *palpebral fissure height* (see Figure 7–8).	A Horner syndrome typically causes only 1–2 mm of ptosis. The degree of ptosis may be highly variable in myasthenia.
Evaluate levator function	Measure upper eyelid excursion in millimeters from extreme downgaze to extreme upgaze, with the brow immobilized by the examiner to prevent any contribution from the frontalis musculature.	Levator function is normal in levator dehiscence, but usually poor in congenital ptosis, myasthenia, or CN III paresis.
Look for lid lag	Present when there is failure of the upper eyelid to follow the downward excursion of the eyeball. A patient who displays *lid lag* will have a higher resting position of the eyelid in relation to the eye in downgaze when compared to the primary gaze (the lid lags behind the eye in downgaze).	Lid lag is often seen in orbital Graves disease and is the result of the decreased elasticity of the levator muscle secondary to muscle fibrosis or infiltration. Lid lag is also a characteristic of congenital ptosis, but not of acquired ptosis.
Measure eyelid crease	Distance from the eyelid margin to the major upper eyelid crease, which is formed by a portion of the levator muscle insertion.	A high, asymmetric, or absent *eyelid crease* is a sign of the loss of attachment of the levator aponeurosis to the tarsus and skin (levator dehiscence), or may occur when levator function is very poor.
Evaluate orbicularis function; look for lagophthalmos	*Lagophthalmos* is the inability of the eyelids to close completely. Weakness of the protractor (orbicularis oculi) or restriction of the retractor (levator palpebrae superioris) may cause lagophthalmos.	CN VII paralysis with weakening of the protractor muscles typically causes a profound lagophthalmos. Poor compliance of the levator muscle such as that seen in congenital ptosis, orbital Graves disease, trauma, or following surgical resection of the levator palpebrae superioris muscle are other potential causes. Lagophthalmos can lead to corneal ulceration and blindness.
Observe ocular motility	Ptosis and an *ocular motility disorder* may be observed in oculomotor paresis, myasthenia gravis, chronic progressive external ophthalmoplegia, or Duane syndrome. Congenital ptosis may be associated with superior rectus dysfunction or Marcus Gunn jaw winking phenomena. Eyelid retraction and a motility disorder suggest orbital Graves disease.	
Observe pupils	Anisocoria: A large *pupil* on the side of the ptosis may indicate a CN III palsy or posttraumatic ptosis associated with iris sphincter injury, and a miotic pupil on the side of the ptosis may indicate an oculosympathetic paresis (Horner syndrome).	

Abbreviations: CN, cranial nerve; MRD, margin-to-light reflex distance.

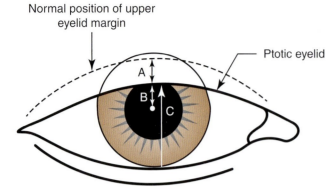

Figure 7–8. Methods for measuring and recording upper eyelid position.
(A) Ptosis (or retraction) is measured (in millimeters) from the normal position of the eyelid, assuming the normal position of the upper eyelid is 1 mm below the upper limbus. **(B)** The *margin-to-light reflex distance* is the distance of the upper eyelid from a central cornea light reflex (produced by having the patient look at the examiner's penlight held centrally, close to the examiner's nose). **(C)** The *palpebral fissure height* is less specific and does not specify the actual position of the eyelid relative to the globe. (Used with permission, from Martin TJ, Yeatts PR. Abnormalities of eyelid position and function. *Semin Neurol* 2000;20(1):33, Fig. 3.)

PTOSIS

Ptosis, or more precisely, *blepharoptosis,* describes an abnormally low resting position of the upper eyelid because of levator insufficiency. True ptosis should be distinguished from dermatochalasis, a condition in which the loose, redundant skin of the upper eyelid droops over the eyelid margin (Figure 7–9). The many causes of ptosis are outlined in Table 7–3 and are addressed in detail in the discussion of specific diseases throughout this book. Two non-neurogenic conditions that commonly cause ptosis deserve special mention: congenital ptosis and involutional ptosis.

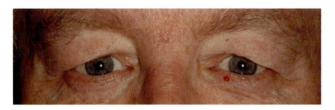

Figure 7–9. Pseudoptosis: dermatochalasis. With aging, the skin of the upper eyelid can become lax and redundant (dermatochalasis), drooping down below the upper eyelid margin and simulating a ptotic upper eyelid. True ptosis is defined by the position of the upper eyelid margin, not the skin draped over the edge of the eyelid.

▶ **TABLE 7–3. DIFFERENTIAL DIAGNOSIS OF ACQUIRED PTOSIS**

Neuropathic
 Oculomotor nucleus/fascicles/nerve palsy
 Oculosympathetic paresis
 Supranuclear ptosis

Neuromuscular junction
 Myasthenia gravis
 Botulism

Myogenic
 Myotonic dystrophy
 CPEO

Aponeurotic (levator dehiscence)
 Involutional ("senile") ptosis
 Contact lens wear
 Following protracted or severe upper eyelid edema
 Trauma

Mechanical
 Eyelid tumors

Pseudoptosis
 Dermatochalasis
 Orbicularis activation (blepharospasm, etc)
 Globe retraction (Duane retraction syndrome, enophthalmos)

Abbreviation: CPEO, chronic, progressive external ophthalmoplegia.

Congenital ptosis refers to a developmental abnormality of the levator palpebrae superioris muscle that results in ptosis. Ptosis may be unilateral or bilateral and can occur as a component of an inherited syndrome (eg, autosomal dominant blepharophimosis syndrome). In congenital ptosis the levator palpebrae superioris muscle contains more fibroblasts than muscle fibers, resulting in both poor contraction and poor relaxation. Therefore, lid lag in downgaze is a characteristic feature of congenital ptosis that is not present in most acquired forms of ptosis. The presence of lid lag also explains why children with either unilateral or bilateral congenital ptosis develop a head position (with chin up) to maintain unobstructed vision.

Involutional ptosis (also called "senile" ptosis) is the result of age-related changes in the levator aponeurosis or levator muscle, and is the most common type of ptosis encountered in clinical practice. Involutional ptosis is commonly the result of *levator dehiscence*, in which aging or other factors cause the levator aponeurosis to become stretched, thinned, or detached from its insertion at the tarsus and skin of the upper eyelid. This results in ptosis, but with normal levator function (excursion). The upper eyelid crease is typically elevated or absent, reflecting loss of the levator insertion. Contact lens wear, recurrent eyelid edema, topical steroid use, and trauma are common causes of

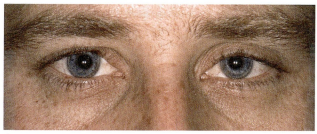

A

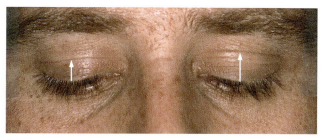

B

Figure 7-10. Elevated eyelid crease in aponeurosis dehiscence.
A 27-year-old man was referred to evaluate a possible neurological cause for left unilateral ptosis. **(A)** There was no associated motility disturbance (to suggest a cranial nerve III paresis), no anisocoria (to suggest a Horner syndrome), and no variability (that would suggest myasthenia). The patient was a contact lens wearer for many years. **(B)** The presence of an elevated eyelid crease on the left (compare arrows) with normal levator function confirmed levator dehiscence as the cause of ptosis.

levator dehiscence that may occur in younger patients (Figure 7–10).

EYELID RETRACTION

Eyelid retraction refers to an abnormally high position of the upper eyelid, giving the appearance of staring. Retraction of the lower eyelid may also contribute to this appearance. Eyelid retraction may give the false impression of exophthalmos, and patients may present with a complaint that their "eye has gotten bigger." Eyelid retraction is common in orbital Graves disease but can be caused by other disorders (Figure 7–11; Table 7–4).

FACIAL NERVE DISORDERS

Hyperactivity (blepharospasm) *or paresis of the orbicularis oculi* (facial nerve disorders) can also affect the position and appearance of the eyelids and ocular fissure. These disorders are discussed in Chapter 12.

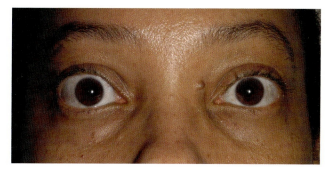

Figure 7-11. Eyelid retraction in orbital Graves disease (thyroid eye disease).
The normal position of the eyelids relative to the limbus is shown in Figure 7–8. The lower eyelid is usually right at the inferior limbus, and the upper eyelid usually covers the superior limbus. Eyelid *retraction* may allow the white of the sclera to be visible between the upper or lower eyelid margin and the limbus (called *scleral show*). This patient with orbital Graves disease has bilateral eyelid retraction with scleral show—this appearance has been called "thyroid stare."

▶ **TABLE 7-4. DIFFERENTIAL DIAGNOSIS OF EYELID RETRACTION**

Graves disease (unilateral or bilateral)
Midbrain disorders (bilateral, but may be asymmetrical)
Aberrant regeneration of the oculomotor nerve

Pseudoretraction
  From contralateral ptosis
  From ipsilateral facial palsy

Levator restriction from trauma or surgery

▶ ORBIT AND ADNEXA

The orbital examination is important in both efferent and afferent disorders because orbital diseases can affect the optic nerve, the ocular motor cranial nerves, the extraocular muscles, and the position of the eye in the orbit. Three key components include inspection, palpation, and auscultation.

INSPECTION

As discussed, the position, laxity, and function of the eyelids should be inspected. The eyelids are also a common site for potentially invasive tumors, such as basal cell carcinoma. Inspection of the conjunctiva may reveal the tortuous vascular arterialization associated with a carotid-cavernous fistula, or a sarcoid granuloma may be found in the inferior fornix. Abnormalities of the position and symmetry of the globes include exophthalmos (orbital Graves disease and orbital tumors), enophthalmos (trauma, scirrhous metastatic breast carcinoma), and globe ptosis (trauma, orbital tumors). Antero-posterior asymmetry is best observed from a "bird's-eye view" and can be measured with exophthalmometry devices (Figure 7–12).

PALPATION

Traumatic fractures of the orbital rim can be identified by gentle palpation with the index and middle fingers. The fingers can also explore the superior orbital sulcus, identifying lacrimal gland tumors or other masses. The examiner can compare the two orbits by *retropulsion*: gently pushing each globe into the orbit (through a closed eyelid) to judge the resistance of retrobulbar structures. Abnormal resistance to compression is often identified in orbital Graves disease and with orbital masses.

AUSCULTATION

In patients with potential arteriovenous malformations (especially after trauma), auscultation of the globe, orbit, or head may reveal audible bruits (Figure 7–13). All

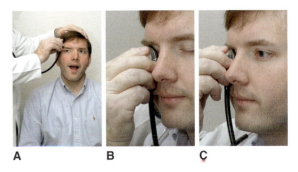

Figure 7–13. **Using the stethoscope to auscultate the eye and head.**
The stethoscope is particularly helpful in the neuro-ophthalmic evaluation in two situations: listening for vascular bruits (embolic and vascular occlusive diseases, and carotid cavernous fistula) and detecting the flutter of superior oblique myokymia. Auscultation over the temporalis muscle (with the bell or diaphragm) should be performed in patients with amaurosis fugax for possible ophthalmic carotid bruits or bruits transmitted from more proximal sources. When auscultating over the temple (where the squamosal bone is the thinnest), the patient should be instructed to open the mouth to inhibit noise from temporalis muscle contraction **(A)**. Both the eyeball and temple should be auscultated when a carotid-cavernous fistula is suspected. When auscultating over the eye, its best to use the diaphragm rather than the bell, as the hole in the bottom of the bell is easily occluded by loose eyelid skin that muffles the sound. When listening over the eye, have the patient close both eyes and then place the diaphragm over the globe **(B)**. Then instruct the patient to open the opposite eye (which will inhibit orbicularis muscle contraction noise in the auscultated eye **(C)**. In superior oblique myokymia, the sound of the fluttering superior oblique muscle can sometimes be heard with auscultation over the globe—sounding like a motorcycle revving up—due to the abrupt starting and stopping of the rapid contractions.

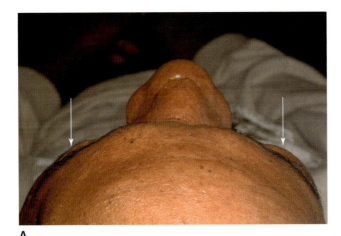

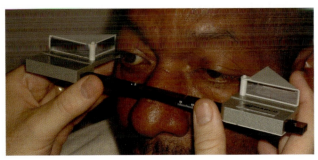

Figure 7–12. **Observing and measuring proptosis.**
The normal anteroposterior position of globes relative to the skull and orbital rim is different among racial groups and can vary significantly among individuals, but is usually the same (symmetric) for an individual's two eyes. **(A)** Asymmetry is best observed by laying the patient back in the chair, with the observer standing above the patient's head (bird's-eye view). The physician can then compare how far each eye protrudes in front of the brow/orbital rim (best with the patient's eyes open, but also works well with eyes closed, as in this example). This patient has proptosis of the right eye—more of the right eye can be seen in front of the brow than the left eye. **(B)** Proptosis can be measured with the Hertel exophthalmometer. The device is adjusted to rest on the lateral orbital rims of the patient. Right-angle prisms in the device redirect the examiner's line of site so a lateral view of the eye is visible with a superimposed millimeter scale.

patients who describe hearing pulsatile noises should be carefully auscultated. Because bruits originating in the neck and precordium can occasionally be transmitted to the head, these areas should also be auscultated when a cranial bruit is found.

▶ ADDITIONAL ASSESSMENTS

CRANIAL NERVE V

Ocular and facial sensation (light touch) can be tested by using a tissue or a cotton-tipped applicator, with the cotton pulled and twisted to a point. This procedure is performed by having the patient close his or her eyes and comparing sensation on the left and right sides of the face above the brow (V_1) and over the cheek (V_2). Pain sensation can be tested by using the sharp point of a broken wooden cotton-tip applicator stick to compare pin-prick sensation in the same areas. The corneal blink reflex allows an element of objectivity because the presence and magnitude of a reflexive blink is used to compare corneal sensation between the two eyes (Box 7–4). Having the patient compare the irritation of eyedrops used during the examination is another way to subjectively evaluate corneal sensation.

The motor component of CN V can be evaluated by observing that the jaw is midline and by testing the strength of the lateral pterygoids by having the patient move his or her jaw sideways against resistance. In addition, the relative bulk of the masseter muscles can be palpated when patients are asked to grit their teeth. Further details on assessing CN V are found in Chapter 13.

CRANIAL NERVE VII

Facial nerve function is assessed by observing the symmetry of the face during the history and examination, especially the brow, nasolabial fold, and corners of the mouth. Orbicularis strength can be tested by having the patient close his or her eyes tightly while the examiner attempts to manually open them, or by using the eyelashes as a relative gauge of orbicularis strength with tight eyelid closure (Figure 7–14). Raising the brows to wrinkle the forehead, puckering the lips, and smiling to show teeth further test facial motor function. Abnormalities of facial nerve function include weakness, episodic spasm, increased tone, or synkinesis (discussed in detail in Chapter 12).

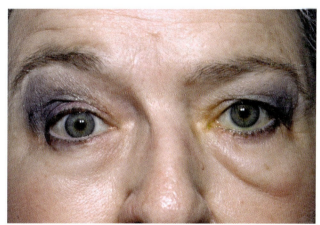

A

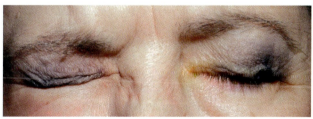

B

Figure 7–14. Evaluating facial nerve weakness.
A 69-year-old woman had a long-standing left facial palsy from a Schwannoma of the left facial nerve. **(A)** At rest, there is no obvious difference in orbicularis tone, and only slight facial asymmetry is apparent (left eyebrow is lower and less wrinkling of the forehead on the left compared to the right). **(B)** The patient can close both eyes, but when asked to squeeze both eyes shut tightly, the eyelashes are "buried" in the right eye, but not on the weaker left side.

▶ BOX 7–4. TESTING CORNEAL SENSATION

Corneal sensation is tested by lightly touching the non-anesthetized conjunctiva and the inferior corneal limbus of each eye in turn with a clean cotton wisp and comparing the magnitude of the (bilateral) blink response. The conjunctiva is less sensitive than the corneal limbus, and testing both conjunctiva and corneal limbus offers two different levels of sensitivity for comparison.

Important points with regard to testing corneal sensation include:

1. Use a fresh cotton wisp, not one that has been used to test the face.
2. If an infectious process is suspected, use a fresh wisp for each eye, or test the uninvolved eye first.
3. Examine the cornea at the slitlamp before this test.
4. Perform this test before topical anesthetic or other drops have been placed in the eyes.
5. Do not test corneal sensation if pharmacologic pupil tests are anticipated.

▶ KEY POINTS

- In pre-verbal/pre-literate children, determination of central, steady, and maintained fixation may be the only clues of central visual function that the examiner can determine.
- The action of the vertically acting muscles is best tested when the eye is in adduction (superior and inferior oblique muscles) or abduction (superior and inferior rectus muscles).
- Convergence should be observed in patients with poor pupillary light reactions, internuclear ophthalmoplegia, and symptoms of convergence insufficiency.
- Pursuit testing can be performed as an integral part of testing ocular versions—observations of how smoothly the patient can track the examiner's moving finger evaluates pursuit, and the ability of each eye to reach the endpoint at extreme gaze evaluates ocular versions.
- An internuclear ophthalmoplegia characteristically causes slow saccades of the adducting eye.
- Slow saccades can be seen in eyes with ocular motor palsies, in contrast to saccades that are abruptly halted in restrictive disorders such as orbital Graves disease.
- Optokinetic stimuli produce a physiological nystagmus that allows observation of saccades and pursuit even in patients who may be incapable of cooperating with other examination techniques.
- Similar to the doll's head maneuver, caloric testing uses vestibular input to drive gaze movement and has application in patients with altered consciousness or who cannot cooperate with other examination methods.
- Graded prisms can be used to quantitate ocular deviations by redirecting the line of sight and neutralizing the deviation observed in tests such as the alternate cover test.
- The secondary deviation (when the palsied eye is fixating) is always greater than the primary deviation (when the normal eye is fixating).
- The three-step test assumes that there is only one palsied vertically acting muscle, which is not always true.
- The single Maddox rod is particularly useful in exploring vertical deviations with the three-step test.
- Using the three-step test, a right superior oblique palsy produces a *right* hypertropia, which is greater in *left* gaze and with a *right* head tilt (mnemonic: right superior oblique palsy is right-left-right, and a left superior oblique palsy is left-right-left).
- Retropulsion of the globes is abnormally stiff in orbital Graves disease and with orbital masses.
- In patients with potential arteriovenous malformations (especially after trauma), auscultation of the globe, orbit, or head may reveal audible bruits.
- Ocular and facial sensation (light touch) can be tested by using a cotton-tipped applicator, with the cotton pulled and twisted to a point; the sharp point of a broken wooden applicator stick can be used to test pin-prick (pain) on the skin of the face.

SUGGESTED READING

Books

Borchert MS: Principles and techniques of the examination of ocular motility and alignment, in Miller NR, Newman NJ (eds): *Walsh and Hoyt's Clinical Neuro-ophthalmology*, Vol. 1, 6th ed. Baltimore, MD: Lippincott Williams & Wilkins; 2005.

Burde RM, Savino PJ, Trobe JD: Diplopia and similar sensory experiences, in *Clinical Decisions in Neuro-ophthalmology*, 3d ed. St. Louis, MO: Mosby; 2002.

Glaser JS: Neuro-ophthalmologic examination: general considerations and special techniques, in Duane TD (ed): *Duane's Clinical Ophthalmology*, Vol. 2, Philadelphia, PA: Lippincott Williams & Wilkins; 1998.

Lee AG, Brazis PW: Diplopia, in *Clinical Pathways in Neuro-ophthalmology, An Evidence-Based Approach*. New York, NY: Thieme; 2003.

Articles

Corbett JJ: The bedside and office neuro-ophthalmology examination. *Semin Neurol* 2003;23(1):63–76.

Martin TJ, Yeatts RP: Abnormalities of the eyelid position and function. *Semin Neurol* 2000;20:31–42.

CHAPTER 8

Ocular Motility Disorders: Extraocular Muscles and the Neuromuscular Junction

- ▶ EXTRAOCULAR MUSCLES 201
  Anatomy and function 201
- ▶ MYOPATHIES 201
  Chronic progressive external ophthalmoplegia 201
  Muscular dystrophies 204
  Orbital inflammatory disorders 204
- ▶ RESTRICTIVE ORBITOPATHIES 206
  Orbital Graves disease 206
  Other restrictive syndromes 210
- ▶ DISORDERS OF THE NEUROMUSCULAR JUNCTION 211
  Myasthenia gravis 211
  Other disorders 215
- ▶ KEY POINTS 215

Disorders of the extraocular muscles and neuromuscular junction can produce a virtually unlimited variety of disordered ocular motility patterns because their clinical manifestations are not limited by the scope of a single cranial nerve or supranuclear process. These disorders are frequently bilateral and often involve the levator palpebrae and orbicularis oculi (but not the pupil), and in some cases can result in total bilateral ophthalmoplegia. Not surprisingly, many of these disorders have systemic manifestations.

Diseases of the extraocular muscles can produce motility disturbances in two ways: (1) the disease process can affect the muscle's ability to contract and thus cause *weakness* and, (2) the muscle may be stiffened by disease, causing a *restriction* of muscle movement by tethering. Occasionally both processes are present to some degree, as weak muscles can become fibrotic and restricted over time. Myasthenia gravis and related disorders cause muscle weakness by affecting transmission at the neuromuscular junction with an otherwise normal nerve and muscle.

▶ EXTRAOCULAR MUSCLES

ANATOMY AND FUNCTION

Six extraocular muscles insert on the globe. In the horizontal plane, the lateral rectus muscle abducts and the medial rectus muscle adducts the eye. Vertical movement is more complicated because two muscles (superior rectus and inferior oblique) elevate the eye, and two muscles (inferior rectus and superior oblique) depress the eye. The actions of the oblique muscles on the globe may seem mysterious, but they are easily remembered with a clear understanding of how they insert on the globe and the direction of their action (Figure 8–1). Table 8–1 lists the primary and secondary actions of the extraocular muscles. Note that the vertically acting muscles also tort the eye, but the torsional forces are balanced when both elevators (superior rectus and inferior oblique) or both depressors (inferior rectus and superior oblique) are active.

▶ MYOPATHIES

Neuromuscular disorders often defy classification as being primarily neural or muscular in origin. For example, the pathological changes in muscle tissue with disorders such as chronic progressive external ophthalmoplegia suggests a muscle disease, but denervation can also cause secondary myopathic changes. With this disclaimer in mind, disorders will be discussed that appear *primarily* to affect the extraocular muscles.

CHRONIC PROGRESSIVE EXTERNAL OPHTHALMOPLEGIA

Chronic progressive external ophthalmoplegia (CPEO) is characterized by symmetric and slowly progressive bilateral ptosis and limitation of eye movements. Ptosis

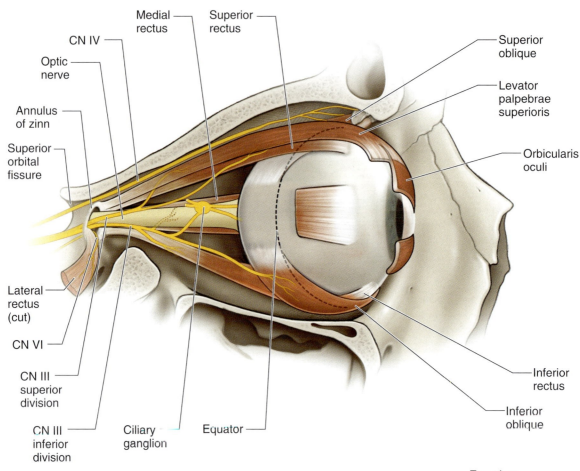
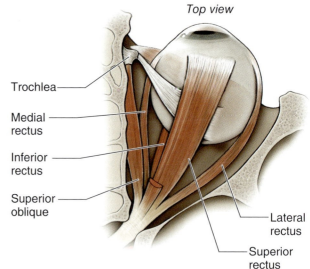

Figure 8–1. **The extraocular muscles and their innervation.** The medial rectus muscle has been sectioned and retracted in this drawing of the right eye to show the position of the extraocular muscles. The course of cranial nerves (CNs) III (*oculomotor*, superior and inferior divisions), IV (*trochlear*), and VI (*abducens*) are shown as they enter the orbit through the superior orbital fissure to innervate the extraocular muscles. Note that CN IV enters the orbit outside of the annulus of Zinn. The action of each of the extraocular muscles is a logical consequence of its insertion on the globe and direction of action. The *medial and lateral rectus muscles* insert anterior to the equator of the globe and pull directly posteriorly, rotating the globe in the horizontal plane. Similarly, the *superior and inferior rectus muscles* move the eye in the vertical plane. However, the superior and inferior rectus muscles insert at a slight angle relative to the visual axis, so they also cause some torsion and adduction of the globe (*inset*). The oblique muscles insert posterior to the equator and pull anteromedially (*inset*). Thus, the superior oblique depresses and the inferior oblique elevates. The torsional forces generated by the oblique muscles should be evident from this diagram.

TABLE 8-1. PRIMARY AND SECONDARY ACTIONS OF THE EXTRAOCULAR MUSCLES[a]

	Extraocular Muscle	Primary Action	Secondary Action	Tertiary Action
Horizontally acting muscles	Lateral rectus	Abducts		
	Medial rectus	Adducts		
Vertically acting muscles	Superior rectus	Elevates	Adducts	Intorts
	Inferior rectus	Depresses	Adducts	Extorts
	Inferior oblique	Extorts	Elevates	Abducts
	Superior oblique	Intorts	Depresses	Abducts

[a]This table should not have to be memorized, but the information should come from a clear mental image of the globe, angle of action, and insertion of the individual muscles as shown in Figure 8–1.

usually precedes the other ocular motility defects. Usually, patients do not complain of diplopia (Figure 8–2). CPEO is a *mitochondrial myopathy*: The muscle disease is the result of dysfunction of the mitochondria in the muscle cells. Light microscopy of limb or extraocular muscle biopsies reveals "ragged red fibers" (with modified Gomori trichrome stain), which consists of subsarcolemmal aggregates of degenerated mitochondria. Electron microscopy shows giant malformed mitochondria and also proliferation of normal-appearing mitochondria. Mitochondrial dysfunction in CPEO is usually the result of mitochondrial DNA deletions, which can be sporadic or heritable in a pattern similar to Leber hereditary optic neuropathy (LHON). There are also autosomal dominant and recessive forms of CPEO, which occur as a result of nuclear DNA mutations that affect production of mitochondrial components. Thus, this clinical entity encompasses a heterogeneous group of sporadic and genetic disorders with different inheritance patterns and presentations, many with systemic signs and symptoms.

In addition to ptosis and ophthalmoplegia, patients with mitochondrial myopathies frequently have weakness of facial and systemic muscles, cardiac conduction abnormalities (potentially fatal), pigmentary retinopathies, and other systemic signs. *Kearns-Sayre syndrome* (KSS) is a type of CPEO associated with a mitochondrial chromosomal defect recognized as a distinct syndrome (Table 8–2). This disorder is most often diagnosed before 20 years of age. Management should include consultation with a cardiologist because KSS is associated with cardiac conduction defects (including heart block and sudden death).

The diagnosis of CPEO or KSS can be made in some patients by genetic testing or muscle biopsy (deltoid or quadriceps muscle). Treatment is largely supportive. Ptosis surgery may be helpful, but the risk of exposure keratopathy must be considered.

Progressive supranuclear palsy (PSP) and ocular myasthenia gravis may be difficult to clinically distinguish from CPEO. However, unlike CPEO, PSP (discussed in Chapter 10) usually occurs in patients 60 years or older, and the oculocephalic reflexes are intact, proving that the extraocular muscles are not the source of the ophthalmoplegia. Patients with myasthenia may have ocular symptoms that vary significantly over time, unlike the steady progression of CPEO.

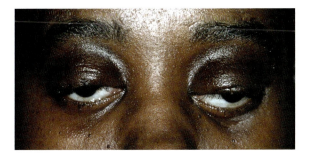

Figure 8–2. Chronic progressive external ophthalmoplegia.
A 27-year-old woman described progressive ptosis over her lifetime. Bilateral ptosis is evident. The patient also had a complete ophthalmoplegia, with inability to move the eyes well in any direction on command or with oculocephalic maneuvers.

TABLE 8-2. KEARNS-SAYRE SYNDROME: DIAGNOSTIC CRITERIA

Must Include
- Progressive ophthalmoplegia, often total, but without diplopia
- Pigmentary retinopathy
- Onset <20 years of age

Plus at Least One of the Following
- Cardiac conduction defect
- Elevated cerebrospinal fluid protein >1 mg/mL
- Cerebellar ataxia
- Short stature
- Neurosensory hearing loss
- Dementia
- Endocrine abnormalities

MUSCULAR DYSTROPHIES

Myotonic dystrophy is an autosomal dominant systemic myopathy that can cause bilateral ptosis and limited ocular motility. Additional ocular signs include a characteristic polychromatic cataract (present in most adults with the disorder) and a pigmentary maculopathy and retinopathy. Visible (and palpable) wasting of the temporalis and sternocleidomastoid muscles, frontal balding, bilateral ptosis, and facial weakness produce a very characteristic and distinctive appearance (Figure 8–3). Systemic findings include diffuse weakness and atrophy of the muscles of the arms and legs, cognitive deficiencies, hearing loss, testicular atrophy, and cardiac abnormalities. Myotonic contraction, typically worsened by cold or excitement, becomes evident before 20 years of age. The presence of *action myotonia* (difficulty voluntarily relaxing a muscle after contraction) and *percussion myotonia* (localized contraction of a muscle when a sharp tap is applied) can distinguish myotonic dystrophy from other myopathies. Clinically, action myotonia may be evident as difficulty releasing after a handshake. With electromyography, the myotonic signature is diagnostic: "Divebomber" discharges demonstrate continued activation of the muscle after attempted relaxation.

Oculopharyngeal dystrophy is a hereditary autosomal dominant condition affecting patients of French-Canadian heritage. Patients usually present between 40 and 60 years of age with progressive bilateral ptosis, limited ocular motility, and weakness of the bulbar musculature with dysphagia. Aspiration pneumonia is common and can be prevented by cricomyotomy.

ORBITAL INFLAMMATORY DISORDERS

Orbital inflammation can be caused by a wide range of infectious, vasculitic, and idiopathic conditions (Table 8–3). The extraocular muscles are often involved, resulting in painful diplopia. Obviously, orbital inflammatory disorders will also frequently involve other orbital structures, causing optic neuropathy, proptosis, and other ocular signs and symptoms.

Idiopathic orbital inflammatory syndrome (IOIS; previously called orbital inflammatory pseudotumor) is characterized by the rapid onset of orbital congestion, proptosis, diplopia, pain, and the lack of identifiable infectious, neoplastic, or other causes (Figure 8–4). IOIS can present as a focal process, primarily affecting the extraocular muscles (orbital myositis), optic nerve, lacrimal gland, or sclera, or may present as a diffuse orbital inflammation (see Table 8–3; subtypes

▶ **TABLE 8–3. ORBTIAL INFLAMMATORY DISORDERS**

Idiopathic Orbital Inflammatory Syndrome (IOIS)
   Diffuse orbital inflammation
   Myositis
   Dacryoadenitis
   Posterior scleritis
   Optic perineuritis
   Sclerosing inflammation

Systemic Vasculitic/Inflammatory Conditions
   Giant cell arteritis
   Granulomatosis with polyangiitis (Wegener granulomatosis)
   Polyarteritis nodosa
   Systemic lupus erythematosus
   Gout
   Psoriatic and rheumatoid arthritis
   Behçet disease
   Sarcoidosis
   Ulcerative colitis
   Crohn disease
   Histiocytic disorders
      Langerhans cell histiocytosis (Eosinophilic granuloma)
      Juvenile xanthogranuloma
      Erdheim-Chester disease
   Necrobiotic xanthogranuloma

Infectious Processes
   Orbital cellulitis
   Syphilis
   Tuberculosis
   Trichinosis

Carotid-Caverous Fistula

Orbital Tumors

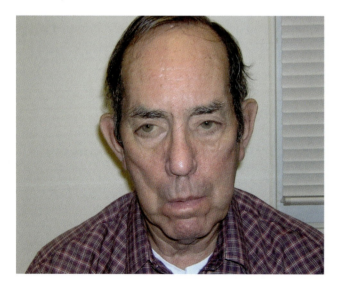

Figure 8–3. **Myotonic dystrophy facial appearance.**
This photoillustration of a patient with myotonic dystrophy type 1 shows characteristic temporal, jaw, and facial muscle atrophy, with frontal balding. (Reproduced, with permission, from Amato A, Russell J: *Neuromuscular Disorders.* New York: McGraw-Hill; 2008.)

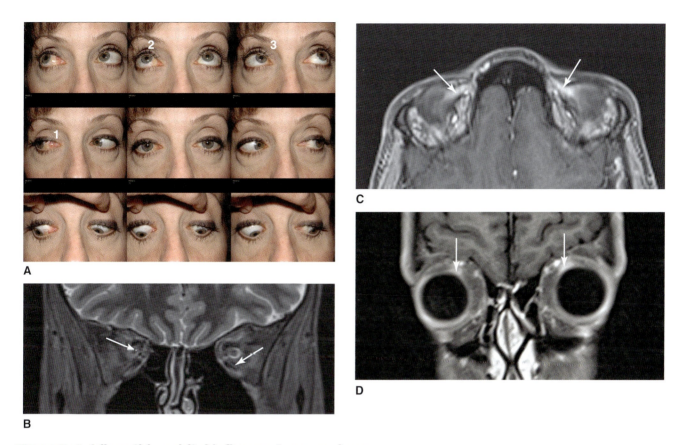

Figure 8–4. **Idiopathic orbital inflammatory syndrome.**
A 48-year-old woman presented with 4 months of bilateral periocular pain. One month prior to presentation she developed diplopia in upgaze and redness of the right eye. Her examination showed normal visual acuities and visual fields, but she had focal injection of the medial bulbar conjunctiva of the right eye and a right hypotropia in upgaze. An extensive evaluation did not reveal any systemic, vasculitic, infectious, or neoplastic cause. The patient's symptoms quickly resolved on oral prednisone, without recurrence after tapering off the medication. **(A)** At presentation, conjunctival injection of the right eye is evident (1). A right hypotropia in upgaze is identified (2),(3). **(B)** Magnetic resonance imaging of the orbit at presentation showed abnormal T2 hyperintensity with reticulation in the retro-orbital fat (*arrows*), seen in this coronal section. **(C)** An axial T1 sequence with contrast shows prominent enhancement of the insertions of the bilateral superior oblique muscles on the globe (*arrows*). **(D)** Coronal view of T1 sequence with enhancement of bilateral superior oblique muscle insertions (*arrows*).

of IOIS). A single extraocular muscle or combination of muscles can be affected. The affected muscles constrict poorly and restrict free movement of the globe. They are usually enlarged on neuroimaging and may enhance with contrast. Systemic vasculitic conditions, sarcoidosis, orbital Graves disease, orbital cellulitis, carotid-cavernous fistulas, and neoplastic processes should be specifically sought and considered because idiopathic orbital inflammatory syndrome is a clinical diagnosis of exclusion (see Table 8–3). The appearance of the tendonous muscle insertion on the globe seen with neuroimaging may help distinguish idiopathic orbital inflammatory syndrome from the muscle enlargement of orbital Graves disease: thickened, involved tendons with IOIS; thin, normal-appearing tendons with orbital Graves disease (although they do sometimes enhance). Patients with IOIS usually experience prompt relief of symptoms with high-dose oral corticosteroids. Failure to respond promptly to corticosteroids should lead the physician to consider other diagnoses with additional testing, such as an orbital biopsy. Patients can usually be successfully tapered off corticosteroids over several months. Recurrence after a slow taper should also prompt reinvestigation of other diagnoses. Nonsteroidal anti-inflammatory agents (NSAIDs) may be effective in less severe cases. Radiation treatment of the orbit and steroid-sparing immunosuppressives (cyclophosphamide, cyclosporine, or methotrexate) are a consideration for patients who recur on repeated attempts to taper corticosteroids. This idiopathic inflammatory condition of the orbit is likely a similar process to the painful inflammatory syndrome of the cavernous sinus—the Tolosa-Hunt syndrome (discussed in Chapter 9).

▶ RESTRICTIVE ORBITOPATHIES

Restrictive myopathies/orbitopathies cause motility disturbances by mechanically restricting globe movement. The most common restrictive processes include trauma (blowout fractures) and orbital Graves disease; less common entities include inflammatory, infiltrating, and space-occupying lesions. In some orbital processes, a combination of neuropathic, myopathic, and restrictive processes are present and are impossible to separate.

ORBITAL GRAVES DISEASE

Orbital Graves disease is a common orbital myopathy that has a confusing number of clinical names: *Graves orbitopathy, Graves ophthalmopathy, thyroid eye disease, thyroid-associated orbitopathy or ophthalmopathy, and dysthyroid myopathy.* Some authorities have reservations regarding the use of the name *thyroid eye disease*, since thyroid abnormalities are not invariably present and this condition is not caused by thyroid dysfunction. The term *Graves disease* is unpopular with those who prefer not to use eponyms, and the orbit disease must be distinguished from Graves disease of the thyroid, since these two disorders do not always occur together. In this book, the term *orbital Graves disease* (or *Graves orbitopathy*) will be used because this term acknowledges that Graves disease of the thyroid and orbital Graves disease likely have the same (immunological) root cause, and it has historic precedent. The use of *orbitopathy* is preferred rather than *ophthalmopathy* because the disease affects the entire orbit, not only the eye.

Description

Orbital Graves disease is an autoimmune disorder characterized by bilateral (but often markedly asymmetric) enlargement of the extraocular muscles and an increase in orbital fat volume, with resultant proptosis, diplopia, ocular congestion, and sometimes a compressive optic neuropathy, usually in patients between 25 and 50 years of age (Figures 8–5 to 8–7). Eyelid retraction occurs independently of the proptosis by an unknown mechanism. The disease begins with an active phase of orbital inflammation causing progressive signs and symptoms that may last months to years, followed by an inactive, quiescent stage with partial reversal of symptoms but usually with permanent sequelae. It is more common in women than men (6:1).

The orbit is one of several anatomic regions affected by systemic Graves disease; other manifestations include diffuse hyperplasia of the thyroid gland and an infiltrative dermatopathy causing localized pretibial myxedema. Orbital Graves disease is frequently (but not always) associated with thyroid dysfunction.

Etiology

The orbital tissues and thyroid gland are *end organs* affected by a poorly understood underlying systemic autoimmune disorder. This is likely due to antigenic similarity between orbital and thyroid tissues. The thyroid abnormalities do not cause the orbital disease. Therefore, thyroid dysfunction is not invariably present with Graves orbitopathy, and normal thyroid function (euthyroid Graves orbitopathy) does not rule out this entity (see Figure 8–5). For the same reason, treatment of thyroid dysfunction does not necessarily improve the course of Graves orbitopathy.

Signs and Symptoms

Patients with Graves orbitopathy may have evidence of systemic hyperthyroidism (90%), but as noted above some patients are euthyroid (6%) or even hypothyroid. Thyroid dysfunction often occurs many years before or after orbital manifestations or may not occur at all. Systemic signs and symptoms of thyroid dysfunction are listed in Table 8–4. Signs and symptoms of Graves orbitopathy fall into three areas: (1) ocular misalignment and diplopia from a restrictive myopathy, (2) exposure keratopathy from proptosis and eyelid retraction, and (3) optic nerve compression at the orbital apex by oversized extraocular muscles.

Involved *extraocular muscles* are diffusely enlarged by lymphocytic infiltration. Any extraocular muscle or combination of muscles in one or both orbits may be involved, but the inferior rectus is the single most commonly involved muscle. The frequency of rectus muscle involvement and the clinical progression of the disease is as follows: inferior rectus, medial rectus, superior rectus, and lateral rectus. The oblique muscles are only occasionally involved. The enlarged muscles lose their compliance and resist passive stretching and relaxation that normally occurs when the antagonist muscle is active. The thickened muscles also do not constrict normally. Eventually, irreversible contracture of the muscle may occur from fibrosis. Thus, a restrictive orbitopathy occurs, with the eye pulled in the direction of the involved muscles. The most common presenting motility disturbance in orbital Graves disease is a consequence of inferior and medial rectus infiltration and restriction: an inability to look up whether the eye is adducted or abducted (often misnamed a "double-elevator palsy") and an esotropia (see Figure 8–6). Medial rectus involvement may simulate cranial nerve (CN) VI palsies, but the restrictive nature of this disorder is evident with forced duction testing. As previously described, restriction can also be identified by measuring an increase in

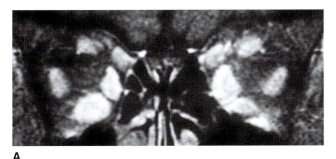

Figure 8–5. Euthyroid orbital Graves disease.
A 61-year-old man presented with the gradual development of vertical diplopia. Thyroid function tests were normal and the patient did not have overt proptosis or eyelid retraction, so the patient was referred to search for a diagnosis other than Graves disease. However, the motility pattern was not suggestive of a cranial neuropathy, and resistance to retropulsion was notable. In addition, the intraocular pressure increased from 10 (in primary position) to 25 mm Hg measured in upgaze, suggesting a restrictive orbitopathy such as orbital Graves disease. **(A)** Magnetic resonance imaging (MRI) of the orbit revealed marked enlargement of the right inferior rectus, with similar but less pronounced involvement of the medial recti and other muscles in both orbits (observe the unusual involvement of the superior oblique muscles bilaterally). **(B)** Ocular versions are most notable for limited elevation of the right eye (*top middle photograph*), correlating with the findings on MRI.

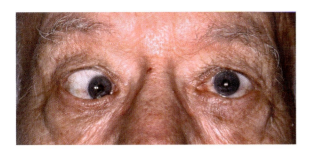

Figure 8–6. Ocular misalignment in orbital Graves disease.
This patient with orbital Graves disease demonstrates a marked vertical deviation and an esotropia—a common appearance due to the predilection of this disorder to cause restriction of the inferior and medial rectus muscles in both orbits asymmetrically. An exodeviation would be unlikely from orbital Graves disease. Note also the presence of eyelid retraction.

intraocular pressure in attempted upgaze or downgaze. (This transient rise in intraocular pressure with extreme gaze does not constitute glaucoma and does not need to be treated.) Occasionally, patients with orbital Graves disease also have myasthenia gravis. The coexistence of multiple autoimmune disorders is not uncommon and suggests an underlying fundamental immune derangement. Concomitant myasthenia should be considered in patients with Graves orbitopathy with atypical or variable ocular misalignment, or in those who have ptosis rather than eyelid retraction.

The most common cause of unilateral or bilateral *proptosis* is Graves orbitopathy. Proptosis results from the expanded volume of the orbital contents (muscles and fat) pushing the globe forward in the orbit. On examination, an involved orbit offers increased resistance to retropulsion: With the patient's eyes closed, the examiner gently pushes the globe toward the apex of the orbit with the thumb and index finger on the patient's eyelid, gauging the amount of resistance to this maneuver in each orbit. The examiner should develop experience with the feel of elastic, compliant retropulsion in the normal eye, so that abnormal resistance to retropulsion can be identified with confidence. Occasionally, proptosis can reach grotesque proportions, resulting in cosmetic deformity and greater risk of exposure keratopathy. The presence of proptosis is in itself an indication for imaging the orbits, because proptosis (and other clinical findings) in orbital Graves disease may be indistinguishable from an orbital mass (Table 8–5). Choroidal folds through the macula, a manifestation of pressure or a mass behind the globe, can also be present.

Eyelid retraction can occur from other disorders but is often specific for orbital Graves disease when accompanied by proptosis and restrictive orbitopathy (see Table 7–4). Retraction of the eyelid is not simply the result of proptosis, as it can occur independently of other orbital signs. Lid lag, or failure of the eyelid to follow the globe in downgaze, is usually present with eyelid retraction. The combination of proptosis, eyelid retraction, and lid lag can produce an exposure keratopathy, causing blurred vision and

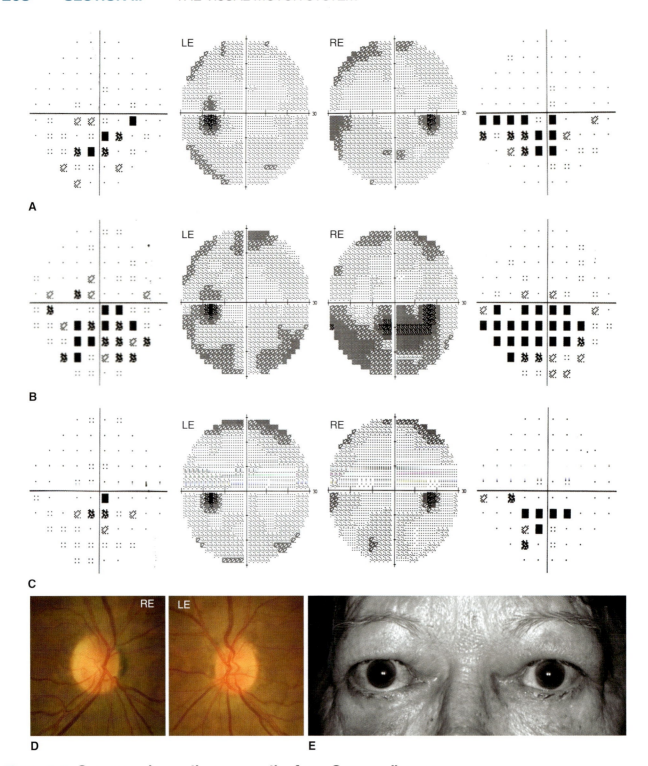

Figure 8-7. **Compressive optic neuropathy from Graves disease.**
An 80-year-old woman with orbital Graves disease had a progressive decline in vision in both eyes from apical compression of the optic nerves by enlarged extraocular muscles and expanding orbital fat. **(A, B)** Automated perimetry shows a progressing inferior-central visual field defect in both eyes over 4 weeks. The defect is best seen in the total deviation plots. **(C)** Marked improvement in the visual fields can be seen after bilateral transantral orbital decompression and bilateral nasal antral windows. **(D)** The optic discs appeared relatively normal throughout the course of the disease despite the decline in vision. **(E)** The patient's preoperative motility examination is typical for Graves orbitopathy, but the orbit does not appear to be particularly "hot" clinically, even in the presence of advancing compressive optic neuropathy. (Case courtesy of Yeatts, RP.)

▶ TABLE 8-4. SYSTEMIC MANIFESTATIONS OF THYROID DYSFUNCTION

Hyperthyroidism	Hypothyroidism
Nervousness and emotional liability	Decreased energy
Sleeplessness and fatigue	Lethargy, sleep apnea
Sweating and heat intolerance	Cold intolerance
Weight loss despite increased appetite	Weight gain
Frequent bowel movements	Constipation
Hyperreflexia	Prolonged relaxation phase of reflexes ("hung-up" ankle jerks)
Tremors	Stiff, cramping muscles with myoedema on muscle percussion
Palpitations (sinus tachycardia atrial arrhythmias)	Bradycardia
Pretibial myxedema	Hair loss and dry skin, periorbital edema, enlarged tongue, carpel tunnel syndrome

▶ TABLE 8-5. DIFFERENTIAL DIAGNOSIS OF PROPTOSIS

Graves disease
Orbital tumors
Arteriovenous malformation of orbit/cavernous sinus
Idiopathic orbital inflammatory syndrome
Congenital or familial proptosis
Pseudoproptosis
    From axial myopia
    From contralateral enophthalmos
Sphenoid wing hypoplasia in type 1 neurofibromatosis

pain. Severe exposure keratopathy can progress to corneal ulceration.

Diffuse bulbar *conjunctival injection* and chemosis are common. Localized conjunctival injection is commonly present over the rectus muscles. The insertion of the extraocular muscles, normally not visible under the conjunctiva, may be prominent.

Compression of the optic nerve can occur in 5% of patients with Graves orbitopathy. Optic nerve compression occurs from oversized rectus muscles and excess orbital fat causing a compartment syndrome at the orbital apex, or less often optic nerve injury due to excessive stretching of the optic nerve from severe proptosis can occur. Any optic-nerve-related visual field defect can occur. Visual loss tends to be slowly progressive but can be fulminant in some patients. The optic disc is often normal initially, with the gradual onset of pallor (see Figure 8–7). Occasionally, optic disc edema is present. Optic nerve function may be difficult to evaluate when a keratopathy is also present. A compressive optic neuropathy can occur even when external signs of orbital Graves disease are minimal or absent. Although the eyes may feel uncomfortable and have a full feeling, pain is distinctly uncommon with compressive optic neuropathy in Graves disease except when corneal epithelial disease is present.

The signs and symptoms of Graves orbitopathy do not occur in a predictable sequential order. Rather, any of the signs and symptoms can be present at any given time in the course of the disease. As discussed above, a treacherous form of Graves orbitopathy occurs in patients who have optic nerve compression without proptosis, eyelid retraction, or ocular motility disturbance.

Evaluation and Differential Diagnosis

The diagnosis of orbital Graves disease can often be made clinically. Close observation of the eyelid position and function may be diagnostic. The restrictive nature of the motility disturbance can be verified by forced duction testing or elevation of intraocular pressure in upgaze. Coronal views of the orbits by computed tomography (CT), fat-suppressed magnetic resonance imaging (MRI), or orbital ultrasound can be used to confirm the presence of thickened muscles, typically sparing the muscle tendon (at the insertion on the globe). Measurement of ocular misalignment, proptosis, and optic nerve function (eg, visual acuity, relative afferent pupillary defect, color vision, visual fields), as well as the presence of any ocular surface disease, should be documented at each visit to follow the disease progression. Progression of proptosis should be followed and measured with Hertel exophthalmometry.

Idiopathic orbital inflammatory syndrome (IOIS) can produce a clinical picture that may be difficult to distinguish from orbital Graves disease, but pain is far more prominent, and orbital imaging reveals characteristic inflammatory thickening of the muscle insertions in IOIS, which are usually spared in Graves orbitopathy (see Figure 8–4). Carotid-cavernous fistulas can produce proptosis, muscle enlargement, conjunctival injection, and motility disturbances similar to orbital Graves disease; however, cranial and orbital bruits, elevated intraocular pressure, and superior ophthalmic vein enlargement on imaging are distinguishing features of this disorder. As previously described, forced duction testing can help separate neurogenic palsies from the restrictive orbitopathy of Graves disease. Because space-occupying orbital lesions can cause proptosis and diplopia (see Table 8–5), imaging of the orbit is an important tool both to confirm the clinical suspicion of orbital Graves disease and to address other orbital processes in the differential diagnosis. Elevated antiperoxidase antibodies, antithyroid antibodies, or thyroid-stimulating immunoglobulins support the diagnosis but are not invariably present. Thyroid dysfunction (when present) can be identified by measuring thyroid-stimulating hormone (TSH), total T4, free T4, and T3.

Treatment

Thyroid abnormalities should be addressed by an endocrinologist, but normalization of thyroid function is unlikely to reliably affect the course of the orbitopathy. In fact, treatment of hyperthyroidism with radioactive iodine is commonly associated with a worsening of the orbitopathy; therefore, oral corticosteroids are recommended for patients with Graves orbitopathy undergoing radioactive iodine therapy for their hyperthyroidism. Graves orbitopathy has no cure; most treatments are directed at palliation of symptoms during the active phase or repair of remaining defects when the active phase is over. Cigarette smoking exacerbates the disease, and patients should be counseled accordingly. The active phase of orbital Graves disease may be mild and may require only supportive measures for ocular surface disease and diplopia. Rarely, patients present with a fulminant acute inflammatory phase that requires early consideration of radiation therapy or short-term corticosteroids.

Virtually all patients require ocular lubricants. The severity of ocular surface disease dictates the intensity of treatment, which may include artificial tears, ointment, moisture shields, taping the eye closed at night, or lateral tarsorrhaphy. Two- to four-inch elevation of the head of the bed at night helps reduce chemosis, which is typically worse in the morning.

Supportive care for diplopia includes ocular occlusion or spectacle prisms in patients with stable myopathy. With time, the extraocular muscles become fibrotic and remain restrictive even when the disease is inactive. Strabismus surgery may help restore fusion in primary position, but this procedure should be considered only when the disease is quiescent, orbital decompression surgery has already been performed or is not anticipated, and the ocular measurements have been stable for at least 6 months. Eyelid surgery can help with the cosmetic and functional effects of eyelid retraction, but should be done after orbital decompression and strabismus surgery if these surgeries are needed.

Optic nerve compression is the most serious potential complication of orbital Graves disease because it can lead to irreversible visual loss. High-dose intravenous or oral steroid therapy may be beneficial in some patients, but is only a temporizing measure, as long-term steroids offer more risk than benefit. A common regimen is to start with 60 to 100 mg of oral prednisone per day, with high-dose oral therapy planned for no longer than 2 weeks, followed by a rapid taper. Patients who do not respond should immediately receive radiation or undergo decompression surgery. Surgical decompression of the orbit can be achieved by transantral (or transeyelid) removal of the orbital floor and/or medial wall, allowing prolapse of the orbital contents into the adjacent sinuses, relieving compression of the optic nerve. Orbital decompression is occasionally performed to reduce extreme proptosis causing exposure keratopathy or to address cosmetic concerns.

Radiation of the orbit is another treatment alternative for optic nerve compression or congestive orbitopathy, especially in patients older than 55 years. A typical dose is 2000 cGy in divided fractions to the orbit (sparing the lens) given over 10 days. Oral steroids are administered simultaneously to reduce radiation-induced orbital inflammation.

OTHER RESTRICTIVE SYNDROMES

Orbital trauma can restrict free movement of the globe. Sudden orbital compression can produce a blowout fracture of the thin orbital floor, entrapping the inferior rectus and other orbital tissue in the fracture (Figure 8–8). Elevation of the eye is restricted by the entrapped muscle or its fascia, and depression of the eye may also be deficient if the muscle cannot constrict normally. Acute (or subsequent) enophthalmos and inferior orbital nerve damage (causing numbness of the cheek) commonly accompany orbital floor fractures. Rarely the ciliary ganglion or ciliary nerve fibers are also damaged in inferior blowout fractures, resulting in a dilated pupil that is fixed to light, which may be mistaken for a Hutchinson pupil from uncal herniation.

A less common variant is a medial wall blowout, where the medial rectus is entrapped in a medial orbital wall fracture, producing an abduction deficit that may mimic a CN VI palsy. Hemorrhage into the extraocular muscles and scarring and fibrosis of the muscles or other orbital tissues also cause restriction as a result of trauma. The myopathic and restrictive consequences of orbital trauma frequently coexist with traumatic injury to the ocular motor cranial nerves, producing a complex motility pattern with both restrictive and paretic components.

Brown tendon sheath syndrome is a restriction of the superior oblique tendon at the trochlea, which

eye fully elevates. Brown tendon sheath syndrome can be distinguished from an inferior oblique palsy by the characteristic downshoot of the eye as it is adducted (Figure 8–9), and by restriction of elevation in adduction on forced duction testing. An acquired tendon sheath syndrome can occur from trauma, sinus or orbital surgery, or (rarely) rheumatoid arthritis. This condition is commonly congenital, and is usually associated with normal binocular vision without amblyopia.

Congenital fibrosis syndromes are often discussed with restrictive myopathies, but the abnormal extraocular muscles are the result of developmental failure due to agenesis of ocular motor neurons in the brainstem. Extraocular muscles (including the levator palpebrae) appear atrophied and fibrotic, with corresponding ophthalmoplegia and ptosis. Amblyopia is common.

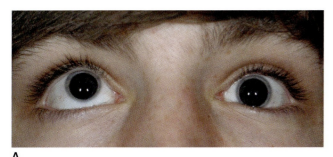
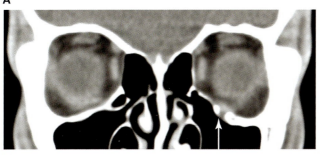

Figure 8–8. **Orbital blowout fracture.**
A 16-year-old patient was punched in the left eye. **(A)** The patient is unable to fully elevate the left eye. **(B)** Computed tomography of the orbit, coronal section, shows a left orbital floor fracture with incarceration of the inferior rectus fascia into the fracture, mechanically restricting elevation of the globe. Young patients with blowout fractures require urgent attention, as prompt surgical relief of an entrapped rectus muscle may be needed to prevent permanent ischemic muscle damage.

prevents the eye from fully elevating in adduction. The superior oblique tendon is thought to hang up in the trochlea. In a few patients, it is intermittent, with an audible snap when the tendon releases and the

▶ **DISORDERS OF THE NEUROMUSCULAR JUNCTION**

MYASTHENIA GRAVIS

Myasthenia gravis is a disorder of the neuromuscular junction that commonly causes weakness of the extraocular muscles (including the levator palpebrae). The disease may affect the extraocular muscles only (*ocular myasthenia*) in some patients, but usually this disorder causes generalized weakness. The designation *gravis* is appropriate for systemic myasthenia, particularly when respiratory muscles are affected or protection of the airway is compromised, resulting in significant morbidity or death. Approximately 50% of patients with myasthenia gravis present with ocular motility signs, and most of the remaining patients develop ocular

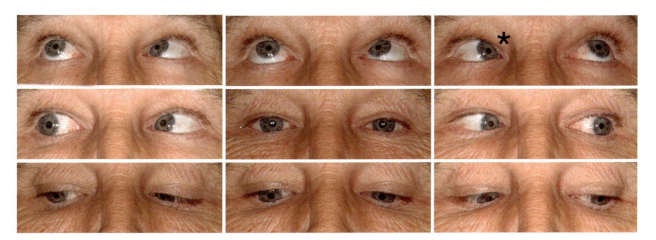

Figure 8–9. **Acquired Brown superior oblique tendon sheath syndrome.**
A 52-year-old man had extensive nasal sinus and skull base surgery followed by radiation, for an invasive carcinoma. This photograph of the patient's ocular motility shows Brown tendon sheath syndrome of the left eye. As the left eye is adducted, the tethered superior oblique tendon gives no slack, forcing the eye to rotate down. This is most evident when the eye is adducted in elevation, with a downshoot as the eye is turned toward the nose (*asterisk*). This patient also has a right abduction deficit.

symptoms during their course. The ophthalmologist, therefore, is important both in the diagnosis and symptomatic treatment of this neurological condition.

Cause

Acetylcholine is the neurotransmitter at the neuromuscular junction in skeletal muscle. Myasthenia is a systemic autoimmune disorder in which postsynaptic receptors for acetylcholine are blocked and inactivated or destroyed by antibodies. The association of myasthenia with abnormalities of the thymus gland suggests that thymus-generated lymphocytes play a role in this immune disorder. Thus, in myasthenia gravis the nerve and muscle are otherwise normal, but the neural signal is unreliably transmitted to the muscle, resulting in variable muscle weakness. Drugs (eg, antibiotics, magnesium-containing medications, beta blockers, calcium channel blockers, anticonvulsants, psychiatric medications) can exacerbate the disease, and several drugs (eg, D-penicillamine and atorvastatin) appear to be causative.

Signs and Symptoms

Clinical characteristics include variable weakness and worsening of symptoms with fatigue. Symptoms may be minimal or absent on arising from sleep, and are usually worse late in the day. Patients often have a long history of unexplained variable diplopia or ptosis. Long periods without symptoms may be interrupted with exacerbations, sometimes triggered by infection or drugs.

Ptosis is present in most patients. In many patients, the ptosis can be seen to worsen during the examination, especially with prolonged upgaze (Figure 8–10). The classic history of an alternating ptosis, in which a ptosis switches sides, is myasthenia until proven otherwise. The *Cogan eyelid twitch sign* is often present but is not entirely specific for myasthenia. This finding is evoked by a rapid saccade from downgaze to primary position and consists of an initial overshoot of the upper eyelid, with slow downward droop. Orbicularis oculi and other facial muscle weakness is common. This can be seen clinically as the *peek sign*: As the patient attempts to keep both eyes closed, a weakening orbicularis causes the eyelids to slowly separate as if the patient were peeking with one or both eyes. The presence of concomitant orbicularis weakness and ptosis can also occur with CPEO, but is otherwise helpful in distinguishing myasthenia from other causes of ptosis.

Diplopia is caused by weakness of the extraocular muscles. Any combination of muscles may be involved, mimicking virtually any motility disorder. However, myasthenia *does not affect the pupil* and so is not likely to be confused with a pupil-involved CN III palsy (or Horner syndrome). Fatigability may manifest as an increasing ocular deviation during the examination.

Systemic symptoms will develop in 80% of patients who present with ocular myasthenia. Systemic symptoms

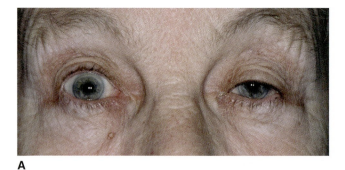

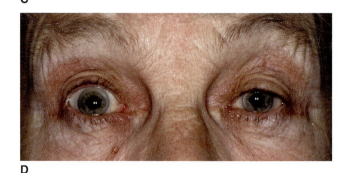

Figure 8–10. **Ocular myasthenia: rest test.** A 63-year-old woman complained of variable ptosis of the left eyelid and intermittent diplopia. The history and clinical examination provided compelling evidence for a diagnosis of ocular myasthenia. **(A)** Ptosis of the left upper eyelid is evident. **(B)** After a period of sustained upgaze, the ptosis is greater. **(C)** With additional eye fatigue, the ptosis is nearly complete. **(D)** However, after closing the eyes and resting for 5 minutes, the ptosis is much improved.

include weakness of arms and legs, and generalized fatigue. Significant morbidity can occur from weakness of the swallowing muscles resulting in aspiration, or involvement in the muscles of respiration. Patients may describe choking, coughing, or regurgitating liquids through the nose when eating or drinking. Dysphonia after extended talking (often deteriorating to a whisper) can occur from weakness of the laryngeal and pharyngeal musculature. Patients with only ocular signs and symptoms of myasthenia after 2 years are less likely to progress to systemic disease.

Evaluation and Differential Diagnosis

Patients with ocular or systemic myasthenia often have intermittent symptoms over many years without a diagnosis. Because myasthenia can produce virtually any motility pattern and/or ptosis, it should be included in the differential diagnosis of every suspected cranial nerve palsy, supranuclear palsy, or other disease causing ocular misalignment or ptosis. Abnormal motility patterns that cannot otherwise be accounted for are highly suspect for myasthenia. Five percent of patients with ocular myasthenia also have orbital Graves disease, which can further confuse the clinical picture.

Variability and fatigability are key clinical diagnostic characteristics. These findings may be evident during a single examination. For example, a ptosis of 1 mm present at the beginning of the examination may measure 5 mm after testing motility. In some patients, variability is evident only between examinations, underscoring the importance of careful and accurate measurement of eyelid function and motility on each encounter. Examinations later in the day, when the patient is more fatigued, are usually more productive than early morning visits.

Simply having the patient close and rest a ptotic eyelid can result in a convincing reversal of ptosis, with a return of the ptosis after further exertion of the eyelid (see Figure 8–10). A 30 minute rest period is suggested in this *sleep test*, but convincing results can often be seen in only 5 minutes. The physician should take advantage of the opportunity presented by children who are napping by observing the patient immediately upon awakening to compare to their state after the fatigue of an examination. The *ice test* involves placing an ice bag over a ptotic eyelid for 2 minutes. Local cooling improves ptosis in myasthenia, but not in other causes of ptosis.

Acetylcholine receptor (binding) antibodies can be serologically identified in about one half of patients presenting with ocular signs alone. Although this test lacks sensitivity in ocular myasthenia, it is helpful because a positive result obviates the need for other tests. Assays for antimuscle-specific kinase (MuSK) antibodies and blocking antibodies may be diagnostic in some patients with a negative acetylcholine receptor antibody test.

Electromyography (EMG) can also assist in the diagnosis. Repetitive nerve stimulation of facial or limb muscles may show the typical *decremental* response in myasthenia, but may be normal in patients with myasthenia. Single-fiber EMG of the frontal muscle is both sensitive and specific in experienced hands, and is especially helpful when other tests fail to confirm a suspected diagnosis of myasthenia gravis.

The short-acting anticholinesterase drug *edrophonium chloride (Tensilon)* can be used as a diagnostic test for myasthenia gravis—the Tensilon test. Anticholinesterase agents block the action of cholinesterase, resulting in an increased amount of acetylcholine available for binding to postsynaptic receptors. In many patients with myasthenia, this action produces a temporary reversal of myasthenic symptoms (Figure 8–11). Patients are incrementally given up to 10 mg of edrophonium chloride intravenously and are observed to see if their ptosis or motility disorder is reversed (Box 8–1). The agent lasts only a matter of minutes, so the motility disturbance or ptosis needs to be significant enough to allow confident appraisal of improvement over just a few minutes of observation. Reversal of ptosis is easily observed, but motility patterns may be more difficult to assess, especially if subtle. Alternate cover testing, or Hess screen testing, may be performed (but must be done quickly) before and after injection of edrophonium to assess motility.

Neostigmine methylsulfate (Prostigmin) is a longer-acting anticholinesterase agent that may be given intramuscularly or orally as a diagnostic test for myasthenia. Atropine is also routinely given with neostigmine to counteract its undesirable systemic cholinergic effects. The longer action of neostigmine allows more formal measurement of ocular deviation. Unlike edrophonium, however, potential undesirable side effects may need to be endured for 2 to 3 hours rather than minutes. Tensilon or Prostigmin testing can be uncomfortable for the patient and is not without risk. Not all patients with myasthenia will have a positive test, and false-positive tests can also occur.

If available, single-fiber EMG testing may be a better choice than Tensilon and Prostigmin testing for patients who need further diagnostic testing for myasthenia. Patients with a diagnosis (or high suspicion) of myasthenia gravis need a neurological evaluation because of the potential for systemic manifestations of this disease. Because 10% of myasthenic patients may harbor a thymus tumor, a CT of the chest is also required.

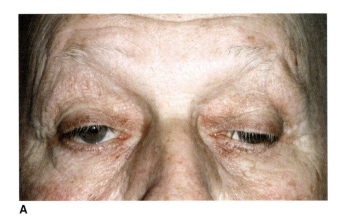

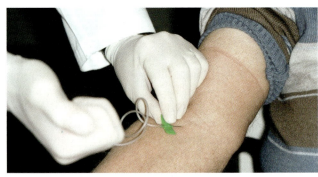

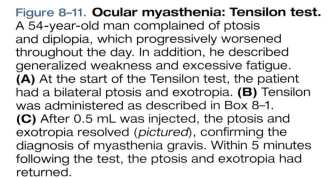

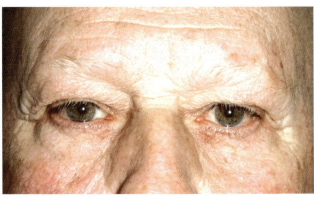

Figure 8–11. Ocular myasthenia: Tensilon test. A 54-year-old man complained of ptosis and diplopia, which progressively worsened throughout the day. In addition, he described generalized weakness and excessive fatigue. **(A)** At the start of the Tensilon test, the patient had a bilateral ptosis and exotropia. **(B)** Tensilon was administered as described in Box 8–1. **(C)** After 0.5 mL was injected, the ptosis and exotropia resolved (*pictured*), confirming the diagnosis of myasthenia gravis. Within 5 minutes following the test, the ptosis and exotropia had returned.

Treatment

The medical treatment options for myasthenia do not cure the disorder but rather treat the symptoms of the disease. Patients who have only mild ocular symptoms may prefer to use an occluder or otherwise tolerate the symptoms rather than take daily medication. Rarely, the ocular misalignment is consistent enough that patients benefit from prism correction in their glasses, or is predictable enough that they have glasses with prism to

---

▶ BOX 8–1. PERFORMING A TENSILON TEST

1. Patient should be advised of potential cholinergic side effects from edrophonium chloride: orbicularis muscle twitching, diaphoresis, lacrimation, abdominal cramping, nausea, vomiting, and salivation. Although serious side effects such as severe bradycardia, respiratory arrest, or syncope are rare, the test should be performed only when emergency life support is available. The patient should be in a comfortable, reclined position to reduce the risk of a fall if syncope should occur.
2. Atropine sulfate (0.4 mg) should be immediately available for intravenous administration for adverse reactions. Some physicians routinely administer atropine prior to Tensilon injection.
3. The patient's pretest ptosis or motility disturbance is carefully observed and measured. Videotaping pretest motility and eyelid function, and the response to Tensilon, adds more objectivity to the test.
4. Ten milligrams of edrophonium chloride (10 mg/mL) is drawn up in a graduated 1-mL syringe (tuberculin syringe) and the syringe is connected to a butterfly intravenous infusion set, with a small amount used to prime the tubing.
5. After venous access is gained (and verified by drawing back on the syringe), a test dose of 2 mg (0.2 mL) is administered, and the patient's ptosis and/or motility is observed.
6. If no severe adverse reaction occurs, and if discernible improvement in function is not noted after 30 to 60 seconds, then the additional 0.8 mL can be administered in increments, or slowly over 30 to 60 seconds. The patient's ptosis or motility is observed or measured during the injection and for 3 to 5 minutes following the dose.
7. If the patient's signs reverse at any point during the infusion of Tensilon, the test is positive and no further injection is necessary.
8. Observation of the waning effects of Tensilon and return of myasthenic signs after 3 to 5 minutes offers further verification of a positive test.

wear when they become symptomatic in the evenings. Even patients with ocular symptoms only still require neurological observation, primarily to look for the development of systemic signs and symptoms.

Pyridostigmine bromide (Mestinon) is a long-acting oral anticholinesterase agent that is effective in relieving symptoms in many patients. The major side effect is gastrointestinal distress and diarrhea. Patients are usually started on 30 mg at 4-hour intervals during the day. The dose is increased until weakness is improved or until side effects become intolerable. Low-dose corticosteroids may be an effective alternative or additional therapy in those patients who are unresponsive to pyridostigmine. Other immunosuppressive agents such as azathioprine (Imuran), mycophenolate mofetil (CellCept), or cyclosporine may be effective, but these agents take weeks or months to demonstrate an effect.

Thymectomy is often effective whether or not there is evidence of thymus enlargement on chest CT, and may be curative. Patients younger than 60 years who have generalized myasthenia that responds poorly to oral therapy may benefit from thymectomy, even when the thymus appears normal on imaging studies. While 80% of patients stabilize or improve following thymectomy, this may not be evident until a year or more after surgery. Plasmapheresis and intravenous immunoglobulin (IVIg) may be needed for acute, life-threatening systemic weakness.

OTHER DISORDERS

Lambert-Eaton syndrome (LES) is a myasthenic-like syndrome with proximal limb weakness, fatigability, dry mouth, and impotence. This disorder only rarely affects the ocular or facial muscles. LES can be a primary or paraneoplastic autoimmune process, with antibodies directed at the *presynaptic* portion of the neuromuscular junction, resulting in an impairment in the release of acetylcholine. Electromyographic findings are the opposite of myasthenia, showing incremental *increased* response to repetitive nerve stimulation. About 70% of patients with Eaton-Lambert syndrome have underlying malignancies, frequently small cell carcinoma of the lung.

Botulism is also a presynaptic neuromuscular disorder, caused by ingestion of food contaminated with *Clostridium botulinum*. This bacterium elaborates botulinum toxin, a neurotoxin that blocks the release of acetylcholine at the neuromuscular junction. Ocular signs include ptosis, ophthalmoparesis, and dilated, poorly reactive pupils. Systemic symptoms include constipation, dizziness, headache, dysphagia, and weakness. Gastrointestinal symptoms may not be prominent.

▶ KEY POINTS

- CPEO is a clinical designation encompassing a group of mitochondrial myopathies that present as symmetric, slowly progressive myopathic bilateral ptosis and limitation of eye movements in all directions.
- Kearns-Sayre syndrome is a type of CPEO resulting from a mitochondrial chromosomal defect and is associated with cardiac conduction defects (including heart block and sudden death).
- *Myotonic dystrophy* is an autosomal dominant systemic myopathy characterized by bilateral ptosis, limited ocular motility, polychromatic cataract, and pigmentary retinopathy; systemic findings include characteristic facies, weakness, action myotonia, and divebomber discharges on EMG.
- Oculopharyngeal dystrophy is a heritable (autosomal dominant) condition affecting adults of French-Canadian heritage between 40 and 60 years of age causing CPEO and weakness of the bulbar musculature.
- Idiopathic orbital inflammatory syndrome causes localized or diffuse inflammation of the orbit without an identifiable infectious, neoplastic, or other systemic cause, presenting as pain with orbital congestion, proptosis, and/or diplopia.
- Common restrictive processes affecting the extraocular muscles include trauma and orbital Graves disease; less common entities include inflammatory, infiltrating, and space-occupying orbital lesions.
- Orbital Graves disease is a common autoimmune disorder that results in enlargement of the extraocular muscles and an increase in orbital fat volume, causing diplopia, eyelid retraction, and proptosis, often with ocular congestion.
- Thyroid dysfunction is not invariably present with Graves orbitopathy, and normal thyroid function does not rule out this entity.
- Symptoms of Graves orbitopathy generally fall into three areas: (1) ocular misalignment and diplopia from a restrictive myopathy, (2) exposure keratopathy from proptosis and eyelid retraction, and (3) potential for optic nerve compression by oversized extraocular muscles at the orbital apex.
- The inferior and medial rectus muscles are commonly involved in Graves disease, causing an esotropia and restricted upgaze.
- The most common cause of unilateral or bilateral proptosis is Graves orbitopathy.
- Compressive optic neuropathy can occur in orbital Graves disease even when the external signs are minimal.
- Brown tendon sheath syndrome is a restriction of the superior oblique tendon at the trochlea, and can be distinguished from an inferior oblique palsy by the characteristic downshoot of the eye

as the eye is adducted, and by restriction of elevation in adduction with forced duction testing.
- Myasthenia gravis is a systemic immunologic disorder of the neuromuscular junction in which the postsynaptic receptors for acetylcholine are blocked and inactivated by antibodies, causing systemic muscular weakness and weakness of the extraocular muscles that can mimic virtually any ocular motility disorder.

SUGGESTED READING

Books

Calvert P: Disorders of neuromuscular transmission, in Miller NR, Newman NJ, Biousse V, et al. (eds): *Walsh and Hoyt's Clinical Neuro-ophthalmology*, 6th ed. Baltimore, MD: Williams & Wilkins; 2005:1041–1108.

Hoffman P: Myopathies affecting the extraocular muscles, in Miller NR, Newman NJ, Biousse V, et al. (eds): *Walsh and Hoyt's Clinical Neuro-ophthalmology*, 6th ed. Baltimore, MD: Williams & Wilkins; 2005:1085–1132.

Leigh RJ, Zee DS: *The Neurology of Eye Movements*, 4th ed. New York, NY: Oxford University Press; 2006.

Smith KH: Myasthenia gravis, in *Focal Points: Clinical Modules for Ophthalmologists*, Vol 21, San Francisco, CA: American Academy of Ophthalmology; 2003:1–14.

Articles

CPEO and IOIS

Mahr MA, Salomao DR, Garrity JA: Inflammatory orbital pseudotumor with extension beyond the orbit. *Am J Ophthalmol* 2004;138:396–400.

Newman NJ: Mitochondrial disease and the eye. *Ophthalmol Clin North Am* 1992;5:405–424.

Graves Orbitopathy

Bradley EA, Gower EW, Bradley DJ, et al: Orbital radiation for Graves ophthalmopathy: a report from the American Academy of Ophthalmology. *Ophthalmology* 2008;115(122):398–409.

Holds JB, Buchanan AG: Graves orbitopathy. Focal points: clinical modules of ophthalmologists. San Francisco: American Academy of Ophthalmology; 2010: module 11.

Kazim M, Goldberg RA, Smith TJ: Insights into the pathogenesis of thyroid-associated orbitopathy. *Arch Ophthalmol* 2002;120:380–388.

Kazim M, Trokel S, Moore S: Treatment of acute Graves orbitopathy. *Ophthalmology* 1991;98:1443–1448.

Trobe JD, Glaser JS, LaFlamme P: Dysthyroid optic neuropathy: clinical profile and rationale for management. *Arch Ophthalmol* 1978;96:1199–1209.

Myasthenia Gravis

Conti-Fine BM, Milani M, Kaminski HJ: Myasthenia gravis: past, present, and future. *J Clin Invest* 2006;116:2843–2854.

Drachman DB: Myasthenia gravis. *N Engl J Med* 1994;330:1797–1810.

Elrod RD, Weinberg DA: Ocular myasthenia gravis. *Ophthalmol Clin North Am* 2004;17:275–309.

Golnik KC, Pena R, Lee AG, et al: An ice test for the diagnosis of myasthenia gravis. *Ophthalmology* 1999;106:1282–1286.

CHAPTER 9

Ocular Motility Disorders: Cranial Nerve Palsies

- ▶ ABDUCENS NERVE:
  CRANIAL NERVE VI   217
  Signs and symptoms   217
  Anatomy: clinical implications   220
  Differential diagnosis and evaluation   222
  Management   223
- ▶ TROCHLEAR NERVE:
  CRANIAL NERVE IV   224
  Signs and symptoms   224
  Anatomy: clinical implications   224
  Differential diagnosis   226
  Evaluation and management   226
- ▶ OCULOMOTOR NERVE:
  CRANIAL NERVE III   228
  Signs and symptoms   228
  Anatomy: clinical implications   228
  Aberrant regeneration   231
  Differential diagnosis   232
  Evaluation and management   232
- ▶ MULTIPLE CRANIAL NEUROPATHIES   234
  Anatomy: clinical implications   234
  Evaluation and differential diagnosis   235
- ▶ KEY POINTS   236

Cranial nerves (CNs) III (oculomotor), IV (trochlear), and VI (abducens) provide motor input to the extraocular muscles. The oculomotor nerve also innervates the levator of the upper eyelid and provides parasympathetic input to the pupillary sphincter. Disorders involving these cranial nerves can cause ocular misalignment and diplopia. Oculomotor palsies can also cause ptosis and anisocoria.

An overview of cranial nerve anatomy is provided in Figure 9–1. The three ocular motor cranial nerves originate as brainstem *motor nuclei*. The motor nuclei receive input from various supranuclear sources to coordinate movement of the eyes. Motor axons traverse the brainstem as *fascicles,* often passing through or near structures that can be simultaneously involved with brainstem disease. The axons then exit the brainstem, forming a *peripheral cranial nerve,* passing through the subarachnoid space and cavernous sinus to innervate the extraocular muscles. The cranial nerves can be affected by many disease processes along their course (Table 9–1). Neighboring structures along the course of each of the cranial nerves may be involved in cranial neuropathies, producing distinctive signs and symptoms that frequently allow localization and characterization of a lesion.

▶ ABDUCENS NERVE: CRANIAL NERVE VI

The abducens nerve (CN VI) innervates the lateral rectus muscle in the ipsilateral orbit. As its name describes, this cranial nerve is responsible for abduction of the eye, and paresis causes an abduction deficit.

SIGNS AND SYMPTOMS

Patients with a CN VI palsy describe horizontal diplopia, worse in gaze toward the palsied muscle. Diplopia may not be a problem at near because convergence moves the eye away from the field of action of the lateral rectus muscle; in other words, the lateral rectus is inhibited with convergence anyway, so a weak lateral rectus is not as likely to cause symptoms with near tasks such as reading.

The measured esotropia in CN VI disorders is incomitant and is much greater in the field of action of the palsied muscle (Figure 9–2). Patients may adopt a head turn posture, with the face turned toward the palsied eye, to minimize the strabismus. A small vertical deviation is often present with lateral rectus weakness, which should not be mistaken for a superimposed skew deviation.

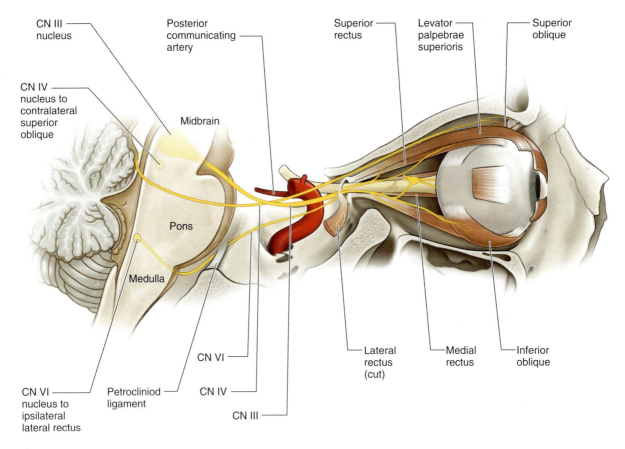
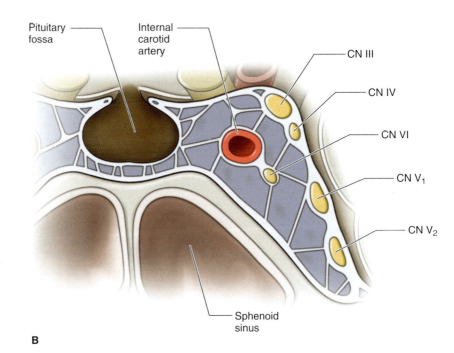

Figure 9-1. **Anatomic overview.**
(A) The nuclei and course of cranial nerves (CNs) III, IV, and VI are shown. CN IV is the only cranial nerve to exit the dorsal brainstem. All three ocular motor nerves travel through the cavernous sinus to enter the orbit.
(B) Cavernous sinus (coronal view). CNs III and IV travel in the lateral wall of the sinus, but CN VI occupies a more vulnerable mid-cavernous route. The first (ophthalmic) branch of the trigeminal nerve (V_1) traverses the length of the sinus to enter the orbit through the superior orbital fissure; the second (maxillary) branch (V_2) exits mid-cavernous sinus; and the third (mandibular) branch (V_3) may variably have a brief appearance in the posterior cavernous sinus (not pictured).

▶ TABLE 9-1. CAUSES BY LOCATION OF OCULAR MOTOR CRANIAL NEUROPATHIES (CN III, IV, VI)

Location	Pathological Processes	Causes
Brainstem (nuclei and fascicles)	Neoplasm	Glioma, metastasis
	Inflammatory/demyelinating	MS, postviral, Miller Fisher variant of Guillain-Barré syndrome
	Vascular	Stroke, hemorrhage, microvascular disease, dolichoectatic basilar arterie, arteriovenous malformation
	Infection	*Toxoplasma gondii*, abscess
	Other	Wernicke encephalopathy
Subarachnoid space	Infection (basilar meningitis)	*Tuberculosis, cryptococcosis*, AIDS, syphilis, and occasionally bacterial infections
	Inflammatory	Sarcoidosis
	Neoplasm	Clivus chordoma, meningioma, carcinomatous meningitis, leukemia, subarachnoid metastasis from ependymomas, medulloblastoma, CNS lymphoma, other neoplasms
	Invasive extracranial neoplasms	Adenoid cystic carcinoma, nasopharyngeal carcinoma
	Trauma	
	Subarachnoid hemorrhage	
	Aneurysm	
Uncertain: subarachnoid space or cavernous sinus	Microvascular (ischemic mononeuropathy)	Diabetes, hypertension, collagen vascular disease, giant cell arteritis, atherosclerosis
Cavernous sinus/superior orbital fissure	Septic thrombosis	Bacterial infection, mucormycosis, *Aspergillus*
	Parasellar tumors	Meningioma, craniopharyngioma, pituitary adenoma, pituitary apoplexy, chordoma, neurilemmoma
	Other neoplasms	Myeloma, lymphoma, metastasis (breast, lung), tumor extension from paranasal sinus, bone tumors
	Vascular abnormalities	Carotid-cavernous fistula, intracavernous aneurysm
Cavernous sinus, superior orbital fissure, or orbital apex	Granulomatous processes	Tolosa-Hunt syndrome, sarcoidosis, herpes zoster
Orbital apex/orbit	Trauma	
	Idiopathic orbital inflammatory syndrome	
	Orbital tumors	
Variable or unknown location	Migraine	

Abbreviations: AIDS, acquired immune deficiency syndrome; CN, cranial nerve; CNS, central nervous system; MS, multiple sclerosis.

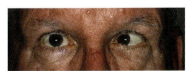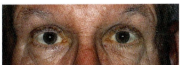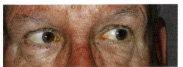

Figure 9-2. **Cranial nerve VI palsy.**
A 62-year-old woman with type 2 diabetes had a sudden onset of horizontal diplopia. The motility examination shows an inability to abduct the right eye.

ANATOMY: CLINICAL IMPLICATIONS

Disorders that can affect CN VI, and the occurrence of associated neurological signs and symptoms, are a direct consequence of the local neuroanatomy.

Nucleus and Fascicles

The paired abducens nuclei are located in the brainstem at the level of the pons and fourth ventricle (Figure 9–3A). The nucleus contains two types of neurons: motor neurons whose axons form the ipsilateral sixth cranial fascicle and nerve, and internuclear neurons. The internuclear neurons send their axons across the midline to ascend in the contralateral medial longitudinal fasciculus (MLF), where they synapse with neurons in the contralateral medial rectus subnucleus to coordinate conjugate horizontal gaze (see Figure 10–2). Therefore, CN VI *nuclear* lesions produce an ipsilateral *gaze palsy*, not just an abduction defect. Involvement of the adjacent paramedian pontine reticular formation (PPRF) and MLF can result in a gaze palsies or a one-and-a-half syndrome (see Figure 10–6). The facial nerve (CN VII) nucleus lies ventrally with fascicles that loop superiorly over the abducens nucleus, forming a bump on the floor of the fourth ventricle (the facial colliculus). This anatomic landmark is useful in identifying the level of the abducens nucleus on axial magnetic resonance imaging (MRI) scans. Disorders affecting the abducens nucleus include brainstem gliomas, metastatic lesions, infarctions, and arteriovenous malformations.

Motor fascicles from the abducens nucleus travel ventrally through the pontine tegmentum toward the pontomedullary junction. Lesions that involve the CN VI fascicles frequently also affect adjacent pontine structures, including the facial nerve nucleus and fascicles, descending oculosympathetic fibers, trigeminal nucleus and fascicles, corticospinal tract, and others. Millard-Gubler syndrome is a CN VI paresis with an ipsilateral CN VII palsy and contralateral hemiparesis, implicating a ventral pontine lesion. Raymond syndrome is a CN VI paresis with contralateral hemiparesis. Foville syndrome occurs from a dorsal pontine lesion and consists of ipsilateral CN V, VII, and VIII palsies, with a horizontal gaze palsy and an ipsilateral Horner syndrome (see Figure 9–3A).

Infarction from vascular disease is the most common lesion involving the abducens fascicles in patients older than 50 years; demyelination from multiple sclerosis (MS) and brainstem gliomas can occur in younger patients. Cerebellar tumors can affect the abducens nucleus or fascicles by compression or extension into the pons.

Subarachnoid Space

CN VI exits the brainstem at the pontomedullary junction approximately 1 cm from the midline, entering the subarachnoid space within the *cerebellopontine angle*. This anatomic space is bounded by the cerebellum and brainstem and includes CN VII and CN VIII. Mass lesions in this area that involve CN VI frequently also affect the neighboring structures, resulting in a CN VI palsy, facial palsy, and hearing loss, frequently with papilledema (see Figure 9–3B). Acoustic neuromas, meningiomas, cerebellar tumors, and nasopharyngeal carcinoma can occur in the cerebellopontine angle.

After exiting the brainstem and traversing the subarachnoid space, CN VI ascends in close association with the dura of the clivus. Metastatic tumors to the clivus (especially prostate), meningiomas, and clivus chordomas can affect CN VI unilaterally or bilaterally in this region. As the nerve ascends toward the top of the clivus, it turns to follow a more level course and enters *Dorello canal*, passing beneath the petroclinoid (Gruber) ligament and over the petrous apex to enter the cavernous sinus. Because the inferior petrosal sinus also shares this confined space, CN VI palsies frequently accompany the venous engorgement that occurs with carotid-cavernous sinus fistulas or cavernous sinus thrombosis.

The subarachnoid portion of CN VI is firmly attached at the pontomedullary junction of the brainstem inferiorly and at Dorello canal in the skull base superiorly. Because of these tether points, the nerve is vulnerable to stretching injury from any downward movement of the brain relative to the skull base, as can occur with intracranial hypertension, as a result of lumbar puncture, or in closed head injury.

Gradenigo syndrome consists of severe facial pain and numbness, unilateral CN VI palsy, facial paresis, and decreased hearing, as the result of severe otitis media involving the petrous apex, where CN VI and CN VII are in close proximity. In the modern antibiotic era, otitis media in children rarely manifests this way. In adults, the syndrome complex suggests a cholesteatoma or nasopharyngeal carcinoma.

Basal skull fractures frequently involve the petrous apex and CN VI, also involving the facial nerve when the temporal bone is fractured. Associated signs include cerebrospinal fluid (CSF) otorrhea, blood in the external auditory meatus, and mastoid ecchymosis (Battle sign).

Cavernous Sinus

CN VI runs through the middle of the cavernous sinus just lateral to the carotid artery, unlike CN III and CN IV, which travel somewhat protected in the lateral wall of the sinus (see Figure 9–1B). This position of CN VI in the cavernous sinus makes the nerve vulnerable, and it is often the first cranial nerve to be affected by cavernous sinus disease processes, such as intracavernous aneurysms, carotid-cavernous fistulas, metastatic tumors, and laterally invasive sellar tumors. Sympathetic fibers from the carotid plexus condense and travel briefly on

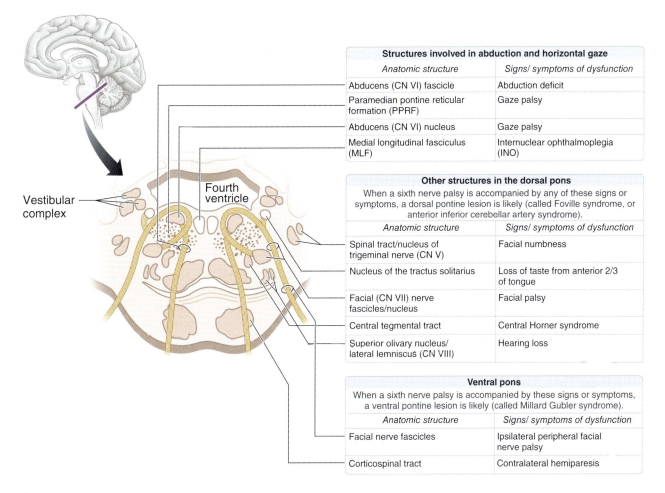

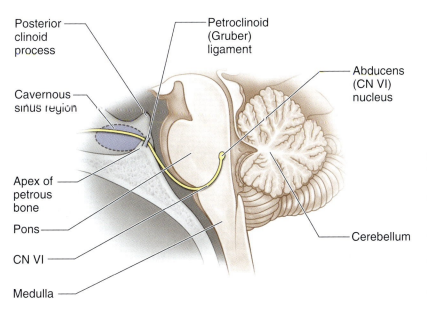

Figure 9-3. **Cranial nerve VI anatomy.**
(A) Brainstem cross section at the level of the cranial nerve (CN) VI nucleus. Neighboring structures and associated signs and symptoms are identified.
(B) Subarachnoid course. CN VI exits the brainstem at the pontomedullary junction into the subarachnoid space and climbs up the clivus, piercing the dura and turning toward the cavernous sinus under the petroclinoid ligament through Dorello canal.

the abducens nerve in the cavernous sinus before joining the first division of CN V to enter the orbit. The combination of an oculosympathetic paresis (Horner syndrome) accompanying a CN VI palsy is highly suggestive of a cavernous sinus process.

Infarction of CN VI (ischemic cranial mononeuropathy) is common with diabetes mellitus, presumably occurring in the cavernous sinus. Associated periorbital pain is most likely caused by ischemia of the adjacent meninges. The nerve is capable of regenerating and regrows along its original course, guided by the myelin tunnel left behind after axonal degeneration. Normal function usually returns within 3 months.

Orbit

CN VI enters the orbit through the superior orbital fissure, inside the annulus of Zinn (and within the muscle cone), and innervates the lateral rectus muscle, entering the muscle on its mesial surface. CN VI, III, and IV can be affected by inflammatory conditions affecting the superior orbital fissure and orbital apex (see Table 9–1).

DIFFERENTIAL DIAGNOSIS AND EVALUATION

Sixth Cranial Nerve Palsy

The sudden onset of an isolated abduction deficit in a patient with known vascular disease or in a patient older than 50 years likely represents an *ischemic mononeuropathy*. The disease process can occur in younger patients, especially with systemic vascular risk factors such as diabetes mellitus or hypertension. Pain can occur but is usually slight and confined to the first week. Because ischemic cranial mononeuropathies can occur with vasculitis, laboratory evaluation should include a sedimentation rate and C-reactive protein. Patients with no known risk factors for ischemic disease should have a medical evaluation for diabetes mellitus, systemic hypertension, hypercholesterolemia, and atherosclerotic disease. Although recovery usually takes 6 weeks or more, reexamination of the patient in the first 2 to 4 weeks after onset is prudent. This follow-up visit is to ensure that the abduction deficit is not progressing and remains isolated, with no signs to suggest involvement of other cranial nerves (suggesting tumor) or variable signs and symptoms (suggesting myasthenia gravis). Most patients have resolution of diplopia by 3 months; those patients with persistent signs and symptoms beyond this time may need additional investigation (such as neuroimaging) for other possible causes.

Compressive lesions of CN VI are characterized by a progressive worsening of the abduction deficit, often with other associated cranial neuropathies or evolving neurological signs. An MRI is indicated if a CN VI palsy is slowly progressing, if the patient has a history of a brain or sinus tumor or potentially metastatic cancer, if other cranial nerves are involved, if the patient is experiencing unrelenting facial pain, or if other neurological symptoms are present. MRI of the brain with contrast allows a detailed view of the brainstem and the course of the nerve, which is not possible with computed tomography (CT) imaging. MRI of the orbit may need to be included if orbital processes (eg, orbital Graves disease) remain in the differential diagnosis.

Children may develop isolated unilateral or bilateral CN VI palsy as a postviral syndrome, presumably autoimmune in origin, with spontaneous recovery. Because brainstem gliomas and cerebellar tumors are a concern in this age group, neuroimaging and close observation for the development of other neurological signs (gaze palsies, cerebellar signs) are required. An otoscopic examination should be performed to address the possibility of middle ear infections.

Unilateral or bilateral CN VI palsies can occur with *elevated intracranial pressure*. The importance of examining the optic discs in this setting is obvious—and is a reminder to the physician of the importance of completing all the basic steps in the neuro-ophthalmic examination, even steps (eg, fundus examination) that appear unrelated to the complaint (eg, diplopia).

Divergence insufficiency is a poorly understood disorder consisting of an esotropia at distance and orthophoria at near in a patient with full ductions, usually identified in patients 60 years or older. Whether this disorder represents a microischemic vascular lesion in a divergence center in the brainstem or is a mild bilateral CN VI paresis is uncertain.

Other Causes of Abduction Deficit

Patients with an abduction deficit should not be immediately labeled as having a *CN VI paresis* (Table 9–2). Restriction of the medial rectus from orbital Graves disease, traumatic medial rectus entrapment, and idiopathic orbital inflammatory syndrome (IOIS) (and other orbital causes) can also cause an abduction deficit. Ocular myasthenia gravis can produce virtually any ocular motility pattern, including an isolated abduction deficit. Congenital esotropia can usually be distinguished from bilateral CN VI palsies because it is comitant and associated with other findings, including latent nystagmus, oblique muscle dysfunction, and amblyopia.

Convergence spasm can mimic bilateral CN VI palsies (Figure 9–4). When this condition occurs with dorsal midbrain syndrome, other signs are invariably present (see Table 10–1). Convergence spasm can be a component of latent hyperopia or presbyopia. Voluntary convergence (functional convergence spasm) is accompanied by miosis and cannot be sustained indefinitely.

Duane syndrome is a congenital condition causing an ocular motility disorder that surprisingly

► **TABLE 9-2. DIFFERENTIAL DIAGNOSIS OF AN ABDUCTION DEFICIT**

Abducens (CN VI) Palsy
  Ischemic mononeuropathy
  Trauma
  Elevated intracranial hypertension
  Compression
  • Brainstem
  • Cerebellopontine angle tumors
  • Clivus tumors
  • Cavernous sinus lesions
  Demyelination (MS)

Orbital/Muscle Causes
  Orbital Graves disease
  Idiopathic orbital inflammatory syndrome
  Traumatic medial rectus entrapment

Congenital
  Duane syndrome
  Möbius syndrome
  Decompensated congenital esophoria

Other
  Convergence spasm
  Ocular myasthenia gravis
  Divergence paralysis

Abbreviations: CN, cranial nerve; MS, multiple sclerosis.

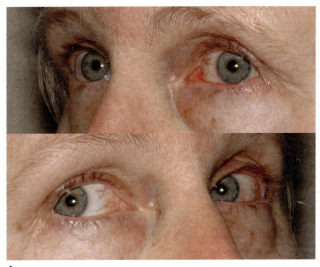

A

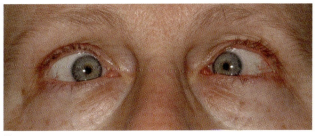

B

Figure 9-4. Convergence (accommodative) spasm.
(A) A patient thought to have intermittent cranial nerve VI palsies is shown to have normal horizontal ocular motility by doll's head maneuver. **(B)** However, attempts to perform ocular versions resulted in marked esotropia, with a pseudoabduction deficit. Note the miotic pupils, confirming that this is an accommodative/convergence spasm.

may not be recognized until adulthood. Patients with an incidentally discovered horizontal strabismus may have Duane syndrome, but the physician must be confident that the patient does not have an acquired strabismus before attributing an abduction deficit to Duane syndrome. Duane syndrome is the result of congenital aplasia or hypoplasia of CN VI nucleus and nerve (unilateral, rarely bilateral), often with anomalous innervation of the lateral rectus muscle by CN III. Characteristics include narrowing of the fissure on attempted abduction from cocontraction and dynamic enophthalmos. Patients may have deficient abduction, adduction, or both (Figure 9-5). Amblyopia is rare. Patients may have a head turn to maintain binocularity.

Möbius syndrome is a congenital malformation that involves multiple brainstem nuclei and results in bilateral abduction or gaze palsies, bilateral hypoglossal paralysis, and bilateral facial palsies (see Figure 12-6).

MANAGEMENT

Treatment of CN VI palsy is determined by the underlying cause. Long-standing palsies that have no potential for spontaneous recovery may benefit from strabismus surgery. Spectacle prisms are occasionally helpful in allowing fusion in primary position when a chronic deviation is small. In traumatic CN VI palsies or other well-defined causes, injection of the antagonist medial rectus muscle with botulinum toxin may (temporarily) permit fusion in primary position and reduce the risk of medial rectus contracture.

Symptomatic relief should be offered to all patients, even when their evaluation is in progress. A spectacle clip-on occluder eliminates diplopia by blocking vision in one eye and is more comfortable and convenient than a pirate patch or voluntarily keeping an eye closed. Patients are usually more comfortable occluding the palsied eye; there is no danger in allowing this occlusion preference for the majority of the time the occluder is used. Suggesting that patients try to use both eyes together part of each day (such as when watching TV) is beneficial. Patients who have diplopia in lateral gaze only may benefit from translucent tape selectively placed over the lateral portion of the spectacle lens in the palsied eye. Placed correctly, the tape blocks vision in one eye in the diplopic field of gaze but allows binocular vision in all other fields of gaze.

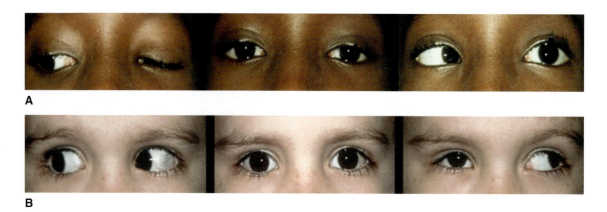

Figure 9-5. Duane syndrome.
(A) Duane type 1 is characterized by an abduction deficit and narrowing of the fissure on adduction, as seen in the left eye of this child. **(B)** Duane type 2 (right eye) is demonstrated in this patient's clinical photographs: an adduction deficit in the right eye, and narrowing of the fissure on attempted adduction of the right eye. Duane type 3 (not shown) has both adduction and abduction deficits.

▶ TROCHLEAR NERVE: CRANIAL NERVE IV

The trochlear nerve (CN IV) innervates only the superior oblique muscle, but this muscle has a complex action: It intorts, depresses, and abducts the eye.

SIGNS AND SYMPTOMS

A CN IV palsy (commonly called a superior oblique palsy) causes a hypertropia of the affected eye (often with a small esotropia), resulting in a vertical or diagonal diplopia. The superior oblique muscle's angle of insertion on the globe is such that the muscle is a strong depressor of the globe when the eye is adducted, but it has little vertical action in abduction. Thus, patients with superior oblique palsies describe a vertical diplopia that is worse when the palsied eye is adducted. The superior oblique muscle also intorts the eye. Paresis causes an excyclotorsion, and patients often volunteer that the double images are tilted with respect to one another. Patients frequently adopt a head tilt position away from the palsied eye and with the chin down, minimizing the misalignment by moving the eye out of the palsied superior oblique muscle's field of action. As discussed in the examination section, the best way to examine superior oblique function is to test how well the eye can look down while adducted. In adduction, the complex actions of the superior oblique are reduced to one main action—depressing the eye—simplifying the assessment (Figure 9-6).

ANATOMY: CLINICAL IMPLICATIONS

Nucleus and Fascicles

The paired CN IV nuclei are located below the periaqueductal gray matter of the dorsal midbrain just behind the CN III nuclei, at the level of the inferior colliculi (Figure 9-7). Each nucleus controls the *contralateral* superior oblique muscle: Motor fascicles travel dorsally and posteriorly from the nucleus and *decussate* in the anterior medullary velum, exit the brainstem dorsally, and sweep around the brainstem to enter the cavernous sinus and eventually innervate the superior oblique muscle.

Brainstem lesions (eg, MS, glioma, infarct) are uncommon causes of a CN IV palsy, primarily because of the extreme dorsal position of the nuclei and very short course of the fascicles within the substance of the brainstem (Figure 9-8 shows an exception). Also, the CN IV nuclei and fascicles are located in an area of the brainstem that is not as "busy" as CN VI and CN III, hence the relative lack of CN IV brainstem syndromes. Adjacent structures that could potentially be involved include the medial longitudinal fasciculus and descending sympathetic fibers, traveling just below the nuclei. A localized lesion involving the CN IV nucleus and the adjacent sympathetic pathway would cause a contralateral superior oblique palsy with an ipsilateral Horner syndrome.

Subarachnoid Space

CN IV exits the dorsal brainstem and curves around the brainstem in the ambient cistern and beneath the free edge of the tentorium, penetrating the edge of the tentorial dura to enter the cavernous sinus. As the longest of the cranial nerves within the subarachnoid space and the only one to exit the brainstem dorsally, CN IV is the most vulnerable to head trauma. Similar to other cranial nerves, ischemic mononeuropathy is common. Tumors, meningitis, and metastatic disease are uncommon causes of CN IV palsies in the subarachnoid space.

Cavernous Sinus and Orbit

CN IV travels in the lateral wall of the cavernous sinus (see Figure 9-1B) and enters the orbit through the superior orbital fissure (outside the annulus of Zinn and the

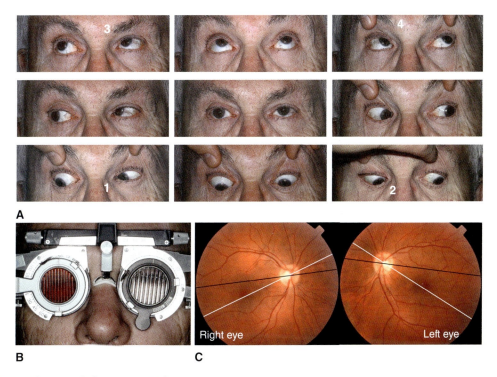

Figure 9-6. **Fourth cranial nerve palsy.**
(A) Ocular versions demonstrate left superior oblique weakness, suggesting a left cranial nerve (CN) IV palsy. The left eye does not depress well in adduction (1). The deficiency is most evident when compared to normal depression of the right eye in adduction (2). Apparent overaction of the left inferior oblique is seen because this muscle acts unopposed by the palsied superior oblique in up gaze (3). Again, comparison with the opposite side is important (4). (B) A total of 12° of excyclotorsion is present as measured by double Maddox rod testing, suggesting that both right and left CN IV may be affected to some extent. (C) Excyclotorsion may be evident on ophthalmoscopy, as seen in a different patient with bilateral CN IV palsies. The dark line shows the normal position of the macula relative to the center of the disc, slightly below horizontal. The white lines show marked excyclotorsion, with rotation of the macula relative to the optic disc.

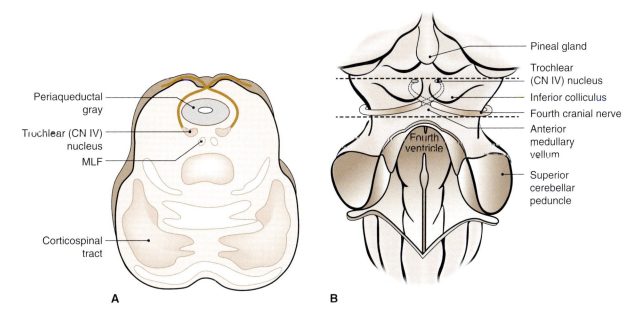

Figure 9-7. **Cranial nerve IV anatomy.**
(A) Brainstem cross section at the level of the cranial nerve (CN) IV nuclei. The nuclei are located dorsally in the brainstem and have only a short course before exiting dorsally. (B) Dorsal view of the brainstem. The left and right CN IVs cross in the anterior medullary vellum, at the anterior extent of the fourth ventricle. Abbreviation: MLF, medial longitudinal fasciculus.

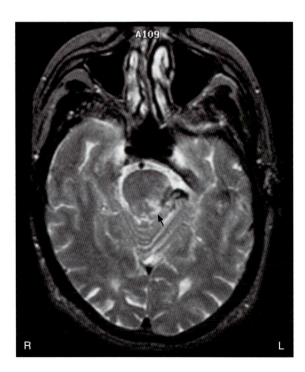

Figure 9-8. Uncommon case: cranial nerve IV palsy from brainstem hemorrhage.
A 65-year-old man, on warfarin (Coumadin) following mitral valve replacement had diplopia following a syncopal episode. This is the same patient shown in Figure 9–6. Magnetic resonance imaging (*pictured*) demonstrated hemorrhage at the level of the inferior colliculus on the left (*arrow*), involving the exiting fascicles of the left trochlear nerve (originating from the right cranial nerve [CN] IV nucleus), but also potentially involving the trochlear nucleus in the left midbrain (the origin of the right CN IV).

muscle cone) to innervate the superior oblique muscle. Lesions in the cavernous sinus and superior orbital fissure are not likely causes of an *isolated* CN IV palsy because multiple cranial nerves are usually affected by lesions in this region (see Table 9–1).

DIFFERENTIAL DIAGNOSIS

A number of entities can cause vertical motility disturbances (Table 9–3). The motility pattern of CN IV palsies can be mimicked by myasthenia. Orbital Graves disease and skew deviations present with vertical tropias but can usually be distinguished from a CN IV palsy. Skew deviations are small vertical misalignments from brainstem disorders (a type of supranuclear palsy).

EVALUATION AND MANAGEMENT

The Bielschowsky three-step test is helpful in confirming the clinical suspicion of a CN IV palsy, as is measurement of ocular torsion with double Maddox rod testing (see Figure 9–6B; see also Figure 7–6). However, with time, CN IV palsies may not obey the classic rules of the three-step test because compensatory adjustments dilute the incomitance (so-called *spread of comitance*).

▶ **TABLE 9-3. DIFFERENTIAL DIAGNOSIS OF VERTICAL DEVIATIONS**

CN IV Palsy
  Traumatic
  Congenital
  Decompensated congenital
  Ischemic (diabetic) mononeuropathy
  Tumor or aneurysm (rare)

CN III Palsy (see Table 9–4)

Orbital
  Orbital Graves disease
  Idiopathic orbital inflammatory syndrome
  Trauma
  • Entrapment (floor fracture)
  • Trochlear trauma
  Postsurgical (cataract)

Neuromuscular Junction
  Ocular myasthenia gravis

Supranuclear
  Skew deviation

Abbreviation: CN, cranial nerve.

Most isolated CN IV palsies are the result of trauma, an ischemic mononeuropathy, or they are congenital in origin. Unilateral or bilateral CN IV palsies in the setting of head *trauma* are very common and are often permanent. The time course of an *ischemic mononeuropathy* of CN IV is similar to the description for ischemic CN VI palsy: (1) the onset is sudden, often with periorbital pain; (2) the ocular deviation is constant for approximately 6 weeks; and (3) most patients recover completely by 3 months. Patients with a presumed ischemic mononeuropathy and known vascular disease usually do not require neuroimaging. Obtaining an erythrocyte sedimentation rate (ESR) and C-reactive protein (CRP) in patients older than 50 years is reasonable to address the (unlikely) possibility of giant cell arteritis as a cause of an ischemic CN IV palsy (or rarely, infarction of the superior oblique muscle).

Congenital CN IV palsies are common. Occasionally, patients may present with an acute decompensation of their hyperphoria, with complaint of new diplopia. Decompensation of a congenital CN IV palsy is a difficult diagnosis to make with certainty. Clinical characteristics include large vertical fusional amplitudes, spread of comitance (discussed above), and lifelong head tilt (identified in old, unposed, family photographs, as in Figure 9–9).

Congenital and traumatic CN IV palsies are frequently bilateral but asymmetric. The bilaterality may not be discovered until the more prominent side is surgically addressed, uncovering the palsy in the other

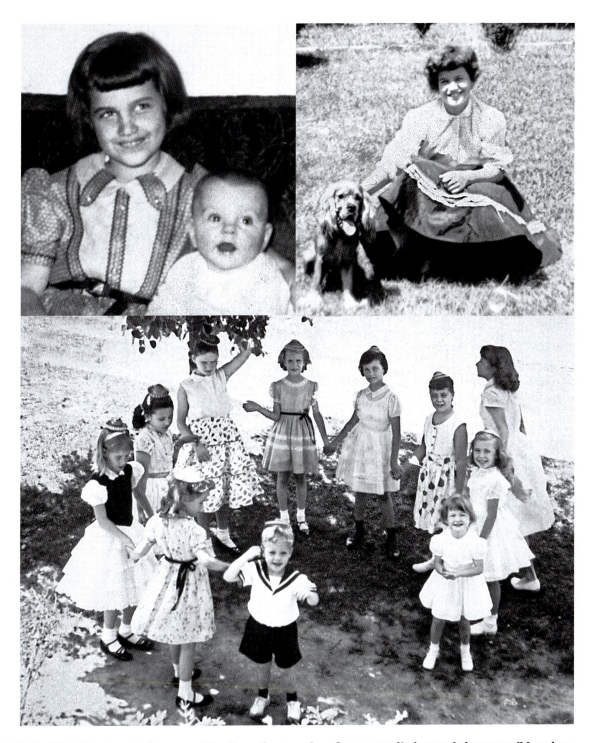

Figure 9–9. **Old photographs provide the diagnosis of congenital cranial nerve IV palsy.** A 39-year-old woman described intermittent diplopia over the previous 2 years. The examination was consistent with a left cranial nerve (CN) IV palsy. Several aspects of the examination suggested that the hypertropia was chronic. Old family photographs provided the final proof of a lifelong, previously compensated left CN IV palsy. The upper photographs show the patient's consistent, compensatory right head tilt present throughout the family album. The lower photograph shows her with a group of friends. Given her characteristic head tilt, the reader should have no difficulty locating the patient in this group.

eye. Bilaterality is likely when a total of greater than 10° of excyclotorsion exists (measured by double Maddox rod, as in Figure 9–6B), or when alternating ipsilateral hypertropias are noted on right and left head tilt.

Isolated CN IV palsy as a result of intracranial tumor or aneurysm is unusual, but an MRI is indicated if new in onset without vascular risk factors, if symptoms are progressing, if the patient has a history of a local or potentially metastatic cancer, if other cranial nerves are involved, or if other neurological symptoms are present.

A clip-on occluder provides symptomatic relief from diplopia. Prisms (stick-on Fresnel prisms or built-in prisms) are only occasionally helpful because prisms cannot correct the torsional component of a superior oblique palsy. Selective fogging of the bifocal of one eye with translucent tape helps those patients who are symptomatic only in downgaze. Surgical therapy can be considered for patients with long-standing, stable superior oblique palsies.

▶ OCULOMOTOR NERVE: CRANIAL NERVE III

The oculomotor nerve (CN III) is complex: It innervates the superior, medial, and inferior rectus muscles; the inferior oblique muscle; and the levator palpebrae muscle (which elevates the eyelids), and provides parasympathetic innervation to the pupillary sphincter and ciliary muscle.

SIGNS AND SYMPTOMS

CN III palsies can cause a ptosis of the upper eyelid and a dilated pupil, in addition to a motility disturbance. The relative degree of pupillary involvement provides important clinical diagnostic clues to guide the investigation. Complete pupillary sphincter paralysis (known as a "blown pupil") causes a very large pupil that is unresponsive to light or near; less involvement creates an anisocoria that may only be evident in bright light. Paresis of innervation to the superior rectus, inferior rectus, medial rectus, and inferior oblique muscles causes a defect in elevating, depressing, and adducting the eye (Figure 9–10). When the oculomotor paresis is profound, the only working extraocular muscles are the lateral rectus and the superior oblique; thus the affected eye is pulled laterally and down. Diplopia with CN III palsies has both vertical and horizontal components that vary with the direction of attempted gaze. Diplopia may not be a prominent complaint when ptosis is sufficient to cover the pupil.

ANATOMY: CLINICAL IMPLICATIONS

Nucleus

The multiple functions served by the oculomotor nerve are represented by individual subnuclei grouped within the oculomotor nuclear complex (Figure 9–11 A).

The right and left components of the CN III straddle the midsagittal plane and are located just beneath the periaqueductal gray matter of the dorsal midbrain (mesencephalon), at the level of the superior colliculi. The central caudal nucleus is midline, and this single nucleus innervates both the right and left levator

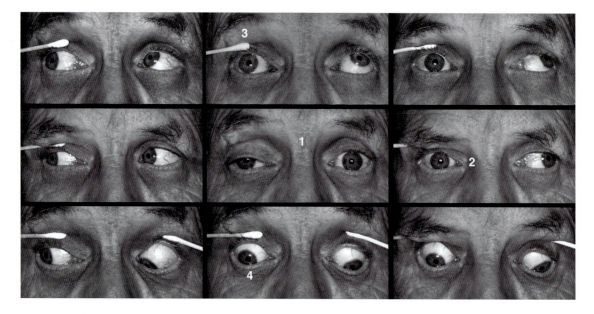

Figure 9–10. Pupil-sparing cranial nerve III palsy in a diabetic patient.
A 50-year-old diabetic man described the onset of right periorbital pain lasting several days. Within 2 days of the onset of pain, diplopia occurred, followed the next day by ptosis. The sedimentation rate was normal, and the clinical presentation was characteristic of an ischemic mononeuropathy. Signs and symptoms cleared within 2 months of onset. The motility examination is pictured. The patient had an incomplete ptosis with no anisocoria (1). The patient cannot fully adduct (2), elevate (3), or depress (4) the right eye.

palpebrae muscles. Thus, a ptosis from a purely nuclear CN III lesion (a rare entity except on neuroophthalmology quizzes) is always bilateral, and on occasion may be an isolated finding with a precisely placed nuclear CN III lesion. Unlike the central caudal nucleus, all other subnuclei in the CN III nuclear complex are essentially paired. The Edinger-Westphal nuclei provide the parasympathetic motor innervation to the pupillary constrictors. This subnucleus, as well as the medial rectus, inferior rectus, and inferior oblique subnuclei, serves the ipsilateral eye. The superior rectus fascicles decussate within the nuclear complex to provide innervation to the contralateral superior rectus muscle. Theoretically, a precisely placed unilateral nuclear CN III lesion could cause contralateral superior rectus weakness with ipsilateral CN III dysfunction, but this point is rarely of clinical importance. Lesions affecting the CN III nuclear complex or its individual components are uncommon but include infarction, demyelination, inflammation (sarcoidosis), and tumor (glioma or metastatic).

Fascicles

The fascicles of CN III travel ventrally through the midbrain tegmentum, passing through the red nucleus and through the medial aspect of the cerebral peduncles. Midbrain lesions affecting the fascicles can occasionally cause isolated CN III palsies that are clinically indistinguishable from peripheral CN III palsies. More frequently, lesions affecting CN III fascicles also involve the red nucleus (Benedikt syndrome) or cerebral peduncles (Weber syndrome) (see Figure 9–11A; Figure 9–12).

Subarachnoid Space

CN III emerges form the brainstem in the interpeduncular fossa, traveling in the subarachnoid space to the cavernous sinus.

CN III has an important relationship to the circle of Willis. The basilar artery ascends on the ventral aspect of the brainstem, giving rise to the paired superior cerebellar arteries, and then the posterior cerebral arteries at the level of the mesencephalon. CN III courses between the superior cerebellar and posterior cerebral arteries as the nerve emerges from the brainstem. The oculomotor nerve then travels adjacent to and lateral to the posterior communicating artery, which connects the posterior cerebral artery and the middle cerebral arteries (forming the posterior half of the circle of Willis). Aneurysms arising at the junction of the posterior communicating and middle cerebral artery can damage the nerve by compression or by inducing

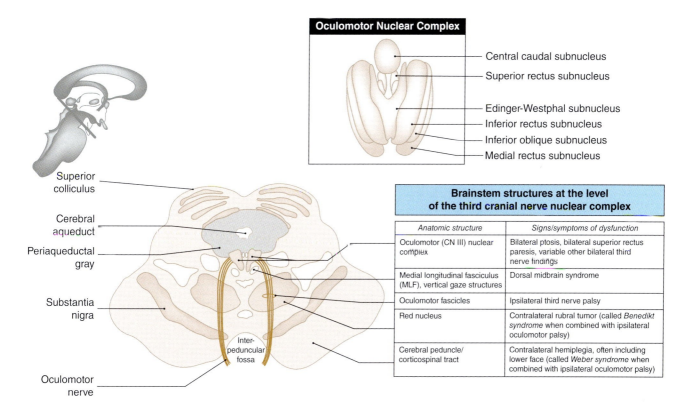

Figure 9–11. Third cranial nerve anatomy.
(A) Brainstem cross section at the level of the cranial nerve (CN) III nuclear complex. The CN III complex consists of individual subnuclei, corresponding to its multiple functions (*inset*). Neighboring structures and associated signs and symptoms are identified.

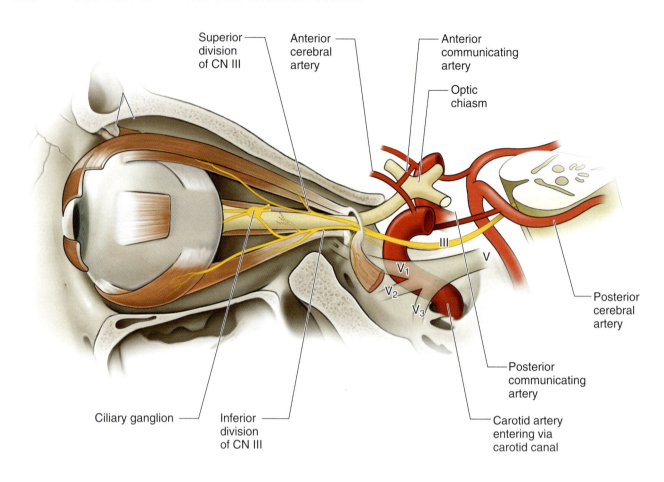

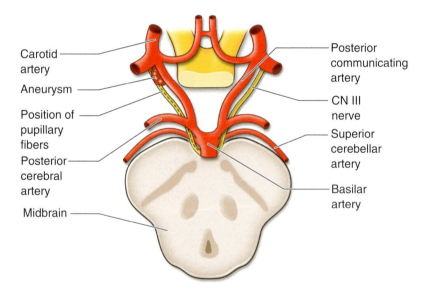

B

Figure 9-11. (Continued)
(B) Subarachnoid course. After exiting the brainstem in the interpeduncular fossa, the nerve runs parallel and adjacent to the posterior communicating artery before entering the cavernous sinus. This position makes it vulnerable to compression from posterior communicating artery aneurysms (*inset*). (Reproduced with permission from Weinstein JM. The pupil. In Slamovits TL, Burde R, associate editors. Neuro-ophthalmology, vol 6. In Podos SM, Yanoff M, editors: Textbook of ophthalmology. St Louis, 1991, Mosby.)

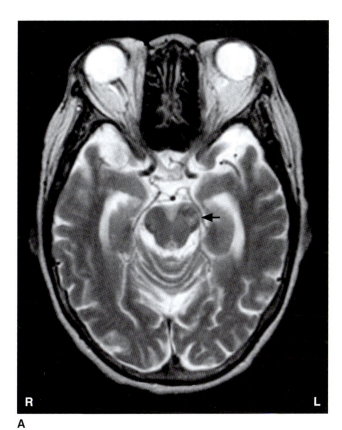

Figure 9–12. Weber syndrome.
A 62-year-old woman had a midbrain stroke. **(A)** Magnetic resonance imaging (T2-weighted axial image) shows an area of infarction in midbrain tegmentum in the region of the left cranial nerve (CN) III fascicles and cerebral peduncle. **(B)** The patient has right upper extremity weakness and a left CN III palsy with a complete ptosis.

intraneural hemorrhage (see Figure 9–11B). Aneurysms in this area can expand suddenly and cause an acute, painful CN III paresis. A subarachnoid hemorrhage can occur when such aneurysms bleed, causing meningismus (headache and stiff neck) and acute neurological dysfunction.

Pupillomotor fibers travel superomedially in the periphery of the nerve. This superficial location makes pupillary involvement more likely as a result of external forces (such as an aneurysm or trauma) than from an ischemic mononeuropathy. Ischemic events tend to affect the central watershed zone of the nutrient arterioles and spare the pupillary axons. Thus, an oculomotor palsy without pupillary involvement is more likely to be ischemic, and those with proportionately more pupillary involvement are much more likely to be compressive, such as from an aneurysm.

Herniation of the uncus of the temporal lobe from an expanding supratentorial mass can stretch CN III or compress it as it courses on the edge of the tentorium cerebelli, usually affecting the peripherally located pupillary fibers first and causing pupillary dilation (Hutchinson pupil).

Cavernous Sinus

CN III passes lateral to the posterior clinoid process and penetrates the cavernous dura to enter the cavernous sinus. In the cavernous sinus, the oculomotor nerve travels relatively protected in the lateral wall, but is susceptible to the same cavernous sinus processes as the fourth, sixth, and ophthalmic division of CN V (see Figure 9–1B, Table 9–1). Ischemic mononeuropathies of CN III likely occur in the region of the cavernous sinus, as discussed for abducens palsy. Before entering the superior orbital fissure, the oculomotor nerve divides into a superior and inferior division. However, isolated palsies in the distribution of the superior or inferior division are not necessarily localizing because they have been reported as the result of lesions anywhere from the brainstem to the orbit.

Orbit

The superior division innervates the superior rectus and levator muscles, with the inferior branch serving the remaining functions: medial rectus, inferior rectus, inferior oblique, and parasympathetic fibers. The parasympathetic component of the inferior division synapses in the ciliary ganglion just behind the globe (see Figure 9–11B). Postganglionic ciliary nerve fibers innervate the pupillary sphincter and the ciliary muscle (more detail in Chapter 11). Trauma and orbital apex syndromes may affect the nerve in the orbit. The inferior division of the nerve and the ciliary ganglion can be involved in orbital floor blowout fractures, and the resultant blown pupil can be mistaken for Hutchinson pupil sign (brain herniation).

ABERRANT REGENERATION

CN III is capable of regenerating after injury. However, after trauma or compression, regenerating axons are

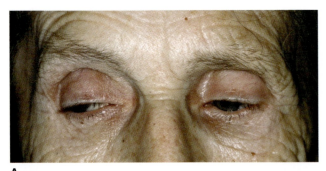
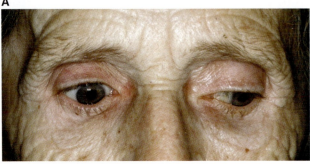

Figure 9–13. Primary aberrant regeneration of the third cranial nerve.
A 75-year-old woman developed a slowly progressive right cranial nerve III palsy from a cavernous sinus meningioma. **(A)** Gaze directed down and to the right shows normal eyelid positions. **(B)** Gaze directed down and to the left causes the right eyelid to elevate because aberrant fibers originally directed to the right medial rectus now innervate the levator.

commonly misdirected and reinnervate the incorrect muscle or muscles. A common syndrome is eyelid elevation on attempted adduction or depression because fibers that originally innervated the medial or inferior rectus muscles aberrantly reinnervate the levator palpebrae (Figure 9–13). Occasionally, the pupillary sphincter (via the ciliary ganglion) receives input that originally was directed to the extraocular muscles, causing an otherwise unresponsive pupil to constrict when the eye is adducted, elevated, or depressed (see Figure 11–14). Other bizarre motility patterns can occur, including globe retraction if opposing muscles receive the same innervation. *Aberrant regeneration never occurs with an ischemic (eg, diabetic) mononeuropathy* and always implies that the nerve has been injured in such a way that the myelin sheath and perineurium have been broached (aneurysm, tumor, or trauma). This condition can rarely occur as a result of ophthalmoplegic migraine. Aberrant regeneration may rarely occur without an antecedent acute CN III palsy. This condition is called *primary aberrant regeneration* and occurs from a slow-growing cavernous sinus mass, such as a meningioma or aneurysm, where there is ongoing damage and aberrant regeneration taking place at the same time.

DIFFERENTIAL DIAGNOSIS

As with all motility disturbances, ocular myasthenia gravis can mimic virtually all components of a CN III palsy except pupillary involvement. Graves disease can affect multiple extraocular muscles, but in Graves disease the eyes are much more likely to be esotropic, rather than exotropic.

EVALUATION AND MANAGEMENT

Common causes of CN III palsy are listed in Table 9–4.

Ischemic mononeuropathies of the oculomotor nerve are very common. Many experts suggest that patients with classic signs and symptoms of an ischemic mononeuropathy—pupil-sparing CN III paresis in a patient with known vascular disease or advanced age—may be simply observed, after eliminating giant cell arteritis (GCA) as a possible cause (by history, ESR, and CRP) and arranging for a medical evaluation as discussed above for ischemic CN VI palsies. But the greater likelihood of aneurysm and other threatening causes with CN III neuropathies (as opposed to CN IV and CN VI) have led some to suggest imaging all CN III palsies.

Patients with a presumed CN III ischemic mononeuropathy should return within a week to ensure that progression to pupil involvement has not occurred and that any associated pain is resolving. Neuroimaging should be performed when patients do not have obvious ischemic risk factors. An ischemic mononeuropathy should recover in 6 to 12 weeks; further investigation is required for those patients who do not recover.

Although less common, the severe morbidity and potential lethality associated with *posterior communicating artery aneurysms* make this condition a universal concern in any patient presenting with a CN III palsy. Although pain is a frequent symptom with CN III palsies caused by aneurysm, pain is also common with ischemic

▶ **TABLE 9–4. CAUSES OF CRANIAL NERVE III PALSIES**

Ischemic (diabetic) mononeuropathy
PComA aneurysm
Trauma
Brainstem/subarachnoid process
- Tumor
- Demyelination
- Infarction
- Meningitis

Cavernous sinus/orbit
- Compression
- Inflammation/infection

Migraine
Congenital

Abbreviation: PComA, posterior communicating artery.

CN III palsies and is therefore not a reliable distinguishing factor. Magnetic resonance angiography (MRA), computed tomography angiography (CTA), or catheter angiography is often necessary to fully explore the possibility of an aneurysm in patients at high risk: younger patients (<45 years) without microischemic risk factors and all patients with relative pupil involvement (Figure 9–14). Note that pupil involvement can evolve several days after the patient first has symptoms, so patients need to be followed carefully to look for this important sign.

Oculomotor palsies can occur from *trauma*, often resulting in aberrant regeneration. However, an oculomotor palsy following minor or trivial trauma suggests the possibility of a preexistent mass lesion.

CN III palsies in children are commonly congenital or traumatic. Less common causes include tumors, aneurysms, meningitis, postinfectious/postvaccination neuropathies, and ophthalmoplegic migraines. Ophthalmoplegic migraine is a rare condition presenting with headache, nausea, and vomiting preceding the development of an oculomotor palsy, usually in a child with a family history of migraine. The headache and nausea may last for days, and the ophthalmoplegia clears anywhere from 1 day to 1 month. Neuroimaging is usually performed even when this diagnosis is suspected because intracranial mass or aneurysm (although rare) cannot be excluded. Cyclic oculomotor palsy is a rare phenomenon in which the signs of CN III paresis transiently reverse in a cyclic fashion: The ptotic eyelid elevates, the dilated pupil constricts, and the depressed exotropic eye is pulled toward primary position. Cyclic palsies are usually associated with congenital oculomotor palsies.

Ptosis with oculomotor palsies may prevent diplopia by acting as an occluder, if sufficient to cover the visual axis. Patients with a resolving CN III palsy may think they are getting worse when diplopia becomes evident as the ptosis improves. The use of an occluder when diplopia is present offers some relief to the patient. Patients with stable residual CN III dysfunction can sometimes be helped with prism in their spectacles, but often the prism prescription is complex with both vertical and horizontal components. Not surprisingly, strabismus surgery for CN III palsy is one of the most challenging situations for the strabismus surgeon.

		Extraocular muscles		
		Total impairment of the extraocular muscles	Partial impairment of the extraocular muscles	No impairment of the extraocular muscles
Intraocular muscles (pupil and accommodation)	Dilated pupil, no light reaction	Highest risk of aneurysm. (Send promptly to neuorology or neurosurgery for evaluation and possible angiography to rule out aneurysm—even if age, gender, and pain do not strongly support the diagnosis.)	Highest risk of aneurysm. (Send promptly to neurology or neurosurgery for evaluation and possible angiography.)	Little risk of aneurysm. In an ambulatory patient, this is almost certainly a peripheral problem (ie, orbital or ocular), and not a third nerve paresis. Atropinic? (1.0% pilo) Adie? (0.1% pilo) Trauma? Angle-closure glaucoma?
	Anisocoria in bright light, weak light reaction	Uncertain risk of aneurysm. This could be an ischemic third nerve palsy on top of preexisting diabetic autonomic neuropathy of the iris sphincter. (Would probably send for studies anyway—especially if age, gender, and pain suggest an aneurysm.)	High risk of aneurysm. This is a partial third nerve palsy without relative sparing of the pupil. (Send promptly to neurology or neurosurgery for evaluation and possible angiography.)	Little risk of aneurysm. In an ambulatory patient, this is almost certainly a peripheral problem (ie, orbital or ocular), and not a third nerve paresis. Atropinic? (1.0% pilo) Adie? (0.1% pilo) Trauma? Angle-closure glaucoma?
	No anisocoria, normal light reaction	Low risk of aneurysm. Very likely an ischemic mononeuropathy. Does the patient have diabetes?	Low risk of aneurysm. Very likely an ischemic mononeuropathy. Does the patient have diabetes?	Not applicable (normal).

Figure 9–14. **The relative risk of an aneurysm as a cause of a cranial nerve III palsy.**
A cranial nerve (CN) III palsy that is caused by compression from a posterior communicating artery aneurysm is more likely to involve the pupillary fibers (that travel superficially in the oculomotor nerve) to a greater degree than an ischemic CN III palsy. The relative risk of an aneurysm as a cause of a CN III palsy, based on the relative involvement of the extraocular and intraocular (pupil) muscles, is shown. (Adapted, with permission, from Kardon RH, Thompson HS: The pupil, in Rosen ES, Thompson HS, Cumming WJK, et al (eds): *Neuro-ophthalmology*. St Louis, MO: Mosby; 1998.)

▶ MULTIPLE CRANIAL NEUROPATHIES

ANATOMY: CLINICAL IMPLICATIONS

Brainstem lesions extensive enough to affect the nuclei or fascicles of cranial nerves III, IV, and VI in combination (eg, Wernicke encephalopathy; see Box 10–1) will likely cause other profound neurological dysfunction. Ocular motor deficits may be the presenting sign of patients with multifocal CNS lesions from *Toxoplasmosis gondii,* a treatable infection primarily seen in immunocompromised patients.

Processes in the *subarachnoid space,* such as carcinomatous or tuberculous meningitis, may cause a sequential march of cranial neuropathies. Head trauma, large midline tumors, or aneurysms are other causes of multiple cranial neuropathies occurring in the subarachnoid space.

Lesions in the *cavernous sinus* are the most common cause of multiple cranial neuropathies because the ocular motor nerves are in close proximity in this space (see Figure 9–1B). Intracavernous lesions (see Table 9–1) can produce various combinations of neuropathies involving CNs II, III, IV, V_1, V_2, VI, or sympathetic nerves (Figure 9–15). Lesions involving the orbital apex can also potentially involve the optic nerve, in addition to CN III, IV, VI, and V_1. Granulomatous inflammatory lesions and meningiomas are common lesions in this area.

Painful ophthalmoplegia is often called *Tolosa-Hunt syndrome.* The implication of this designation is that the patient has an idiopathic inflammatory condition of the cavernous sinus or orbital apex. All such patients obviously require a rigorous evaluation for infectious or neoplastic processes (Table 9–5). Idiopathic inflammation of the cavernous sinus or orbital apex generally responds rapidly to steroids, but the chronicity of the disease generally requires steroid-sparing drugs for long-term management. This condition is likely a variant of idiopathic orbital inflammatory syndrome (IOIS), only located more posteriorly.

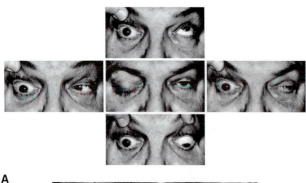

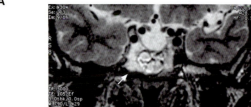

Figure 9–15. Multiple cranial neuropathies from pituitary apoplexy.
A 43-year-old man had an acute event, characterized by retro-orbital pain, right ptosis, and an inability to move the right eye. **(A)** A complete ptosis is present in the right eye. Ocular versions show an abduction deficit in right gaze, as well as an inability to elevate, depress, or adduct the right eye. The findings are consistent with a right cranial nerve III and VI palsy. Lack of torsion when the right eye is depressed suggests that the right fourth nerve is also involved.
(B) Magnetic resonance imaging (T2 coronal image) revealed a necrotic sellar mass extending into the right cavernous sinus (*arrow*), most consistent with acute hemorrhage into a previously undiscovered pituitary adenoma.

▶ TABLE 9–5. PAINFUL OPHTHALMOPLEGIA

Orbit
    IOIS
    Contiguous sinusitis
    Mucormycosis or other fungal infections
    Tumors: local, metastatic
    Lymphoma

Superior Orbital Fissure and Anterior Cavernous Sinus
    Nonspecific granulomatous inflammation (Tolosa-Hunt syndrome)
    Metastatic tumor
    Nasopharyngeal carcinoma
    Lymphoma
    Carotid-cavernous fistula
    Cavernous sinus thrombosis

Parasellar Area
    Pituitary adenoma
    Intracavernous aneurysm
    Metastatic tumor
    Nasopharyngeal carcinoma
    Sphenoid sinus mucocele
    Meningioma, chordoma
    Petrositis (Gradenigo syndrome)

Aneurysm
    Posterior communicating artery aneurysm
    Basilar artery aneurysm (rare)

Miscellaneous
    Ischemic (diabetic) cranial mononeuropathy
    Ophthalmoplegic migraine
    GCA
    Herpes zoster

Abbreviations: GCA, giant cell arteritis; IOIS, idiopathic orbital inflammatory syndrome.

EVALUATION AND DIFFERENTIAL DIAGNOSIS

Neuroimaging of the brain, cavernous sinus, and orbits is required when multiple simultaneous cranial neuropathies are present because mass lesions are commonly identified. Orbital Graves disease, idiopathic orbital inflammatory syndrome, myasthenia gravis, myopathies (chronic progressive external ophthalmoplegia), and supranuclear palsies frequently produce complex ocular motility disturbances that may be difficult to discriminate from multiple cranial neuropathies (Table 9–6). Clues that suggest these alternate diagnoses include the presence of orbital signs, bilateral motility disturbances, and variability of signs and symptoms. Forced duction testing, Tensilon testing, electromyography (EMG) of the limb muscles, and single-fiber EMG of the frontalis muscles are sometimes required to sort through the differential diagnosis.

CN II to VIII must be individually and specifically evaluated when a cranial neuropathy is suspected. As previously discussed, the differential diagnosis and management of cranial neuropathies is different if more than one nerve is involved. Evaluation of the first (V_1) and second (V_2) branches of CN V (corneal and facial sensation) is helpful in localizing lesions to the cavernous sinus. Involvement of the optic nerve indicates a large parasellar tumor or an orbital apex lesion. Facial nerve involvement suggests a systemic polyneuropathy, myasthenia, sarcoidosis, or lymphoma, whereas CN VIII dysfunction may indicate a cerebellopontine angle tumor.

Simultaneous unilateral involvement of CN III and VI is usually readily apparent clinically because their fields of action do not overlap. Diagnosis of a CN IV paresis in the setting of a dense CN III palsy is more challenging because the eye cannot be fully adducted to test CN IV function in the standard manner. In this situation, CN IV function can be assessed by the degree of incyclotorsion induced from upgaze to downgaze (Figure 9–16).

▶ **TABLE 9–6. MOTILITY DISORDERS THAT DO NOT CONFORM TO ISOLATED CRANIAL NERVE PATTERNS**

Orbital
    Graves disease
    IOIS
    Trauma
    Orbital mass
    Myopathy (CPEO)
    Carotid-cavernous fistula

Neuromuscular Junction
    Myasthenia gravis

Cranial Nerves
Multiple Cranial Neuropathies
    Cavernous sinus lesions
    Orbital apex syndrome
    Herpes zoster
    GCA (and other vasculitis)
    Basilar meningitis/carcinomatosis
    Systemic neuropathies (Miller-Fisher variant)
Aberrant Regeneration of Third Cranial Nerve
Spread of Comitance from Isolated Cranial Neuropathy

Supranuclear
    Gaze palsy
    One and a half syndrome

Congenital
    Duane syndrome
    Möbius syndrome

Abbreviations: CPEO, chronic progressive external ophthalmoplegia; GCA, giant cell arteritis; IOIS, idiopathic orbital inflammatory syndrome.

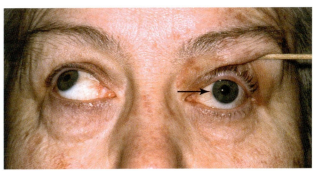
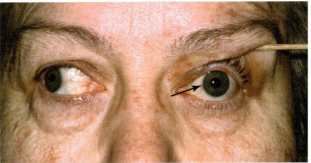
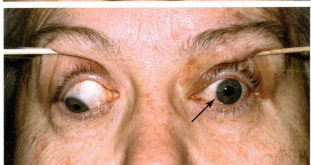

Figure 9–16. Evaluating cranial nerve IV function when a cranial nerve III palsy is present.
Incyclotorsion, showing normal left cranial nerve (CN) IV function, is present in this patient with a left CN III palsy. Observe how the conjunctival vessels in the left eye (*arrow*) move from upgaze to downgaze, showing intact incyclotorsion of the left eye.

The Miller-Fisher variant of Guillain-Barré syndrome is an acute inflammatory demyelinating polyneuropathy affecting cranial and peripheral nerves. The classic triad consists of ataxia and areflexia, in addition to a rapidly progressive, bilaterally symmetric ophthalmoplegia. Variable involvement of CN III, IV, and VI can produce complex motility disturbances. Bilateral facial palsies are commonly present.

▶ KEY POINTS

- The abducens nerve (CN VI) innervates the lateral rectus muscle in the ipsilateral orbit.
- A lesion affecting the abducens nucleus produces a gaze palsy because the nucleus contains two types of neurons: (1) motor neurons forming the abducens nerve, and (2) internuclear neurons that communicate with the contralateral medial rectus subnucleus.
- CN VI can be injured with minimal shifts in brain position that may occur in intracranial hypertension, following lumbar puncture (therapeutic, diagnostic, and spinal anesthesia), with trauma, and with intracranial hypotension (CSF leaks).
- Most isolated CN VI palsies are ischemic mononeuropathies or traumatic.
- An abduction deficit can be caused by disorders other than an abducens palsy, such as orbital Graves disease, traumatic medial rectus entrapment, and myasthenia gravis.
- The trochlear nerve (CN IV) innervates only the superior oblique muscle, but this muscle has a complex action: It intorts, depresses, and abducts the eye.
- Motor neurons in the CN IV nucleus innervate the *contralateral* superior oblique muscle.
- CN IV has the longest subarachnoid course of the ocular motor nerves and is the only one to exit the brainstem dorsally.
- Most isolated CN IV palsies are traumatic, ischemic mononeuropathies or are congenital.
- The oculomotor nerve (CN III) innervates the superior, medial, and inferior rectus muscles; the inferior oblique muscle; and the levator palpebrae (which elevates the eyelids), and provides parasympathetic innervation to the pupillary sphincter and ciliary muscle.
- Aberrant regeneration of CN III never occurs from an ischemic mononeuropathy and always implies that the nerve has undergone disruption of the myelin sheath and perineurium caused by an aneurysm, tumor, or trauma.
- MRA and CTA demonstrate many but not all aneurysms—cerebral (catheter) angiography is the gold standard at present.
- Ocular myasthenia gravis can mimic all isolated or combined ocular motor cranial neuropathies, except a dilated pupil in a CN III palsy.
- Similar to CN III palsy, orbital Graves disease can affect multiple extraocular muscles, but in orbital Graves disease the eyes are more likely to be esotropic, rather than exotropic as with a CN III palsy.
- An MRI is indicated to evaluate ocular motor cranial nerve palsies (1) if the cranial nerve palsy is progressing, (2) if the patient has a history of a local tumor or potentially metastatic cancer, (3) if other cranial nerves are involved, (4) if other neurological symptoms or signs are present, (5) if there are no evident ischemic risk factors.
- An MRI of the brain with contrast allows a detailed view of the brainstem and course of the ocular motor cranial nerves, that is superior to CT imaging.
- Ischemic mononeuropathy caused by microvascular disease is a common cause of an *isolated* palsy of CN III, IV, or VI: characteristically sudden in onset, with mild initial pain, and complete recovery in 8 to 12 weeks.
- Multiple (simultaneous) cranial neuropathies are much less likely to be the result of microvascular disease, and inflammatory or neoplastic disease should be sought.
- Unilateral, multiple ocular motor cranial neuropathies suggest cavernous sinus or orbital apex lesions.

SUGGESTED READING

Books

Glaser JS, Siatkowski RM: Infranuclear disorders of eye movements, in Duane TD (ed): *Duane's Clinical Ophthalmology*, Vol. 2. Philadelphia, PA: Lippincott Williams & Wilkins; 1998.

Leigh RJ, Zee DS: *The Neurology of Eye Movements*, 4th ed. New York, NY: Oxford University Press; 2006:385–474.

Newman SA: Disorders of ocular motility, in Slamovits TL, Burde R (assoc eds): *Neuro-ophthalmology*, Vol. 6, in Podos SM, Yanoff M (eds): *Textbook of Ophthalmology*. St Louis, MO: Mosby; 1991.

Seargent JC: Nuclear and infranuclear ocular motility disorders, in Miller NR, Newman NJ (eds): *Walsh and Hoyt's Clinical Neuro-ophthalmology*, Vol. 1, 6th ed. Philadelphia, PA: Lippincott Williams & Wilkins; 2005:969–1040.

Sedwick LA: The efferent visual system, in Slamovits TL, Burde R (assoc eds): *Neuro-ophthalmology*, Vol. 6, in Podos SM, Yanoff M (eds): *Textbook of Ophthalmology*. St Louis, MO: Mosby; 1991.

Articles

Brazis PW: Localization of lesions of the oculomotor nerve: recent concepts. *Mayo Clin Proc* 1991;66:1029–1035.

Brazis PW: Palsies of the trochlear nerve: diagnosis and localization—recent concepts. *Mayo Clin Proc* 1993;68:501–509.

Brazis PW, Lee AG: Binocular vertical diplopia. *Mayo Clin Proc* 1998;73:55–66.

Jacobson DM: Relative pupil-sparing third nerve palsy: etiology and clinical variable predictive of a mass. *Neurology* 2001;56(6):797–798.

Jacobson DM, Trobe JD: The emerging role of magnetic resonance angiography in the management of patients with third cranial nerve palsy. *Am J Ophthalmol* 1999;128:4–96.

Peters GB, Bakr SJ, Krohel GB: Cause and prognosis of nontraumatic sixth nerve palsies in young adults. *Ophthalmology* 2002;109:1925–1928.

Richards BW, Jones FR Jr, Younge BR: Causes and prognosis in 4278 cases of paralysis of the oculomotor, trochlear, and abducens cranial nerves. *Am J Ophthalmol* 1992;113:489.

Sibony PA, Lessell S, Gittinger JW Jr: Acquired oculomotor synkinesis. *Surv Ophthalmol* 1984;28:382–390.

Trobe JD: Isolated third nerve palsies. *Semin Neurol* 1986;6(2):135–141.

Warwick R: Representation of the extraocular muscles in the oculomotor nuclei of the monkey. *J Comp Neurol* 1953;98:449–503.

CHAPTER 10
Supranuclear Visual Motor System and Nystagmus

- ▶ INTERNUCLEAR ORGANIZATION:
  GAZE CENTERS 239
  Horizontal gaze 239
  Vertical gaze 242
- ▶ SUPRANUCLEAR PATHWAYS
  AND DISORDERS 244
  Saccades 244
  Pursuit 249
  Vestibulo-ocular reflex 249
  Optokinetic reflex 250
  Vergence 250
  Fixation reflex 251
- ▶ NYSTAGMUS 251
  Classification and terminology 252
  Physiological nystagmus 252
  Other forms of nonpathological
    nystagmus 253
  Congenital nystagmus and nystagmus
    in children 253
  Recognizable forms of acquired
    nystagmus 254
  Other nystagmus-like oscillations 256
  Nystagmus treatment 257
- ▶ KEY POINTS 257

Six systems coordinate and stabilize eye movements. The systems are termed *supranuclear* because they are higher in the chain of command than the ocular motor nuclei. *Internuclear* pathways connect the ocular motor nuclei to coordinate conjugate movement of yoke muscles and provide a common pathway for supranuclear systems. Disorders of supranuclear or internuclear pathways can cause conjugate gaze palsies or ocular misalignment. Supranuclear disorders can also cause nystagmus or nystagmus-like oscillations, which are unwanted eye movements that can degrade vision or cause oscillopsia.

▶ INTERNUCLEAR ORGANIZATION: GAZE CENTERS

Gaze centers are premotor nuclei that organize and relay supranuclear commands to the appropriate individual motor nuclei of yoked muscles to move the two eyes together in the same direction. Separate systems exist for horizontal and vertical eye movements.

HORIZONTAL GAZE

To achieve horizontal gaze, motor neurons innervating the lateral rectus and the contralateral medial rectus subnucleus need to receive equal and simultaneous activation.

Organization

The *paramedian pontine reticular formation* (PPRF) is the horizontal gaze center. This nucleus is adjacent to the abducens (cranial nerve [CN] VI) nucleus in the pons (Figure 10–1). The PPRF activates the abducens nucleus in response to supranuclear gaze commands. As discussed in Chapter 9, the abducens nucleus contains two sets of neurons: (1) motor neurons whose axons innervate the ipsilateral lateral rectus muscle, and (2) internuclear neurons with axons that decussate to the contralateral *medial longitudinal fasciculus* (MLF) and travel to the medial rectus subnucleus (Figure 10–2). Thus, activation of the PPRF in turn activates the two populations of cells in the CN VI nucleus and produces conjugate gaze (to the ipsilateral side).

Disorders

Internuclear Ophthalmoplegia Lesions of the MLF interrupt the pathway from the abducens nucleus to the medial rectus subnucleus. Thus, a lesion of the *left MLF* causes a *left internuclear ophthalmoplegia (INO)*: an isolated *adduction deficit of the left eye* on attempted *right* gaze, with normal left gaze (Figure 10–3). In many patients, the eye on the affected side does not adduct past midline. In less severe instances, the adduction deficiency is seen only by observing the horizontal saccades:

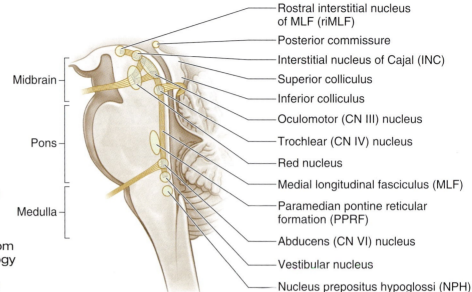

Figure 10-1. **Key brainstem nuclei involved in eye movement control and neighboring structures.** (Modified with permission from Kline LB: Neuro-ophthalmology Review Manual, 7th edition. Thorofare, NJ SLACK, 2013.)

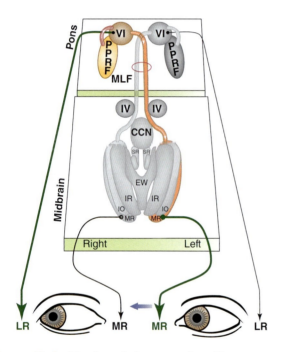

Figure 10-2. **Horizontal gaze circuits.** This rendering of the brainstem circuitry involved in eye movements is drawn from the examiner's view of a patient. The drawing is not to scale. The example shown is right gaze in a normal subject: Right gaze is initiated by the right paramedian pontine reticular formation, activating the right cranial nerve (CN) VI nucleus. The right lateral rectus is activated via CN VI. The left medial rectus subnucleus is activated by an internuclear pathway originating from cells within the CN VI nucleus, whose axons cross to the left medial longitudinal fasciculus to reach the CN III nuclear complex. CCN, central caudal nucleus; EW, Edinger-Westphal nucleus; IO, inferior oblique; IR, inferior rectus; IV, fourth cranial nerve nucleus; MR, medial rectus; PPRF, paramedian pontine reticular formation; LR, lateral rectus; SR, superior rectus; VI, sixth cranial nerve nucleus.

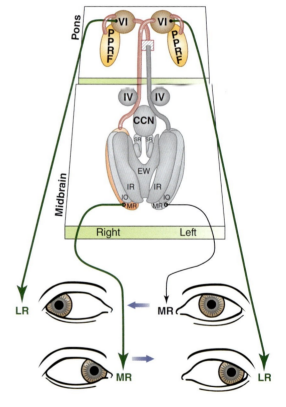

Figure 10-3. **Internuclear ophthalmoplegia.** A lesion affecting the left medial longitudinal fasciculus (*cross-hatched square*) will cause an adduction deficit of the left eye in right gaze; left gaze is unaffected. CCN, central caudal nucleus; EW, Edinger-Westphal nucleus; IR, inferior rectus; IO, inferior oblique; MR, medial rectus; SR, superior rectus; LR, lateral rectus; PPRF, paramedian pontine reticular formation; IV, fourth cranial nerve nucleus; VI, sixth cranial nerve nucleus.

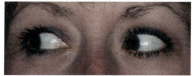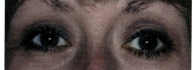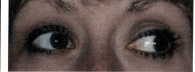

A

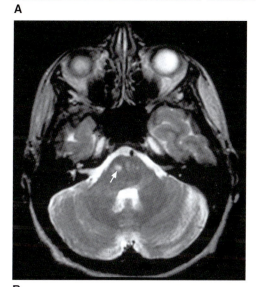

B

Figure 10–4. Internuclear ophthalmoplegia from multiple sclerosis.
A 48-year-old woman presented with blurred vision and diplopia worse with left gaze, and numbness and weakness of her right leg. **(A)** Ocular versions show an adduction deficit in the right eye (in left gaze). The condition was most evident with horizontal saccades: The right eye moved slowly with leftward saccades, and transient nystagmus of the left eye was also observed with saccades to the left. **(B)** Magnetic resonance imaging (axial T2-weighted image) shows one of several white matter lesions in the brainstem (*arrow*) affecting the right medial longitudinal fasciculus. Periventricular white matter lesions were also seen in other images, consistent with a diagnosis of multiple sclerosis.

The adducting eye moves more slowly as it slides into position, lagging behind the faster-moving abducting eye (Figure 10–4). The abducting eye commonly displays a dissociated horizontal jerk nystagmus. Adduction *with convergence* is spared if the MLF lesion is in the pons, but may be affected if the lesion is anterior in the MLF (in the midbrain) where convergence input to the medial rectus subnucleus may be interrupted as well.

Common causes of INO include multiple sclerosis (MS) (in patients 50 years old or younger) or brainstem vascular disease (in patients older than 50 years). An INO can be differentiated from a CN III palsy by the lack of ptosis, anisocoria, or other CN III–mediated motility disturbances, as well as the preservation of adduction with convergence (in most cases). Myasthenia gravis can precisely mimic the clinical findings of an INO (including the abducting nystagmus).

A bilateral INO can cause a large exotropia referred to as *WEBINO syndrome* ("wall-eyed" bilateral INO). This condition likely results from a lesion that involves the MLF on both sides (Figure 10–5). As discussed for unilateral INO, adduction with convergence is spared unless the lesion is anterior, also involving the medial rectus subnuclei.

Gaze palsy Lesions that affect the PPRF produce a gaze palsy to the ipsilateral side. Lesions that affect the abducens (CN VI) nucleus also produce a gaze palsy (not just an abduction deficit) because the nucleus activates both the ipsilateral lateral rectus muscle and the contralateral medial rectus subnucleus. The resulting gaze palsy may not be easily differentiated from lesions in cortical areas of supranuclear gaze initiation, such as the frontal eye fields. Vestibular input occurs at the level of the CN VI nucleus, so the vestibulo-ocular reflex is

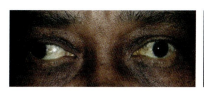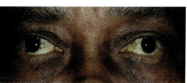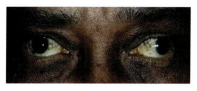

Figure 10–5. "Wall-eyed" bilateral internuclear ophthalmoplegia syndrome.
A 66-year-old woman with diabetes, hypertension, and a history of multiple strokes described difficulty focusing after being hospitalized for a syncopal episode. Family members commented that since that time her eyes "splay out." Neurological evaluation and magnetic resonance imaging confirmed a brainstem stroke. The patient's horizontal versions (*pictured*) show that the left eye does not adduct in right gaze and the right eye does not adduct in left gaze: a bilateral internuclear ophthalmoplegia. In primary position the eyes are markedly exotropic, thus the designation wall-eyed bilateral internuclear ophthalmoplegia, or WEBINO. This condition results from brainstem lesions extensive enough to include the medial longitudinal fasciculus on both sides.

unaffected by PPRF or supranuclear lesions. Therefore, oculocephalic or caloric tests should be normal in PPRF or supranuclear palsies, but will be abnormal if the abducens nucleus or more distal CN VI pathway is affected.

One-and-a-half syndrome Lesions that involve the PPRF or CN VI nucleus can also involve the adjacent ipsilateral MLF. The condition produces a gaze palsy to the ipsilateral side and an INO in contralateral gaze. The gaze palsy to the ipsilateral side is the "one" and the INO in contralateral gaze is the "half." The only normal movement remaining in the horizontal plane is abduction of the contralateral eye (Figures 10–6 and 10–7). Similar to INO, demyelinating disease and brainstem infarction are common causes of one-and-a-half syndrome. Wernicke encephalopathy is another brainstem process that can cause a variety of horizontal gaze disturbances (Box 10–1).

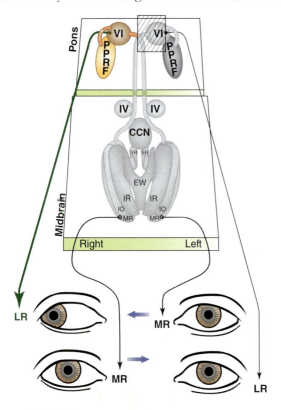

Figure 10–6. One-and-a-half syndrome.
A lesion large enough to include the left cranial nerve VI nucleus/paramedian pontine reticular formation and the adjacent medial longitudinal fasciculus (*cross-hatched area*) would produce a left gaze palsy (the "one") and an internuclear ophthalmoplegia on attempted right gaze (the "half"). Observe that innervation of the right lateral rectus is the only horizontal action unaffected by such a lesion. An ipsilateral facial nerve palsy is also commonly present. CCN, central caudal nucleus; EW, Edinger-Westphal nucleus; IR, inferior rectus; IO, inferior oblique; MR, medial rectus; SR, superior rectus; LR, lateral rectus; PPRF, paramedian pontine reticular formation; IV, fourth cranial nerve nucleus; VI, sixth cranial nerve nucleus.

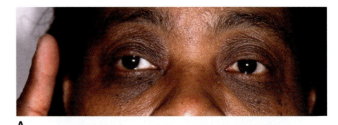

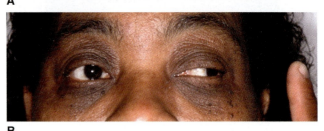

Figure 10–7. One-and-a-half syndrome: clinical case.
A 59-year-old African American woman has a diagnosis of multiple sclerosis. There is a gaze palsy to the right **(A)** and an adduction deficit (internuclear ophthalmoplegia) in the right eye on left gaze **(B)** consistent with a lesion in the right pons. This is a *right* one-and-a-half syndrome (a *left* one-and-a-half syndrome is illustrated in Figure 10–6).

▶ BOX 10–1. WERNICKE ENCEPHALOPATHY

Wernicke encephalopathy is a disorder caused by a thiamine (vitamin B_1) deficiency that occurs most frequently with alcoholism or chronic vomiting. Lesions occur throughout the midline brainstem tegmentum, the thalamus, the hypothalamus, and in the cerebellum. The classic triad of symptoms includes (1) ophthalmoplegia, (2) mental confusion, and (3) gait ataxia. Neuro-ophthalmic manifestations include cranial nerve palsies, horizontal gaze palsies with gaze-evoked nystagmus, abnormal pursuit and saccades, internuclear ophthalmoplegia (INO), abnormal vestibulo-ocular responses, and vertical (usually upbeat) nystagmus. Additional manifestations include cognitive defects and ataxia. Treatment with thiamine reverses many, but not all, of the signs and symptoms of Wernicke encephalopathy. A prompt diagnosis of Wernicke encephalopathy is crucial because the disorder is treatable and reversible in its early stages. Korsakoff syndrome is a more severe form of thiamine-deficiency encephalopathy, with severe memory loss and permanent ocular motor abnormalities.

VERTICAL GAZE

Organization

The *rostral interstitial nucleus of the MLF (riMLF)* is the vertical gaze center. These paired nuclei are located in the pretectum anterior to the mesencephalon near

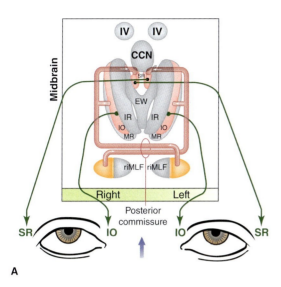
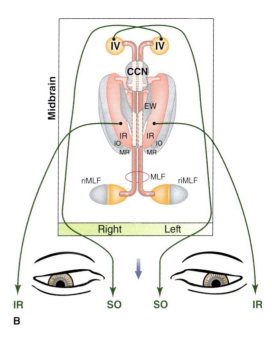

Figure 10-8. **Vertical gaze circuits.**
(A) Upgaze is coordinated by the lateral rostral interstitial nucleus of the medial longitudinal fasciculus (riMLF) with pathways that cross at the level of the cranial nerve (CN) III nucleus. **(B)** Downgaze is coordinated by the medial riMLF, utilizing the MLF to activate the inferior rectus subnucleus and the CN IV nucleus. CCN, central caudal nucleus; EW, Edinger-Westphal nucleus; IR, inferior rectus; IO, inferior oblique; MR, medial rectus; SR, superior rectus; riMLF, rostral interstitial nucleus of the medial longitudinal fasciculus; IV, fourth cranial nerve nucleus.

the CN III complex (see Figure 10–1). The lateral portion of the riMLF mediates upgaze; outflow crosses to the contralateral side and communicates with both inferior oblique and superior rectus subnuclei. These motor nuclei control yoked muscles in opposite eyes (remember that the superior rectus fascicles decussate) that elevate the eyes (Figure 10–8A). The medial portion of each riMLF mediates downgaze; outflow travels down the MLF to the ipsilateral inferior rectus subnucleus and fourth nerve (CN IV) nucleus (see Figure 10–8B). These motor nuclei control yoked muscles in opposite eyes that are depressors (remember that CN IV decussates). Vertical gaze is initiated by *bilateral* activation of the medial or lateral portions of the riMLF.

Disorders

Dorsal midbrain syndrome (also known as Parinaud syndrome, sylvian aqueduct syndrome, or dorsal mesencephalic syndrome) is a constellation of signs and symptoms caused by lesions of the dorsal midbrain that affect the vertical gaze centers and the CN III nuclear complex, their interconnections, and midbrain pupillary circuits (Table 10–1). Upgaze disturbances are the hallmark, with convergence-retraction nystagmus on attempted upgaze, and a light-near dissociation of the pupils is frequently present (discussed in Chapter 11). Convergence-retraction nystagmus is a nystagmus-like

▶ **TABLE 10–1. SIGNS AND SYMPTOMS OF DORSAL MIDBRAIN SYNDROME**

Vertical gaze disturbance (especially upgaze)
Convergence-retraction nystagmus (on attempted upward saccades)
Light-near dissociation of the pupils
Lid retraction (Collier sign)
Spasm or paresis of convergence
Spasm or paresis of accommodation
Skew deviation

oscillation that occurs from co-contraction of the extraocular muscles innervated by CN III on attempted upgaze, without inhibition of the remaining muscles (Figure 10–9). Attempted upward saccades cause retraction of the globes into the orbits, best seen when viewing the patient's globes from the side. At the same time, the eyes make a convergence movement. A downward-moving optokinetic stimulus produces repeated upward saccades, allowing the best opportunity to observe the phenomenon.

Lesions in the dorsal midbrain include caudal aqueductal stenosis, stroke, MS, arteriovenous malformations, trauma, and compression from tumor. Pinealomas cause the dorsal midbrain syndrome by extrinsic compression of the dorsal mesencephalon, usually in young patients.

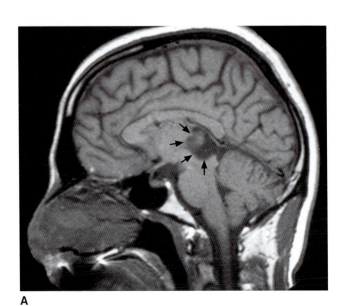
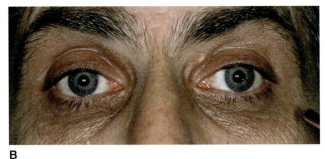
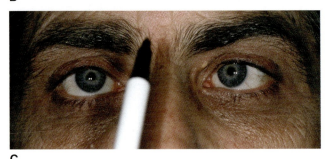

Figure 10–9. **Dorsal midbrain syndrome.**
A 49-year-old man with a cystic pineal mass presented with increasing difficulty focusing, especially when looking up (which was frequently required in his occupation as an electrician). Ocular versions showed limited vertical gaze and prominent convergence-retraction nystagmus on attempted upgaze (best seen with a downward-moving optokinetic stimulus). **(A)** Magnetic resonance imaging (sagittal T1-weighted image) shows a large cystic mass in the pineal region indenting and deforming the dorsal midbrain. **(B)** The pupils are mid dilated and only sluggishly reactive to light. **(C)** Prompt pupillary constriction (greater than with a light stimulus) occurs with the near response.

▶ SUPRANUCLEAR PATHWAYS AND DISORDERS

There are two basic types of eye movements: (1) *fast* eye movements to reposition the eyes, in which afferent visual information is suppressed, and (2) *slow* eye movements to keep the eyes on an object of regard despite movement of the world view or observer. Six systems of eye movement control the fast or slow eye movements to coordinate the eyes. Four of the systems coordinate types of conjugate gaze: *saccade, smooth pursuit, vestibulo-ocular,* and *optokinetic* systems. The *vergence* system controls the disconjugate movement of convergence and divergence for far and near binocular fixation. The *fixation* system keeps the eyes relatively still and continuously trained on objects of interest. Table 10–2 is an overview and summary of the systems and pathways, each of which is discussed in the following sections.

SACCADES

Saccades are phasic fast eye movements (rotational velocities of 300 to 500° per second) that redirect the eyes to a new fixation object. Saccades occur voluntarily, but they can be involuntary: a normal reflexive response to the sudden appearance of a new visual, auditory, or tactile stimulus; a part of the optokinetic or vestibulo-ocular reflex; or may be intrusive and unwanted in certain disease states. Saccades can occur in any direction, but the pathways for saccades in the horizontal plane are better understood than vertical saccades.

Synthesis of a Saccade

The production of a horizontal saccade involves more than just activating the PPRF for horizontal gaze. To generate a horizontal saccade, a strong *pulse* is needed to overcome orbital viscous forces and get the eyes started moving, followed by a *step* up in the baseline firing rate to the muscles to keep the eye in its new position. Specialized cells in the PPRF and other adjacent areas produce the key components of the pulse and step for horizontal saccades. Burst cells in the PPRF provide the strong (high-frequency) *pulse* signal to initiate the saccade (Figure 10–10). The strength of the signal is proportional to the size of the intended saccade. Pause cells (in nucleus raphe interpositus) hold the burst cells in check, discharging continuously except immediately before and during a saccade to allow burst cells to fire. Neural integrator cells in the nucleus prepositus hypoglossi (NPH) and medial vestibular nucleus (see Figure 10–1) also receive the burst cell pulse signal and generate a proportional step signal to hold the eye at

TABLE 10-2. EYE MOVEMENT SYSTEMS AND PATHWAYS

Eye Movement Type	Description	Basic Pathways	Comments
Saccade	Fast eye movement to redirect gaze	Contralateral frontal eye fields	May be voluntary or reflexive.
Smooth pursuit	Slow eye movement to track a moving object	Ipsilateral occipito-temporal-parietal junction	
Vergence	Slow disconjugate eye movement to achieve binocular fixation on near and distant objects	Midbrain, pons	
Fixation and gaze holding	Keep eye steady on object of interest	Cerebellum and associated areas	
Vestibulo-ocular	Slow eye movement to compensate for head movement	Inner ear labyrinthine organs and vestibular nuclei, utilizes pursuit pathway	With continuous rotation, saccades reset the eyes and a physiological nystagmus develops.
Optokinetic	Slow eye movement to stabilize movement of the visual field	Occipito-parietal pursuit area, utilizes pursuit pathway	Physiological nystagmus develops as pursuit movement tracks continuous visual field movement, and saccades reset gaze.

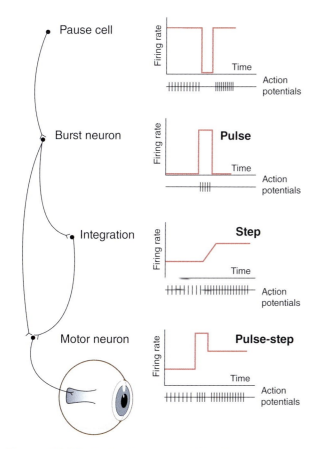

Figure 10-10. **Pulse/step synthesis.** (Reproduced with permission from Flitcroft DI: Neurophysiology of eye movements, in Rosen ES, Thompson HS, Cumming WJK, et al. (eds): *Neuro-ophthalmology.* St Louis, MO: Mosby; 1998.)

the new position. The larger the saccade, the larger the pulse signal, and the larger the step (firing rate) required to hold the eyes in a new eccentric position. Thus, the pulse portion of the saccadic signal is generated by the PPRF, and the step portion is calculated by the neural integrator in the NPH. The combined (pulse-step) signal drives the two populations of cells in the abducens nucleus: motor neurons for ipsilateral CN VI and intercalated neurons that connect to the contralateral medial rectus subnucleus. The result is a coordinated saccadic movement (and holding) of both eyes toward the side of the activating PPRF and abducens nucleus.

Pathways for Horizontal Saccades

The frontal eye field and superior colliculus, on the side contralateral to the direction of gaze, are the major supranuclear initiators of horizontal saccadic movement. These areas have direct connections to the contralateral PPRF (Figure 10-11). Other contributors to saccadic control include the supplementary eye fields, dorsolateral prefrontal cortex, areas of the parietal lobe, and the *ipsilateral* frontal eye fields.

Pathways for Vertical Saccades

Supranuclear pathways for vertical saccades originate from either both frontal eye fields or both superior colliculi. These areas provide their input to the riMLF, which generates the vertical pulse, similar to the role of the PPRF in producing horizontal gaze (Figure 10-12). The interstitial nucleus of Cajal (INC) is the vertical step integrator that is analogous to the NPH for horizontal gaze (Table 10-3).

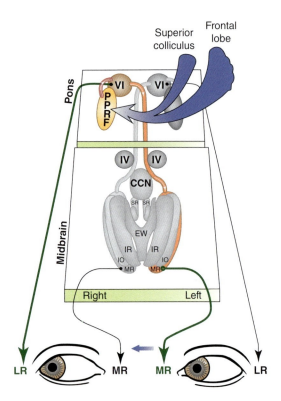

Figure 10-11. Supranuclear control of horizontal saccades.
The paramedian pontine reticular formation is activated by the contralateral frontal eye fields and contralateral superior colliculus. CCN, central caudal nucleus; EW, Edinger-Westphal nucleus; IR, inferior rectus; IO, inferior oblique; MR, medial rectus; SR, superior rectus; LR, lateral rectus; IV, fourth cranial nerve nucleus; VI, sixth cranial nerve nucleus.

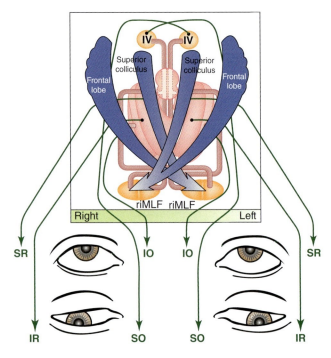

Figure 10-12. Supranuclear control of vertical saccades.
Vertical saccades originate from bilateral supranuclear input to both rostral interstitial nuclei of the medial longitudinal fasciculus. IR, inferior rectus; IO, inferior oblique; SR, superior rectus; riMLF, rostral interstitial nucleus of the medial longitudinal fasciculus; IV, fourth cranial nerve nucleus.

▶ **TABLE 10-3. ANATOMIC LOCATION OF THE COMPONENTS OF GAZE SYNTHESIS**

	Supranuclear Origin	Pause Cells	Pulse (Burst) Cells	Step (Neural Integrator) Cells	Premotor Nucleus	Motor Nucleus
Horizontal saccades	Contralateral frontal eye fields (FEF) and contralateral porterior parietal cortex through superior colliculus (SC)	Omnipause neurons (OPNs) located in nucleus raphe interpositus	PPRF	Nucleus propositus hypoglossi (NPH) and medial vestibular nucleus (MVN)	PPRF	Abducens nucleus (neurons for CN VI and internuclear connection to contralateral medial rectus subnucleus)
Vertical saccades	Bilateral FEF or bilateral SC	Nucleus raphe interpositus	riMLF	Interstitial nucleus of Cajal (INC)	riMLF	Yolked vertically acting nuclei of CN III and IV

Abbreviations: CN, cranial nerve; PPRF, paramedian pontine reticular formation. ; riMLF, Rostral interstitial nucleus of the medial longitudinal fasciculus

Saccadic Disorders

Abnormalities of the saccadic system include the inability to produce voluntary saccades (ocular motor apraxia), saccades that are too slow, saccades that overshoot (hypermetric saccades) or undershoot (hypometric saccades), or unwanted saccades (saccadic intrusions).

Frontal lobe lesions Injury to the frontal eye fields can cause difficulty in generating horizontal saccades to the contralateral side, creating a preferential gaze to the ipsilateral side. Pursuit, optokinetic, and vestibulo-ocular (oculocephalic or caloric) responses are intact, demonstrating the supranuclear nature of the lesion. Over several weeks, the patient regains the ability to generate bilateral saccades, even after permanent frontal lobe injury. This recovery results from activation of secondary projections from the intact contralateral frontal eye field to the PPRF on the same side (ipsilateral projection), allowing the remaining frontal lobe to initiate saccades to both sides.

Congenital oculomotor apraxia This is a condition in which the patient cannot initiate normal voluntary horizontal saccades. Vertical saccades are normal. An optokinetic stimulus moves the eyes to the side (with a normal pursuit) where they remain because no saccades are generated to move the eyes back. An interesting compensatory head movement develops in infancy to redirect gaze. Because a horizontal saccade is not possible, the infant turns its head to place the (still fixating) eyes in extreme lateral gaze. Because the eyes cannot move any farther in the horizontal plane, additional turning of the head forcibly drags the eyes away from the original fixation object to a new fixation point, after which the head re-centers in the new direction of gaze. These *head thrusts* are characteristic and recognizable, and are clinically diagnostic of oculomotor apraxia (Figure 10–13). As these children grow older, much smaller head movements are required to break fixation, and the head thrusts become less noticeable.

Acquired ocular motor apraxia This disorder can occur from bilateral parieto-occipital lesions in which voluntary, visually guided saccades and pursuit are affected, but reflexive saccades remain intact (thus an apraxia rather than palsy). This finding, when combined with optic ataxia and simultanagnosia, constitutes Balint syndrome (discussed in Chapter 5). If the frontal eye fields are also involved bilaterally, saccade generation is severely impaired, and patients may develop compensatory head thrust similar to congenital oculomotor apraxia. Acquired oculomotor apraxia can be seen in ataxia-telangiectasia, inherited spinocerebellar ataxias, Joubert syndrome, Gaucher disease, and Niemann-Pick

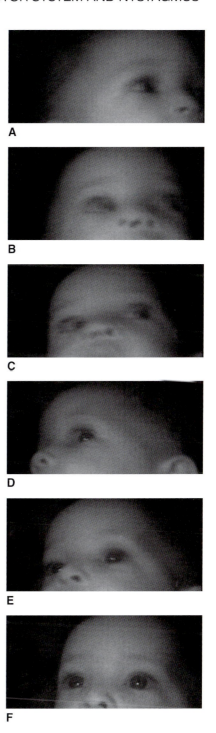

Figure 10–13. Oculomotor apraxia.
This sequence of video frames of a child with congenital oculomotor apraxia shows the characteristic "head thrust" movement used to refixate the eyes, given an inability to generate a saccade. **(A)** The child is looking left when a squeaking toy to the right gets his interest. **(B, C)** The child "drags" his leftward fixed eyes by moving his head to the right until his eyes are lined up on the toy. **(D)** Now that fixation is achieved, his eyes will stay on the target as he turns his head back to the left to re-center his head **(E, F)**.

disease. A curious type of acquired ocular motor apraxia can rarely occur following cardiac surgery (aortic valve surgery most often) that may be related to intraoperative cardiopulmonary bypass and hypothermia.

Progressive supranuclear palsy This is a degenerative neurological condition that causes a progressive slowing of saccades in all directions, gradually diminishing the amplitude of saccadic eye movements to the point that all voluntary movement is lost. The supranuclear origin of the disorder is evident because oculocephalic and caloric movements are retained until the terminal stages of the disease. Downgaze is usually affected early in the disease course. Associated neurological symptoms include progressive nuchal and axial rigidity, dementia, and dysarthria, usually leading to death within several years of diagnosis. Neck rigidity makes it difficult for patients to compensate for loss of saccades by moving their head.

Oculogyric crisis This condition is an acute, often painful and dramatic dystonic upward deviation of the eyes that can last for hours. Originally described as a component of postencephalitic parkinsonism, oculogyric crisis is now primarily seen as a reaction to neuroleptics, although it can occur in other neurological disorders. Acute cases are treated with intravenous or intramuscular benztropine or diphenhydramine.

Spinocerebellar ataxias This group of disorders present in early adulthood with ataxia, slurred speech, and dementia. Histopathologically, atrophy of the cerebellar cortex, basis pontis, and inferior olivary nucleus is identified in affected patients (historically this was called olivopontocerebellar degeneration). Eye movements in all directions are progressively affected, eventually leading to total ophthalmoplegia. Associated ocular findings include optic atrophy and pigmentary retinopathy. Other central nervous system (CNS) disorders associated with paretic saccades are listed in Table 10–4.

Cerebellar disease The cerebellum contributes heavily to the coordination of eye movements. Cerebellar disease commonly causes ocular dysmetria. When a *hypometric* saccade fails to get the eye to the new target, additional saccades in the same direction are required. *Hypermetric* saccades frequently cause an oscillation around the new fixation point because the initial overshoot is corrected by a saccade in the opposite direction that is also hypermetric.

Saccadic intrusions In addition to affecting voluntary saccades, cerebellar disease can cause spontaneous involuntary saccades. Square-wave jerks, ocular flutter, and opsoclonus are types of saccadic intrusions.

Square-wave jerks are named for their appearance on eye movement recordings (Figure 10–14). They consist of

▶ **TABLE 10–4. CAUSES OF SLOW SACCADES**

CNS Degenerative Disorders
  Spinocerebellar ataxia (SCA), especially olivopontocerebellar degeneration (SCA2)
  Other hereditary ataxias (eg, ataxia telangiectasia)
  Progressive supranuclear palsy
  Huntington disease
  Alzheimer disease
  Parkinson disease
  Wilson disease
  Amyotrophic lateral sclerosis (ALS)

Paramedian Pontine Reticular Formation Lesions
  Demyelination
  Infarct, hematoma
  Neoplasm

Drugs
  Anticonvulsants
  Benzodiazepines

Peripheral Ocular Motility Disorders
  Ocular motor cranial nerve palsy
  Graves orbitopathy
  Chronic progressive external ophthalmoplegia
  Myasthenia gravis

Infections
  Acquired immune deficiency syndrome (AIDS)
  Whipple disease
  Tetanus

Lipidosis
  Tay-Sachs
  Gaucher (horizontal saccades)
  Niemann-Pick (vertical saccades)

Paraneoplasitic Syndromes

Abbreviation: CNS, central nervous system. Data from Leigh RJ, Zee DS: *The Neurology of Eye Movements,* 4th ed. Contemporary Neurology Series. New York: Oxford University Press; 2006: 598–686.

sporadic saccades that take the eyes off the fixation point but promptly return to fixation after a brief interval of 100 to 200 milliseconds. Small square-wave jerks are a normal component of the fixation reflex. Square-wave jerks greater than 1° are usually pathological. Macrosquare-wave jerks are greater than 10°. Square-wave jerks are nonspecific and nonlocalizing, but are commonly associated with cerebellar disease. Greater than 10 per minute is a nonspecific indicator of CNS disease.

Ocular flutter consists of intermittent brief volleys of rapid horizontal ocular oscillations around fixation that are a common companion of dysmetria. Unlike square-wave jerks, these back-to-back saccades have no intersaccadic interval. *Opsoclonus* is similar, but the chaotic saccades occur randomly in any direction (called "saccadomania"). Both ocular flutter and opsoclonus can occur from cerebellar disease or postviral encephalopathy. Opsoclonus (as well as ataxia and myoclonus) can occur as a paraneoplastic

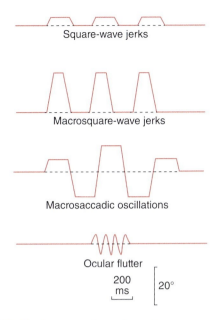

Figure 10–14. **Saccadic intrusion waveforms.** The horizontal line represents primary position, with deflections to the right shown above the line, and to the left below. Square-wave and macro square-wave jerks take the eyes off fixation for a short interval. Macrosaccadic oscillations and ocular flutter oscillate around fixation, but in ocular flutter there is no intersaccadic interval (back-to-back saccades). (Reproduced with permission from Leigh RJ, Zee DS: *The Neurology of Eye Movements,* 4th ed. Contemporary Neurology Series. New York: Oxford University Press; 2006. Figure 10–14 on page 523.)

sign, associated with neuroblastoma in children or visceral carcinoma in adults. Opsoclonus has also been associated with amitriptyline, haloperidol, and lithium use, and toxins such as chlordecone (an insecticide).

PURSUIT

Smooth pursuit mechanisms permit the eyes to conjugately track a moving visual target (rotational velocities of 20 to 50° per second). This tracking movement keeps the object of regard stabilized in the visual axis. The pursuit mechanism is integrated with the vestibular system and head rotation to allow smooth tracking with combined head and eye rotation. Nonvisual proprioceptive conditions, such as having the patient follow his or her own moving finger in darkness, will also generate a pursuit movement.

Pursuit Pathways

The organization of the pursuit system is not entirely understood, but it begins with neurons in the primary visual cortex of the occipital lobes that are sensitive to movement in the visual field. Extrastriate visual areas in the parietal-temporal-occipital junction are responsible for integrating the movement data. The pathway proceeds through the deep parietal lobe and sequentially through the dorsal pontine nuclei, the flocculus and dorsal vermis of the cerebellum, and the vestibular nuclei to premotor areas for vertical and horizontal gaze. From the vestibular nuclei, the horizontal pursuit pathway feeds directly to the abducens nucleus, rather than through the PPRF as for horizontal saccades. Vertical pursuit appear to be mediated by the interstitial nucleus of Cajal (INC), rather than the riMLF as described for vertical saccades (see Figure 10–1). Like saccades, pursuit begins with a rapid acceleration for the first 100 milliseconds, followed by a slower rotational velocity that attempts to match the movement of the object.

Pursuit Disorders

Pursuit abnormalities may be more difficult to appreciate clinically than saccadic abnormalities. Eye movement recordings demonstrate low gain pursuit (the eyes fall behind the target) in Parkinson disease, in progressive supranuclear palsy (PSP), with certain CNS active drugs, or as a manifestation of aging. Low gain pursuit manifests clinically as a choppy "saccadic" pursuit in which catch-up saccades are generated to keep up with the moving target. Deep parietal lobe lesions produce pursuit abnormalities toward the side that is *ipsilateral* to the lesion. The response is best identified clinically as an abnormal optokinetic nystagmus (OKN) response when the stimulus is moved toward the side of the lesion.

VESTIBULO-OCULAR REFLEX

Connections between the vestibular and ocular motor systems allow coordination of eye movements with head movement, permitting continued fixation on an object despite head rotation. This system is an involuntary, reflexive, eye movement system that produces a slow pursuit-like conjugate movement of eyes in a direction opposite that of head rotation or translation. If rotation is continuous (as in a Barany chair), a repeating cycle of a slow, compensatory pursuit and a reset saccade develops, a condition known as *physiological vestibular nystagmus*.

The position and movement of the head in space are monitored by the bilateral labyrinthine organs of the middle ear consisting of the three semicircular canals, which monitor rotational acceleration, and the utricle and saccule, which monitor linear acceleration and the direction of gravity. The vestibular portion of the vestibulocochlear nerve (CN VIII) conveys this information to the vestibular nuclei in the brainstem. The vestibular nuclei have direct connections to the cranial nerve nuclei and the premotor nuclei. This circuitry results in a short latency (<16 milliseconds) between the start of a head movement and the beginning of a compensatory eye movement.

Rotational acceleration of the head is detected by movement of the fluid endolymph within the semicircular canals. This information is conveyed to the vestibular nuclei by a modulation of the resting baseline (~100 spikes per second) of the corresponding vestibular nerve. Inertial movement of fluid in one direction increases the frequency of the discharge; movement in the opposite direction decreases the frequency of the signal. Each of the three semicircular canals is paired with its complement in the opposite inner ear that lies in the same plane of rotation; rotation of the head in this plane produces opposite effects on the signal from each ear that codes the direction of the spin. Three orthogonal planes are represented by this complementary pairing so that complex rotations in a plane can be accurately computed. The horizontal semicircular canals are tilted back 30° with respect to the axial plane, and the anterior and posterior canals are angled relative to the sagittal plane.

Lesions in the inner ear, vestibular nerve, or central connections disrupt this carefully balanced system, simulating continuous head rotation even when the head is still. This erroneous information causes *pathological vestibular nystagmus*. The patient may perceive that the world (or self) is spinning or moving (vertigo), a sensation that is often accompanied by nausea and vomiting.

The vestibule-ocular reflex is tested clinically with doll's head maneuver (slow turning of the patient's head), head impulse test (rapid turning of the patient's head), rotation of the patient, and less often with cold/warm calorics.

Two otolith organs in the inner ear, the utricle and saccule, detect linear acceleration and the direction of gravity. A head tilt to the right or left is conveyed by these organs for central vestibular processing to produce compensatory reflexes: counter roll (torsion) of the eyes (to keep the eyes as level with the world as possible), a correction movement to return the head to upright, and a rudimentary disconjugate vertical movement to elevate the lower eye and depress the higher eye. This reflex is relatively unimportant clinically except when it goes awry: Disruption of the peripheral or central utricle pathway or the connected components can cause a skew deviation or the full manifestation of the ocular tilt reaction.

Skew Deviation

Skew deviation is a small vertical tropia that is the pathological manifestation of the disconjugate vertical eye movement described above with head tilt. It can occur with utricle and vestibular lesions and also from nonspecific brainstem or cerebellar injury. The deviation is usually relatively comitant, and the hypotropic eye is often on the side of the lesion. Skew deviations from lesions outside of the midbrain in the pons, medulla, and cerebellum are a reminder that the conjugate gaze schematics previously discussed are greatly simplified; many complex connections exist between the vestibular nuclei, cerebellum, and cerebral cortex that coordinate eye movements.

Ocular tilt reaction (OTR) is the logical consequence of erroneous information from unbalanced input from the utricles. If the signals inform the brain that the head is tilted when it is upright, the reflex will tilt the head to the opposite side and cyclotort the eyes the "wrong" way relative to the manifest tilt (away from the true horizontal) with a skew deviation. OTR may occur as a result of lesions in the peripheral vestibular pathways, vestibular nuclei, cerebellum, and in the midbrain.

OPTOKINETIC REFLEX

The slow conjugate eye movement of the optokinetic reflex is similar to smooth pursuit because it matches eye movement to movement in the visual field. However, it differs from smooth pursuit because it is involuntary and moves the eyes to follow movements of the visual field as a whole, rather than a small moving object in a stationary visual field. The optokinetic reflex is evident by observing the eye movements of a subject who is observing the landscape from a moving vehicle. A large portion of the observer's visual field is continuously moving. The eyes slowly track the moving landscape until the eyes are in far horizontal gaze, then a fast saccadic movement resets the eyes to allow another pursuit-like movement. This reflex stabilizes the moving visual field, preventing an otherwise continuous blur from constant relative motion of the visual field. Similar to smooth pursuit, the afferent limb originates in the visual cortex, which contributes information about motion in the visual field. The efferent limb utilizes the standard smooth pursuit and saccadic systems as previously described. For this reason, testing with an optokinetic stimulus is an effective way to evaluate both the saccadic and smooth pursuit systems (see Figure 7–2).

VERGENCE

The vergence system produces slow *disconjugate* movements of the eyes to track or fixate on objects in near or more distant three-dimensional space. Refixation from a distant object to a near object requires convergence of the eyes to maintain binocular fixation. The reverse process requires a divergence movement of the eyes: from an eso-position of the visual axes to a more parallel position. Refixation by vergence movement has a longer latency (~160 milliseconds) and is much slower (20° per second) than conjugate saccades or pursuit.

Vergence is part of the *near synkinetic triad,* which also includes accommodation (of the lens) and pupillary miosis. Without activation of the near synkinetic reflex, an object approaching the nose would appear double and blurred. Not surprisingly, double images and visual blurring are strong stimulators of convergence.

Although not as intuitive as convergence and divergence, vergence also technically includes the small disconjugate vertical and torsion movements of the eyes with head tilt as discussed above.

Organization

Supranuclear control of vergence is not fully understood, but structures important to vergence coordination are likely located in the mesencephalon near the CN III nuclei. Vergence disturbances are a prominent component of the dorsal midbrain syndrome.

Disorders of the Vergence System

High accommodative convergence-to-accommodation ratio As previously discussed, activation of convergence and accommodation are linked as components of the near synkinetic reflex. In some cases of childhood strabismus, activation of these two components may not be balanced. For instance, in patients with a high accommodative convergence-to-accommodation (AC/A) ratio, the amount of accommodation required to focus a near object may result in too much convergence, causing an esotropia at near.

Convergence insufficiency This condition is essentially the result of a low AC/A ratio, where convergence is not adequate despite normal accommodative tone. Patients are exophoric or exotropic at near and often present with vague discomfort with reading (asthenopia) or diplopia with near tasks. Convergence insufficiency is usually a benign condition when it occurs in isolation, but it can occur following head injury. Convergence exercises ("pencil push-ups") may help strengthen convergence.

Divergence insufficiency This term is ascribed to patients who are orthophoric at near, esotropic at distance, but who have full ocular ductions. Patients with divergence insufficiency are often elderly with microvascular disease, suggesting the possibility of a lacunar infarct involving a yet-unidentified divergence center. This condition is difficult to differentiate from mild bilateral CN VI palsies, and neuroimaging may be required to address possible causes of isolated, bilateral CN VI palsies, such as a clivus lesion. Divergence insufficiency can also occur with head trauma, PSP, brainstem stroke, and cerebellar lesions.

Spasm of the near reflex This condition may rarely occur from seizures or following head injury, but it may also be a voluntary (nonorganic) finding. Patients are esotropic and may appear to have bilateral CN VI palsies. However, if the pupils are miotic, the findings are likely a result of continued, voluntary activation of the near reflex (see Figure 9–4).

FIXATION REFLEX

The eyes are in constant motion, even when they are locked on an object of interest. Slow, small angle drifts off the fixation object are corrected with microsaccades. These normal eye movements are approximately 0.1° and are not evident clinically (but may be detected with ophthalmoscopy).

The conjugate eye movement systems (saccades, pursuit, vestibulo-ocular, and optokinetic) combine an eye velocity component with an eye position-holding component, as previously discussed with saccades. The initial velocity component is different for slow and fast eye movements, but all systems use the same *neural integrator* to produce the step up in innervation that allows the eyes to *fixate* in a new position. The neural integrator is located in the medial vestibular nuclei and the nucleus propositus hypoglossi (caudal pons and upper medulla). These areas are responsible for calculating the final position of the eye from the strength of the saccadic pulse and for changing the level of sustained innervation to hold the eye in the new position.

Fixation disorders occur when the integrator is "leaky" and unable to hold fixation in a new position, causing a (large-angle) slow drift back toward primary position. To maintain gaze position, a corrective saccade is generated to reposition the eye. The repeating cycle of slow drift and correcting saccade produces a gaze-evoked nystagmus, described in more detail in the following sections.

▶ NYSTAGMUS

Ophthalmologists are often uncomfortable when evaluating nystagmus, perhaps because this finding is usually a sign of neurological disease rather than eye disease. In addition, nystagmus presents in many forms, often changing depending on the direction of gaze; the physician may be unsure how to describe and characterize the findings and uncertain of the significance. However, only a few types of nystagmus are likely to be encountered in clinical practice, many with easily defined characteristics.

The following discussion addresses the descriptive characteristics of nystagmus so that clinical findings can be accurately described, recorded, and used to define a differential diagnosis. Clinically distinct types of nystagmus are also described.

CLASSIFICATION AND TERMINOLOGY

Nystagmus is a rhythmic to-and-fro movement of the eyes. The ocular oscillations are either jerk or pendular. In *jerk nystagmus*, the eye drifts away from fixation in a pursuit-like movement and returns with a fast, saccadic movement. Jerk nystagmus is named for the direction of the fast component, for example, "right-beating jerk nystagmus." However, it is the slow component that is the manifestation of disease (or the primary action in physiological nystagmus); the quick saccadic component can be thought of as a corrective movement to get the eye back on target. Jerk nystagmus usually becomes more prominent with gaze toward the side of the fast component, a clinical dictum known as *Alexander law*. For example, when the gaze-holding mechanism is deficient in right gaze, the eyes drift back toward the left, generating a saccade to drive the eye back to the right. This right-beating jerk nystagmus will have greater amplitude the farther the patient looks to the right, and the nystagmus will likely be absent in left gaze. *Pendular nystagmus* consists of oscillations that have equal speed in both directions. Therefore, pendular nystagmus is defined by a *plane* (such as the horizontal plane) rather than a direction.

Nystagmus is not confined to the vertical or horizontal planes. *Oblique* nystagmus may be thought of as a vector summation of coincident horizontal and vertical nystagmus. *Circular or elliptical* nystagmus results if the horizontal and vertical vectors are out of phase. In this case, the visual axis of the eye describes a continuous, repeating circular or elliptical path. *Torsional* nystagmus occurs as a to-and-fro rotation (cyclotorsion) around the visual axis.

Both jerk and pendular nystagmus have a frequency and amplitude of oscillation. The *frequency* is the number of oscillations per second and is often clinically graded as high, medium, or low. *Amplitude* describes the size of the ocular rotation, with common clinical descriptors including fine, medium, and coarse.

Most forms of nystagmus are conjugate: Both eyes move in the same direction. In disconjugate nystagmus the trajectory is different between the two eyes. In dissociated nystagmus the amplitude differs between the two eyes, the extreme of which is a purely unilateral nystagmus.

The *waveform* of nystagmus in eye movement recordings offers additional diagnostic information (Figure 10–15).

Precipitating factors offer important diagnostic clues. Nystagmus may be present only in certain positions of gaze. Latent nystagmus only occurs when one eye is covered. Intermittent nystagmus precipitated by head movement suggests a peripheral vestibular mechanism (inner ear).

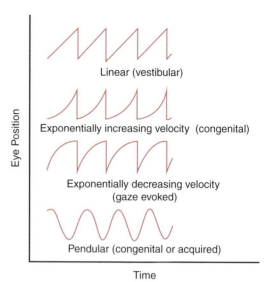

Figure 10–15. **Nystagmus waveforms.** In true nystagmus, the slow phase is from the disease, and the saccade (if there is one) is corrective (to get the eye back on target). Vestibular nystagmus causes a slow drift of the eyes off fixation of a constant velocity (linear waveform) with a refixation saccade that produces a saw-toothed waveform (*top*). Other forms of decelerating or accelerating slow phases with corrective saccades are shown. Pendular nystagmus is a slow to-and-fro movement and has no saccadic component. (Reproduced with permission from Leigh RJ, Zee DS: *The Neurology of Eye Movements,* 4th ed. Contemporary Neurology Series. New York: Oxford University Press; 2006. Figure 10–1 on page 476.)

PHYSIOLOGICAL NYSTAGMUS

Some forms of nystagmus are normal. As discussed above, the nystagmus generated by the optokinetic and vestibulo-ocular reflexes plays an important physiological role in stabilizing vision with movement of the visual field or movement of the head, and can be induced by the physician for diagnostic purposes.

Optokinetic Nystagmus

Optokinetic nystagmus is a normal physiological response to a continuously moving visual panorama. It can be observed in subjects looking out a car window at the scenery as it moves by, and can be induced in the clinic with OKN drum or tape (or OKN smartphone app!). This reflex allows the physician to observe and compare saccades and pursuit in different directions in an objectively induced fashion.

Vestibulo-ocular Nystagmus

Vestibulo-ocular nystagmus is induced by actual or simulated continuous head rotation. As discussed earlier in this chapter, a slow compensatory eye movement is generated by the vestibular apparatus in the direction opposite of the head rotation to allow stabilization of the visual field. With continued rotation, the eyes are reset by a saccade to allow a new smooth pursuit to be generated, with the repeating cycle generating nystagmus. Rotation of a subject's head induces eye movements mediated by the semicircular canals. In a Barany chair, continuous spinning induces a normal, physiological jerk nystagmus with the fast phase in the same direction as the rotation. Vestibulo-ocular nystagmus is useful in evaluating the eye movements of infants; the examiner can hold the patient and spin, observing the induced nystagmus.

As discussed in Chapter 7, irrigation of the ear with cold or warm water (caloric testing) induces movement of labyrinthine fluids, simulating rotational nystagmus and producing vestibular nystagmus (see Box 7–3).

OTHER FORMS OF NONPATHOLOGICAL NYSTAGMUS

Endpoint Nystagmus

A few beats of jerk nystagmus in the direction of eccentric gaze may be a normal finding. Characteristics of normal end-point nystagmus include low amplitude, irregular frequency, and symmetry in the opposite direction. The amplitude of nystagmus may be slightly greater in the abducting eye. The physician can greatly increase his or her confidence in determining when nystagmus is normal or abnormal by observing end-point nystagmus in all patients, especially patients with a normal examination.

Prolonged eccentric gaze can produce a sustained physiological jerk nystagmus in some normal patients, presumably from fatigue in maintaining eccentric gaze. *Gaze-evoked* and *gaze-paretic* nystagmus are abnormal forms of nystagmus that are of greater amplitude than end-point nystagmus, occurring with much less eccentricity of gaze.

Voluntary "Nystagmus"

This phenomenon is a high-frequency, low-amplitude, horizontal, pendular-appearing oscillation that can only rarely be sustained for greater than 30 seconds. This "party trick" consists of back-to-back saccades without a slow component and therefore is not a true nystagmus. Although often startling to the examiner, voluntary nystagmus can usually be differentiated from ocular oscillations caused by organic disease.

CONGENITAL NYSTAGMUS AND NYSTAGMUS IN CHILDREN

Nystagmus resulting from a primary disorder of the efferent visual system is known as a *motor nystagmus*. Children or adults with poor vision can develop nystagmus secondarily because of loss of vision, called *sensory deprivation nystagmus*. However, the distinction between motor and sensory nystagmus is not always clear cut; a motor nystagmus in infancy can cause amblyopia and subnormal vision, and poor vision from any cause can result in nystagmus.

Congenital Nystagmus

Congenital motor nystagmus is a jerk or pendular nystagmus that is present at birth or shortly thereafter and remains throughout life. It can be heritable or sporadic. The nystagmus may be associated with poor vision (as in oculocutaneous albinism), but most congenital nystagmus is thought to be a primary motor disorder. Differentiating congenital motor nystagmus from acquired types is important because a diagnosis of congenital nystagmus in an adult may avert a needless extensive neurological evaluation. Some adult patients are not aware that they have had lifelong congenital nystagmus; their vision may be excellent and the nystagmus may be of small amplitude or be manifest only when one eye is covered for an eye examination (see latent nystagmus discussion below).

Congenital nystagmus is binocular and conjugate (the same in both eyes). Unlike many acquired forms of nystagmus, patients with congenital nystagmus do not complain of oscillopsia. The nystagmus is *uniplanar,* meaning that the orientation of the nystagmus is the same in all positions of gaze. For example, the vast majority of the time, congenital nystagmus is horizontal and will remain horizontal in up or downgaze, even though the *direction* of the nystagmus changes with horizontal gaze. Even in those cases in which the nystagmus appears to be pendular in primary position, horizontal jerk nystagmus (in the direction of gaze) can be seen in eccentric gaze. Frequently, a *null point,* a position of gaze at which the nystagmus is minimized, is present. Gaze to the right of the null point induces a right-beating nystagmus and gaze to left induces a left-beating nystagmus. The null point is not necessarily in primary position, and patients frequently adopt a head position to keep the position of gaze near the null point. Congenital nystagmus is usually damped by convergence and extinguished in sleep. Patients may have an associated head oscillation.

The waveform in congenital nystagmus is distinct. The slow component in congenital jerk nystagmus shows an increasing velocity waveform, as if the eyes are driven away from fixation (unlike the decreasing velocity drift of gaze-paretic nystagmus). Distinctive foveation periods, in which the eyes are briefly still, may allow good central vision despite the otherwise constant movement of the eyes.

Approximately two-thirds of patients with congenital nystagmus may display an inverted response to an optokinetic stimulus. When an optokinetic stimulus is presented at the null position of gaze, or in the presence of a pendular nystagmus, a jerk nystagmus is induced that is opposite in direction from the expected normal response. This peculiar response is diagnostic of congenital nystagmus when present.

Latent nystagmus is not present under binocular viewing conditions but only occurs when one eye is covered. It is frequently discovered incidentally when examining the fundus with the ophthalmoscope. The induced jerk nystagmus is present in both eyes and has a fast component toward the side of the uncovered eye. Latent nystagmus is congenital and may exist in a pure form or may be superimposed on congenital nystagmus as previously described. When visual acuity is measured by covering one eye, the presence of latent nystagmus may reduce the measured acuity considerably—the visual acuity of both eyes together is much better than each eye alone. The use of a high-plus lens to fog, but not totally occlude, the nontested eye may allow monocular visual acuity measurement without inducing latent nystagmus.

The term *manifest latent nystagmus* appears at first glance to be an oxymoron, but it is an accurate descriptive label for patients with latent nystagmus with monocular amblyopia or suppression. Because these patients are viewing monocularly, their latent nystagmus is always manifest. This diagnosis can be confirmed by covering the preferred eye and observing a reversal of the jerk nystagmus. Making a diagnosis of latent or manifest latent nystagmus is important clinically because these conditions are congenital and are not associated with acquired CNS disease.

Acquired Nystagmus in Children

Acquired nystagmus in children may be the result of vision- or life-threatening disease and must be differentiated from congenital nystagmus. As previously discussed, nystagmus can result from afferent visual loss. This sensory deprivation nystagmus is typically pendular and damped by convergence. Obviously, nystagmus associated with progressive visual loss, optic nerve pallor or edema, or other neurological signs suggests an intracranial tumor or other process affecting the afferent visual system and requires neuroimaging. Differentiating congenital nystagmus from nystagmus acquired in infancy may be impossible in many patients, necessitating neuroimaging when the diagnosis is uncertain.

Spasmus nutans is an acquired nystagmus of infancy. This horizontal or vertical pendular nystagmus is of high frequency and low amplitude; it is bilateral but asymmetric, or may appear entirely monocular. The classic triad consists of (1) nystagmus, (2) head nodding, and (3) head turn (torticollis). Spasmus nutans appears in children before 2 years of age and disappears before 10 years. Although this condition is benign, neuroimaging is usually performed because spasmus nutans cannot be differentiated clinically from similar nystagmus resulting from CNS disease, particularly chiasmal/hypothalamic glioma.

RECOGNIZABLE FORMS OF ACQUIRED NYSTAGMUS

Most forms of nystagmus can be identified clinically without eye movement recordings. The nystagmus *type* (jerk or pendular), *amplitude, frequency,* and *plane or direction* in each cardinal position of gaze, as well as the time course and associated signs and symptoms, are distinguishing features. Classifying the type of acquired nystagmus is very important; the type of nystagmus determines the most likely location of the lesion (Table 10–5) and pathologic process involved.

Periodic Alternating Nystagmus

Periodic alternating nystagmus (PAN) is a horizontal jerk nystagmus that changes direction throughout a cycle of 2 to 3 minutes. In primary position, a right-beating nystagmus may be observed to decrease in amplitude, stop, and then become a left-beating nystagmus of increasing amplitude, followed by a similar transition back to right-beating. The cycle repeats continuously. The nystagmus is horizontal and uniplanar, and thus remains horizontal even in upgaze. Unless the examiner is patient and observant, the cyclic nature of the nystagmus (and the diagnosis of PAN) will be missed.

Horizontal versions during the cycle reveal that this nystagmus is bidirectional with a null point that slowly cycles in the horizontal plane. Some patients are observed to have a slowly cycling compensatory head turn, in an attempt to keep eyes in the ever-changing null position of gaze. PAN may be congenital. Acquired forms are associated with craniocervical junction anomalies, MS, spinocerebellar degenerations, bilateral blindness, or toxicity from anticonvulsant therapy. Baclofen (Lioresal) is often effective in suppressing the nystagmus.

Downbeat Nystagmus

To qualify as downbeat nystagmus, the nystagmus must be present in primary position (not just in downgaze). The amplitude is greatest when gaze is directed down and to

▶ **TABLE 10-5. LOCALIZATION OF LESIONS CAUSING NYSTAGMUS AND NYSTAGMUS-LIKE CONDITIONS**

Nystagmus or Nystagmus-Like Condition	Most Common Anatomic Location of Lesion
Periodic alternating nystagmus	Craniocervical junction, cerebellum
Downbeat nystagmus	Craniocervical junction (vestibulocerebellum)
Upbeat nystagmus	Posterior fossa (medulla, also pons and midbrain)
See-saw nystagmus	Parasellar/diencephalon
Gaze-evoked nystagmus	Cerebellum and brainstem, but most often from medications
Rebound nystagmus	Posterior fossa
Vestibular nystagmus	Central or peripheral (inner ear) vestibular areas
Dissociated nystagmus with INO	MLF
Acquired pendular nystagmus (APN)	Different locations and mechanisms
Oculopalatal myoclonus	*Mollaret triangle* (red nucleus, inferior olive, and contralateral dentate nucleus)
Flutter/opsoclonus	Cerebellum/pons
Ocular bobbing	Pons
Convergence-retraction nystagmus	Dorsal mesencephalon

Abbreviations: INO, internuclear ophthalmoplegia; MLF, medial longitudinal fasciculus.

the side (a variant of Alexander law). Impaired downward pursuit is invariably present. Downbeat nystagmus is characteristic of disorders of the vestibulocerebellum and brainstem connections, including Arnold-Chiari malformation, basilar invagination, MS, spinocerebellar degeneration, brainstem stroke, hydrocephalus, metabolic disorders, familial episodic ataxia, drug toxicity (lithium, anticonvulsants), and Wernicke encephalopathy. However, the majority of patients older than 70 years with downbeat nystagmus have no clinically evident causative diagnosis. 4-Aminopyridine and 3, 4-diaminopyridine are potassium channel blockers that can be effective in suppressing downbeat nystagmus. Clonazepam may also be effective.

Upbeat Nystagmus

Upbeat nystagmus in primary position is associated with lesions of the medial medullary tegmentum, ventral pontine tegmentum, and cerebellar vermis. Causes include MS, stroke, and tumors, as well as drug toxicity and Wernicke encephalopathy. Similar to downbeat nystagmus, the clinical designation upbeat nystagmus implies that the nystagmus is present in primary position (not just gaze-evoked nystagmus in upgaze).

See-Saw Nystagmus

See-saw nystagmus is a pendular (but occasionally jerk) form of nystagmus in which one eye elevates and intorts while the other eye depresses and extorts. This peculiar form of nystagmus is associated with third ventricle tumors and bitemporal hemianopia, trauma, MS, and brainstem vascular disease. A congenital form exists with variable torsional features that may or may not have associated bitemporal visual field loss.

Gaze-Evoked Nystagmus

Gaze-evoked nystagmus is similar to physiological end-point nystagmus, but it is of greater amplitude and occurs with less eccentricity of gaze. Any disorder affecting the initiation or maintenance (position holding) of conjugate gaze can produce gaze-evoked nystagmus. The most common causes include the effect of medications (anticonvulsants, sedatives) and cerebellar or brainstem disease. *Gaze-paretic nystagmus* is a type of gaze-evoked nystagmus caused by a paresis of the gaze initiation mechanism in the brainstem or hemispheres. In cerebellar disease, gaze-evoked nystagmus is likely the result of a defective neural integrator, in which the step component of the pulse-step signal is not sufficient to hold the eyes in eccentric gaze, causing a large-amplitude, low-frequency nystagmus.

Rebound Nystagmus

Rebound nystagmus is a transient, rapid, horizontal jerk nystagmus initiated by eccentric gaze, which first beats in the direction of gaze and then quickly reverses direction after several seconds. Rebound nystagmus can also be seen as the eyes return to primary position from eccentric gaze as a transient jerk nystagmus that beats in an opposite direction. This form of nystagmus is associated with cerebellar or other posterior fossa lesions.

Vestibular Nystagmus

Diseases affecting any of the components of the vestibular system (eg, brainstem nuclei, CN VIII, or inner ear vestibular organs) can cause nystagmus that is usually associated with imbalance or vertigo. Lesions in the vestibular pathway simulate continuous head rotation, resulting in vestibular nystagmus. The nystagmus is usually a horizontal or horizontal-rotary jerk nystagmus, with specific characteristics that help

▶ TABLE 10-6. VESTIBULAR NYSTAGMUS

Sign or Symptom	Peripheral (Inner Ear)	Central (Brainstem)
Type of nystagmus	Mixed horizontal-torsional	Purely vertical, torsional, or horizontal, but can be mixed
Direction of nystagmus	Unidirectional, fast phase opposite lesion	Unidirectional or can reverse with gaze change
Visual fixation	Inhibits nystagmus and vertigo	No inhibition
Severity of vertigo	Marked	Mild
Direction of spin	Toward fast phase	Variable
Direction of pastpointing	Toward slow phase	Variable
Direction of Romberg fall	Toward slow phase	Variable
Effect of head-turning	Changes Romberg fall	No effect
Duration of symptoms	Finite (minutes, days, weeks) but recurrent	May be chronic
Tinnitus of deafness	Often present	Usually absent
Common causes	Infection (labyrinthitis), Meniere disease, neuronitis, vascular disorders, trauma, toxicity	Vascular, demyelinating, and neoplastic disorders

Data from Dell'Osso LF, Daroff RB: Nystagmus and saccadic intrusions and oscillation, in Duane TD (ed): *Duane's Clinical Ophthalmology*, Vol 2. Philadelphia, PA: Lippincott Williams & Wilkins; 1998.

differentiate central (brainstem) from peripheral (inner ear, labyrinthine disease). These differences are summarized in Table 10–6. *Peripheral (inner ear) disorders* may be associated with tinnitus or hearing loss and include infections (labyrinthitis), Meniere disease, vascular disorders, trauma, and drug toxicities. *Central (brainstem/cerebellar) vestibular disorders* include MS, tumors, vascular disorders, and encephalitis.

Acquired Pendular Nystagmus

Acquired pendular nystagmus (APN) is most commonly seen in patients with MS. The plane, amplitude, and phase is usually mixed and complex. The nystagmus is not conjugate: It may be unilateral, and is usually very different in the two eyes when present bilaterally. Patients may experience blur or oscillopsia. Causes other than MS include cerebellar degeneration and toluene abuse. Some patients respond to gabapentin. In children, APN can occur with leukodystrophies such as Pelizaeus-Merzbacher disease.

Dissociated Nystagmus with INO

The dissociated nystagmus that occurs with an INO was previously discussed. The abducting eye demonstrates a jerk nystagmus of much greater amplitude than the poorly adducting eye, which may have no nystagmus at all.

Oculopalatal Myoclonus

A pendular, vertical nystagmus that occurs synchronous with contractions of the palate (palatal myoclonus), face, pharynx, diaphragm, or limb can result from lesions in *Mollaret triangle* (triangular area composed of the red nucleus, ipsilateral inferior olive, and contralateral dentate nucleus). The myoclonus usually begins several months after a posterior circulation stroke and may be mistaken for a new event. Once established, myoclonic movement persists even during sleep. Gabapentin and memantine are occasionally effective in suppressing the nystagmus.

OTHER NYSTAGMUS-LIKE OSCILLATIONS

In pathological nystagmus, it is the slow component that is the manifestation of disease. Saccadic intrusions (including macro square wave jerks, ocular flutter, and opsoclonus), ocular bobbing, convergence retraction "nystagmus," and superior oblique myokymia are characterized by an abnormal saccade as the pathological eye movement, and thus cannot be categorized as true nystagmus, and are often called *nystagmoid* or *nystagmus-like*.

Ocular Bobbing

Ocular bobbing is a conjugate eye movement with fast downward movements and a slow drift up, similar to a fishing bob on the water. Ocular bobbing is usually identified in a comatose patient with an extensive pontine lesion, obstructive hydrocephalus, or metabolic encephalopathy. Inverse bobbing with an upward fast phase is seen in similar circumstances.

▶ TABLE 10-7. DRUGS USED IN TREATING ACQUIRED NYSTAGMUS

	First-Line Drugs	Second-Line Drugs
Periodic alternating nystagmus	Baclofen	Memantine
Downbeat nystagmus	4-Aminopyridine, 3,4-diaminopyridine	Clonazepam
Upbeat nystagmus	Memantine, 4-aminopyridine, baclofen	
See-saw nystagmus	Clonazepam, gabapentin, memantine	
Acquired pendular nystagmus (APN)	Gabapentin, memantine	
Torsional nystagmus	Gabapentin	

Data from Thurtell MJ, Leigh RJ: Therapy for nystagmus. *J Neuroophthalmol* 2010;30:361–371.

Superior Oblique Myokymia

Superior oblique myokymia is an episodic rapid twitching (buzzing) of the superior oblique muscle causing monocular oscillopsia. Episodes occur sporadically but can sometimes be induced by moving the eye in and out of the field of action of the involved superior oblique muscle. The twitch is high frequency and low amplitude and may only be appreciated with high magnification at the slit lamp, or with auscultation (see Figure 7–13). In primary position, the oscillation is torsional and best appreciated using a conjunctival blood vessel to watch the rotary movements. In adduction, the movement is primarily vertical. Myokymia may occasionally also cause sustained tonic spasm of the superior oblique muscle, resulting in intermittent vertical diplopia. This disorder is idiopathic and generally benign and may remit spontaneously. Patients may respond to carbamazepine (Tegretol), baclofen (Lioresal), or by limiting caffeine intake. Some physicians advocate surgical weakening of the superior oblique muscle in patients with long-standing, intolerable symptoms.

NYSTAGMUS TREATMENT

A clear diagnosis is the key step in considering treatment options for nystagmus and other abnormal eye movements. Eliminating the cause rather than treating the symptom only is obviously the best treatment. Because there is no general treatment for symptomatic nystagmus, a clear diagnosis is crucial for determining potential treatment options.

As discussed above, there are medications that have been shown to be effective in suppressing specific types of nystagmus, most notably baclofen in acquired PAN, 4-aminopyridine for downbeat nystagmus, and gabapentin for acquired pendular nystagmus. Memantine may also be of some help in PAN, APN, and upbeat nystagmus (Table 10–7).

Optical aids can sometimes suppress nystagmus or reduce blur and oscillopsia. Contact lenses may provide clearer vision than glasses for patients with congenital nystagmus. Using base-out prisms to induce convergence may help in those forms of nystagmus that dampen with convergence. Combining high-minus contact lenses with high-plus spectacles can optically reduce oscillopsia, but only monocularly and when the patient's head is stationary.

Surgical options are limited, as weakening the extraocular muscles to reduce nystagmus also eliminates the useful and purposeful movements of the eye, resulting in diplopia and limited eye movements. However, superior oblique muscle tenotomy with recession of the inferior oblique muscle can be very effective with limited undesirable effects in intractable superior oblique myokymia. The Anderson-Kestenbaum procedure is performed on patients with an eccentric null point and head turn, by operating on the horizontally acting muscles to move the null-point to primary position. Cüppers divergence procedure creates a divergence that induces convergence to suppress nystagmus, much like base-out prisms.

Botox can be used to weaken the extraocular muscles and reduce nystagmus, but is only temporary in effect and results in diplopia and immobility of the eyes.

▶ KEY POINTS

- The paramedian pontine reticular formation (PPRF) acts as the horizontal gaze center, activating the abducens (CN VI) nucleus in response to supranuclear gaze commands.
- The abducens nucleus contains two classes of neurons: (1) motor neurons whose axons innervate the ipsilateral lateral rectus, and (2) internuclear neurons with axons that immediately cross to the contralateral MLF and travel to the medial rectus subnucleus (CN III nucleus).
- Lesions of the abducens nucleus produce an ipsilateral gaze palsy, not just an ipsilateral abduction defect.
- A lesion of the right MLF causes a right internuclear ophthalmoplegia (INO), consisting of an isolated adduction deficit of the right eye on attempted left gaze, with normal right gaze.
- Lesions that involve the PPRF (or CN VI nucleus) and the ipsilateral MLF cause a "one-and-a-half" syndrome, a gaze palsy to the ipsilateral side and an INO (of the ipsilateral eye) in contralateral gaze.

- The riMLF is the vertical gaze center, analogous to the PPRF in horizontal gaze.
- Pinealomas and intrinsic midbrain lesions can cause dorsal midbrain syndrome: vertical gaze disturbances, convergence-retraction nystagmus, light-near dissociation of the pupil, and vergence abnormalities.
- The six systems of eye movement control are saccade, smooth pursuit, vestibulo-ocular, optokinetic, vergence, and fixation systems.
- Saccades are fast eye movements (rotational velocities of up to 500° per second) that redirect the eyes to a new fixation object.
- The frontal eye field and superior colliculus, on the side contralateral to the direction of gaze, are the major supranuclear initiators of horizontal saccadic movement.
- The supranuclear pathway for vertical saccades originates from the bilateral frontal eye fields or bilateral superior colliculi.
- Injury to a frontal lobe causes a transient ipsilateral gaze preference from loss of contralateral saccades; recovery occurs as the functioning contralateral frontal lobe utilizes a secondary pathway to normalize gaze function.
- In congenital ocular motor apraxia, voluntary horizontal saccades are absent and head thrusts are used to refixate.
- Progressive supranuclear palsy (PSP) is a degenerative neurological condition that causes a progressive slowing of saccades in all directions (downgaze affected first).
- Cerebellar disease can cause ocular dysmetria and saccadic intrusions (square wave jerks, ocular flutter, opsoclonus).
- Opsoclonus (saccadomania) can occur as a paraneoplastic manifestation of neuroblastoma in children or visceral carcinoma in adults.
- Pursuit mechanisms permit the eyes to conjugately track a slowly moving visual target and keep the object of regard stabilized in the visual axis.
- Deep parietal lobe lesions produce ipsilateral pursuit abnormalities that are best identified as a diminished OKN response when the stimulus is moved toward the side of the lesion.
- The vestibular nuclei have direct connections to the ocular motor nuclei and the premotor nuclei, resulting in a short latency (<16 milliseconds) from the start of a head movement to the beginning of a compensatory eye movement.
- The optokinetic reflex stabilizes a moving visual field, preventing an otherwise continuous blur from constant relative motion of the visual field.
- The afferent limb of the optokinetic reflex originates in the visual cortex; the efferent limb utilizes the standard smooth pursuit and saccadic systems.
- Convergence is part of the near synkinetic triad, which also includes accommodation and miosis.
- Both fast and slow eye movements combine an eye velocity component with an eye position-holding component synthesized by the neural integrator in the medial vestibular nuclei and the nucleus propositus hypoglossi.
- A "leaky" neural integrator is unable to hold fixation in a new position, producing a gaze-evoked nystagmus: a slow drift back toward primary position alternating with a repositioning saccade.
- Congenital nystagmus is a uniplanar, conjugate jerk or pendular nystagmus that is present at birth or shortly thereafter and continues throughout life.
- Making a diagnosis of latent or manifest latent nystagmus is important clinically because these conditions are always congenital and are not associated with acquired CNS disease.
- Differentiating congenital nystagmus from acquired nystagmus in infancy may be impossible in many patients, necessitating neuroimaging when the diagnosis is uncertain.
- Spasmus nutans is an acquired nystagmus of infancy consisting of a high-frequency, low-amplitude, asymmetric (or monocular) nystagmus, associated with head-nodding and torticollis.
- Although spasmus nutans is benign, neuroimaging is usually performed because this condition cannot always be clinically differentiated from nystagmus resulting from CNS disease (particularly chiasmal/hypothalamic glioma).
- Unless the examiner is patient and observant, the cyclic nature of periodic alternating nystagmus (PAN) will be missed, depriving the patient of an accurate diagnosis and potential treatment.
- PAN is associated with craniocervical junction anomalies, MS, bilateral blindness, or toxicity from anticonvulsant therapy, or may be congenital.
- To qualify *downbeat* or *upbeat nystagmus*, nystagmus must be present in primary position.
- *Down*beat nystagmus is characteristic of disorders *down* in the brainstem at the craniocervical junction.
- Upbeat nystagmus is caused by lesions of the anterior vermis and lower brain stem, as well as drug intoxication and Wernicke encephalopathy.
- See-saw nystagmus is associated with third ventricle tumors and bitemporal hemianopia, trauma, and brainstem vascular disease.
- Gaze-evoked nystagmus results from any disorder affecting the initiation (brainstem or hemisphere) or position-holding (neural integrator, cerebellum) mechanisms of conjugate gaze.

- Lesions in the vestibular pathway simulate head movement, resulting in pathological vestibular nystagmus.
- Oculopalatal myoclonus causes a pendular, vertical nystagmus that is synchronous with contractions of the face, palate, pharynx, diaphragm, or extremity from lesions in Mollaret myoclonic triangle.
- Superior oblique myokymia is an idiopathic rapid twitching of the superior oblique muscle, causing intermittent monocular oscillopsia and vertical diplopia.

SUGGESTED READING

Books

Supranuclear Disorders

Leigh RJ, Daroff RB, Troost BT: Supranuclear disorders of eye movements, in Duane TD (ed): *Duane's Clinical Ophthalmology*, Vol. 2 Philadelphia, PA: Lippincott Williams & Wilkins; 1998.

Leigh RJ, Zee DS: *The Neurology of Eye Movements*, 4th ed. Contemporary Neurology Series. New York, NY: Oxford University Press; 2006.

Zee DS, Newman-Toker DE: Supranuclear and internuclear ocular motility disorders, in Miller NR, Newman NJ (eds): *Walsh and Hoyt's Clinical Neuro-ophthalmology*, Vol. 1, 6th ed. Philadelphia, PA: Lippincott Williams & Wilkins; 2005:907–967.

Nystagmus

Dell'Osso LF, Daroff RB: Nystagmus and saccadic intrusions and oscillations, in Duane TD (ed): *Duane's Clinical Ophthalmology*, Vol. 2. Philadelphia, PA: Lippincott Williams & Wilkins; 1998.

Leigh RJ, Rucker JC: Nystagmus and related ocular motility disorders, in Miller NR, Newman J (eds): *Walsh and Hoyt's Clinical Neuro-ophthalmology*, Vol. 1, 6th ed. Philadelphia, PA: Lippincott Williams & Wilkins; 2005:1133–1173.

Walker MF, Kline LB: Nystagmus and related ocular oscillations, in Kline LB (ed): *Neuro-ophthalmology Review Manual*, 7th ed. New Jersey, NJ: Slack; 2013.

Articles

Supranuclear Disorders

Brodsky MC, Donahue SP, Vaphiades M, et al: Skew deviation revisited. *Surv Ophthalmol* 2006;51:105–128.

Cogan DG: Congenital ocular motor apraxia. *Can J Ophthalmol* 1966;1:253–260.

Sharpe JA, Rosenberg MA, Hoyt WF, et al: Paralytic pontine exotropia. *Neurology* 1974;24:1076–1081.

Nystagmus

Digre KB: Opsoclonus in adults: report of three cases and review of the literature. *Arch Neurol* 1986;43:1165–1175.

Straube A: Therapeutic considerations for eye movement disorders. *Dev Ophthalmol* 2007;40:175–192.

Thurtell MJ, Leigh RJ: Nystagmus and saccadic intrusions. *Handb Clin Neurol* 2011;102:333–378.

Thurtell MJ, Leigh RJ: Therapy for nystagmus. *J Neuroophthalmol* 2010;30:361–371.

CHAPTER 11

The Pupil

- ▶ ANATOMY AND OVERVIEW OF PATHOPHYSIOLOGY 261
  - The iris 261
  - Sympathetic innervation of the pupil 262
  - Parasympathetic innervation of the Pupil 262
  - The afferent pupillary pathway and midbrain connections 265
- ▶ AFFERENT DISORDERS: THE RELATIVE AFFERENT PUPILLARY DEFECT 266
- ▶ MIDBRAIN DISORDERS AFFECTING THE PUPILS 267
  - Light-near dissociation 267
  - Midbrain relative afferent pupillary defects 267
- ▶ THE PUPIL AND EFFERENT DISORDERS OF THE VISUAL SYSTEM 268
  - Pupil states without anisocoria 268
  - Anisocoria 268
  - The iris and local factors 269
  - Oculosympathetic paresis (Horner syndrome) 269
  - Parasympathetic disorders of the pupil: oculomotor nerve 277
  - Parasympathetic disorders of the pupil: tonic pupil 278
  - The pharmacologically dilated pupil 281
  - Transient pupillary dilation 281
  - Clinical evaluation of anisocoria: overview 283
- ▶ KEY POINTS 284

The pupils constrict relative to the amount of light perceived by the eye; therefore, the pupil can be used as a measure of *afferent* visual function. This principle is the basis of the relative afferent pupillary defect (RAPD) test. When the pupillary *efferent* system is normal, the pupils in the right and left eye are clinically the same size as each other, even though their size is constantly changing in response to ambient light and accommodative tone, and to other factors such as mood and state of alertness.

Pupil size is ultimately determined by the balance of *efferent* sympathetic and parasympathetic flow to the pupil musculature. Disorders involving these autonomic systems can cause an asymmetry in pupil size (anisocoria). The pupil, therefore, is particularly important in neuroophthalmology because it is affected in both afferent and efferent disorders of the visual system.

▶ ANATOMY AND OVERVIEW OF PATHOPHYSIOLOGY

Pupillary signs in neuro-ophthalmic disorders can be mastered by understanding the afferent and efferent systems that control the pupil. The neuroanatomic discussion begins with the iris and efferent pupillary systems followed by discussion of the pupillary light reflex and midbrain connections. Disease processes are briefly mentioned at pertinent points in the initial discussion of the neuroanatomy, but will be addressed in detail in the remainder of the chapter.

THE IRIS

The iris stroma readily contracts and expands in response to the forces generated by the intrinsic iris musculature (Figure 11–1). The *pupillary constrictor muscle* (iris sphincter) consists of a band of muscle fiber bundles encircling the pupillary aperture. Activation causes the diameter of the sphincter (and the pupil) to constrict (miosis). The muscle fiber bundles of the sphincter are segmentally innervated by parasympathetic autonomic nerves that travel from the midbrain to the orbit as part of the third cranial nerve (CN III).

The *dilator muscle* fiber bundles are radially oriented. The muscle fibers are anchored at the iris root and stretch centrally toward the papillary aperture. Constriction of these muscle fibers causes the iris to retract toward the iris root, dilating the pupil (mydriasis). The

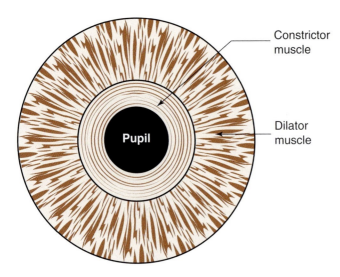

Figure 11-1. Location and orientation of iris musculature.
The parasympathetically innervated pupillary constrictor muscle runs circumferentially around the pupillary aperture at the pupillary margin. The pupillary dilator muscle is sympathetically innervated and consists of radially oriented muscle fibers.

dilator muscle of the iris is segmentally innervated by sympathetic autonomic nerves.

Similar to most opposing muscle systems in the body, there is dynamic sympathetic and parasympathetic pupillary tone at all times. The balance of the two efferent systems determines the pupil size at any given moment. However, the iris sphincter muscle is much stronger than the dilator muscle, so the parasympathetic innervation of the pupil plays the dominant role in controlling pupil size.

SYMPATHETIC INNERVATION OF THE PUPIL

The oculosympathetic chain begins with *first-order neurons* located in the posterolateral hypothalamus, with axons that descend through the brainstem and into the intermediolateral cell column of the spinal cord. These axons synapse at the *ciliospinal center (of Budge)* located at the C8 to T2 level in the spinal cord (Figure 11-2). Axons from these *second-order (preganglionic) neurons* then exit the spinal column primarily at the T1 level in the chest cavity, arch over the apex of the lung, and travel under the subclavian artery (ansa subclavia) to ascend with the cervical sympathetic plexus associated with the carotid arteries. These second-order axons pass through the stellate ganglion and ascend to synapse in the superior cervical ganglion located at the carotid bifurcation, at the level of C3/C4 and the angle of the jaw. From the superior cervical ganglion, most *third-order (post-ganglionic) axons* travel with the internal carotid artery through the cavernous sinus and eventually to the eye, with the remainder following the external carotid to supply vasomotor and sudomotor (sweat gland) innervation to the face. Therefore, asymmetric facial flushing and sweating are important accompanying clinical signs with localizing value.

Sympathetic nerves bound for the eye travel as a plexus surrounding the internal carotid artery. When the third-order axons reach the cavernous sinus they condense, briefly traveling with the sixth cranial nerve (CN VI) before entering the orbit through the superior orbital fissure with the nasociliary branch of the ophthalmic division of the trigeminal nerve.

The sympathetic fibers enter the eye via the long ciliary nerves, which pierce the sclera and travel in the suprachoroidal space to innervate individual segments of the radially oriented dilator muscle. Sympathetic nerves in the orbit also travel to the upper and lower eyelids. In the upper eyelid, a small sympathetically innervated accessory muscle called *Müller muscle* provides 1 to 2 mm of lift to the upper eyelid. A similar but more rudimentary muscle is also found in the lower eyelid.

An oculosympathetic palsy, therefore, causes the affected pupil to be smaller (miotic) than the unaffected pupil because the parasympathetic tone to the constrictor is unopposed, and also causes an ipsilateral ptosis of the upper eyelid of 1 to 2 mm. In some patients, a slight elevation of the lower eyelid is also present, further narrowing the palpebral fissure (which contributes to the impression of enophthalmos, without being truly present).

The clinical implications of the long circuitous route of the oculosympathetic chain should be evident: Diseases in the spinal cord, chest, and neck (remote from the eye) can present with a purely ocular sign—Horner syndrome.

PARASYMPATHETIC INNERVATION OF THE PUPIL

The pupillary constrictor muscle is innervated by the parasympathetic component of CN III. Parasympathetic pupillomotor fibers originate from the midline but paired Edinger-Westphal nuclei, which occupy the most dorsal position in the CN III nuclear complex. Fascicles from this parasympathetic motor nucleus join other fascicles from the CN III nuclear complex and traverse the midbrain tegmentum, exiting the brainstem at the interpeduncular cistern to form CN III. As described in Chapter 9, this nerve has a short but

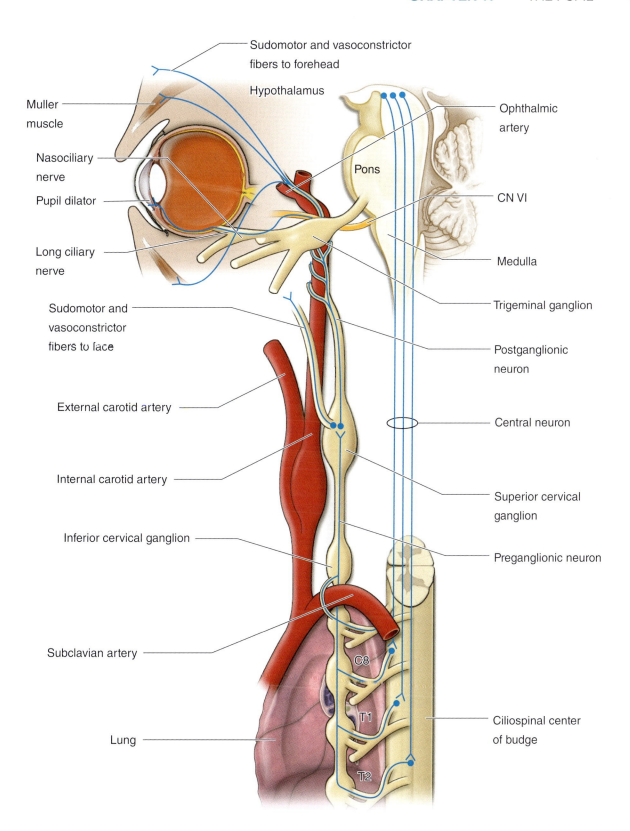

Figure 11–2. **Oculosympathetic pathway.**
The origin and course of first-order (central), second-order (preganglionic), and third-order (postganglionic) components of the oculosympathetic pathway are diagrammed. (Modified with permission from Weinstein JM. The pupil. In Slamovits TL, Burde R, associate editors. Neuro-ophthalmology, vol 6. In Podos SM, Yanoff M, editors: Textbook of ophthalmology. St Louis, 1991, Mosby.)

eventful course in the subarachnoid space, passing between the superior cerebellar and posterior cerebral arteries to travel both adjacent and parallel to the posterior communicating artery (see Figure 9–11B). The pupillary fibers occupy a superficial position in the nerve and are more vulnerable to external compression of CN III (eg, aneurysm or uncal herniation). CN III traverses the cavernous sinus, entering the orbit through the superior orbital fissure where the nerve bifurcates. The parasympathetic pupillary axons travel in the inferior division of the oculomotor nerve, along with fibers innervating the inferior oblique muscle. As the inferior division courses along the lateral border of the inferior rectus, the parasympathetic fibers exit midway as the *motor root of the ciliary ganglion*, to synapse in the ciliary ganglion (Figure 11–3). The motor root is short because the ciliary ganglion lies close to the inferior division of CN III and adjacent to the inferior rectus muscle. The ciliary ganglion is the origin of axons that enter the posterior aspect of the globe as *the short posterior ciliary nerves*, traveling in the suprachoroidal space to innervate both the pupillary sphincter (for pupillary constriction) and the ciliary muscle within the ciliary body (for accommodation). Many more postganglionic axons innervate the ciliary muscle than the pupillary sphincter (ratio of 30:1); this fact is important in the discussion of Adie tonic pupil later in this chapter.

Interruption of the parasympathetic pupillary pathway produces a paresis of pupillary constriction and hence a dilated pupil. As discussed in Chapter 9, a dilated pupil is a very important clinical sign when it

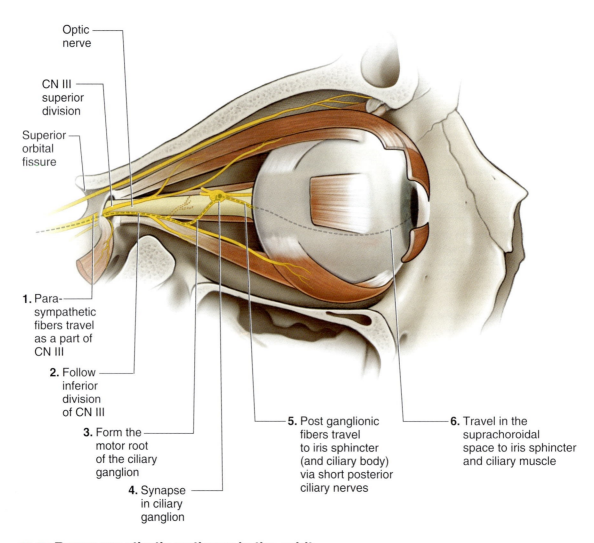

Figure 11-3. **Parasympathetic pathway in the orbit.**
Parasympathetic fibers travel as part of cranial nerve III, inferior division, synapsing in the ciliary ganglion. From the ciliary ganglion, postganglionic fibers enter the eye as short posterior ciliary nerves, traveling in the suprachoroidal space to innervate the iris sphincter.

accompanies the motility disturbances produced by a CN III palsy.

THE AFFERENT PUPILLARY PATHWAY AND MIDBRAIN CONNECTIONS

The response of the photoreceptors to a light stimulus is processed in the retina and conveyed to the brain by the retinal ganglion cell axons. There is a specialized subset of retinal ganglion cells that send their output directly to the pupillary centers in the midbrain. Evidence suggests these pupillomotor ganglion cells are melanopsin-containing, and have some intrinsic ability to respond to light on their own, in addition to input from the photoreceptors. Axons from these specialized ganglion cells travel along with axons carrying visual information in the optic nerve, chiasm, and optic tract. Similar to the axons subserving vision, the pupillary fibers undergo a slightly uneven hemidecussation in the chiasm, with a few more fibers crossing (from each nasal hemiretina) than those remaining ipsilateral (from each temporal hemiretina). This asymmetry of pupillary input is the reason that an optic tract lesion can cause a contralateral RAPD: A tract lesion disrupts input from the ipsilateral temporal hemiretina but also from the more powerful contralateral nasal hemiretina. Thus, an RAPD is present in the contralateral eye (the eye with the temporal visual field defect). Pupillary axons leave the optic tract before it terminates at the lateral geniculate nucleus (LGN), exiting via the brachium of the superior colliculus to synapse in the midbrain pretectal olivary nucleus. The pretectal olivary nuclei provide input to the parasympathetic motor nuclei (the Edinger-Westphal nuclei) (Figure 11–4).

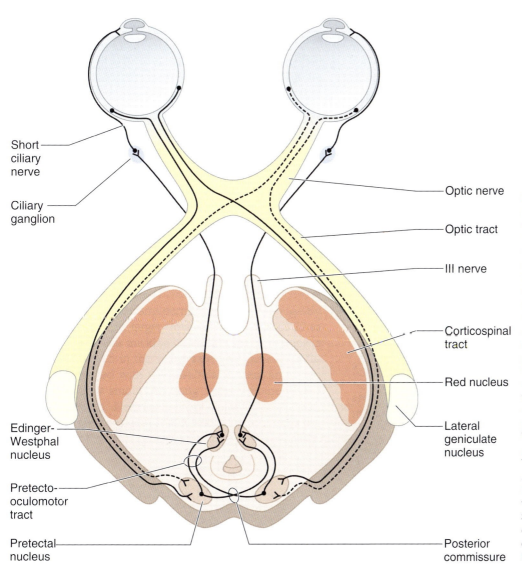

Figure 11-4. **The pupillary light reflex.** The pupillary light reflex consists of the afferent limb from the retina to the midbrain pretectal nuclei and midbrain interconnections, with parasympathetic innervation of the pupillary sphincter (via the oculomotor nerve) serving as the efferent limb. (Reproduced with permission from Weinstein JM. The pupil. In Slamovits TL, Burde R, associate editors. Neuro-ophthalmology, vol 6. In Podos SM, Yanoff M, editors: Textbook of ophthalmology. St Louis, 1991, Mosby.)

Each Edinger-Westphal nucleus receives innervation from both the contralateral and ipsilateral pretectal nuclei. Input from the contralateral pretectal nucleus decussates at the posterior commissure. Thus, the pupillary light reflex undergoes a *double hemidecussation*—fibers from the right and left eyes undergo a hemidecussation at the chiasm, and fibers from each pretectal nucleus hemidecussate in the midbrain—ensuring a fairly equal distribution of light stimulation to each of the Edinger-Westphal nuclei regardless of the eye of origin. Consequently, in the normal state, the right and left pupils are essentially the same size, moving equally in concert with each other regardless of any difference in light input to each eye. *Therefore, visual loss in an eye (or any other afferent visual disorder) does not cause a difference in pupil size.* Anisocoria is always the result of uneven efferent (motor) innervation of the pupil. The other clinical implication of the double hemidecussation of the pupillary light reflex pathway is that light shone in one eye alone will cause equal constriction of both the ipsilateral pupil (the direct pupillary response) and the contralateral pupil (the consensual pupillary response).

The afferent pupillary pathway provides input to the Edinger-Westphal nuclei, which in turn (via the parasympathetic portion of the oculomotor nerve) drives the pupillary sphincter. This circuit constitutes *the pupillary light reflex*, in which the pupils constrict (in concert) with an amplitude that is proportional to the amount of light perceived by the afferent limb of the light reflex (see Figure 11–4).

▶ AFFERENT DISORDERS: THE RELATIVE AFFERENT PUPILLARY DEFECT

The pupillary light reflex is the basis of the RAPD test: A light stimulus is alternated between the two eyes, and the pupillary response serves as a "light meter" to compare the light sensitivity of each eye. Details for performing the RAPD test are given in Figures 2–26 and 2–27.

As discussed in Chapter 2, the RAPD test is a powerful, *objective* clinical test. Unlike most tests of afferent visual function, the patient is not required to consciously respond during RAPD testing, and only a minimal degree of cooperation is required.

One would anticipate finding an RAPD in any disorder that causes a significant *difference* in visual function between the eyes, essentially any unilateral or asymmetric bilateral disorder of the optic nerve or retina. Comparing the relative difference in visual field defects between the eyes is the best predictor of the presence and magnitude of an RAPD. However, optic nerve disorders tend to produce RAPDs of relatively greater magnitude than retinal disorders.

Disorders of the ocular media (corneal scars, cataract, and vitreous hemorrhage) usually do not cause an RAPD despite poor vision, because the scattered light still reaches the retina and participates in the light reflex. In fact, a unilateral cataract distributes the stimulus light more effectively than a clear lens, producing a small apparent RAPD (usually <0.6 log unit [LU]) in the eye without cataract (Table 11–1).

▶ **TABLE 11–1. CONDITIONS OTHER THAN AFFERENT VISUAL LOSS THAT CAN CAUSE A RELATIVE AFFERENT PUPILLARY DEFECT**

Condition	Observation	Explanation
Cataract in one eye, clear media in the other	Small (0.6 LU) RAPD in the eye opposite the cataract	Cataract scatters the light and illuminates more of the retina than the eye with clear media.
Ptotic eyelid or patched eye	Transient RAPD in the uncovered eye; will recover after both eyes equilibrate to the same light exposure	Retinal sensitivity is increased in a light-deprived eye.
Unilateral exposure to a bright light	Transient RAPD in the dazzled eye; will recover after both eyes equilibrate to the same light exposure	A bright light will temporarily bleach the photoreceptors, reducing sensitivity.
Marked anisocoria	Small RAPD in the eye with the larger pupil	The eye with the smaller pupil is relatively light deprived (develops greater sensitivity).
Midbrain or brachium of superior colliculus lesion	RAPD in the eye opposite the lesion	Asymmetric disruption of midbrain input from the right and left eyes.

Abbreviations: LU, log unit; RAPD, relative afferent pupillary defect.

Visual field loss from disorders of the chiasm may produce a RAPD when the visual field defects are asymmetric. Optic tract lesions may produce a small RAPD in the eye with the temporal visual field loss because the nasal retina provides greater pupillary input than the temporal hemiretina. One would not anticipate a RAPD in LGN or retrogeniculate disorders because they do not participate in the pupillary reflex arc. Why developmental amblyopia occasionally produces a small RAPD is unclear because amblyopia is considered to be of cortical origin.

▶ MIDBRAIN DISORDERS AFFECTING THE PUPILS

LIGHT-NEAR DISSOCIATION

In addition to the pupillary light reflex afferents, the Edinger-Westphal nuclei receive input from other midbrain nuclei that coordinate the near synkinetic reflex triad of convergence, accommodation, and miosis. Accommodation and miosis are mediated by the Edinger-Westphal nucleus, which innervates both the iris sphincter (miosis) and the ciliary muscle (accommodation) via the ciliary ganglion. The third function, convergence, is mediated by the medial rectus subnucleus.

Midbrain lesions in the region of the posterior commissure can disrupt the dorsally located pupillary light pathway by affecting the pretectal nuclei and their communication with the Edinger-Westphal nuclei, without disturbing the more ventral near-reflex fibers as they travel to the Edinger-Westphal nuclei. These disorders result in a bilateral light-near dissociation, in which the pupillary constriction to light is poor or absent, but the pupil still constricts normally to a near stimulus (Box 11–1). Examples of this condition include the dorsal midbrain syndrome and Argyll Robertson pupils. In the dorsal midbrain syndrome, the pupils are mid-dilated, and the associated findings are invariably present (see Table 10–1). Argyll Robertson pupils are small and irregular, and are a manifestation of neurosyphilis. Given the variable manifestations of neurosyphilis, testing for syphilis should be performed whenever a light-near dissociation is present. Diabetes, chronic alcoholism, encephalitis, and extensive panretinal photocoagulation can also produce Argyll Robertson–like pupils.

Blindness is another cause of a light-near dissociation, resulting in poor pupillary response to light but pupillary constriction when attempting to look at a near object (eg, the patient's own finger). Other causes of light-near dissociation are the result of aberrant regeneration: Adie tonic pupil and aberrant regeneration of the oculomotor nerve, discussed in a later section (Table 11–2).

MIDBRAIN RELATIVE AFFERENT PUPILLARY DEFECTS

Rarely, unilateral or asymmetric midbrain lesions that interfere with the pupillary axons after they leave the optic tract, the pretectal nuclei, or the interconnections between the pretectal nuclei and the Edinger-Westphal nuclei can cause an apparent RAPD. This RAPD can occur in the absence of any visual field defect or other evidence of afferent visual loss (see Table 11–1). Similar to tract lesions, the RAPD is usually on the side opposite the midbrain lesion. Other signs of dorsal midbrain

---

> ▶ **BOX 11–1. HOW TO LOOK FOR A LIGHT-NEAR DISSOCIATION**
>
> 1. The pupil's response to light is best tested by having the patient look at a distant target with both eyes open, first in dim lighting, then with bright light. If the patient is noted to have a poor pupillary response to light in one or both eyes, the pupil response to a near stimulus should be observed. A light-near dissociation may be unilateral or bilateral.
>
> 2. To gauge the pupil response to near, the patient is asked to focus on a visual target (with both eyes) at reading distance. The goal is to have the patient invoke the near synkinetic reflex triad of accommodation, convergence, and miosis. Therefore, it is best if an accommodative stimulus is used, such as text, or a picture, or toy for younger patients.
>
> 3. A proprioceptive stimulus, such as having a patient look at his or her own thumb, may be needed for the patient with poor vision.
>
> 4. The patient who generates a greater degree of miosis with near focus than with a bright light is said to have a light-near dissociation.
>
> 5. Getting the patient to generate an adequate near focus is entirely effort dependent: It may require a great deal of encouragement and several attempts. Thus, a poor near pupillary response may only mean poor patient effort.
>
> 6. If the pupils respond normally to light, there is no need to test pupillary reaction to a near stimulus.

TABLE 11-2. CAUSES OF A LIGHT-NEAR DISSOCIATION OF THE PUPIL

Disorder	Pupil Appearance	Associated Signs and Symptoms	Pathophysiology
Blindness (de-afferented pupil)	Bilateral normal-sized to large, no anisocoria	Poor vision, RAPD if asymmetric	Poor afferent visual input to midbrain nuclei, intact near-response input.
Dorsal midbrain lesion	Bilateral mid-dilated to large, anisocoria possible	Other components of dorsal midbrain syndrome	Afferent pupillary input to E-W nucleus (dorsal) interrupted in midbrain; near response input to E-W (ventral) is spared.
Argyll Robertson pupils	Bilateral small, irregularly shaped	Signs and symptoms of neurosyphilis	Afferent pupillary input to E-W nucleus interrupted (as above) by neurosyphilis (rarely MS, sarcoidosis).
Tonic (Adie pupil)	Anisocoria with affected pupil larger than unaffected (over time the pupil can become small)	Blurred vision from accommodative abnormalities; hyporeflexia in some patients	Aberrant regeneration from ciliary ganglion. Accommodative fibers reinnervate iris sphincter.
Aberrant regeneration of CN III	Anisocoria, affected pupil can be smaller or larger	Other signs of CN III dysfunction, aberrant regeneration of the eyelid common	Aberrant regeneration of peripheral CN III. Medial rectus fibers reinnervate pupillary sphincter (via the ciliary ganglion), activated with convergence (or horizontal gaze).
Autonomic neuropathy	Irregularly shaped pupils	Other evidence of autonomic neuropathy	Diabetes, retinal photocoagulation (affecting the neurovascular bundle travelling in the suprachoroidal space).

Abbreviations: CN, cranial nerve; E-W, Edinger-Westphal nucleus; MS, multiple sclerosis; RAPD, relative afferent pupillary defect.

involvement are typically present, such as vertical gaze disturbance.

THE PUPIL AND EFFERENT DISORDERS OF THE VISUAL SYSTEM

PUPIL STATES WITHOUT ANISOCORIA

Normal pupil size can vary over a broad range: The pupils are large when subjects are frightened or anxious (sympathetic effect), and can become quite small with near tasks such as reading (parasympathetic component of the near synkinetic triad). The average pupil size tends to become smaller with age. Abnormally small (miotic) pupils can occur with pontine hemorrhage and opiate intoxication. Pilocarpine eyedrops for glaucoma cause a marked miosis, but this medication is now only rarely used as treatment for chronic glaucoma. Bilaterally large pupils can occur from topical or systemic drugs with anticholinergic properties such as atropine or tricyclic antidepressants.

ANISOCORIA

A difference in the pupil sizes of the eyes is called anisocoria. As previously discussed, clinically significant anisocoria is always caused by an efferent (motor) disorder, not by a difference in vision between the eyes. The examiner's task in the patient with anisocoria is to determine if the pupillary inequality is clinically significant, to discover which pupil (or both) is abnormal, to derive a differential diagnosis, and to plan an appropriate evaluation.

When the pupils are different sizes, the larger pupil may be abnormal or the smaller pupil may be abnormal. When the larger pupil is abnormal (does not constrict well), the anisocoria is greatest in bright light. When the smaller pupil is abnormal (does not dilate well), the anisocoria is greatest in darkness (Figure 11–5).

CHAPTER 11   THE PUPIL   269

and may even switch sides. This condition can be distinguished from pathological states because the degree of anisocoria remains relatively constant in light and dark (see Figure 11–5D).

THE IRIS AND LOCAL FACTORS

Any disorder that physically damages the mechanical compliance of the iris or the iris musculature can result in a pupil abnormality. Eye trauma can cause visible tears in the pupillary margin and constrictor muscle. Such pupils constrict poorly or irregularly. Intraocular inflammation (uveitis) can cause a relative miosis or can cause adhesions of the iris to the lens or cornea (synechiae), creating abnormally shaped pupils or an iris that is immobile. Neovascularization of the iris in diabetic eye disease or in ocular ischemic disorders also can cause a "stiff" pupil. Acute glaucoma can cause irreversible ischemic damage to the iris musculature, often causing focal atrophy of the pupillary constrictor, resulting in spiraling of the radially oriented iris elements seen with the slitlamp. The chronic use of topical miotic medications (used in the treatment of glaucoma) can permanently affect the pupil's ability to dilate. Iris malformations and iris atrophy from any cause can also affect the pupil's size and function. Cataract surgery (and other intraocular procedures) commonly affects pupil size and function.

Events that could potentially cause iris damage and anisocoria should be sought in the history and may be evident on examination. The ophthalmologist may be in a position to avert an extensive neurological evaluation by identifying iris structural abnormalities as the cause of anisocoria.

OCULOSYMPATHETIC PARESIS (HORNER SYNDROME)

A pupil that does not dilate well (one that is too small) may be the result of an interruption of the sympathetic innervation of the pupillary sphincter—a Horner syndrome. Although the signs and symptoms of Horner syndrome may seem unimpressive, this condition may be the first manifestation of life-threatening disease.

Signs and Symptoms

The classic triad of signs described by Friedrich Horner in 1869 include (1) miosis, (2) ptosis and, (3) facial anhidrosis. Many patients with an oculosympathetic paresis do not have anhidrosis (unilateral lack of facial sweating), but the term *Horner syndrome* has come to be synonymous with oculosympathetic paresis even when this component of the classic triad is not present. Additional signs that can occur acutely include conjunctival injection and a transient relative hypotony.

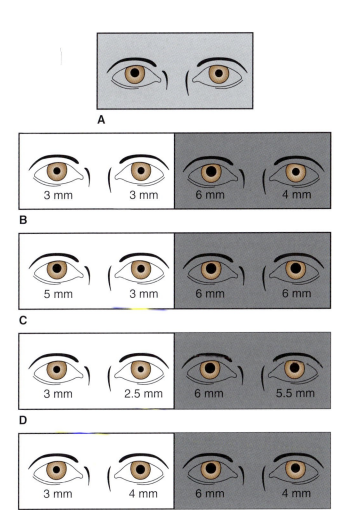

Figure 11–5. **Determining the abnormal pupil.** Observing an anisocoria in darkness and in bright light can determine which pupil is abnormal. **(A)** In this illustration, an anisocoria is observed in room light with the right pupil larger than the left. **(B)** If the smaller (left) pupil is the abnormal one, both pupils will constrict well in bright light. In darkness, the left pupil will not dilate well, maximizing the anisocoria. **(C)** If the larger (right) pupil is the abnormal one, both pupils will dilate well in darkness. In bright light, the anisocoria is maximized by the right pupil's failure to constrict. **(D)** In an *essential anisocoria*, a small amount of anisocoria is present in both dark and light, and an abnormal pupil cannot clearly be determined. **(E)** A pupil that will not dilate or constrict is usually obvious. The anisocoria can be made to reverse, depending on the lighting conditions.

Essential, or physiological, anisocoria is a difference in pupillary size (generally <0.5 mm) that may be present in normal individuals. A pupil difference of 0.3 mm is clinically noticeable, and 20% of the normal population may have at least this amount of anisocoria at any given time. In essential anisocoria, the pupillary inequality changes from day to day

Miosis Because some sympathetic and parasympathetic tone is present virtually at all times, interruption of the oculosympathetic pathway results in a smaller pupil on the affected side because the parasympathetic tone to the constrictor is unopposed. The resultant anisocoria is most evident by observing the pupils as they are *in the process of dilating* in darkness. Because innervation to the pupillary sphincter is unaffected in an oculosympathetic paresis, little or no anisocoria is apparent in bright light. In darkness, the pupil with normal sympathetic innervation dilates quickly because the dilator muscles are activated and the pupillary sphincter is inactivated. The eye with the oculosympathetic paresis *will dilate*, but more slowly. Dilation occurs because the passive structural forces of the iris pull the pupil open even without the help of the dilator muscle when parasympathetic tone to the constrictor muscle is turned off. The anisocoria is greatest after approximately 5 seconds in darkness, when the normal pupil is about as large as it will become and the affected pupil is just beginning to dilate. After this time, the anisocoria slowly diminishes as the sympathetically denervated pupil continues to slowly dilate, approaching the size of the maximally dilated normal pupil. This *dilation lag* is characteristic and virtually diagnostic of an oculosympathetic paresis (Figure 11–6).

Ptosis An upper eyelid ptosis, limited to 1 or 2 mm, results from paresis of Müller muscle. Most of the lift to the upper eyelid is supplied by the levator palpebrae with innervation by CN III; therefore, a ptosis greater than 1 to 2 mm cannot be the sole result of an oculosympathetic paresis. In some patients, the lower eyelid may be slightly elevated (an *upside-down ptosis*) from paresis of a rudimentary sympathetically innervated lower eyelid analog of Müller muscle.

Sudomotor and vasomotor deficiency Patients who have interruption of the sympathetic pathway at the level of the superior cervical ganglion (or more proximally) may also interrupt vasomotor and sudomotor innervation to the face, resulting in unilateral facial anhidrosis. Because sudomotor innervation to the forehead travels with postganglionic fibers, anhidrosis isolated to this area can occur with postganglionic lesions (see Figure 11–2). In an ideal setting, beads of perspiration may be observed to be confined to the unaffected side of the face. But in the temperature-controlled environment of the clinic or hospital, the presence of anhidrosis is usually not readily evident. Women may note a difference between the two sides of the face in these areas when they apply makeup.

Rarely, a difference in facial flushing between the right and left sides of the face is noted as a consequence of interruption of unilateral sympathetic vasomotor innervation to the face. The condition sometimes manifests

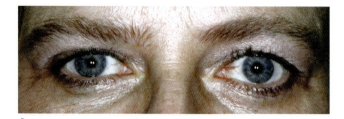
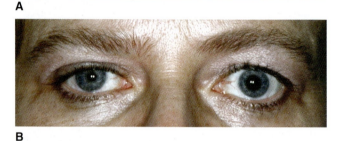
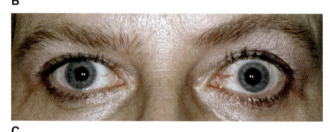

Figure 11–6. Dilation lag in Horner syndrome. A 46-year-old woman with periodic headache presented with drooping of the right upper eyelid. The history suggested cluster headache, and the examination confirmed the presence of a right Horner syndrome. **(A)** A 1-mm upper eyelid ptosis and miotic pupil is evident in the right eye. Also observe the "upside-down ptosis": the lower eyelid is higher (relative to the corneal limbus) in the right eye than the left eye. **(B)** After 5 seconds in darkness the anisocoria is maximized because the normal pupil is almost fully dilated and the affected pupil is slow to dilate. **(C)** After 15 seconds in darkness the anisocoria is less because the affected pupil continues to gradually dilate.

as a lack of hemifacial blushing. In other patients, vasomotor instability may cause the affected side only to appear flushed at times. The *harlequin baby syndrome* is hemifacial flushing that strikingly respects the vertical midline in infants with a sympathetic paresis.

Causes of Oculosympathetic Paresis

Given the long, circuitous course of the oculosympathetic chain, a variety of lesions at many diverse anatomic locations can cause an oculosympathetic paresis.

First-order neuron First-order neurons (or *central neurons*) are affected by lesions of the brainstem and cervical or upper thoracic spinal cord. In these patients,

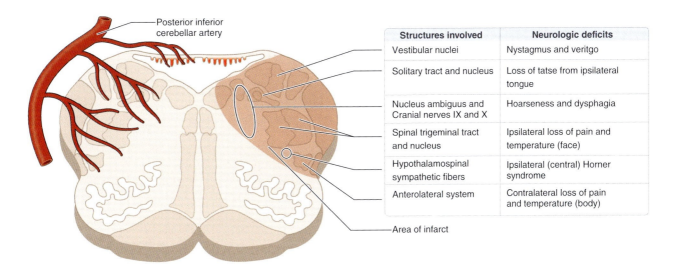

Figure 11-7. Wallenberg syndrome.
Illustration of a cross section of the medulla showing the structures affected in Wallenberg syndrome (lateral medullary syndrome) and the resultant clinical manifestations. The distribution of the posterior inferior cerebellar artery is shown (*left*), and for clarity the area of infarction is shown on the opposite side (*right*). (Modified with permission from Haines, Duane E., and M. D. Ard. *Fundamental neuroscience for basic and clinical applications.* Philadelphia, PA: Elsevier/Saunders, 2013.)

a Horner syndrome is often incidentally noted among other more evident neurological signs and symptoms. *Wallenberg lateral medullary syndrome* is the result of infarction of the lateral medulla, typically from occlusion of the vertebral or posterior inferior cerebellar artery. A central oculosympathetic paresis occurs from involvement of the descending (first-order) sympathetic fibers (Figure 11-7). Spinal cord trauma or tumors affecting the first-order sympathetic pathway generally show associated long-tract signs (Table 11-3).

Second-order neuron The second-order component of the sympathetic chain is also called *preganglionic* because it is proximal to the terminal neurons originating in the superior cervical ganglion. The classic second-order neuron lesion is the *Pancoast tumor*, which is an apical lung tumor presenting as a unilateral Horner syndrome (see Figure 11-9A). Compression of the brachial plexus is usually also present, causing arm or hand pain. Other paraxial tumors, such as neuroblastoma in children, can present with metastases to the

▶ **TABLE 11-3. ANATOMONIC LOCATION AND PATHOLOGICAL PROCESSES IN HORNER SYNDROME**

	Anatomic Location	Disease Process
First order	Hypothalamus, mesencephalon, pons	Tumor, hemorrhage, infarction
	Medulla	Lateral medullary stroke (Wallenberg syndrome)
	Spinal cord	MS, syringomyelia, trauma, infarction, tumor
Second order	Thoracic cavity	Pancoast tumor, metastases, mediastinal mass, chest surgery, thoracic aortic aneurysms, central vascular access
	Neck	Trauma, abscess, lymphadenopathy, thyroid neoplasm, thyroidectomy, radical neck surgery, central vascular access
Third order	Carotid artery plexus, superior cervical ganglion	Carotid artery dissection or thrombosis, trauma (including intraoral)
	Cavernous sinus, superior orbital fissure, orbit	Carotid-cavernous fistula, nasopharyngeal carcinoma
	Other or unknown	Cluster headache, microvascular ischemia, giant cell arteritis, autonomic neuropathies

Abbreviation: MS, multiple sclerosis.

sympathetic system in the neck or thorax. Trauma to the neck or chest is a common cause of preganglionic oculosympathetic paresis. About 25% of the time, a preganglionic oculosympathetic paresis is due to a malignancy (see Table 11–3).

Third-order neuron Lesions affecting the third-order, or *postganglionic*, oculosympathetic axons arise in the neck, skull base, cavernous sinus, or orbit. *Carotid artery dissection* occurs when intimal tears allow blood to dissect into the arterial wall, narrowing the lumen and occluding arterial branches. Acute pain in the neck, throat, face (eye, ear, teeth), or head is characteristic and may migrate from one area to another. The sympathetic nerves form a rete around the circumference of the carotid artery and may be damaged by the rapid expansion of the arterial diameter or by ischemia, owing to loss of nutrient vessels damaged by the dissection. In proximal common carotid artery dissection, a preganglionic oculosympathetic paresis may result. Dissection in the internal carotid system produces a postganglionic Horner syndrome.

Cluster headaches frequently cause transient postganglionic Horner syndrome associated with bouts of excruciating hemicranial headache (discussed further in Chapter 13). With repeated attacks, the oculosympathetic paresis may become permanent (see Figure 11–6).

Tumors of the skull base causing an oculosympathetic paresis frequently involve the trigeminal ganglion, causing associated chronic facial pain and hypesthesia in the distribution of the trigeminal nerve. Tumors or aneurysms in the cavernous sinus inevitably cause other cranial nerve dysfunction (especially CN VI). The combination of a CN III paresis and a Horner syndrome produces a middilated pupil that does not constrict well in bright light or dilate well in darkness.

Horner syndrome in children Sympathetic tone is important in the development of iris melanocytes, which determine iris color. Patients with an oculosympathetic paresis in the perinatal period or early childhood may have a lighter-colored iris on the affected side. Horner syndrome present at birth is usually idiopathic, but less often it may be associated with a brachial plexus injury from birth trauma, and rarely it can be caused by an intrauterine neuroblastoma. An *acquired* oculosympathetic paresis in a young child suggests a neuroblastoma involving the sympathetic chain or other mediastinal malignancy until proven otherwise.

Differential Diagnosis

Pseudo-Horner syndrome occurs when other causes of ptosis and anisocoria mimic an oculosympathetic paresis. For example, the combination of an essential anisocoria and a ptosis from any cause may look similar to an oculosympathetic paresis. The examination and history may reveal a non-neurological explanation for the ptosis (such as levator dehiscence or a history of trauma) or miosis (essential anisocoria, history of ocular surgery, trauma, or uveitis). A ptosis greater than 2 mm (and certainly a ptotic eyelid that covers the visual axis) cannot be fully explained by an oculosympathetic palsy. The pupil examination and pharmacologic tests (described below) should effectively differentiate between an oculosympathetic paresis and other causes of a small pupil (Table 11–4A).

Pharmacologic Testing

Not infrequently, the examiner can diagnose an oculosympathetic paresis with confidence on the basis of the history and examination. However, pharmacologic tests are helpful: (1) cocaine or apraclonidine testing evaluates whether an oculosympathetic paresis exists at all, and (2) hydroxyamphetamine (Paredrine) testing helps differentiate between preganglionic (or central) and postganglionic lesions.

Cocaine testing Norepinephrine is the neurotransmitter at the neuromuscular junction of the sympathetic

▶ **TABLE 11–4A. DIFFERENTIAL DIAGNOSIS OF ANISOCORIA WITH ABNORMALLY SMALL PUPIL**

Horner syndrome (oculosympathetic paresis): 1 to 2 mm ptosis virtually always present, occasionally facial anhidrosis identified

Iris damage: trauma, iritis, angle-closure glaucoma, eye surgery

Long-standing Adie pupil

Aberrant regeneration of CN III involving the pupil

Pharmacologic: glaucoma medications

Abbreviation: CN, cranial nerve.

▶ **TABLE 11–4B. DIFFERENTIAL DIAGNOSIS OF ANISOCORIA WITH ABNORMALLY LARGE PUPIL**

Third nerve (CN III) palsy: associated with ptosis and motility disturbance

Tonic (Adie) pupil

Pharmacologic: atropinic or adrenergic mydriasis

Iris damage: trauma, iritis, angle-closure glaucoma, eye surgery

Cocaine

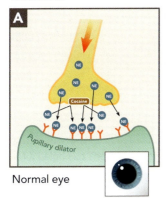
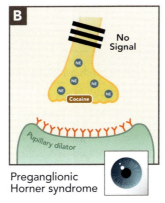
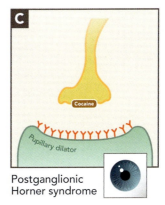

Figure 11-8. Cocaine test in Horner syndrome.
Cocaine blocks the normal reuptake of norepinephrine (NE), allowing NE to accumulate in the synaptic cleft, dilating a normal pupil **(A)**. In preganglionic Horner syndrome, little or no NE is released, so blocking the reuptake has no effect, and the pupil fails to dilate **(B)**. In postganglionic Horner syndrome, cocaine has no effect because the presynaptic terminal not functional **(C)**.

third-order neuron and the iris dilator muscle. In the normal state (when all three neurons are connected), norepinephrine is continuously released from the presynaptic terminal because of baseline sympathetic tone. The neurotransmitter is continuously degraded by reuptake by the presynaptic nerve terminal. Topical *cocaine* blocks this reuptake of norepinephrine, causing a rapid accumulation of the neurotransmitter in the synapse, which produces dilation of a normal pupil. If sympathetic tone is lacking and little or no norepinephrine is released, then cocaine is an ineffective dilator (Figure 11–8). *Thus, topical cocaine can be used to detect a deficiency of oculosympathetic tone caused by a defect at any point in the sympathetic chain.*

The test is performed by placing one 10% cocaine eyedrop in each eye. The cocaine eyedrops must be placed in both eyes because the normal eye serves as the control. After 45 minutes, the amount of dilation in each eye is assessed: If the affected eye fails to dilate as well as the normal eye (resulting in an anisocoria of at least 1 mm), then an oculosympathetic paresis is likely present (Figure 11–9). If both pupils dilate equally well, then an oculosympathetic paresis is unlikely. Because the same neurotransmitter is involved at the junction of the sympathetic nerves and Müller muscle, a slight reversal of the ptosis may be noted with cocaine eyedrops, but this finding is usually so subtle that it is not clinically useful.

Apraclonidine Apraclonidine is a direct α-adrenergic receptor agonist that is commercially available as a topical agent for lowering intraocular pressure. Its pressure-lowering effect is due to a strong affinity for α_2 receptors that downregulate production of aqueous by the ciliary body. Apraclonidine is also a weak α_1 agonist that has little or no effect on pupil size in the normal eye. However, apraclonidine will dilate the pupil in an eye with a Horner syndrome, due to upregulation of postjunctional adrenergic receptors in the sympathetic-denervated pupillary dilator muscles (Figure 11–10). This supersensitivity to apraclonidine has proven to be an excellent clinical test for Horner syndrome. Apraclonidine 0.5% instilled in both eyes will cause a reversal of the anisocoria in Horner syndrome, as the affected smaller pupil dilates from denervation supersensitivity, and the larger normal pupil is relatively unaffected. *The reversal of the anisocoria with apraclonidine is a much more distinct and convincing endpoint than the criteria for a positive cocaine test* (Figure. 11–11).

While there appear to be a number of practical advantages of apraclonidine over cocaine as a clinical test for Horner syndrome (Table 11–5), the sensitivity and specificity of apraclonidine for diagnosing Horner syndrome has not been fully determined, thus cocaine remains the gold standard at present. Also, unlike cocaine, apraclonidine is not helpful in the acute setting, as it may take weeks for upregulation of receptors (and subsequent supersensitivity to apraclonidine) to occur.

Hydroxyamphetamine Hydroxyamphetamine hydrobromide (Paredrine) acts by forcing the release of norepinephrine from presynaptic vesicles into the synaptic cleft at the neuromuscular junction. This action causes pupillary dilation independent of any neural signal as long as the third-order neuron is intact. If the third-order

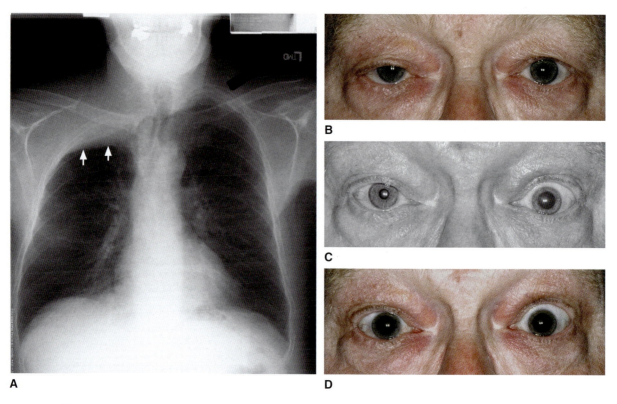

Figure 11-9. Pharmacologic testing of a patient with preganglionic Horner syndrome.
A 77-year-old man with small cell carcinoma in the right lung apex had right arm pain and a right Horner syndrome. **(A)** Chest radiograph shows a mass in the apex of the right lung (*arrows*). **(B)** Right ptosis and miosis. **(C)** After instillation of 10% cocaine, the affected pupil does not dilate as well as the normal pupil, confirming the presence of an oculosympathetic paresis. **(D)** After instillation of hydroxyamphetamine, the affected pupil dilates as well as the unaffected pupil, consistent with a preganglionic lesion.

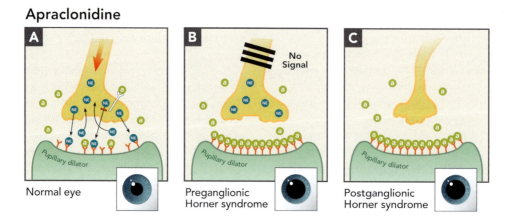

Figure 11-10. Apraclonidine test in Horner syndrome.
Apraclonidine (*a* in the illustration) is primarily an α_2 agonist that acts on the presynaptic bulb to decrease norepinephrine (NE) production, thus tending to weaken dilation of a normal pupil. Its weak postsynaptic α_1 action (which tends to dilate the pupil) is negligible in the normal state **(A)**. However, in Horner syndrome, the lack of sympathetic tone results in an upregulation of postsynaptic adrenergic receptors, resulting in a supersensitivity to apraclonidine for dilation of the pupil in both preganglionic **(B)** and postganglionic **(C)** Horner syndrome. Therefore, the affected pupil dilates and the normal pupil does not change much—reversing the anisocoria.

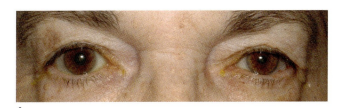
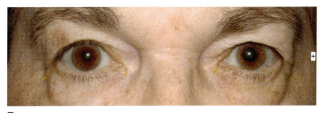

Figure 11-11. Apraclonidine testing of a patient with Horner syndrome.
(A) A 57-year-old man with a left Horner syndrome has a ptosis of the left upper eyelid (and lower eyelid) with a smaller left pupil and resultant anisocoria. **(B)** Apraclonidine 0.5% was instilled in each eye, and after 45 minutes the anisocoria is reversed—the Horner pupil has dilated, and the normal pupil is little changed (appears smaller in this patient). Also note reversal of the left ptosis.

neurons or their axons are damaged, the presynaptic bulb degenerates and no norepinephrine vesicles are available to respond to hydroxyamphetamine, and hence no dilation occurs with this agent (Figure 11–12).

For this test to be effective, sufficient time for axonal atrophy to occur is required. The test is generally considered accurate after the symptoms have been present for 3 to 4 weeks.

▶ **TABLE 11-5. APRACLONIDINE COMPARED WITH COCAINE AS A DIAGNOSTIC TEST FOR HORNER SYNDROME**

	Apraclonidine	**Cocaine**
Advantages of apraclonidine compared with cocaine	Commercially available as stable, multiuse, preserved eyedrops	Must be made in a compounding pharmacy; has a short shelf life, and is a controlled substance that must be kept under lock and key.
	No stigma	Patients may be reluctant to have an "illicit drug" put in their (or their child's) eye. Patients may test positive in urine drug screening for several days after a cocaine test.
	Currently available in most ophthalmology offices	Not widely available and is not an option in some healthcare settings.
	Positive (mydriatic) action in an affected eye	Lack of dilation to cocaine could be secondary to local iris factors (eg, iris neovascularization).
	Could potentially be diagnostic in bilateral cases	Requires a normal control pupil.
	Endpoint (reversal of anisocoria) clinically obvious and is the opposite situation from the starting point	Control pupil may not convincingly dilate. Endpoint (anisocoria or 1 mm present) is more subject to measurement error, is dependent on lighting conditions, and is not substantially different from the starting point.
Disadvantages of apraclonidine compared with cocaine	False negatives can occur in recently acquired Horner syndrome	Should work immediately, even in acute cases.
	Sensitivity and specificity yet to be determined	Gold standard in pharmacologic diagnosis of Horner syndrome; long track record.

Reproduced with permission from Martin TJ: Horner's syndrome, pseudo-Horner's syndrome, and simple anisocoria. *Curr Neurol Neurosci Reports* 2007; 7(5): 397–406. Table 2 on page 403.

Hydroxyamphetamine

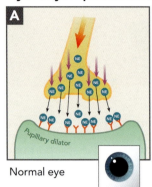
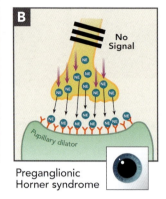
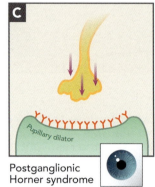

Figure 11–12. Hydroxyamphetamine test in Horner syndrome.
Hydroxyamphetamine forces the release of norepinephrine (NE) from presynaptic vesicles into the synaptic cleft independent of any neural signal **(A)**. This action will dilate a normal pupil or a pupil with a Horner syndrome, but only if the third-order neuron presynaptic bulb is intact. Therefore, hydroxyamphetamine will dilate the pupil in preganglionic **(B)**, *but not in postganglionic Horner syndrome* **(C)**.

Similar to cocaine testing, hydroxyamphetamine is placed in both eyes, with the unaffected eye serving as a control. The pupil in the normal eye dilates in response to the release of norepinephrine into the synaptic cleft. An eye with a central or preganglionic lesion also dilates because the third-order neuron is intact (see Figure 11–9D). Failure to dilate suggests a lesion involving the third-order neuron—from the superior cervical ganglion to the eye (see Figure 11–13).

A rational sequence of eyedrop testing to confirm and differentiate Horner syndrome would thus include (1) apraclonidine and/or cocaine testing to confirm the presence of an oculosympathetic paresis, and (2) if Horner syndrome is confirmed, hydroxyamphetamine testing is performed (no sooner than 48 hours) to localize the lesion. If the pupil in question does not dilate in any of the pharmacologic tests, it may be that the pupil is incapable of dilating from iris damage or other local factors. In this situation, performing a third pharmacologic test by placing 2.5% phenylephrine in each eye to see if the affected pupil is capable of dilating at all, is helpful (see Figure 11–18A). Obviously, local mechanical factors that prevent dilation invalidate the pharmacologic tests for Horner syndrome.

Small variations in the amount of apraclonidine, cocaine, or hydroxyamphetamine absorbed in each eye should not affect the tests because these drugs are given in doses that basically saturate the system. The effect of phenylephrine *does* depend on the amount of drug given in each eye. Care should be taken to distribute diagnostic eyedrops evenly between the eyes and to control factors that affect topical drug absorption. Thus, do not place other medications in the eye (such as topical anesthetics) or touch the cornea (with a tonometer or ocular sensory testing) before administering any of the test eyedrops (Box 11–2).

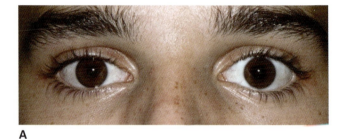

A

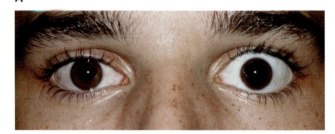

B

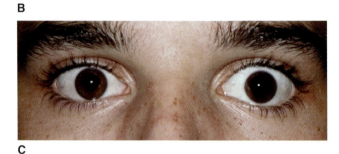

C

Figure 11–13. Pharmacologic testing of patient with postganglionic Horner syndrome.
A 27-year-old man with a history of closed head trauma had a long-standing right ptosis since his injury. **(A)** Right ptosis (observe both upper and lower eyelids) and miosis. **(B)** After instillation of 10% cocaine, the affected pupil does not dilate as well as the normal pupil. **(C)** After instillation of hydroxyamphetamine, the affected pupil again fails to dilate as well as the unaffected pupil, consistent with a postganglionic lesion.

▶ BOX 11–2. GENERAL PRINCIPLES IN PHARMACOLOGIC TESTING FOR HORNER SYNDROME

1. Concentration and availability of diagnostic agents
   a. Cocaine eyedrops are usually a 10% concentration. Lesser concentrations have been used but 10% has been the standard.
   b. Apraclonidine (Iopidine) has been studied in 1.0% and 0.5% concentrations and both concentrations appear to be effective. The 0.5% concentration is convenient, since this is the typical strength already available in the ophthalmologist's office.
   c. Hydroxyamphetamine was commercially available as a 1% solution but is no longer available. It may be obtained from compounding pharmacies.
2. Cocaine, hydroxyamphetamine, and apraclonidine work by saturating the receptors, so one does not have to precisely match the dose in each eye, as long as there is sufficient drug to permit saturation of the system. However, eyedrop testing should be performed before the cornea permeability is disturbed with other eyedrops or by applanation tonometry. Typically, one eyedrop is placed in the inferior conjunctival cul-de-sac of each eye, with a second eyedrop placed about 1 minute later. Systemic absorption can be minimized by having the patient keep both eyes closed for 2 to 3 minutes after instillation of diagnostic eyedrops.
3. Following placement of the eyedrops, one should wait approximately 45 minutes to evaluate the endpoint.
4. Pupil photography (especially 1:1 digital photos of both pupils in the same frame) is valuable for documentation before and after pharmacologic testing.
5. Wait at least 2 days (preferably longer) between eyedrop tests.

Evaluation and Management

An important factor in deciding how to evaluate a Horner syndrome depends on the length of time it has been present. An isolated postganglionic Horner syndrome that has been present for greater than 1 year may not need further evaluation. Sometimes patients are uncertain about the duration of their symptoms, particularly if their ptosis and anisocoria were noted during a routine examination. One very effective method of gauging how long an oculosympathetic paresis has been present is to look at old photographs (see Box 1–3). Even a driver's license sometimes reveals enough detail to show the presence of ptosis or an anisocoria. Patients can be instructed to bring family photos with them for their follow-up visits. A 20-diopter indirect lens or the slitlamp can be used for magnification when examining printed photographs to assess the pupil size and degree of ptosis.

Patients who are suspected of having a central or preganglionic (first-or second-order neuron) defect could harbor lesions in the brain, neck, and upper chest; magnetic resonance imaging (MRI) of the brain, and computed tomography (CT) scan of the chest and neck should be obtained. As previously discussed, malignancies are not uncommon in patients with preganglionic oculosympathetic pareses, and this possibility must be fully evaluated.

Although isolated postganglionic lesions are more likely to be benign or idiopathic, an MRI of the brain and orbits with and without contrast is often needed in acute and subacute cases, especially when the patient has ongoing pain or other associated symptoms. Careful scrutiny for the presence or development of cranial neuropathies is required when an oculosympathetic paresis is present.

The pharmacologic tests are helpful, but should not be the only factor in determining the diagnosis and location of Horner syndrome. In practice, most patients presenting with new symptoms suggestive of a Horner syndrome get imaging of the full oculosympathetic pathway regardless of pharmacologic testing: MRI of brain, CT of chest and neck, with additional studies such as carotid ultrasound or CT angiography (CTA) as directed by the history and examination. Apraclonidine and cocaine testing are helpful in uncertain cases, but strong clinical suspicion should outweigh the results of pharmacologic testing. Hydroxyamphetamine is often not readily available (some authorities suggest that phenylephrine 1% can be used instead), but these tests are not foolproof in their ability to localize lesions.

PARASYMPATHETIC DISORDERS OF THE PUPIL: OCULOMOTOR NERVE

Lesions affecting the parasympathetic component of CN III are one cause of an anisocoria from an abnormally large pupil (see Table 11–4B).

Pathophysiology

Any lesion that affects the nuclear complex or course of the oculomotor nerve can cause a dilated pupil that is poorly reactive to light and near. The right and left motor components of the Edinger-Westphal subnuclei are adjacent at the midline, essentially creating a single midline subnucleus. Therefore, in the rare instance of a true *nuclear* CN III palsy, both pupils are dilated, if the pupils are affected at all.

As discussed in detail in Chapter 9, compressive lesions are more likely than ischemic disorders to affect the peripherally situated pupillary fibers of the oculomotor nerve. Pupil involvement in a CN III palsy is an important sign that suggests the possible presence of an expanding intracranial aneurysm, which requires immediate attention (see Figure 9–14). A dilated pupil from a CN III palsy is almost invariably associated with other signs of CN III dysfunction (ptosis, motility disturbance). A dilated pupil in isolation is very unlikely to be a CN III palsy, but it warrants serial observation and careful scrutiny for the development of other signs of oculomotor nerve dysfunction. As discussed in Chapter 9, a unilateral dilated pupil in a comatose patient may be the only sign of a unilateral expanding supratentorial mass, with entrapment and compression of the oculomotor nerve across the tentorial edge by herniation of the uncus (Hutchinson pupil).

Aberrant Regeneration

Pupillary involvement in an acute CN III palsy produces a pupil that responds poorly to light and near. However, with aberrant regeneration of the oculomotor nerve, the pupil may develop a *light-near dissociation*: a near response even though the light reaction remains poor (see Box 11–1). When aberrant regeneration occurs, CN III motor fibers that were originally destined for the extraocular muscles (usually the medial rectus) can end up innervating the pupillary sphincter (via the ciliary ganglion). In this circumstance, the pupil may not respond to light but can constrict with attempted activation of the medial rectus muscle. Because medial rectus activation is part of the near response, the pupil constricts with near effort but not to light, similar to an Adie tonic pupil (discussed in the following section). However, unlike an Adie pupil, the pupil in aberrant regeneration of CN III will also constrict with medial rectus activation in horizontal gaze (Figure 11–14).

PARASYMPATHETIC DISORDERS OF THE PUPIL: TONIC PUPIL

A tonic pupil is an abnormally large pupil with poor or absent light reaction and a slow, sustained (tonic) constriction to near effort. The unique clinical characteristics are caused by aberrant regeneration resulting from damage to the ciliary ganglion. When this condition occurs in isolation, it is considered idiopathic and is called an *Adie tonic pupil*. Adie pupil is most common in women aged 20 to 40 years. In many patients, the pupillary abnormality is associated with diminished deep tendon reflexes, yielding the designation *Adie (Holmes-Adie) pupillary syndrome*.

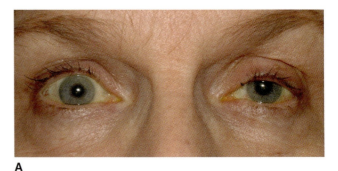

A

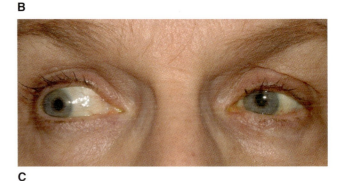

B

C

Figure 11–14. Aberrant regeneration of cranial nerve III.
A 46-year-old woman developed aberrant regeneration of the left oculomotor nerve several months after a coiling procedure for a carotid-cavernous fistula. **(A)** In primary position, the left pupil is larger than the right. A left ptosis is also evident. The patient had deficient supraduction, infraduction, and adduction of the left eye. **(B)** In left gaze, the anisocoria is unchanged. **(C)** In right gaze, the pupil (which is unresponsive to bright light) constricts and even becomes smaller than the normal right pupil. The constriction of the pupil in adduction is due to misdirected fibers—axons that originally innervated the medial rectus now go to the pupillary sphincter (via the ciliary ganglion).

Pathophysiology

Acutely, damage to the ciliary ganglion causes a dilated pupil, which does not constrict well to either light or near, and a paresis of accommodation. Within weeks of injury and axonal degeneration, the ciliary ganglion regrows postganglionic axons. Attempts at regeneration scramble

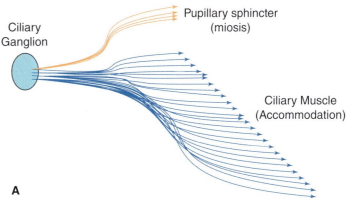

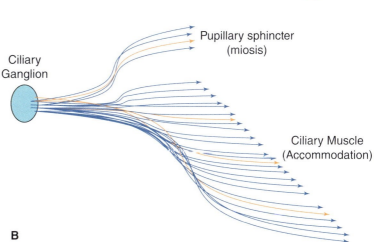

Figure 11–15. **Aberrant regeneration in Adie pupil syndrome.**
(A) In the normal state, the vast majority of fibers from the ciliary ganglion innervate the ciliary muscle for accommodation, with the remaining few innervating the pupillary sphincter. **(B)** Given this overwhelming ratio, it is no surprise that with aberrant regeneration originating at the ciliary ganglion, the pupillary sphincter would be reinnervated primarily by fibers originally serving accommodation. Therefore, there are likely to be a only several random segments of the pupillary sphincter that are correctly reinnervated and respond to light, with much of the pupil responding to accommodative tone instead.

the original destination of axons, with many of those originally serving accommodation ending up reinnervating the pupil, and some pupillary axons reinnervating the ciliary muscle. Given the overwhelming number of accommodation fibers, the pupillary sphincter is likely to be reinnervated by a high percentage of misdirected axons (that are suppose to innervate the ciliary muscle) (Figure 11–15). The result is a light-near dissociation: The pupillary response to light is poor because pupillary axons innervating the pupillary sphincter are now in the minority, but a near stimulus results in pupillary constriction from activation of the misdirected accommodation axons now innervating the pupillary sphincter.

Signs and Symptoms

Tonicity Tonicity describes the behavior of the pupil after a sustained near effort: The pupil becomes appropriately miotic with attempted near focus, but it is very slow to redilate when gaze is redirected from near to distance (Figure 11–16). Accommodation (near focus) may be achieved only (if at all) by a sustained effort, which is also very slow to relax for distance focus. Thus, prepresbyopic patients may present with a chief complaint of unilateral blurred vision at near or transient blurring with refocusing from distance to near and vice versa. Tonicity of accommodation can be tested by measuring the time required to refocus and read the distance acuity chart after sustained near effort in each eye. Accommodation (but not light reaction) may improve with time following the onset of an Adie pupil, with approximately 50% of patients recovering their age-appropriate accommodation after 2 years.

Vermiform movements The segmental innervation of the pupillary sphincter is evident with the aberrant regeneration in the tonic pupil: Some segments respond to accommodation, a few may respond to a light stimulus, and some segments do not respond at all (Figure 11–17). Grossly, this situation may be evident as an irregularity in the pupil shape on constriction with light or the near response. At the slitlamp, the uncoordinated innervation may cause an undulating wormlike movement of the iris margin known as a *vermiform* movement. The small number of pupillary axons that are misrouted to the ciliary muscle are of little clinical consequence (though the theoretical possibility of light-induced astigmatism is intriguing).

Pupil size The tonic pupil is usually large and does not constrict well, causing some patients to complain of

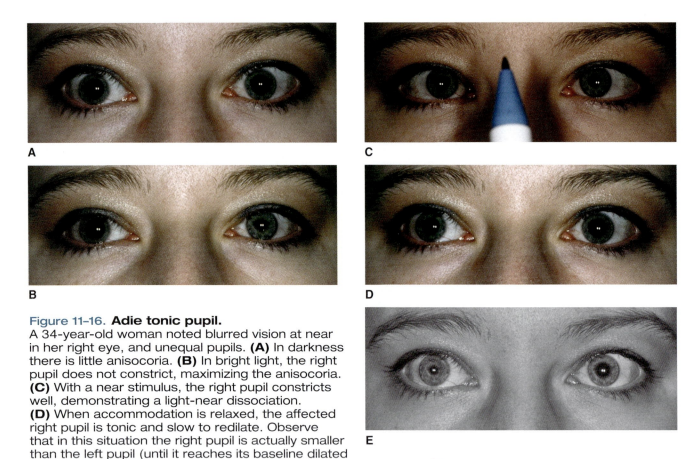

Figure 11–16. **Adie tonic pupil.**
A 34-year-old woman noted blurred vision at near in her right eye, and unequal pupils. **(A)** In darkness there is little anisocoria. **(B)** In bright light, the right pupil does not constrict, maximizing the anisocoria. **(C)** With a near stimulus, the right pupil constricts well, demonstrating a light-near dissociation. **(D)** When accommodation is relaxed, the affected right pupil is tonic and slow to redilate. Observe that in this situation the right pupil is actually smaller than the left pupil (until it reaches its baseline dilated state). **(E)** Dilute pilocarpine (0.1%) causes maximal constriction of the affected pupil, demonstrating denervation supersensitivity; the normal left pupil is not significantly affected by this dilute agent.

photosensitivity. Over time the pupil can become small, even smaller than the normal pupil. The small tonic pupil can still be recognized by its characteristic tonicity, light-near dissociation, and supersensitivity to pilocarpine.

Causes

By far, idiopathic Adie pupil is the most common type of tonic pupil. The underlying mechanism is unknown but appears to be systemic because it is associated with decreased deep tendon reflexes and an increased risk of occurrence in the fellow eye (risk increases at a rate of ~4% per year). Infectious and inflammatory disorders of the orbit, orbital trauma (including orbital surgery), and orbital tumors can cause a tonic pupil. These orbital processes only rarely affect the ciliary ganglion or the short ciliary nerves in isolation—other orbital signs are invariably present.

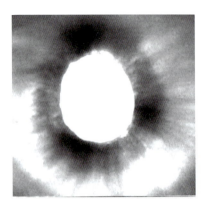

Figure 11–17. **Segmental reinnervation of the iris sphincter in Adie tonic pupil.**
Transillumination iris photograph showing a patient with an Adie tonic pupil. The dark bands show segments where the pupillary sphincter is constricting, with atonic intervening segments. (Reproduced, with permission, from Kardon RH, Corbett JJ, Thompson HS: Segmental denervation and reinnervation of the iris sphincter as shown by infrared videographic transillluminaton, Ophthalmology Feb;105(2):313–321 1998.)

Differential Diagnosis and Evaluation

A unilaterally dilated pupil can be the result of local iris factors, a CN III paresis, pharmacologic dilation, or a tonic pupil (see Table 11–4B).

A careful examination for signs of CN III dysfunction is required to differentiate Adie pupil from the mydriasis of a CN III palsy. As previously discussed, an isolated dilated pupil is unlikely to be the result of an oculomotor nerve paresis, but patients should be seen back after a short interval to ensure that CN III signs do not emerge.

A light-near dissociation can be caused by other conditions, but these disorders usually can be clinically distinguished from Adie pupil (see Table 11–2). Patients with a pharmacologically dilated pupil do not have the characteristic signs of an Adie tonic pupil, and these two conditions can be differentiated by pharmacologic testing.

Pharmacologic Testing

The neurotransmitter at the parasympathetic nerve/pupillary constrictor neuromuscular junction is acetylcholine. Even with reinnervation, the pupillary sphincter muscle in Adie pupil still receives only a small percentage of its normal neural tone. The decrease in synaptic activity causes a significant increase in the number of postsynaptic receptors, greatly increasing sensitivity to exogenous cholinergic agents.

To test for supersensitivity, dilute (0.1%) pilocarpine is placed in each eye. This direct-acting cholinergic agonist has a small but negligible effect on the normal pupil but is a potent constrictor in an affected eye that has developed supersensitivity. The pupils are observed 45 minutes after the instillation of eyedrops. Similar to sympathetic pharmacologic tests, the eyedrops should be placed in both eyes so the normal eye can serve as a control. The test is positive when the anisocoria is reversed, with the affected pupil now smaller than the pupil in the normal eye (see Figure 11–16E). In bilateral processes, the physician's confidence in interpreting pilocarpine testing is diminished. Dilute solution supersensitivity tests rely on delivery of an equal dose to each eye and are unreliable if the cornea or tear film has been disturbed. Be aware that the pupil in CN III palsy can also exhibit denervation supersensitivity, limiting the diagnostic specificity of this test (Figure 11–18B).

Management

A confident diagnosis of an Adie tonic pupil is crucial because it can avert an extensive neurological or neurosurgical evaluation and unnecessary anxiety. Some patients with an isolated, unilaterally dilated pupil have needlessly undergone cerebral angiography in search of a nonexistent aneurysm. The keys to confident diagnosis include the characteristic clinical signs previously discussed, the lack of cranial nerve signs or other neurological dysfunction (except decreased deep tendon reflexes), and confirmatory pharmacologic testing for supersensitivity. The presence of orbital signs or other cranial nerve dysfunction requires imaging and further investigation.

THE PHARMACOLOGICALLY DILATED PUPIL

Pharmacologic dilation of a pupil presenting as an anisocoria of unknown origin can occur in several settings: mydriatic eyedrops accidentally (or purposely) placed in the eye or exposure of the eye to an agent with mydriatic properties from contaminated fingers or other means. Sinus decongestants, cardiac medications, scopolamine patches for motion sickness, and naturally occurring jimsonweed are common potential contaminants causing mydriasis. Patients who use eyedrops or who wear contact lenses have the greatest opportunity to introduce such substances into the eye.

The pupils of patients who have mydriasis from the effect of an *anticholinergic* medication do not constrict well with a direct-acting cholinergic agent such as pilocarpine 1% because the postsynaptic receptors on the pupillary sphincter are effectively blocked. This property of pharmacologic blockage helps distinguish this condition from other causes of a unilateral dilated pupil: A dilated pupil from a CN III palsy should respond normally to pilocarpine or even exhibit a degree of supersensitivity; a tonic pupil (Adie pupil) is supersensitive, constricting maximally to even dilute pilocarpine (see Figure 11–18B).

Mydriasis from accidental topical *adrenergic* agents is less common. The pupil's response to pilocarpine testing in this situation is less definitive. Adrenergic drugs dilate the pupil by activating the pupillary dilator muscle. Because the pupillary sphincter is much stronger than the dilator, pilocarpine 1% constricts the pupil to a variable degree in this circumstance.

Patients suspected of having a pharmacologically dilated pupil should be carefully examined for any CN III dysfunction (ptosis or ocular motility disorder) or neurological signs, and reexamined after a short interval—anisocoria from a pharmacological mydriasis should resolve over days or weeks depending on the agent (unless the agent is reapplied).

TRANSIENT PUPILLARY DILATION

Transient sectoral dilation of the pupil resulting in an irregular *tadpole-shaped pupil* can occur in healthy individuals with a history of migraine. The phenomenon

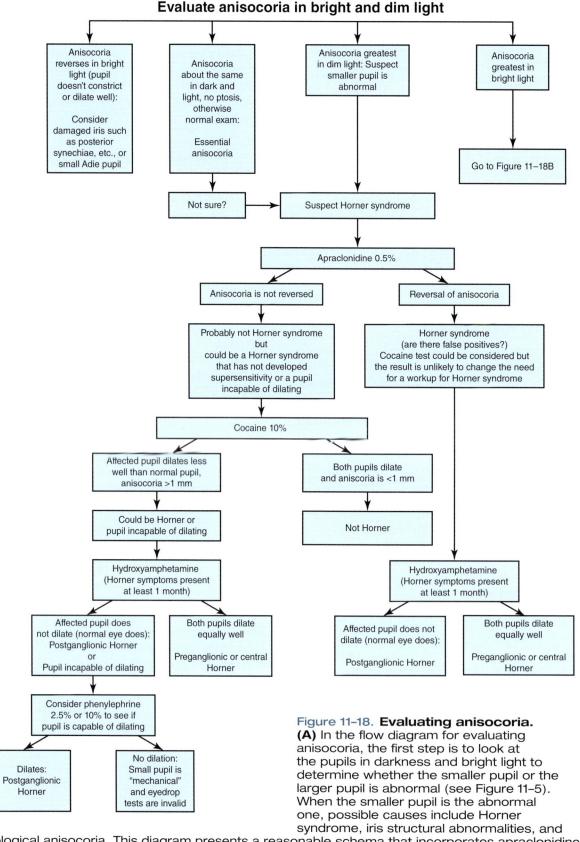

Figure 11–18. **Evaluating anisocoria.** **(A)** In the flow diagram for evaluating anisocoria, the first step is to look at the pupils in darkness and bright light to determine whether the smaller pupil or the larger pupil is abnormal (see Figure 11–5). When the smaller pupil is the abnormal one, possible causes include Horner syndrome, iris structural abnormalities, and physiological anisocoria. This diagram presents a reasonable schema that incorporates apraclonidine as a diagnostic agent for Horner syndrome without abandoning the well-vetted cocaine test. (Adapted, with permission, from Martin TJ: Horner's syndrome, pseudo-Horner's syndrome, and simple anisocoria. *Curr Neurol Neurosci Reports* 2007;7(5):397–406.)

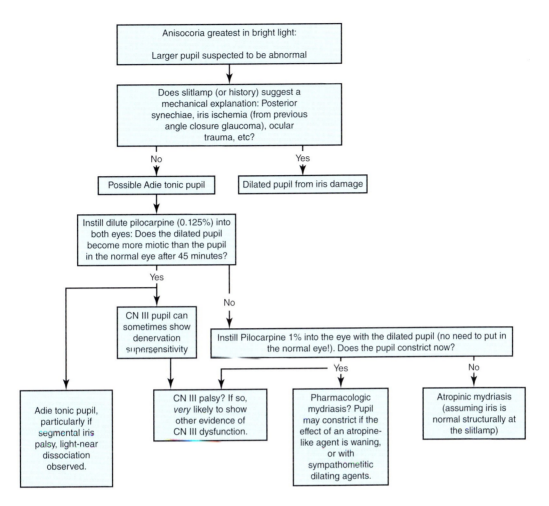

Figure 11-18. *(Continued)*
(B) If the anisocoria is greatest in bright light, the larger pupil is the abnormal one and the differential diagnosis commonly includes Adie tonic pupil, cranial nerve (CN) III palsy, and atropinic mydriasis.

lasts for a only few minutes, occurring several times over several weeks followed by spontaneous remission, then the cycle recurs months later. Similarly, benign episodic pupillary dilatation, known as a *springing pupil*, has been described in migraineurs, characterized by unilateral dilation for minutes to hours with blurred vision and periocular discomfort, followed by headache.

CLINICAL EVALUATION OF ANISOCORIA: OVERVIEW

The first step in the evaluation of an anisocoria is to determine whether the larger or smaller pupil is abnormal by observing the degree of anisocoria in bright light and darkness. If the degree of anisocoria is small and remains relatively constant in light and dark, an essential (or physiological) anisocoria is likely (see Figure 11–5).

If the smaller pupil is abnormal, the possibility of oculosympathetic paresis should be addressed first. Other causes of a small pupil are far less threatening, such as a long-standing Adie pupil or local iris factors. Non-neurological, structural abnormalities of the iris as a cause of anisocoria are usually evident at the slitlamp (see Figure 11–18A).

If the larger pupil is abnormal, the most concerning potential cause is a compressive CN III palsy. This condition is unlikely in the absence of other signs of CN III dysfunction. Next, an Adie tonic pupil and pharmacologic dilation should be considered. The history and examination usually identifies these entities, but pharmacologic testing with pilocarpine 0.1% for supersensitivity is helpful. This test can be immediately followed by pilocarpine 1% to test for the presence of an anticholinergic agent (see Figure 11–18B).

▶ KEY POINTS

- Pupillary axons leave the optic tract before its termination at the LGN, exiting via the brachium of the superior colliculus to synapse in the midbrain pretectal nuclei.
- The pupillary light reflex undergoes a *double hemidecussation,* ensuring a fairly equal distribution of light stimulation to both motor nuclei regardless of the eye of origin; *therefore, afferent visual loss does not cause a difference in pupil size.*
- Anisocoria is the result of an abnormality of the *efferent* (motor) innervation of the pupil, or local iris factors.
- Monocular optic nerve disorders tend to produce relative afferent pupillary defects of greater magnitude than monocular retinal disorders.
- Midbrain disorders that disrupt the afferent portion of the pupillary light reflex, without disturbing the (more ventral) near-reflex, cause a bilateral light-near dissociation: Examples include dorsal midbrain syndrome and syphilis (Argyll Robertson pupils).
- Other causes of light-near dissociation are the result of aberrant regeneration syndromes (Adie pupil and aberrant regeneration of the oculomotor nerve) or blindness.
- When the larger pupil is abnormal (does not constrict well), the anisocoria is greatest in bright light; conversely, when the smaller pupil is abnormal (does not dilate well), the anisocoria is greatest in darkness.
- The iris sphincter muscle has a mechanical advantage over the dilator muscle and is much stronger given equal innervation.
- The classic triad in Horner syndrome includes (1) miosis, (2) a 1- to 2-mm ptosis, and (3) facial anhidrosis; additional signs that occasionally occur acutely include conjunctival injection and hypotony.
- *Wallenberg lateral medullary syndrome* is caused by infarction of lateral medulla, resulting in a central (*first-order*) Horner syndrome (oculosympathetic paresis), ipsilateral facial anesthesia, contralateral hemianesthesia below the neck, and variable involvement of CN IX to XII.
- A Pancoast tumor is an apical lung tumor that can present as unilateral *preganglionic* (*second-order*) Horner syndrome and is often associated with arm or hand pain.
- Carotid artery *dissection* can cause a *postganglionic* (*third-order*) Horner syndrome associated with acute pain in the neck or face.
- Cluster headaches can cause transient Horner syndrome that may become permanent with repeated episodes.
- *Essential anisocoria* may account for an anisocoria of 0.5 mm or less (and occasionally larger).
- An abnormally small pupil may be caused by an interruption of the oculosympathetic chain anywhere in its course—from the hypothalamus through the spinal column, chest, neck, carotid plexus, and orbit.
- The combination of an essential anisocoria and a ptosis from any cause may mimic a Horner syndrome.
- Pharmacologic testing with topical cocaine helps the examiner determine if an oculosympathetic paresis exists: If the affected eye fails to dilate as well as the normal eye (resulting in an anisocoria of at least 1 mm) a Horner syndrome is likely present.
- Apraclonidine can be used (similar to cocaine) to help the examiner determine if a Horner syndrome exists. The endpoint is distinct: The anisocoria reverses.
- Pharmacologic testing with topical hydroxyamphetamine is used to differentiate a central or preganglionic oculosympathetic paresis from a postganglionic paresis: If the affected eye fails to dilate as well as the normal eye, a postganglionic lesion is likely present.
- The presence of a central or preganglionic Horner syndrome is more likely to be associated with a malignancy than a postganglionic Horner syndrome.
- Pupil involvement in a CN III palsy is an important sign that may suggest the presence of an expanding intracranial aneurysm.
- A tonic pupil is an abnormally large pupil caused by aberrant regeneration from a damaged ciliary ganglion; characteristics include a poor response to light, good response to a near stimulus, and supersensitivity to dilute pilocarpine.
- An Adie pupil is an idiopathic tonic pupil commonly affecting women 20 to 40 years of age, often associated with decreased tendon reflexes (Adie pupillary *syndrome*).
- Pharmacologic testing with topical pilocarpine is useful in sorting out pupils that are too large: A tonic pupil (Adie pupil) is supersensitive and constricts maximally to even dilute pilocarpine (0.1%), whereas a pupil that is dilated by an anticholinergic agent does not constrict well even with pilocarpine 1%.

SUGGESTED READING

Books

Burde RM, Savino PJ, Trobe JD: *Clinical Decisions in Neuro-ophthalmology,* 3d ed. St Louis, MO: Mosby; 2002:246–271.

Kardon RH: Anatomy and physiology of the autonomic nervous system, in Miller NR, Newman NJ (eds): *Walsh* and Hoyt's Clinical Neuro-ophthalmology, Vol 1, 6th ed. Philadelphia, PA: Lippincott Williams & Wilkins; 2005:649–714.

Lowenstein IE: *The Pupil: Anatomy, Physiology, and Clinical Application.* Detroit, MI: Wayne State University Press; 1993.

Slamovits TL, Glaser JS: The pupils and accommodation, in Glaser JS (ed): *Neuro-ophthalmology,* 3d ed. Philadelphia, PA: Lippincott Williams & Wilkins; 1999:527–552.

Articles

Relative Afferent Pupillary Defect

Thompson HS, Corbett JJ, Cox TA: How to measure the relative afferent pupillary defect. *Surv Ophthalmol* 1981;26:39–42.

Anisocoria

Lam BL, Thompson HS, Corbett JJ: The prevalence of simple anisocoria. *Am J Ophthalmol* 1987;104:69–73.

Thompson JS, Pilley SFJ: Unequal pupils: a flow chart for sorting out anisocorias. *Surv Ophthalmol* 1976;21:45–48.

Oculosympathetic Paresis (Horner syndrome)

Almog Y, Gepstein R, Kesler A: Diagnostic value of imaging in Horner syndrome in adults. *J Neuroophthalmol* 2010;30:7–11.

Cremer SA, Thompson HS, Digre KB, et al: Hydroxyamphetamine mydriasis in Horner's syndrome. *Am J Ophthalmol* 1990;110:66–70.

Freedman KA, Brown SM: Topical apraclonidine in the diagnosis of suspected Horner syndrome. *J Neuroophthalmol* 2005;25:83–85.

Kardon RH, Denison CE, Brown CK, et al: Critical evaluation of the cocaine test in the diagnosis of Horner's syndrome. *Arch Ophthalmol* 1990;108:384–387.

Maloney NR, Liu GT, Menacker SJ, et al: Pediatric Horner syndrome: etiologies and roles of imaging and urine studies to detect neuroblastoma and other responsible mass lesions. *Am J Ophthalmol* 2006;142(4):651–659.

Maloney WF, Young BR, Moyer NJ: Evaluation of the causes and accuracy of pharmacological location of Horner's syndrome. *Am J Ophthalmol* 1980;90:394–402.

Martin TJ: Horner's syndrome, pseudo-Horner's syndrome, and simple anisocoria. *Curr Neurol Neurosci Reports* 2007;7(5):397–406.

Thompson BM, Corbett JJ, Kline LB, et al: Pseudo-Horner's syndrome. *Arch Neurol* 1982;39:108–111.

Trobe J: The evaluation of Horner syndrome. *J Neuroophthalmol* 2010;30:1–2.

Weinstein JM, Zweifel TJ, Thompson HS: Congenital Horner's syndrome. *Arch Ophthalmol* 1980;98:1074–1078.

Tonic Pupil

Thompson HS: Adie's syndrome: some new observations. *Trans Am Ophthalmol Soc* 1977;75:587–626.

Aberrant Regeneration of Cranial Nerve III

Czarnecki JSC, Thompson HS: The iris sphincter in aberrant regeneration of the third nerve. *Arch Ophthalmol* 1978;96:1606–1610.

CHAPTER 12

The Facial Nerve

- ▶ NEUROANATOMY 287
  - Supranuclear (upper motor neuron) pathways 287
  - Facial nucleus and fascicles (lower motor neuron) 288
  - Subarachnoid space 288
  - Temporal bone and peripheral course 288
- ▶ ASSESSMENT OF FACIAL NERVE FUNCTION 291
  - Facial motor function 291
  - Taste 291
  - Tear function 292
  - Hearing 292
- ▶ FACIAL NERVE PALSIES 292
  - Bell palsy 292
  - Herpes zoster oticus 292
  - Other infectious diseases 293
  - Acute inflammatory demyelinating polyradiculopathy 293
  - Trauma 293
  - Other causes 294
- ▶ EXPOSURE KERATOPATHY 294
  - Risk factors 294
  - Management 295
- ▶ FACIAL NERVE DISORDERS: HYPERACTIVITY 295
  - Blepharospasm 295
  - Hemifacial spasm 296
  - Facial myokymia 297
  - Benign eyelid myokymia 297
- ▶ KEY POINTS 298

The *facial nerve* is the seventh cranial nerve (CN VII). CN VII is of major importance to ophthalmologists for at least two reasons. First, the facial motor pathways are in close anatomic proximity to the ocular motor pathways; therefore, the evaluation of facial motor function may offer important clues in the diagnosis and localization of lesions that cause ocular motility disorders. Second, CN VII controls eye closure (orbicularis oculi). Weakness of eye closure can lead to exposure keratopathy and visual loss.

▶ NEUROANATOMY

SUPRANUCLEAR (UPPER MOTOR NEURON) PATHWAYS

Corticobulbar Pathway

Volitional (voluntary) facial movements originate in the precentral gyrus of the frontal lobe cortex. Fibers descend within the corticobulbar tract through the internal capsule and cerebral peduncles to synapse in the facial motor nuclei located in the pons. Cortical fibers controlling the lower face decussate to innervate the contralateral facial nucleus. Fibers innervating the upper face (forehead muscles and orbicularis oculi) originate from both the ipsilateral and contralateral facial nuclei (Figure 12–1). Thus, a unilateral hemispheric lesion that affects the supranuclear pathway (upper motor neuron) produces a contralateral lower facial paresis; voluntary eye closure and forehead movement are relatively spared because the upper face can be controlled by either hemisphere.

Other neurological signs and symptoms frequently accompany a facial palsy from upper motor neuron disease. The portion of the precentral motor gyrus that serves the hand and fingers lies immediately superior to the facial motor area, and motor control for the tongue lies adjacent inferiorly (see Figure 12–1). Therefore, hemispheric lesions in this area may produce contralateral weakness of the lower face, hand, and tongue, as well as other hemispheric signs.

Limbic (Extrapyramidal) Pathway

Patients with upper motor neuron disease involving the corticobulbar pathway may be unable to smile voluntarily or close their eyes on command, but periodic blinking or emotional facial responses (such as a smile in response to a funny story) may still occur.

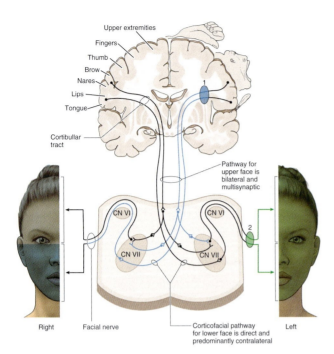

Figure 12-1. Corticobulbar (supranuclear) facial pathway.
Observe that the upper face has bilateral supranuclear input. Thus, a left supranuclear lesion (1) produces a right facial palsy that spares the upper face. However, a left facial nerve lesion (2) would likely affect both the upper and lower left face. (Modified, with permission, from Sibony PA, Evinger C: Anatomy and physiology of normal and abnormal eyelid position and movement. In Miller NR, Newman NJ, editors. Walsh and Hoyt's clinical neuro-ophthalmology, ed 5. Vol 1, Baltimore, 1998, Lippincott, Williams & Wilkins.)

This preservation of emotional facial expression occurs because another supranuclear motor pathway with input to the facial nucleus—the *limbic* (or *extrapyramidal*) *pathway*—controls involuntary and automatic facial movements. This pathway involves the basal ganglia, thalamus, and brainstem. Selective damage to the limbic supranuclear input to the facial nucleus leaves volitional facial movement intact but affects emotional facial expression. For example, Parkinson disease interferes with the limbic pathway, and affected patients have a relatively expressionless face with infrequent blinking ("reptilian stare"). Because the corticobulbar pathway is intact in Parkinson disease, affected patients can still produce facial movements on command. *Hyperactivity* of the limbic facial pathway produces *Meige syndrome* consisting of blepharospasm with dystonic buccal and nuchal facial movements.

Because both supranuclear systems require an intact lower motor neuron, lesions of the facial nucleus, its fascicles, or the facial nerve affect both voluntary and involuntary facial expression. Lesions involving the supranuclear pathways have less effect on baseline facial tone; therefore, asymmetry of the face at rest is not nearly as noticeable than with lower motor neuron disease.

FACIAL NUCLEUS AND FASCICLES (LOWER MOTOR NEURON)

The facial nucleus is located in the pons, inferior and lateral to the abducens nucleus (see Figure 9–3A). The motor axons exit the nucleus and travel dorsally and medially, where they loop over the abducens nucleus before taking a more ventral course to exit the lateral aspect of the caudal pons. As the CN VII fascicles sweep over the abducens nucleus (the facial genu), they form a bump on the floor of the fourth ventricle called the *facial colliculus*. The *superior salivatory nucleus* is located just rostral to the facial nucleus. This parasympathetic motor nucleus controls the sublingual, submandibular, and lacrimal glands via the *nervus intermedius,* which joins CN VII in the subarachnoid space (Figure 12–2).

Important adjacent structures at this level of the brainstem include the cochlear nuclei, the spinal tract and the trigeminal (CN V) nucleus, the abducens (CN VI) nucleus, and descending sympathetic fibers. Thus, potential associated symptoms with a nuclear or fascicular CN VII palsy include ipsilateral facial numbness, Horner syndrome, deafness, or CN VI palsy (see Figure 9–3A). Lesions in this area are frequently the result of demyelination, ischemic infarct, or intrinsic brainstem tumors (Table 12–1).

SUBARACHNOID SPACE

CN VII and the nervus intermedius exit the lateral aspect of the pons close together, and close to the point that the eighth cranial nerve (CN VIII) enters the brainstem, in a region of the subarachnoid space known as the *cerebellopontine angle*. The nervus intermedius merges with CN VII in the subarachnoid space shortly after exiting the brainstem. Tumors in the area can affect CN VIII (hearing and balance), CN VII, and the nervus intermedius. Large tumors in this area can also affect CN V and CN VI, as well as the brainstem and cerebellum. Cerebellopontine angle tumors include meningiomas, acoustic neuromas, facial neuromas, and epidermoid tumors (see Table 12–1).

Within the subarachnoid space, CN VIII and CN VII are separated by the anterior inferior cerebellar artery. Irritation of CN VII by the anterior inferior cerebellar artery or other vascular structures in this area can cause hemifacial spasm (discussed below).

TEMPORAL BONE AND PERIPHERAL COURSE

CN VII and associated nervus intermedius enter the temporal bone with the vestibulocochlear nerve (CN VIII) through the internal auditory meatus. On entering this

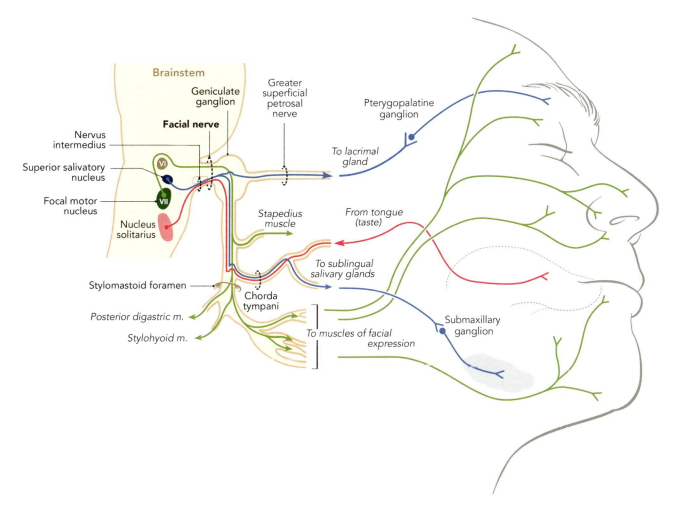

Figure 12-2. **Facial nerve anatomy.**
Origin and distribution of the seventh cranial nerve.

bony foramen, CN VII/nervus intermedius separates from the vestibuloacoustic nerve and enters the *fallopian canal*. The fallopian (or facial) canal carries CN VII nearly 3 cm through a complex, descending Z-shaped course within the temporal bone. Trauma involving the temporal bone is a common cause of CN VII injury. Bony metastasis can also affect CN VII as it courses in the fallopian canal.

The first segment of the fallopian canal contains the geniculate ganglion and the first branch of CN VII, the *greater superficial petrosal nerve*. This nerve contains fibers that will travel via the vidian nerve to synapse in the sphenopalatine ganglion, eventually supplying the lacrimal gland. Much of the course of the greater superficial petrosal nerve is in the middle cranial fossa, and tumors or inflammatory processes in this area may impair reflex tear secretion (often with accompanying CN V and CN VI dysfunction). Additional branches of CN VII include the nerve to the stapedius muscle and the chorda tympani. The *chorda tympani* (so called because it courses across the inferior border of the tympanic membrane) is the terminal branch of fibers that began as the nervus intermedius, supplying parasympathetic motor input to the submandibular and sublingual glands. The chorda tympani also carries afferent taste fibers from the anterior two-thirds of the tongue (see Figure 12–2).

CN VII exits its bony course through the stylomastoid foramen and immediately gives off branches to innervate the digastric, stylohyoid, and posterior auricular muscles. The facial nerve then enters the substance of the parotid gland, where it spreads out like a goose's foot (the *pes anserinus*), dividing into a superior temporofacial and inferior cervicofacial trunk. Although some variability exists, the superior trunk provides temporal, malar, and infraorbital nerves, and the inferior trunk divides into buccal, mandibular, and cervical portions. Parotid gland tumors (mucoepidermoid and adenoid cystic carcinoma), trauma to CN VII during parotid gland surgery, and parotid

TABLE 12-1. CAUSES OF FACIAL NERVE PALSY BY LOCATION

Location		Disease Processes	Notes
Supranuclear	Corticobulbar pathway	Infarction, tumor	Upper face and involuntary movement spared; adjacent regions (tongue and hand) may also be affected.
	Limbic (or extrapyramidal)	Parkinson disease; Infarction, AVM, or tumor of basal ganglia	Dull, expressionless face; volitional movement intact.
Nucleus and fascicles	Pons	Infarction, glioma, metastasis, hemorrhage, demyelination, infection	Possible involvement of CNs V, VI, VIII; oculosympathetics (Horner syndrome); corticospinal tract.
Peripheral nerve	Cerebellopontine angle	Acoustic schwannoma, meningioma, metastasis, cerebellar tumors, cholesteatoma, glomus jugulare, facial schwannoma	Lesions of CN VII at this point would also affect sensory fibers from the external ear, motor fibers to the stapedius muscle (hyperacusis), the nervus intermedius (loss of taste on the anterior two-thirds of the tongue, decreased tearing/salivation). Neighboring structures including CN VIII (hearing loss), cerebellum (nystagmus), brainstem (gaze palsy) are frequently involved. CNs IX, X, XI affected by large tumors.
	Subarachnoid space	Glomus jugulare, carcinomatous meningitis, leukemia, diphtheria, tuberculosis.	Multiple or sequential cranial nerve palsies.
	Temporal bone	Bell palsy, trauma, schwannoma, meningioma, cholesteatoma, hemangioma, AVM, herpes zoster oticus (geniculate ganglion), acute suppurative otitis media	CN VII components affected, but no other neurological deficits.
	Extracranial course	Facial trauma, parotid surgery, parotid gland tumor, sarcoidosis	Isolated facial motor paralyses (nervus intermedius and nerve to stapedius not affected).
Not site specific		Sarcoidosis, Guillain-Barré syndrome, mononucleosis, metastatic disease, Melkersson-Rosenthal syndrome	

Abbreviations: AVM, arteriovenous malformation; CN, cranial nerve.

infiltration/inflammation (from disorders such as sarcoidosis) can affect CN VII as it courses within the parotid gland (see Table 12–1).

Because CN VII has multiple functions and many branches, a variety of aberrant regeneration syndromes can result from the misdirection of regenerating axons following injury. *Crocodile tears* result when parasympathetic fibers that were originally destined for the salivary gland are misdirected to the lacrimal gland, causing tearing associated with eating. Lesions that cause this syndrome must involve CN VII at or above the geniculate ganglion, before the greater superficial petrosal nerve arises. Other aspects of aberrant regeneration involving CN VII motor function include eye closure (orbicularis activation) on attempted smiling or puckering. A common form of aberrant regeneration (often following Bell palsy) is lower face movement or dimpling over the chin with eye closure.

The vascular supply of CN VII is abundant. Within the fallopian canal, at least three sources are present. The anterior inferior cerebellar artery enters the internal auditory meatus; the petrosal branch of the middle meningeal artery accompanies the greater petrosal nerve; and the stylomastoid branch of the posterior auricular artery enters the facial canal at the stylomastoid foramen. Despite this rich blood supply, ischemia may be a common factor in CN VII palsies because the narrow confines of the bony facial canal can severely restrict perfusion in the presence of edema. The narrowest portion of the interosseous canal is at the level of the geniculate ganglion; the facial nerve is especially vulnerable at this point.

▶ ASSESSMENT OF FACIAL NERVE FUNCTION

Clinical testing of the multiple functions of CN VII makes localization possible, although such testing is tedious. For example, lesions of CN VII in the subarachnoid space tend to impair all functions of CN VII. Distal lesions may involve only a few CN VII functions because more proximal branches may be spared. However, pontine lesions can affect the motor, sensory, or autonomic functions in isolation because the superior salivatory nucleus and CN VII nucleus exist as separate nuclei in the brainstem with axons that converge after exiting the brainstem (see Figure 12–2).

FACIAL MOTOR FUNCTION

The evaluation of facial motor function begins as soon as the examiner encounters the patient. Asymmetries of the face may be evident during the history, before a formal examination. In *acute* upper or lower motor neuron disease, the nasolabial fold may be flattened, the palpebral fissure may be wider, and spontaneous blinks may be incomplete on the affected side. However, following recovery of a lower motor neuron facial palsy, facial tone actually is *increased* and the face looks "tight" on the affected side, even though on formal testing the muscles may not be as strong as normal.

Formal examination of CN VII functions should be carried out by a systematic fractionation of facial muscle function. Motor function of the upper face is evaluated by asking the patient to raise his or her eyebrows to wrinkle the forehead. Orbicularis oculi function is tested by asking the patient to close the eyes as tightly as possible and noting the degree to which the eyelashes are buried (see Figure 7–14). In addition, the examiner can attempt to open tightly closed eyelids to note weakness or asymmetry between eyes. Using a cotton wisp to check the corneal reflex also evaluates efferent innervation of the orbicularis muscle through the corneal-blink reflex arc (see Box 7–4). The examiner can ask the patient to pucker in order to evaluate the orbicularis oris. Asking the patient to smile and to show his or her teeth are effective methods to evaluate the lower face (Figure 12–3). By asking the patient to show a "million dollar smile," the examiner invariably brings out both motor and limbic smiles.

The anatomic substrate for the clinical characteristics of supranuclear facial disorders—the dissociation of voluntary facial movements and emotion-related facial expression and the tendency to spare the upper face—was previously discussed. Peripheral CN VII disorders would obviously cause weakness both in volitional and involuntary facial movements and involves both the upper and lower face. However, the spatial distribution of fibers that serve different portions of the face is preserved in the facial nucleus and in CN VII itself. Therefore, lower motor neuron lesions (such as parotid tumors) may occasionally spare the upper face.

TASTE

CN VII (via the chorda tympani) carries taste from the anterior two-thirds of the tongue. Although evaluation

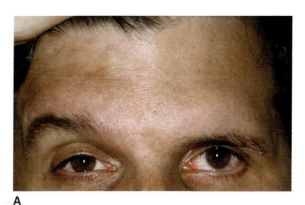

A

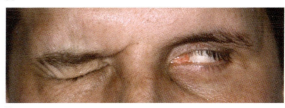

B

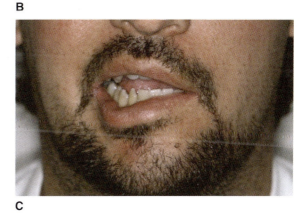

C

Figure 12–3. **Examining facial nerve function.** The patient pictured sustained a peripheral left seventh cranial nerve palsy from trauma. **(A)** Elevation of the brow is weak on the left side and manifests as poor wrinkling of the left forehead. **(B)** Lack of left orbicularis strength is evident. Observe that the patient has a good Bell phenomenon. **(C)** The command, "Smile and show your teeth," reveals lower face weakness.

of taste is rarely performed in the clinical setting, it may be useful in characterizing facial nerve lesions in special circumstances.

TEAR FUNCTION

Although one would suspect that looking for decreased lacrimation would be helpful in evaluating CN VII dysfunction, a number of confounding factors prevent it from being a useful sign. For example, tearing may be increased because of irritation from exposure keratopathy or decreased from the defective corneal sensation that can accompany an exposed cornea.

HEARING

Hyperacusis may result from paresis of the facial nerve branch to the stapedius muscle. This muscle normally functions to dampen loud sounds by tightening the tympanic membrane. However, hearing tests are far more useful in detecting *decreased* hearing that may occur from CN VII lesions that involve the adjacent vestibulocochlear nerve (CN VIII) than documenting hyperacusis.

▶ FACIAL NERVE PALSIES

BELL PALSY

Bell palsy is the most common facial neuropathy (Figure 12–4). This condition is usually described as an idiopathic facial paralysis, but there may be a link to herpes simplex type one virus (HSV-1) infection. Bell palsy occurs with a higher incidence in patients with diabetes mellitus, during pregnancy, and in those with a family history of Bell palsy.

Signs and Symptoms

Facial weakness in Bell palsy generally develops rapidly. A facial paresis that continues to progress after 2 to 3 weeks is more suggestive of a compressive neuropathy (tumor) than a Bell palsy. Pain (usually retroauricular) is common and may antedate the onset of paralysis by hours or days. Additional signs and symptoms include a sensation of facial and tongue numbness, decreased tearing, altered taste, and dysacusis. In many patients, Bell palsy is associated with a viral prodrome, which supports the proposal of a possible viral cause.

Greater than 80% of patients have a satisfactory recovery. Improvement usually begins within 3 weeks of onset and continues for 3 to 4 months; improvement is not expected beyond this point. Poor prognostic signs for recovery include advanced age and the presence of dysacusis or impaired lacrimation at presentation. Electromyography performed early in the course of a facial palsy can also provide helpful prognostic information. Even when recovery is relatively complete, subtle signs of facial motor aberrant regeneration can be noted by an observant examiner.

Treatment

The treatment recommendations for Bell palsy continue to evolve. Ninety percent of patients with Bell palsy treated with prednisone have a complete recovery within 60 days, compared to 75% without. Because of evidence indicating that HSV-1 may be a cause, antiviral agents (such as acyclovir or famciclovir) are often used but have not been proven to be of benefit. Treatment is also required for a potentially devastating complication of orbicularis weakness with Bell palsy—exposure keratopathy and its sequelae (discussed later in this chapter).

HERPES ZOSTER OTICUS

In *herpes zoster oticus* (also called *Ramsay Hunt syndrome*), the signature of herpes zoster is readily

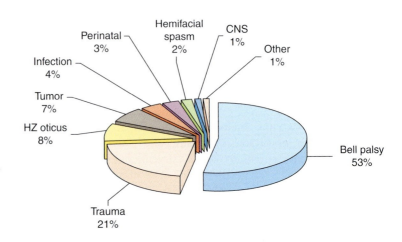

Figure 12–4. **Causes of facial nerve disorders.**
Data from 2406 patients seen over 24 years. Abbreviations: CNS, central nervous system; HZ, herpes zoster. (Data from May M, Galetta S: The facial nerve and related disorders of the face, in Glaser JS (ed): *Neuro-ophthalmology*, 2d ed. Philadelphia: Lippincott; 1990.)

apparent by the presence of severe pain and cutaneous vesicles in addition to facial weakness. Pain is primarily around the ear and upper neck. Vesicles may be noted in any areas supplied by sensory portions of CN VII including the posterior aspect of the external auditory canal, over the tympanic membrane, on the pinna, or on the tongue, the buccal mucosa, or the lateral neck. Other nerves that communicate with CN VII may also be involved. Associated involvement of CN VIII, with associated sensorineural hearing loss and vestibular dysfunction, is common. The prognosis for recovery is poorer than with idiopathic Bell palsy, and the course of the disease is frequently excruciatingly painful. Postherpetic neuralgia occurs often.

OTHER INFECTIOUS DISEASES

Cranial neuropathies occur frequently with Lyme disease, including unilateral or bilateral facial palsies. *Lyme disease* is an infection caused by the tick-borne spirochete *Borrelia burgdorferi*. Following a tick bite, a skin lesion develops that expands, forming a target or "bull's-eye" lesion consisting of an erythematous ring of inflamed skin with central clearing as it expands. Systemic symptoms include fatigue, headache, nausea, and vomiting. Secondary complications include meningopolyneuritis and arthritis. Lyme disease can be detected by the enzyme-linked immunosorbent assay (ELISA) test for antibodies to *B. burgdorferi*. However, in many endemic areas of the country, serologic titers may be high in unaffected individuals. Although the prognosis for recovery of CN VII function with Lyme disease is good even without treatment, diagnosis and appropriate treatment is important to prevent other systemic, neurological, and arthritic complications of the disease.

An isolated CN VII palsy can be the presenting sign of acquired immunodeficiency syndrome (AIDS). Human immunodeficiency virus (HIV) testing should be considered when patients with facial paralysis have risk factors for HIV or present with opportunistic infections.

Inner ear infections can involve the temporal bone and CN VII. In the preantibiotic era (and in rare cases today), infections that extend to the petrous apex from complicated otitis media can involve the trigeminal (CN V), abducens (CN VI), and facial nerves (CN VII) (*Gradenigo syndrome*). Although acute otitis media is a frequent infection, antibiotic treatment is effective and cranial nerve complications from bacterial ear infections are uncommon. Currently, Gradenigo syndrome is more likely to occur from invasive nasopharyngeal tumor, squamous cell carcinoma, or cholesteatoma than from infection.

ACUTE INFLAMMATORY DEMYELINATING POLYRADICULOPATHY

Guillain-Barré syndrome, or acute inflammatory demyelinating polyradiculopathy (AIDP), is an immune-mediated inflammatory disease that affects motor and cranial nerves. In many patients, symptoms begin in the legs and ascend in a cephalad direction, with progression over 3 to 4 weeks. One-half of patients develop CN VII paralysis, often bilateral. Ophthalmoplegia, ptosis, optic neuritis, and papilledema can also occur.

The *Miller-Fisher variant of Guillain-Barré syndrome* causes ophthalmoplegia, areflexia, and ataxia with bilateral facial palsies (Table 12–2). This condition appears to be a postinfectious autoimmune disorder that targets neuronal elements, following *Campylobacter jejuni* infectious gastritis. Greater than 90% of patients have antibodies to ganglioside GQ1b, which cross-reacts with antigens in the cell wall of the organism. Examination of the cerebrospinal fluid reveals elevated protein with a normal cell count. The prognosis for a complete recovery is excellent.

TRAUMA

Given the long interosseous course of CN VII in the skull base, it is not surprising that head trauma (particularly if accompanied by basilar skull fracture) is a frequent cause of facial palsies. Fractures of the temporal bone that run parallel to the axis of

▶ **TABLE 12–2. CAUSES OF BILATERAL FACIAL WEAKNESS: FACIAL DIPLEGIA**

Guillain-Barré syndrome (AIDP, Miller-Fisher syndrome)
Brainstem trauma, glioma, or stroke (basilar artery stroke)
Möbius syndrome
Meningeal carcinomatosis
Leukemia
HIV infection
Lyme disease
Polio
Diphtheria
Sarcoidosis
Porphyria
Melkersson-Rosenthal syndrome
Myotonic dystrophy
Myasthenia gravis

Abbreviations: AIDP, acute inflammatory demyelinating polyradiculopathy; HIV, human immunodeficiency virus.

the petrous bone usually spare CN VII, but fractures across the long axis produce facial palsies in approximately 50% of patients. A key accompanying sign is ecchymosis of the skin over the mastoid (Battle sign), resulting from extravasation of blood from a skull-base fracture. Other signs that accompany traumatic CN VII palsy from basilar skull fracture include tympanic membrane rupture, cerebrospinal fluid (CSF) otorrhea, and hemotympanum. Another potential site for CN VII trauma is at the stylomastoid foramen, where the CN VII exits the skull base. In some patients, surgical exploration is indicated in traumatic CN VII paralyses, particularly if displaced fractures are seen on neuroimaging.

OTHER CAUSES

The wide variety of *tumors* that can affect CN VII along its course from the brainstem through the cerebellopontine angle, fallopian canal, and parotid gland were discussed in the preceding neuroanatomy section (see Table 12–1).

Sarcoidosis is an idiopathic inflammatory condition that can involve many organ systems (see Box 4–4). CN VII palsy can occur when sarcoidosis involves the parotid gland. Parotid infiltration is invariably bilateral, although asymmetric facial palsies are the rule with sarcoidosis. CN VII is the most common cranial nerve affected by sarcoidosis.

Melkersson-Rosenthal syndrome is a rare idiopathic disorder characterized by facial swelling and a transversely fissured tongue, accompanied by unilateral or bilateral facial paralysis.

Möbius syndrome is a congenital disorder of nuclear agenesis that consists of bilateral facial palsies, bilateral CN VI palsies, deafness, palatal and lingual palsies, and defects of the extremities. This rare disorder produces rather characteristic facies (Figure 12–5) with muscular atrophy corresponding to affected motor cranial nerves. *Birth trauma* (especially from forceps) can also cause a facial paralysis.

Myasthenia gravis, discussed in detail in Chapter 8, is an autoimmune disorder of the neuromuscular junction. This disorder frequently affects the facial muscles, especially the orbicularis oculi, and can mimic CN VII paresis. Orbicularis weakness may manifest during sustained forceful closure of the eyes as the "peek sign," in which the eye gradually opens slightly from fatigue of the orbicularis oculi.

▶ EXPOSURE KERATOPATHY

Preventing the potentially serious sequelae of exposure keratopathy is critical in caring for patients with facial palsies. Exposure keratopathy leads to epithelial breakdown with corneal erosion and the potential for corneal ulceration, corneal perforation, and endophthalmitis (Figure 12–6).

RISK FACTORS

Patients with orbicularis weakness, a poor Bell phenomenon, and/or decreased corneal sensation are at risk for exposure keratopathy and its sequelae. The vision-destroying potential of these predisposing conditions is commonly unrecognized and underappreciated. Comatose or obtunded inpatients (eg, those in intensive care units) with the potential for exposure keratopathy are at high risk, and topical lubrication may be sight saving. The degree of *orbicularis weakness* is the primary determinant of corneal exposure risk. The risk parallels the degree of abnormal eye closure, which is obviously greatest when there is a complete inability to close the eye, and less so when there is an adequate but asymmetric blink.

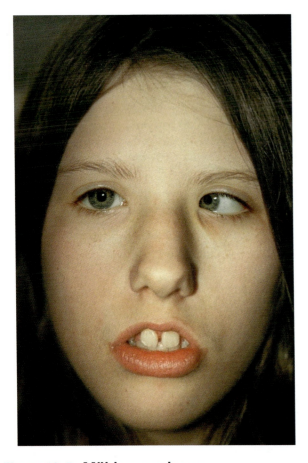

Figure 12–5. **Möbius syndrome.** Patients with Möbius syndrome have a characteristic "mask-like" facies due to bilateral facial weakness. Esotropia is also often present due to bilateral sixth cranial nerve palsies, as pictured in this photo illustration. (Courtesy of Richard Gray Weaver Jr., MD.)

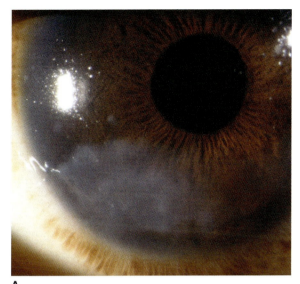

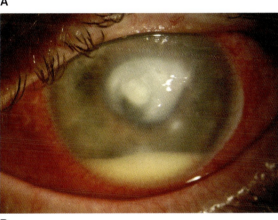

Figure 12-6. **Sequelae of exposure keratopathy.**
(A) Chronic exposure keratopathy in a patient with a chronic facial nerve palsy has resulted in scarring of the inferior cornea. **(B)** In a different patient, exposure keratopathy progressed to a corneal ulcer with hypopyon. The patient's blind, painful eye subsequently required enucleation.

Bell phenomenon is a reflexive upper rotation of the eyes on eye closure, and when present helps to protect the cornea when the orbicularis oculi are weak (see Figure 12–3B). This normal reflex is most apparent when facial (orbicularis) weakness keeps the eye from closing completely, because the reflexive upward rotation of the eye is not visible with normal eye closure. The presence and intensity of this reflex ocular rotation varies widely among normal individuals. When a Bell reflex is present in a patient with orbicularis weakness, the upward rotation of the eye under the upper eyelid on attempted blinking offers at least intermittent relief for the exposed cornea; when absent, there is a greater risk of complications from exposure keratopathy.

Relative *corneal anesthesia* in the presence of a facial palsy can occur from concomitant involvement of the trigeminal nerve or from exposure hypoesthesia (decreased sensation from corneal adaptation to constant exposure). Even in the absence of orbicularis weakness, corneal anesthesia is a serious threat to the eye, leading to neurotropic corneal breakdown that is difficult to treat. Thus, disorders that affect both sensation (CN V_1) and eye closure (CN VII) present the greatest challenge.

Evaluation of three factors—(1) orbicularis weakness, (2) Bell phenomenon, and (3) corneal sensation—as well as anticipated recovery time, will determine how aggressive the treatment must be to protect the eye.

MANAGEMENT

Supportive care of the ocular surface includes topical artificial tears at regular intervals throughout the day and ointment at night. In more severe cases, patients may need to be taught how to tape their eyelid closed during the night for protection. Tape splints that support and elevate the lower eyelid, or that prevent the upper eyelid from fully retracting, are helpful when applied correctly. Punctal plugs may be helpful. Occasionally, a partial or complete tarsorrhaphy is required, especially in patients who develop poorly healing corneal epithelial defects from exposure keratopathy. Injection of the levator palpebrae muscle with botulinum toxin or placement of gold weights in the upper eyelid are alternatives therapies. The management of corneal ulceration and other manifestations of severe keratopathy require specialized care and are beyond the scope of this book.

Regardless of the treatment method used, reevaluation of the patient with exposure keratopathy at frequent intervals is important because poor corneal sensation may allow dangerous progression of the corneal disease without significant pain.

▶ FACIAL NERVE DISORDERS: HYPERACTIVITY

Lesions involving the supranuclear facial motor pathways or CN VII can produce irritative states causing overactivity, including blepharospasm, hemifacial spasm, and other abnormal movements.

BLEPHAROSPASM

Benign essential blepharospasm (BEB) is an idiopathic condition in which intermittent spasm of the orbicularis oculi occurs bilaterally. The unwanted spasms of eye closure can severely disable patients, making activities such as driving, ambulating, and reading difficult or impossible. This condition is most common in patients aged 40 to 60 years. BEB is thought to be related to dysfunction of the limbic (extrapyramidal) supranuclear facial motor system. *Meige syndrome* is blepharospasm associated with other facial movements such as grimacing, torticollis, and retrocollis.

Differential Diagnosis

Secondary blepharospasm can be caused by ocular surface disease. A careful slitlamp examination and evaluation of the tear film and cornea is therefore necessary in all patients with blepharospasm. Rarely, blepharospasm can be caused by intraocular inflammation or from meningeal irritation associated with intracranial lesions. Photophobia, regardless of the cause, may be the source of blepharospasm.

Blepharospasm can be a manifestation of tardive dyskinesia, resulting from neuroleptic drugs, and can occur in extrapyramidal disorders such as Parkinson disease, Huntington chorea, and basal ganglia infarction.

Treatment

Secondary blepharospasm is best addressed by treating the underlying disorder, if possible. Symptomatic photophobia can be treated with FL-41 tinted glasses as well as gabapentin, sometimes with remarkable success in reducing blepharospasm (see Figure 13–9).

Medical therapy for BEB is generally disappointing. Local injection of botulinum toxin (Botox) into the orbicularis oculi to weaken the muscle is a temporary but effective treatment for blepharospasm. The injection sites and the amount of drug injected can be titrated in individual cases. Repeat injections are necessary because the effect lasts only several months at best. Surgical procedures to weaken CN VII or to remove the orbicularis oculi are complex and fraught with complications.

HEMIFACIAL SPASM

Intermittent spasm involving the upper and lower face on one side is a hemifacial spasm (Figures 12–7 and 12–8). The condition can begin subtly, involving only the periocular muscles initially, but over time both the upper and lower face becomes involved. The spasms are intermittent and may abate or recur spontaneously. CN VII function is otherwise normal. Spasms can be reliably induced clinically by having the patient pucker his or her lips.

Causes

Most investigators agree that hemifacial spasm is caused by irritation and intermittent compression of CN VII by the anterior inferior cerebellar artery or other branches

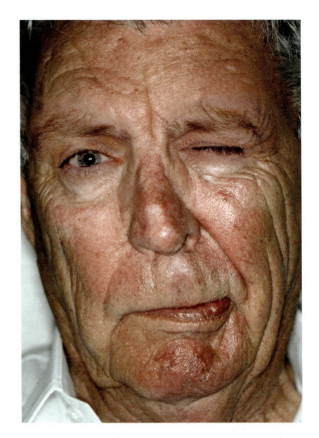

Figure 12–7. **Hemifacial spasm.** This photo illustration is representative of a 65-year-old man who developed hemifacial spasm following head trauma 20 years previously. Spasms involve the entire left side of the face (*pictured*). Between spasms, the facial asymmetry is mild.

of the basilar artery in the subarachnoid space. Trauma resulting in CN VII injury is a potential cause. Tumors or other lesions in the cerebellopontine angle may rarely cause hemifacial spasm and are usually accompanied by facial weakness or other neurological signs.

Differential Diagnosis

Hemifacial spasm can be differentiated from facial tics: Unlike hemifacial spasm, tics can be suppressed voluntarily for a period of time and typically begin in childhood. Focal epilepsy involving the face is rare and is usually followed by postictal facial paralysis (*Todd paralysis*).

Evaluation and Treatment

Patients with typical hemifacial spasm that has been present for several years may not require neuroimaging if they do not have any other associated neurological or ophthalmic signs and symptoms. Patients with hemifacial spasm who also have facial weakness must be imaged because this combination of signs is suggestive

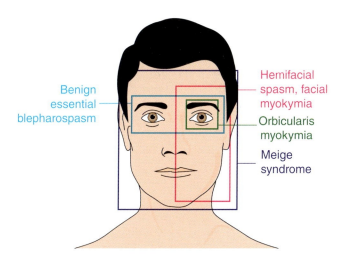

Figure 12-8. Facial spasms and hyperactive states.
The regions of the face involved in common facial spastic conditions are shown.

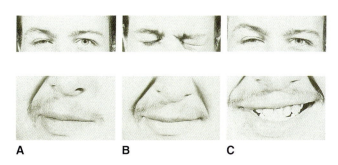

Figure 12-9. Spastic paretic facial contracture.
This patient has spastic paretic facial contracture with facial myokymia due to a brainstem glioma. The clinical photographs demonstrate how a contracture (hyperactivity) and paresis can be present at the same time. **(A)** *Spastic facial contracture* is evident on the right side. Note also the narrowed right palpebral fissure, elevated right eyebrow, and prominent right nasolabial fold. The contracture is continuous (not intermittent as seen in hemifacial spasm). **(B)** Paradoxically, the right side of the face is also *paretic*: The orbicularis oculi muscle on the affected side squeezes closed less completely on forced lid closure, and the patient is unable to "bury" the lashes on the affected side, whereas the lashes bury completely on the unaffected side. **(C)** A *paretic* right side is also demonstrated with smiling: The smile is asymmetric and the right nasolabial fold is less prominent than the left. (Courtesy Dr. James Corbett.)

of a compressive lesion such as a cerebellopontine angle tumor.

Medical treatment of hemifacial spasm has included baclofen, carbamazepine (Tegretol), clonazepam, and gabapentin (Neurontin), but is rarely helpful. Botulinum toxin injection is often effective, although repeat injections are required as with blepharospasm treatment. Neurosurgical exploration of CN VII root and placement of a sponge between CN VII and impinging vascular structures has been successful in many patients, but the surgical risks of suboccipital craniotomy (including stroke and deafness) must be considered.

FACIAL MYOKYMIA

Unlike the rapid jerking of hemifacial spasm, facial myokymia is a continuous, (usually) unilateral undulating and twitching movement of the facial muscles. The abnormal movement often seems to begin at a fixed point and then ripple across the face. This disorder may involve the orbicularis oculi muscles only initially, but over time tends to involve all of the unilateral facial muscles and is occasionally bilateral. In advanced cases, the myokymia progresses to a continuous tonic hemifacial contracture that is associated with facial paralysis. This condition is called *spastic paretic facial contracture and facial myokymia* (Figure 12–9).

Facial myokymia is generally caused by lesions immediately rostral to or involving the facial nucleus and its fascicles within the pons. The most common causes are multiple sclerosis in adults and pontine glioma in children or young adults. Facial myokymia has also been associated with extramedullary brainstem compression, brainstem infarction, a tuberculous abscess, Guillain-Barré syndrome, toxins, anoxia, and obstructive hydrocephalus. Neuroimaging is required in all patients with facial myokymia.

In most cases, the underlying cause cannot be definitively eliminated, but carbamazepine (Tegretol), baclofen, or clonazepam may offer limited symptomatic relief of the myokymia.

BENIGN EYELID MYOKYMIA

Benign eyelid (orbicularis) myokymia consists of an annoying unilateral twitching movement of the upper or lower eyelids, and is a common complaint in otherwise normal individuals. The twitching is rapid and episodic, lasting hours or even days at a time, and it does not involve any other portions of the face. Associated factors include stress, fatigue, and caffeine and nicotine use. This benign disorder can be differentiated from hemifacial spasm and blepharospasm by the lack of involvement of any other portion of the face or opposite eye (see Figure 12–8), by the absence of any other neurological or neuro-ophthalmic findings, and by its self-limited course.

▶ KEY POINTS

- Two supranuclear systems innervate the facial motor nucleus: (1) the corticobulbar pathway for voluntary facial movement originating in the precentral gyrus of the frontal lobe cortex, and (2) the *limbic (extrapyramidal pathway)* that controls involuntary and automatic facial movements.
- Corticobulbar axons serving voluntary movement of the lower face descend from the precentral gyrus and cross to innervate the contralateral facial nucleus; fibers representing the upper face are distributed to both the ipsilateral and contralateral facial nuclei.
- A unilateral hemispheric lesion produces a contralateral lower facial paresis with sparing of the upper face; facial nerve (CN VII) lesions tend to involve both the upper and lower face.
- Patients with disease involving the supranuclear corticobulbar pathway may not be able to smile or close their eyes on command, but periodic blinking or emotional facial responses may still occur.
- In diseases that affect the limbic (extrapyramidal) supranuclear facial pathways (eg, Parkinson disease), patients have a dull, expressionless face with weakness of emotional smiling, but can produce facial movement (a normal smile) on command.
- Hyperactivity of the extrapyramidal facial pathway produces Meige syndrome: blepharospasm with dystonic facial movements.
- The CN VII nucleus is located in the pons, inferior and lateral to the CN VI nucleus.
- CN VII fascicles loop over the CN VI nuclei before exiting the lateral pons, forming the facial collicului in the floor of the fourth ventricle.
- Fascicles from the superior salivatory nucleus (innervating the sublingual, submandibular, and lacrimal glands) form the nervus intermedius, which joins CN VII in the subarachnoid space.
- Important structures adjacent to the nucleus of CN VII in the pons include the cochlear nuclei, the spinal tract and nucleus of the trigeminal nerve (CN V), the CN VI nucleus, and the descending sympathetic fibers.
- In the cerebellopontine angle, CNs VII and VIII (and sometimes CNs V and VI) can be affected by meningiomas, acoustic neuromas, facial neuromas, and trauma.
- The facial nerve (CN VII) enters the temporal bone and travels for 3 cm in the fallopian (facial) canal: a complex Z-shaped passage through the temporal bone, particularly prone to trauma.
- The course of CN VII within the parotid gland gives rise to two potential etiologies for CN VII palsies: (1) parotid gland tumors that involve CN VII, and (2) trauma to CN VII during parotid gland surgery.
- Aberrant regeneration following CN VII injury is common and includes misdirection of fibers to facial muscles and misdirection of parasympathetic fibers (crocodile tears).
- Despite a rich blood supply, ischemia may be a common factor in CN VII palsies because the narrow confines of the bony fallopian canal can severely restrict perfusion in the presence of edema.
- Bell palsy is a common idiopathic facial paralysis (potentially related to HSV-1) with rapid onset and improvement beginning within 3 weeks of onset, but often with incomplete recovery.
- Herpes zoster oticus (Ramsay Hunt syndrome) causes a painful CN VII palsy; acutely, vesicles may be noted in any area supplied by sensory portions of CN VII. These patients often have severe postherpetic neuralgia.
- CN VII palsy is common in acute inflammatory demyelinating polyradiculopathy (AIDP), sarcoidosis, and trauma, and in infectious diseases such as Lyme disease, AIDS, and fulminant otitis media.
- Myasthenia gravis commonly affects the facial muscles, especially of the orbicularis oculi.
- Patients with profound orbicularis weakness, a poor Bell phenomenon, or decreased corneal sensation are at high risk for exposure keratopathy and its sequelae.
- Benign essential blepharospasm (BEB) is an idiopathic condition causing intermittent spasm of the orbicularis oculi bilaterally, thought to be related to dysfunction of the basal ganglia and limbic (extrapyramidal) supranuclear facial motor system.
- The differential diagnosis of blepharospasm includes ocular surface disease, tardive dyskinesia, and extrapyramidal disorders such as Parkinson disease, Huntington chorea, and basal ganglia infarction.
- Hemifacial spasm is intermittent spasm involving the upper and lower face on one side with otherwise normal CN VII function, usually caused by dolichoectatic vessels compressing or pulling on CN VII.
- Facial myokymia is a continuous unilateral undulating movement of the facial muscles associated with lesions involving the facial nucleus or fascicles within the pons.
- Benign eyelid myokymia is an irritating unilateral twitching movement of the upper or lower eyelids in otherwise normal individuals.

SUGGESTED READING

Books

Liu GT, Volpe NJ, Galetta SL: Eyelid and facial nerve disorders, in *Neuro-ophthalmology, Diagnosis and Management*, 2d ed. Philadelphia: Saunders Elsevier; 2010, Chapter 14.

Patel BCK, Anderson RL: Essential blepharospasm and related diseases, in *Focal Points: Clinical Modules for Ophthalmologists*. San Francisco, CA: American Academy of Ophthalmology; 2000, module 5.

Articles

Facial Palsies

Adour KK, Ruboyianes JM, van Doerston PG, et al: Bell's palsy treatment with acyclovir and prednisone compared with prednisone alone: a double-blind, randomized, controlled trial. *Ann Otol Rhino Laryngol* 1996;105:371–378.

Hughes RA, Cornblath DR: Guillain-Barré syndrome. *Lancet* 2005;366:1653–1666.

Rahman I, Sadiq SA: Ophthalmic management of facial nerve palsy: a review. *Surv Ophthalmol* 2007;52(2):121–144.

Schirm J, Mulkens PS: Bell's palsy and herpes simplex virus. *APMIS* 1997;105(11):815–823.

Sullivan FM, Swan IR, Donnan PT, et al: Early treatment with prednisolone or acyclovir in Bell's palsy. *N Engl J Med* 2007;357(16):1598–1607.

Hyperactivity of the Facial Nerve

Auger R, Peipgras D, Laws E: Hemifacial spasm: results in microvascular decompression of the facial nerve in 54 patients. *Mayo Clin Proc* 1986;61:650.

Ben Simon GJ, McCann JD: Benign essential blepharospasm. *Int Ophthalmol Clin* 2005;45(3);49–75.

Digre K, Corbett JJ: Hemifacial spasm: differential diagnosis, mechanism, and treatment. *Adv Neurol* 1988;49:151–176.

Grandas F, Elston J, Quinn N, et al: Blepharospasm: a review of 264 patients. *J Neurol Neurosurg Psych* 1988;51:767–772.

Mauriello JA, Coniaris H, Haupt EJ: Use of botulinum toxin in the treatment of one hundred patients with facial dyskinesias. *Ophthalmology* 1987;94:976–979.

SECTION IV

Additional Topics

Section IV addresses issues that do not fit easily into the categories defined by Sections I to III. Although pain syndromes and the trigeminal nerve (Chapter 13) are sensory (afferent) concerns, these topics deserve a forum separate from discussions of the optic nerve and sensory visual system. Neurovascular and neurocutaneous diseases (Chapter 14) affect both the afferent and efferent visual systems.

CHAPTER 13

Pain and Sensation

- ▶ THE TRIGEMINAL NERVE 303
  - Neuroanatomy 303
  - Clinical testing 304
  - Symptoms of trigeminal nerve dysfunction 305
- ▶ FACIAL NUMBNESS 305
- ▶ CAUSES OF FACIAL PAIN AND HEADACHE 306
  - Migraine 307
  - Tension-type headache 311
  - Cluster headache 311
  - Ocular causes of pain 311
  - Orbital and cavernous sinus disease 312
  - Giant cell arteritis 312
  - Intracranial disorders 312
  - Carotid dissection 313
  - Neurogenic pain 313
  - Sinus and dental disease 315
  - Pain of unknown origin 315
- ▶ PHOTOPHOBIA 315
- ▶ KEY POINTS 316

Given the ubiquitous (but mistaken) belief that headaches are usually caused by eye problems, ophthalmologists will see many patients with headache as the chief complaint. Therefore, the ophthalmologist needs to be familiar with common primary headache syndromes. The neurologist, on the other hand, has broad experience in the area of primary headaches, but needs to be well-versed in ocular, orbital, and other secondary causes of headache and face pain.

Pain and sensation from the eye and face, as well as intracranial structures, are mediated by the trigeminal nerve, which is directly or indirectly involved in all pain syndromes of neuro-ophthalmic interest. After exploring trigeminal neuroanatomy and its clinical implications, clinical conditions causing facial numbness, headache, and other head and ocular pain are discussed.

▶ THE TRIGEMINAL NERVE

NEUROANATOMY

The trigeminal nerve (cranial nerve [CN] V) is a mixed cranial nerve: In addition to its major sensory function, CN V provides motor innervation to the muscles of mastication. At its origin CN V does not contain autonomic fibers; however, parasympathetic innervation to the lacrimal gland and sympathetic fibers to the pupillary dilator travel briefly with peripheral segments of the nerve.

The trigeminal system also innervates cranial blood vessels (the trigeminovascular system), and in this role has the unusual ability to act as an effector as well as a sensor. Trigeminally innervated cranial blood vessels dilate after a nociceptive stimulus by way of chemical mediators released from the same *sensory* terminals that were activated by the stimulus; in this circumstance trigeminal nerves are serving as both the afferent and efferent limbs of a reflex. It is referred to as the *trigeminovascular reflex* and is believed to play an important role in the pathogenesis of primary headache syndromes such as migraine.

Nuclear Complex

The sensory portion of the trigeminal nucleus is markedly elongated and stretches from the midbrain to the upper cervical segments in the spinal cord where it blends with the root entry zone of the spinal cord (Figure 13–1). The trigeminal nucleus is a major sensory integration area and receives input from more than CN V; it has afferent connections with the somatosensory cortex above, with spinal cord afferents below, from the reticular formation and red nucleus, in addition to sensory input from other cranial nerves (CNs VII, IX, and X).

In the mesencephalon, the upper aspect of the nuclear complex (*rostral or mesencephalic nucleus*) receives proprioceptive and deep sensation afferents from the tendons and muscles of mastication. The pons contains the section known as the *principal (or chief) sensory nucleus,* serving light touch from skin and mucous membranes of the face. The lower extension of the nuclear complex is the *spinal nucleus* that receives pain and temperature afferents. The spinal nucleus is divided into segments that correspond to dermatomes that are

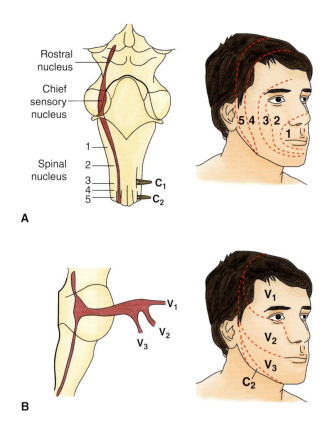

Figure 13–1. **Central and peripheral trigeminal representation of facial sensation.**
(A) The central organization of the trigeminal nucleus corresponds to dermatomes that are concentric around the mouth.
(B) The divisions of the peripheral nerve are represented by longitudinal bands across the face. Observe that the angle of the mandible is not innervated by the trigeminal nerve.

concentric around the mouth (see Figure 13–1A). This central representation of the face is different from the trigeminal nerve's peripheral distribution that divides the face into three longitudinal regions (see Figure 13–1B). Thus, the distribution of facial numbness or paresthesia is helpful in determining whether sensory deficits are central or peripheral in origin. For example, brainstem ischemia or demyelination is likely to cause concentric perioral numbness or paresthesia, whereas lesions affecting the peripheral nerve cause a band of numbness in the trigeminal nerve's cutaneous distribution.

Fibers from the chief sensory nucleus travel in the contralateral medial lemniscus to the ventral posteromedial nucleus of the thalamus. A smaller uncrossed projection also exists, as well as more diffuse pathways through the reticular formation.

The motor nucleus of CN V is medial to the chief sensory nucleus in the pons. Axons from the motor nucleus join the sensory fibers to form CN V and travel with the mandibular division of the nerve to innervate the muscles of mastication.

Peripheral Nerve

The trigeminal nerve enters the brainstem at the level of the pons from the gasserian ganglion. The *gasserian (or trigeminal) ganglion* is the point at which the ophthalmic, maxillary, and mandibular divisions of CN V converge (Figure 13–2). This structure relays sensory information from the three major divisions of CN V to the trigeminal nuclear complex. The gasserian ganglion is located in *Mekel cave*, a concavity in the base of the temporal bone, inferolateral to the sella turcica.

The *ophthalmic division* (V_1) extends through the cavernous sinus and the superior orbital fissure into the orbit, receiving sensory information from three branches: the frontal, lacrimal, and nasociliary branches (see Figure 13–2). The ophthalmic division and its branches carry sensation from the eye, upper eyelid, and forehead. The branches of the nasociliary nerve receive sensation from the eye, the skin on the tip and side of the nose, and the medial canthus. Vesicular eruption from herpes zoster ophthalmicus in these cutaneous areas is ominous because involvement of the nasociliary branch represents a serious threat to the eye.

A tentorial-dural branch joins the ophthalmic division in the cavernous sinus, receiving sensory innervation from much of the intracranial dura, arteries at the skull base, and major venous structures. It is understandable why pain from intracranial diseases is commonly referred to the eye and orbit, given the common sensory pathway through the ophthalmic division.

The *maxillary division* (V_2) passes through the inferior cavernous sinus for a variable extent, and extends through the foramen rotundum and then into the inferior orbital fissure, traveling in the infraorbital canal along the floor of the orbit (see Figure 13–2). The nerve and its branches receive sensory innervation from parts of the mouth, nasopharynx, teeth, and maxillary sinus, as well as the lower eyelid and cutaneous areas of the cheek. Blowout fractures of the orbital floor commonly damage the infraorbital nerve, resulting in numbness of the cheek and other areas supplied by this nerve.

The *mandibular division* (V_3) contains both sensory and motor components, exiting the skull ventrally through the foramen ovale in the floor of the middle cranial fossa (see Figure 13–2). Motor branches supply the muscles of mastication (Table 13–1). The sensory distribution includes the area of the mandible (but not the angle of the mandible), lower lip, tongue, and external ear.

CLINICAL TESTING

Testing pain and light touch over the face is best performed by having the patient compare one side of the face to the other, as discussed in Chapter 7. The corneal blink reflex consists of an involuntary

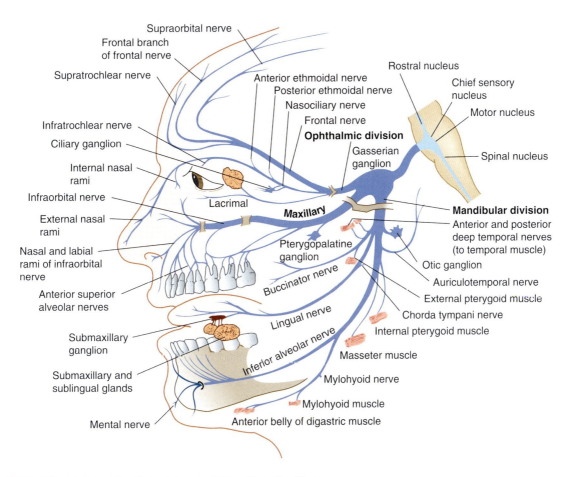

Figure 13–2. The trigeminal nerve and its distribution.
(Reproduced, with permission, from Waxman SG: *Clinical Neuroanatomy*, 26th ed. New York, NY: McGraw-Hill; 2010, Figure 8–11.)

bilateral blink in response to light touch to the cornea, and thus offers a more objective assessment of sensory function. The ophthalmic division of the trigeminal nerve provides the afferent limb. The efferent response is activation of both orbicularis oculi via the facial nerves. The test is performed by lightly touching the unanesthetized conjunctiva and corneal limbus of each eye in turn with a clean cotton-tip or tissue wisp, and by comparing the magnitude of the bilateral blink response (see Box 7–4).

The motor component of the trigeminal nerve is assessed by palpating and comparing the bulk of the masseter muscles on each side as the patient grits his or her teeth. Lateral pterygoid function is evaluated by having the patient push his or her jaw laterally against resistance, comparing each side. Weakness to one side suggests contralateral pterygoid weakness.

SYMPTOMS OF TRIGEMINAL NERVE DYSFUNCTION

Numbness and paresthesias are common symptoms of disorders that affect the trigeminal nerve or nucleus. Pain can also be caused by disorders of CN V, such as trigeminal neuralgia or herpes zoster ophthalmicus.

▶ FACIAL NUMBNESS

Facial numbness and paresthesias caused by disorders affecting the brain are usually accompanied by other significant neurological deficits. Thalamic lesions cause hemi-body and hemifacial numbness on the same side, while medullary lesions such as Wallenberg syndrome cause a crossed sensory loss, with facial numbness on the side opposite the body numbness. As discussed above and in Figure 13–1, the distribution of numbness and paresthesias on the face will show whether the lesion is central or peripheral.

The location of a lesion affecting the trigeminal nerve may be evident by concomitant signs and symptoms, such as ocular motor palsies from cavernous sinus or orbital apex lesions. Table 13–2 lists potential causes of decreased sensation from trigeminal nerve disorders by division.

Decreased corneal sensation from lesions affecting the ophthalmic division of the trigeminal nerve

TABLE 13–1. THE TRIGEMINAL NERVE AND ITS BRANCHES

Division	Major Branches	Terminal Branches	Areas Served
Ophthalmic (V$_1$)	Frontal	Tentorial-dural	Supplies much of the dura, including dural sinuses, falx cerebri, tentorium cerebelli, and other intracranial structures
		Supraorbital	Medial upper eyelid, conjunctiva, forehead, scalp, frontal sinuses
		Supratrochlear	Conjunctiva, medial upper eyelid, forehead, side of nose
	Lacrimal		Conjunctiva, skin over lacrimal gland (Parasympathetic fibers to lacrimal gland join this branch.)
	Nasociliary	Nasal nerves	Mucosa of nasal septum, lateral nasal wall
		External nasal	Nose tip
		Infratrochlear	Medial canthus: skin, conjunctiva, lacrimal sac
		Long ciliary	Ciliary body, iris, cornea (Sympathetic fibers to iris dilator join this branch.)
		Sensory root of ciliary ganglion	Globe
Maxillary (V$_2$)	Superior alveolar		Upper teeth, maxillary sinus, nasopharynx, tonsils, roof of mouth
	Infraorbital	Zygomaticofacial	Side of cheek
		Inferior palpebral	Lower eyelid
		Nasal	Side of nose
		Superior labial	Upper lip
Mandibular (V$_3$)	Motor branches		Pterygoid, masseter, temporalis
	Sensory branches		Mandible, lower lip, tongue, external ear, tympanum

Data from Glaser J: *Neuro-ophthalmology,* in Duane TO (ed): *Duane's Clinical Ophthalmology,* Vol. 2. Philadelphia, PA: Lippincott Williams & Wilkins; 1998.

---

can cause a *neurotrophic cornea*, a keratopathy that can progress to corneal ulceration, and ultimately to a blind, painful eye. The trigeminal nerve provides the afferent limb of the corneal blink reflex, and loss of this reflex can lead to corneal injury. In addition, trigeminal innervation is important in maintaining the tear film and corneal integrity. A neurotrophic cornea is notoriously difficult to manage, often requiring tarsorrhaphy, as treatment with topical lubricants alone is often not sufficient. This condition can occur in the setting of cerebellopontine angle surgery, or as a result of surgery to relieve trigeminal-mediated pain (such as a trigeminal rhizotomy for trigeminal neuralgia).

Numb chin syndrome (mental neuropathy) presents as isolated numbness of the chin and lower lip that respects the midline. This condition is caused by boney lesions affecting the mental foramen, which is the passage for terminal branches of the mandibular division of CN V. Numb chin syndrome is rare but deserves mention, because this syndrome is frequently caused by mass lesions, such as metastatic cancer.

▶ CAUSES OF FACIAL PAIN AND HEADACHE

Headaches are classified as *primary* (migraine, tension-type, and cluster) or *secondary* (eg, from ocular disease). The clues to a headache's origin may be revealed during a neuro-ophthalmic history and examination, even when the headache is not secondary to eye and orbit disease. A working knowledge of both primary and secondary headache syndromes is necessary to develop a differential diagnosis and make appropriate referrals when indicated. The history is particularly important when pain is the patient's chief complaint, because in many cases few physical findings are present (Table 13–3).

▶ **TABLE 13-2. DIFFERENTIAL DIAGNOSIS OF FACIAL NUMBNESS/PARESTHESIA IN THE DISTRIBUTION OF THE TRIGEMINAL NERVE**

Isolated corneal hypesthesia
Viral keratopathy
- Herpes simplex virus
- Herpes zoster

Ocular surgery
Cerebellopontine angle tumors
Dysautonomia
Congenital

Ophthalmic division
Neoplasm
- Orbital apex
- Superior orbital fissure
- Cavernous sinus
- Middle cranial fossa

Intracavernous aneurysm

Maxillary division
Orbit floor fractures
Maxillary antrum carcinoma
Perineural spread of skin carcinoma
Other neoplasm
- Foramen rotundum
- Sphenopterygoid fossa

Mandibular division
Neoplasm
- Nasopharyngeal tumor
- Middle fossa tumor

Skull base mass (often metastasis)
- Numb chin syndrome
- Numb cheek syndrome

All divisions affected
Neoplasm
- Nasopharyngeal carcinoma
- Cerebellopontine angle tumors
- Middle fossa or Meckel cave tumor
- Tentorial meningioma

Brainstem lesions (dissociated sensory loss)
Multiple sclerosis
Benign sensory neuropathy
Trigeminal neurofibroma
Toxins (trichloroethylene)

Data from Glaser JS. *Neuro-ophthalmology*. 2nd ed. Philadelphia, PA: Lippincott:1999:51-55.

▶ **TABLE 13-3. CLINICAL FINDINGS IN CONDITIONS CAUSING FACE AND HEAD PAIN**

LIKELY TO BE REVEALED BY THE EYE EXAMINATION

Ocular disease
  Local eyelid, conjunctival, and anterior segment disease
  Ocular inflammation
  Dry eye and tear deficiency syndromes
  Ocular ischemic syndrome
  Angle-closure glaucoma
Herpes zoster ophthalmicus
Orbital disease
Intracranial disorders causing papilledema, cranial neuropathies of CN II to VII

LIKELY TO BE REVEALED BY GENERAL OR NEUROLOGICAL EXAMINATION

Dural pain from tumors and infarction (often referred to the eye)
Medullary lesions
Sinusitis
Nasopharyngeal carcinoma
Dental disease and TMJ syndrome
Trigeminal neuralgia
"Salt and pepper" face pain
Herpes zoster
Giant cell arteritis (GCA)

LIKELY TO HAVE A NORMAL NEURO-OPHTHALMIC EXAMINATION

Asthenopia
Migraine
Cluster headache
Tension-type headache
Posttraumatic headache
Atypical facial neuralgias

Abbreviation: TMJ, temporomandibular joint.

MIGRAINE

Migraine headaches are common in the general population (15–18% of women; 5–6% of men), and there is a strong familial tendency. The term *migraine* is derived from Greek, *hemicrania*, describing the tendency of migraine headache to lateralize to one side of the head. The headache is frequently described as "throbbing" and is commonly associated with nausea, vomiting, photophobia, phonophobia, and osmophobia. Children may have episodes of abdominal pain (*abdominal migraine*) and night terrors as manifestations of migraine.

Migraine headache usually lasts 4 to 24 hours. Many individuals experience a period of fatigue for 24 to 48 hours following the headache. Rarely, individuals have a continuous headache lasting greater than 72 hours (*status migrainosus*).

Patients with migraine often have head or face pain for many years, but frequently deny having "migraine headaches," convinced that their pain is from sinus disease, allergies, or some other self-diagnosis. Migraine patients are more prone to experience motion sickness than individuals without migraine.

Migraine headaches in men and women typically begin in puberty and cease or change in character in women after menopause. Migraine headaches in some premenopausal women occur only during menses.

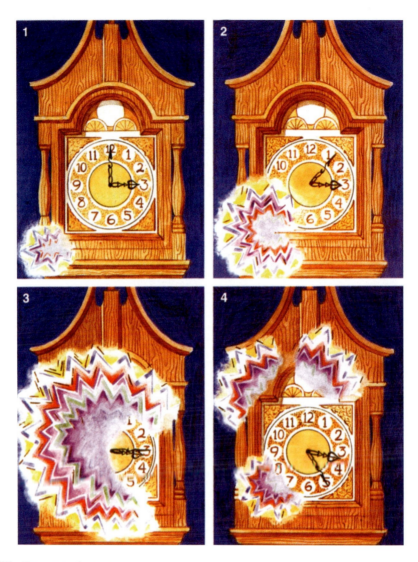

Figure 13–3. **Scintillating scotoma.**
The most common migraine aura is a *scintillating scotoma* (also called a *fortification spectra*): an expanding, angulated, advancing perimeter of shiny, often colorful lights (positive visual component), with a scotoma in its center (negative visual component). This illustration shows how it often starts as a small, angulated "c" shape (1) that enlarges over 20 to 30 minutes (2, 3) (note the time on the clock), eventually dissipating with clearing of the central scotoma (4). This phenomenon is homonymous, though this fact is not usually obvious to the patient. The onset of the migraine headache is usually after the aura has resolved. (Reproduced, with permission, from Hupp SL, Kline LB, Corbett JJ: Visual disturbances of migraine. *Surv Ophthalmol* 1989; 33:221–236.)

It has been suggested that migraine is caused by cerebrovascular constriction and dilation, but recent research has demonstrated a far more complex origin. Specific sites in the brain (such as the serotonin-rich raphe nuclei in the brainstem), circulating vasoactive agents (such as substance P), and other modulators of the trigeminovascular system play a role in the complex pathogenesis of migraine.

Migraine With Visual Aura

Approximately 20% of individuals with migraine have an aura of transient neurological dysfunction (<60 min duration) just before the onset of headache. Visual auras are the most common, originating from the occipital cortex. The visual aura is therefore a homonymous phenomenon that appears on the side opposite of the affected visual cortex. Visual auras can be positive (visual scintillations), negative (hemianopia, scotoma), or both. The classic *scintillating scotoma* consists of black and white or colored pulsating, jagged lines that begin as a small paracentral arc. Over the next 15 to 30 minutes, the angulated boundary enlarges and progresses toward the peripheral visual field, leaving a scotoma in its wake (Figure 13–3). The time course and evolution of this visual phenomenon reportedly corresponds to a slow, spreading wave of depression of activity over the surface of the occipital cortex (moving 3-5 mm/minute). Patients often do not understand the homonymous nature of the aura, and are often insistent that the aura occurred only in one eye (on the side of the homonymous visual phenomenon). Other common descriptions of migraine aura include a "heat wave" visual effect or a visual distortion similar to water running down a windowpane. A variably severe, unilateral, throbbing headache (on the side opposite the visual aura) usually follows.

Visual Aura Without Headache (Acephalgic Migraine)

Patients (usually >50 years) may describe a visual aura without headache, termed *acephalgic migraine*. Acephalgic migraine occurs more commonly in men than in women. Most patients have a previous history of migraine headaches with or without aura. The visual aura may be positive or negative and must be differentiated from amaurosis fugax or other causes of transient visual loss (Table 13–4, see Table 1–3).

Arteriovenous malformations of the occipital lobes can cause headache and incite a migraine-like visual aura. Magnetic resonance imaging (MRI) of the brain with gadolinium is indicated in patients whose visual phenomena are atypical in duration or progression, whose visual aura continue into the headache phase, who have other neurological signs and symptoms, or who have persistent visual field defects (Table 13–5). A visual aura that alternates sides is more likely to be caused by migraine rather than by an occipital lobe lesion (see Table 13–4).

Migraine With Other Aura

In addition to visual aura, migraine aura can manifest as transient focal neurologic dysfunction in a variety of

▶ **TABLE 13–4. CLINICAL EVIDENCE THAT SUPPORTS MIGRAINE AURA AS THE CAUSE OF TRANSIENT VISION LOSS**

Presence of a classic scintillating scotoma

Duration 5–45 min (occasionally longer)

Confirmation of the homonymous nature of the visual aura

Lack of other neurological signs and symptoms

Known history of migraine headaches

Family history of migraine

Normal visual fields

Homonymous aura has occurred on both right and left sides

▶ **TABLE 13–5. OMINOUS SIGNS AND SYMPTOMS IN A PATIENT WITH HEADACHE**

Abrupt onset	Acute hemorrhage into subarachnoid space (aneurysm), brain (AVM, hemorrhagic stroke), or brain tumor; posterior fossa mass with developing hydrocephalus; ischemic event (stroke, arterial dissection)
Relentless progression	Mass lesion, subdural hematoma
Systemic symptoms (fever, rash, neck stiffness, jaw or tongue pain)	GCA or other systemic vasculitis, collagen vascular disease, systemic infection causing meningitis or encephalitis
Focal neurological symptoms or signs	Stroke, brain tumor, AVM
Papilledema	Elevated ICP from brain tumor, IIH, hemorrhage, dural venous sinus thrombosis, meningitis, or encephalitis
Precipitated by cough, exertion, Valsalva maneuver, or rapid head/neck movements	Carotid or vertebral dissection, elevated intracranial pressure, brain tumor (especially with impending herniation), subarachnoid hemorrhage
Affected by postural changes	Conditions causing intracranial hypertension or hypotension
Onset during pregnancy and peripartum period	Idiopathic intracranial hypertension, venous sinus thrombosis, carotid dissection, pituitary apoplexy
New headache in patients with cancer, HIV, infectious diseases	Metastasis, opportunistic infection and lymphoma, or meningoencephalitis

Abbreviations: AVM, arteriovenous malformation; GCA, giant cell arteritis; HIV, human immunodeficiency virus; ICP, intracranial pressure; IIH, idiopathic intracranial hypertension. (Modified, with permission, from Kline LB: *Neuro-ophthalmology Review Manual*, 7th ed. Thorofare, NJ: SLACK; 2013:216.)

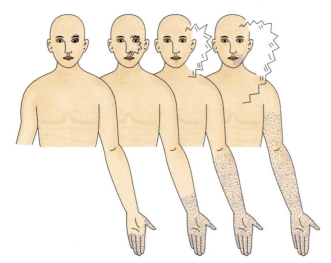

Figure 13–4. Cheiro-oral migraine.
This is a depiction of a patient who had simultaneous onset of a scintillating scotoma and *cheiro-oral* migraine (shown developing over time). Cheiro (Gr. *extremity*)-oral migraine is a migraine with a somatosensory aura consisting of spreading paresthesias of the face and upper extremity (*dotted areas*). Involved areas of the brain include the thalamus, parietal cortex, and brainstem, and these areas may show evidence of injury on neuroimaging. (Courtesy of Dutch Migraine Genetic Research Group.)

other ways. For example, patients with *ophthalmoplegic migraine* have a transient CN III palsy preceded by days of severe unilateral headache. On MRI, the affected CN III enhances with contrast. Another type is *cheiro-oral migraine*, characterized by numbness that starts in the fingers of one hand and ascends to the elbow, also involving the corner of the mouth on the same side (Figure 13–4). Hemiparesis, hemisensory loss, confusion, and transient global amnesia may also occur as migraine aura. Transient dysfunction of higher cortical visual areas may accompany migraine, resulting in *central achromatopsia* (loss of color vision), *prosopagnosia* (loss of face recognition), *alexia* (inability to read), or *transient global amnesia*. Children (and some adults) experience *Alice in Wonderland syndrome,* consisting of illusions with distortion in size and shape (macropsia, micropsia, and telopsia), particularly when going to sleep. Combinations of these manifestations may also occur. *Basilar-type migraine* is a form of complicated migraine affecting the brainstem and base of the hemispheres. Neurological dysfunction includes visual loss, diplopia, vertigo, tinnitus, hearing loss, dysarthria, ataxia, facial numbness, and altered consciousness.

In most cases, the neurological disturbances of the migraine aura develop gradually over 5 to 20 minutes and last for less than 60 minutes, but may persist for days (Figure 13–5), and rarely can be permanent from migrainous infarction.

Retinal or ocular migraine involves the retinal or choroidal vasculature and therefore produces a true monocular, rather than homonymous, visual disturbance. Episodes of transient monocular visual loss may last minutes to hours and may not be temporally related to headache symptoms. Patients with this condition are

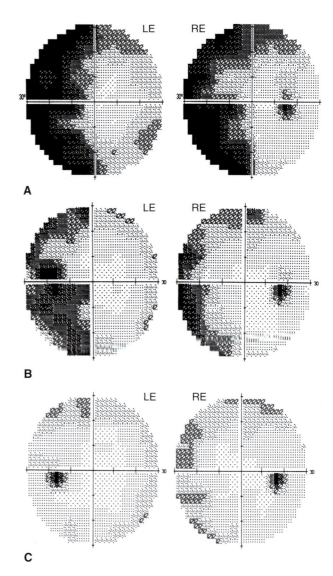

Figure 13–5. Persisting homonymous visual field defect with migraine.
A 43-year-old man with a history of migraine with aura had a particularly severe headache associated with left homonymous visual field loss. Unlike his typical visual aura, the visual loss in this case occurred at some point during the headache, was not associated with positive visual phenomena, and did not resolve quickly. Magnetic resonance imaging did not show a discrete infarct, but showed nonspecific, scattered ischemic changes. **(A)** Visual fields 1 day after onset demonstrate dense left homonymous visual field loss. **(B)** One week later the visual field loss was still present, but improved. **(C)** Within 2 weeks, the visual fields had almost normalized.

usually younger than 50 years and often have a history of other manifestations of migraine. Other causes of transient visual loss must be considered in the differential diagnosis. Severe or repeated events can cause permanent visual field defects from retinal artery occlusion or rarely from anterior ischemic optic neuropathy.

Migraine Treatment

Although the ophthalmologist plays an important role in the evaluation of patients with headache, the treatment of chronic headache should be referred to a neurologist or other headache specialist.

The treatment of migraine depends on how its manifestations interfere with the patient's life. Some patients are tolerant of their symptoms but are worried that their symptoms may indicate a serious disease. With these patients, a thorough evaluation and reassurance (when warranted) may be all that is wanted or needed.

In some cases, the patient may be able to *modify behavior* to alleviate headaches. Medications or toxins (eg, dipyridamole or smoking), or foods (eg, chocolate, alcohol, cheese) may trigger headaches. Many headache specialists advocate that patients keep a diary of their diet, activities, and headache symptoms to help discern precipitating or aggravating factors. Other nonpharmacologic measures include physical therapy and biofeedback.

The *medical treatment* of migraine headache comes in two forms: (1) *acute therapy* (also called abortive therapy) to help suppress a headache once it starts, and (2) *prophylactic therapy* to decrease the frequency, duration, and intensity of recurrent headaches. Medications used for acute therapy include barbiturate and narcotic analgesics, nonsteroidal anti-inflammatory drugs (NSAIDs; mainly naproxen sodium), ergot alkaloids, dihydroergotamine (DHE 45), and especially triptans (selective 5-HT$_1$ receptor agonists). Antiemetic and sedative medications, as well as local heat or ice are supportive measures. Prophylactic medications include beta blockers (propranolol, metoprolol), calcium-channel blockers (verapamil), low-dose nocturnal tricyclic antidepressants (amitriptyline, nortriptyline), serotonin agonists and reuptake inhibitors (trazodone), and anticonvulsants (valproic acid, topiramate, gabapentin).

TENSION-TYPE HEADACHE

Tension-type headache (muscle contraction headache, stress headache) causes a dull, steady pain often described as a band or vise around the head, and is reported to affect 80% of individuals. The muscles of the head or neck seem tight and may be tender to touch. Tension headache differs from migraine in that the pain with tension headache is dull rather than throbbing and is less severe; is more likely to be bilateral; and is usually not associated with nausea, vomiting, or photophobia. Tension-type headache can, however, trigger a migraine.

CLUSTER HEADACHE

Cluster headache is characterized by a sequence of abrupt-onset, short-lived episodes (60–90 min) of excruciating unilateral (side-locked) periorbital pain grouped temporally in "clusters." This type of headache is more common in men (6:1 male-to-female ratio) aged 20 to 50 years. Alcohol is a common trigger, and patients commonly have a history of cigarette smoking and peptic ulcer disease.

Typically, cluster headaches occur episodically over 2 to 3 months of the year, with lengthy symptom-free intervals. Unlike migraine sufferers, who seek a dark and quiet room for sleep, patients with cluster headache tend to pace restlessly around the room and hold the affected side of the head. The severe retro-orbital pain often occurs nocturnally, awakening the sufferer after 2-3 hours of sleep, and is characterized by accompanying ipsilateral autonomic signs: tearing, rhinorrhea, and conjunctival injection. The headache ends as abruptly as it begins and could be characterized as a "square-wave headache." A transient Horner syndrome on the affected side may also occur, which may become permanent with repeated bouts (see Figure 11–6).

Treatment is usually unsatisfying and only partially successful. Verapamil and lithium are used as prophylactic measures. Acute (abortive) treatments include oxygen inhalation, sumatriptan (subcutaneous or intranasal), DHE 45 (intranasal or intravenous), intranasal lidocaine, and oral corticosteroids.

Cluster headache is one type of *trigeminal autonomic cephalgia,* a category that includes the paroxysmal hemicranias, and SUNCT syndrome (short-lasting, unilateral, neuralgiform headache with conjunctival injection and tearing). Unlike cluster headache, paroxysmal hemicranias are more common in women, and are further differentiated from the other trigeminal autonomic cephalgias by a dramatic resolution with indomethacin.

OCULAR CAUSES OF PAIN

Although most headaches are not related to eye disease, the ophthalmologist can perform a valuable service by systematically looking for ocular disorders that can cause pain.

Ocular Diseases

It is important that acute glaucoma, uveitis (iritis, episcleritis, scleritis), ocular ischemic syndrome, ocular surface disease, and other ocular abnormalities be searched for in patients with pain in or around the eye. Intermittent or subacute angle-closure glaucoma may cause paroxysms of severe pain. During episodes, the patient's eye is red (perilimbal *ciliary flush*) and the vision is blurred. The eye examination may appear relatively normal between episodes, but a careful slitlamp examination and gonioscopy may reveal the diagnosis.

Eye Strain

Refractive errors, ocular misalignment, and other causes of "eye strain" may result in mild discomfort but are almost never the source of severe headache. The mild, bilateral, persistent ache above the eyebrow that can occur in these settings is often referred to as *asthenopia,* but the term means "weakness of vision" and so is not particularly meaningful or clinically useful. Such headaches are associated with extended and persistent visual tasks and do not occur immediately with a visual challenge. Latent hyperopia and convergence insufficiency are the most common causes of true eye-strain headaches. Patients with headache should have the benefit of a proper refraction, but corrective lenses are unlikely to have a significant effect on most common headaches.

ORBITAL AND CAVERNOUS SINUS DISEASE

Orbital cellulitis usually presents with impressive external findings proportional to the pain, but other infectious processes such as mucormycosis may have pain without notable clinical signs. *Idiopathic orbital inflammatory syndrome* (discussed in Chapter 8) causes pain, usually accompanied by a motility disturbance, proptosis, or ocular injection. However, the clinical spectrum of this disorder includes conditions that cause orbital or facial pain even in the presence of a "quiet" eye. *Myositis* is inflammation of one or more extraocular muscles, usually presenting with pain worsening on eye movement. *Trochleitis* is characterized by point tenderness over the trochlea in the absence of other orbital disease. The *Tolosa Hunt syndrome* is an idiopathic inflammatory disorder of the orbital apex or cavernous sinus, causing cranial nerve dysfunction and a painful ophthalmoplegia. Sarcoidosis and other granulomatous diseases can present in a similar manner (see Table 9–5).

GIANT CELL ARTERITIS

Giant cell arteritis (GCA) should always be considered in patients with new or different headache who are older than 50 years. As discussed in Chapter 4, GCA is a vasculitis, causing tenderness over involved arteries or ischemic regions of the scalp. Typically, the headache in GCA manifests as tenderness over the temporal area. Jaw claudication is commonly present and consists of pain in the jaw muscles with chewing caused by ischemia to these muscles. Other signs and symptoms include systemic weakness, malaise, and aches and pains of the proximal limbs. Prompt diagnosis and treatment are required to prevent blindness from anterior ischemic optic neuropathy or other ischemic events.

INTRACRANIAL DISORDERS

The headache from elevated intracranial pressure (ICP) is often worsened with coughing or Valsalva maneuver and is usually worse in the morning. Additional findings with elevated ICP include papilledema and occasionally CN VI palsies. *Idiopathic intracranial hypertension* typically occurs in young, obese women, and headache is often the presenting complaint. Other causes of elevated intracranial hypertension, such as intracranial tumor or venous sinus thrombosis, are usually evident with MRI of the brain (see Chapter 4).

Intracranial *hypo*tension can also cause headache, and is most commonly seen after a lumbar puncture. Obviously, persistent intracranial hypotension can be a complication of any procedure that violates the dura, but this condition can also occur spontaneously. The headache is worse when upright and improves with lying down. Diffuse enhancement of the dura can be seen on neuroimaging (Figure 13–6).

A severe, sudden headache may signal a *subarachnoid hemorrhage* (SAH) from a ruptured aneurysm. The pain is usually severe and abrupt in onset. Accompanying signs include changes in mental status and focal neurological signs such as cranial nerve palsies. A stiff neck is further evidence of blood in the subarachnoid space. This condition is a true emergency and requires immediate neurological and neurosurgical treatment in a hospital setting. A vitreous hemorrhage can occur with SAH (*Terson syndrome*) causing visual loss.

Acute *meningitis* causes severe headache that can be differentiated from primary headache by associated neurological symptoms. Photophobia, pain with eye movement, back pain, as well as neck stiffness and pain with neck flexion are findings suggesting meningeal inflammation. However, chronic meningitis (eg, cryptococcal meningitis) may present in an outpatient setting with chronic headache and papilledema, with few other neurological findings. Papilledema in patients with chronic fungal and tuberculous meningitis may be long standing, but should be treated as a neuro-ophthalmic emergency since the chronicity and severity of the optic disc edema has the potential to cause blindness.

Although the brain parenchyma does not have sensory (pain) innervation, the dura, venous sinuses, and the proximal intracranial vasculature do.

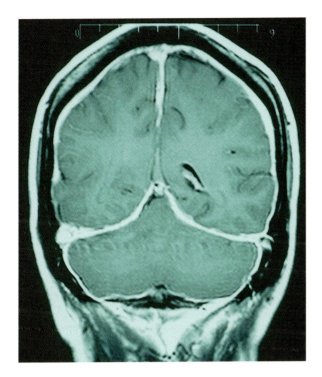

Figure 13–6. Dural enhancement from intracranial *hypo*tension.
A patient with a spontaneous cerebrospinal fluid leak presented with headache when sitting up or standing, relieved by lying down. Diffuse meningeal enhancement is seen in this magnetic resonance imaging scan of the brain (T1 sequence with contrast).

The tentorial-dural branch of the ophthalmic division of the CN V innervates much of the intracranial dura. Inflammation, neoplasm, or ischemia involving intracranial structures may cause pain, often referred to the ipsilateral eye, eyebrow, forehead, and orbit.

CAROTID DISSECTION

A carotid dissection occurs when a tear in the intima of the carotid artery allows blood to dissect into the arterial wall, narrowing the lumen. This condition is usually the result of trauma or traction injury to the neck, but may occur spontaneously in patients with degenerative vascular disease, fibromuscular dysplasia, Ehler-Danlos syndrome, and Marfan syndrome. The pain in an internal carotid dissection involves the face, neck, and retroauricular areas on the side of the injury and usually subsides within 3 to 4 days of onset. Pain may be the only symptom, but a postganglionic Horner syndrome is present in greater than 50% of cases. Additional neurological symptoms can occur from thrombosis and occlusion of the internal carotid and its branches or from thromboembolism, causing cranial nerve dysfunction, stroke, and transient ischemic attacks. MRI and magnetic resonance angiography (MRA) of the carotid system are often diagnostic, but arteriography may be required for a firm diagnosis.

Other conditions previously discussed that are associated with facial or ocular pain include pain with eye movement in optic neuritis and headache with microvascular cranial neuropathies.

NEUROGENIC PAIN

Herpes Zoster Ophthalmicus

Similar to herpes zoster (shingles) elsewhere in the body, herpes zoster ophthalmicus is caused by reactivation of latent herpes varicella-zoster virus (VZV). In this case, latent VZV residing in the gasserian ganglion is reactivated and travels along the first (ophthalmic) division of the trigeminal nerve to the tissues it innervates. Severe, burning pain occurs initially, followed several days later by a vesicular rash in the dermatomal distribution of the ophthalmic division of the trigeminal nerve (see Figure 13–1). The cause of the patient's pain may not be evident until the vesicular rash finally erupts. Rarely, a patient can have herpes zoster pain without the vesicles (so-called *herpes sine herpete*). Keratouveitis (with additional ocular pain) can occur when the nasociliary branch is involved. The significance of vesicles on the side of the nose or medial canthus in this regard was previously discussed. Herpes zoster can cause a local vasculitis which, in turn, can result in ocular motor cranial neuropathies (CNs III, IV, or VI) (Figure 13–7), or less likely an optic neuropathy or orbital myositis. Early intervention with antiviral medication (acyclovir, famciclovir) can significantly reduce the incidence and severity of ocular involvement. Prior to the availability of antivirals, ocular involvement frequently led to blindness and phthisis bulbi.

The severe pain from herpes zoster usually resolves in 1 to 2 weeks, but approximately 10% of patients develop *postherpetic neuralgia*: a deep, burning pain that persists after the vesicles resolve. In addition to chronic baseline pain, the patients develop a superimposed painful sensitivity to even the lightest touch. The persistent pain is difficult to manage and is usually accompanied by severe depression. Gabapentin (Neurontin), pregabalin (Lyrica), carbamazepine, or tricyclic antidepressants may be helpful. The risk of developing postherpetic neuralgia (and its intensity) can be reduced with early aggressive treatment of the acute episode with acyclovir or famciclovir. Adding corticosteroids to the antiviral regimen has also been advocated, but there is currently insufficient evidence of its efficacy and safety.

Reactivation of latent VZV infection is likely due to a transient failure in immune surveillance,

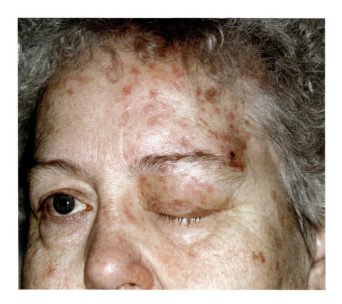

Figure 13–7. Third cranial nerve palsy following herpes zoster ophthalmicus.
A 71-year-old woman developed pain and vesicles in the distribution of the first division of the left trigeminal nerve. An acute, profound left third cranial nerve palsy occurred 2 weeks after the onset of pain, when the vesicles were healing. A complete ptosis is evident in this clinical photograph, along with the healing vesicles. (This patient's motility examination is shown in Figure 9–16.)

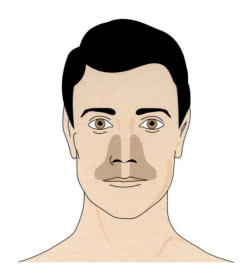

Figure 13–8. Trigeminal neuralgia trigger zones.
Patients with trigeminal neuralgia tend to "nurse" the regions around the nose (shaded areas). Although paroxysms of pain may be triggered when the regions are touched, patients alternately stroke and protect these areas.

so is more common in older patients, but can occur in younger patients who may be immunocompromised. A vaccine to boost immunity to VSV (recommended for patients >60 years) is effective in reducing the incidence of herpes zoster.

Neuralgias

Trigeminal neuralgia causes recurrent, excruciating, stabbing facial pain that lasts for seconds. The pain usually originates in the distribution of the maxillary or mandibular division of the trigeminal nerve and only rarely is confined to the ophthalmic division. Attacks of pain may be precipitated by activities such as eating and brushing teeth, or more commonly by touching certain areas of the face. Patients with trigeminal neuralgia protect these trigger zones from inadvertent contact, but peculiarly also tend to stroke and nurse these areas (Figure 13–8). Trigeminal neuralgia usually occurs in individuals older than 60 years. Most cases are idiopathic, but some are caused by vascular compression of the intracranial portion of the trigeminal nerve. The signs and symptoms of trigeminal neuralgia can also occur from multiple sclerosis (in patients 20 to 40 years) or from CN V compression by a posterior fossa mass, but unlike trigeminal neuralgia, these conditions are usually associated with abnormal facial sensation. Patients with trigeminal neuralgia should be evaluated with an MRI of the brain with gadolinium, with special attention to the posterior fossa. Medical treatment includes gabapentin, pregabalin, carbamazepine, baclofen, clonazepam, or valproate. In severe cases that are resistant to medication, rhizotomy or surgical decompression of the trigeminal nerve may be indicated. A serious condition called *anesthesia dolorosa* can occur as a complication of procedures used to treat trigeminal neuralgia. Damage to the trigeminal nerve causes partial or complete numbness, but also constant excruciating pain over the cheek and into the orbit that is recalcitrant to treatment.

Similar syndromes can occur involving other sensory nerves. *Glossopharyngeal neuralgia* causes paroxysms of pain in the larynx, the base of the tongue, the tonsil, and the ear and may be precipitated by swallowing; this condition can occur in multiple sclerosis (MS). *Greater occipital neuralgia* causes unilateral pain that begins in the occiput and may radiate to the eye.

Central Pain Mechanisms

Damage to the thalamus or trigeminal nucleus and its central projections can cause *thalamic or central pain*, referred to any part of the body. Although demyelination, neoplasms, or inflammation are potential causes, infarction of the thalamus (Dejerine-Roussy syndrome) or medulla (Wallenberg syndrome) are the most common causes. A rare but important pain syndrome characterized as "salt and pepper" facial and eye pain may be a premonitory symptom of lateral pontine ischemic infarction.

SINUS AND DENTAL DISEASE

Dental disorders involving the upper teeth can cause pain referred to the eye or upper face. Eating usually exacerbates the pain. *Temporomandibular joint (TMJ) syndrome* is pain in the jaw, ear, or face precipitated by jaw movement that is caused by derangement of the TMJ. Other findings may include tenderness over the joint on palpation (anterior to the tragus) and crepitus during jaw opening. TMJ and dental pain that occurs with eating is usually present as soon as chewing begins, whereas jaw claudication from GCA gradually develops over time as the patient chews.

PAIN OF UNKNOWN ORIGIN

In cases of unexplained eye or face pain, the physician should appreciate that the phenomenon of referred pain can cause diagnostic conundrums. It is worth repeating that intracranial diseases can refer pain *to the eye*, and such disorders should be considered in the differential diagnosis of eye pain when the eye examination is found to be normal. In addition, pathology far from the eye, such as cardiac ischemia and lung cancer, can refer pain to the face.

Some patients who complain of pain in the eye, face, or head do not have a definable diagnosis despite a thorough and extensive evaluation. Often termed *atypical face pain*, this diagnosis does not mean that the pain is not "real." Because most well-known pain syndromes do not exhibit objective findings, the physician has no objective way to differentiate psychogenic or functional pain from atypical manifestations of real disorders. Suspicion of a non-organic disorder may be raised when the pain or accompanying symptoms do not seem to be consistent with known anatomic or physiological principles. However, caution is urged because there are patients with atypical face pain who eventually are found to have disorders such as nasopharyngeal cancer, squamous cell carcinoma, or other serious disease.

The search for a diagnosis in the case of atypical facial pain is likely to involve a multidisciplinary team, including ophthalmologists, neurologists, dentists, otolaryngologists, and other specialists. Lack of a firm diagnosis after an appropriate evaluation does not preclude treatment. Such patients may require the services of a neurologist or an anesthesiologist with expertise in pain control.

▶ PHOTOPHOBIA

Photophobia is a common symptom. Although there may be a functional component in some patients, photophobia is a real symptom associated with real diseases, most commonly dry eye syndrome, migraine, depression, blepharospasm, and progressive supranuclear palsy (PSP) (see Table 1–6). Technically, photophobia is a broad term that encompasses a multitude of states in which there is an aversion to light, not all of which may be painful. For example, patients with posterior subcapsular cataract, central achromatopsia, or retinal cone dystrophy may avoid light because it makes their vision worse. However, most commonly, the term *photophobia* is used to describe light-induced eye pain. *Photo-oculodynia* has been suggested as a more accurate and specific label for *pain or discomfort from normally innocuous light*.

The neural pathways responsible for photophobia are complex. As discussed above, sensation from the eye and orbit is carried by the ophthalmic (V_1) portion of the trigeminal nerve. This is the pathway for painful stimuli (trauma, inflammation, ischemia) in this region. But what about light? There are no known trigeminal afferents in the retina. Likewise, the optic nerve makes no contribution to V_1. One possible pathway involves melanopsin-containing intrinsically photosensitive retinal ganglion cells (IPRGCs; unique in that they can detect light without any input from the photoreceptors) that project directly to thalamic nuclei associated with pain and somatosensation. Another pathway involves the visual afferents from the retina that follow the pupillary pathway to the olivary pretectal nuclei, and from there to the superior salivatory nucleus. The superior salivatory nuclei then activate parasympathetic efferents (trigeminoautonomic pathway) that evoke ocular vasodilation and activation of nociceptors on the blood vessels, transmitted as pain via V_1.

The evaluation and treatment of photophobia is shown in Table 13–6. The first step in evaluating photophobia is to identify any underlying central nervous system (CNS) or ocular disease. The history and examination may aid in diagnosing migraine or benign essential blepharospasm (BEB). Treatment of the inciting disorder whenever possible is obviously the most direct approach to treating photophobia. Light adaptation, lightly tinted lenses (FL-41 tint), and rarely medication (sedatives) may offer limited

▶ TABLE 13–6. CLINICAL EVALUATION AND MANAGEMENT OF PHOTOPHOBIA

Accompanying Signs/ Symptoms	Suspected Conditions	Evaluation	Treatment or Disposition
Eye pain, red eye, blurred vision	Dry eye, uveitis, keratopathy, blepharitis	Slitlamp examination, corneal staining, Schirmer testing. Photophobia may transiently improve with topical anesthetic or dilation during the examination.	Treat inflammation, dry eyes (topical lubricants, punctal plugs), blepharitis.
Bilateral excessive blinking, involuntary closure to light	Benign essential blepharospasm	Evaluate for inciting conditions: dry eye, keratopathy.	Botulinum toxin, medications, FL-41 tint in glasses.
Headache, phonophobia, nausea, vomiting; history of migraine	Migraine	Exclude other CNS causes. Screen for anxiety and depression.	Prophylactic and abortive treatment for migraine, FL-41 tint in glasses, antidepressants.
Focal neurological signs, visual field defects	Meningitis, PSP, other CNS disorders	Neuroimaging and other studies (lumbar puncture, laboratory studies).	Address underlying problem.
Poor vision, hemeralopia, nyctalopia	Cone dystrophy, retinitis pigmentosa	Electroretinogram, genetic studies.	Help patients understand why and how their vision is affected.

Abbreviations: CNS, central nervous system; PSP, progressive supranuclear palsy.

symptomatic relief of photophobia when a causative process cannot be identified or eliminated.

▶ KEY POINTS

- The trigeminal nerve (CN V) is a mixed nerve recieving sensory innervation from much of the head and face and providing motor innervation to the muscles of mastication.
- The distribution of facial numbness is helpful in determining whether trigeminal nerve lesions are central or peripheral.
- The ophthalmic, maxillary, and mandibular divisions of the trigeminal nerve converge to form the gasserian ganglion in Meckel cave before entering the brainstem.
- The ophthalmic division of the trigeminal nerve (V_1) carries sensation from the eye, upper eyelid, and forehead.
- Vesicular eruption from herpes zoster ophthalmicus on the tip or side of the nose or the medial canthus is worrisome because it implies involvement of the nasociliary branch of the ophthalmic division, which also supplies the eye.
- Because the tentorial-dural branch arises from the ophthalmic division, pain from intracranial diseases can be referred to the eye and orbit.
- The maxillary division of the trigeminal nerve (V_2) receives sensory innervation from the mouth, the maxillary sinus, and the lower eyelid and cutaneous areas of the cheek.
- Blowout fractures of the orbital floor commonly damage the infraorbital nerve, causing numbness of the cheek and other areas supplied by this nerve.
- The mandibular division of the trigeminal nerve (V_3) contains both sensory and motor components, supplying the muscles of mastication and serving sensation over the mandible, lower lip, tongue, and external ear.
- The corneal blink reflex consists of an involuntary bilateral blink in response to light touch to the cornea and thus offers an objective assessment of sensory function.
- The history is particularly important when pain is the patient's chief complaint, because in many cases few physical findings are present.
- The classic scintillating scotoma preceding a migraine headache consists of iridescent, pulsating, jagged lines that begin as a small paracentral arc and progress for 15 to 30 minutes in a homonymous fashion.
- Patients aged 50 to 70 years may report a migraine visual aura without headache, termed *acephalgic migraine*.

- Retinal or ocular migraine involves retina or choroidal vasculature, and therefore causes true monocular rather than homonymous visual disturbances.
- The manifestations of basilar artery migraine include visual loss, vertigo, tinnitus, hearing loss, dysarthria, ataxia, and altered consciousness.
- Treatment of migraine includes behavior modification to eliminate migraine triggers, daily prophylactic medications to reduce the frequency and intensity of migraine, and abortive therapies used once a headache has begun.
- Cluster headache is common in men aged 20 to 30 years and is characterized by a sequence of short episodes (60–90 min) of excruciating, unilateral pain grouped temporally in clusters.
- Tension-type headache differs from migraine in that the former is less severe, and pain is dull rather than throbbing, is more likely to be bilateral, and is usually not associated with nausea, vomiting, or photophobia.
- Refractive errors, ocular misalignment, and eye strain may result in a mild discomfort commonly called *asthenopia*; however, these conditions are almost never the source of severe headache.
- Acute glaucoma, uveitis, ocular surface disease, and other ocular abnormalities must be searched for in patients with pain in the eye, orbit, or head.
- The headache from elevated ICP is often made worse with coughing or Valsalva maneuver, and is often worse in the morning.
- The pain from carotid dissection can involve the face, neck, and retroauricular areas, and usually subsides within 3 to 4 days of onset; a postganglionic Horner syndrome is present in greater than 50% of cases.
- Herpes zoster ophthalmicus causes severe, burning pain followed several days later by a cutaneous vesicular rash in the distribution of the ophthalmic division of the trigeminal nerve.
- Approximately 10% of patients with herpes zoster (shingles) develop postherpetic neuralgia: a persistent, burning pain with a superimposed painful sensitivity to even the lightest touch, usually accompanied by depression.
- Trigeminal neuralgia is an idiopathic, recurrent, severe facial pain lasting seconds in the distribution of the maxillary or mandibular division of CN V, occurring in individuals over 60 years of age.
- When evaluating photophobia, possible underlying disorders must be considered, including CNS disease, ocular surface disorders, uveitis, retinal disorders, BEB, or migraine. Symptomatic treatment includes addressing any underlying disorders, consideration of FL-41 tinted spectacles, light adaptation, and rarely medication (sedatives).

SUGGESTED READING

Books

Liu GT: The trigeminal nerve and its central connections, in Miller NR, Newman NJ (eds): *Walsh and Hoyt's Clinical Neuro-ophthalmology*, Vol 1, 6th ed., Philadelphia, PA: Lippincott Williams & Wilkins; 2005:1233–1274.

Siberstein SD, Lipton RB, Dodick DW (eds): *Wolff's Headache and Other Head Pain*, 8th ed. New York, NY: Oxford University Press; 2007.

Van Stavern GP: Headache and facial pain, in Miller NR, Newman NJ (eds): *Walsh and Hoyt's Clinical Neuro-ophthalmology*, Vol 1, 6th ed. Philadelphia, PA: Lippincott Williams & Wilkins; 2005:1275–1311.

Articles

Bousser M-G, Biousse V: Small vessel vasculopathies affecting the central nervous system. *J Neuroophthalmol* 2004;24(1):56–61.

Conforto AB, Martin MG, Ciriaco JG, et al: "Salt and pepper" in the eye and face: a prelude to brainstem ischemia. *Am J Ophthalmol* 2007;144(2):322–325.

Corbett JJ: Neuro-ophthalmic complications of migraine and cluster headaches. *Neurol Clin* 1983;1:973–995.

Digre KB, Brennan KC: Shedding light on photophobia. *J Neuroophthalmol* 2012;32:68–81.

Goadsby PJ: Recent advances in the diagnosis and management of migraine. *BMJ* 2006;332(7532):25–29.

Goadsby PJ, Lipton RB, Ferrarai MD: Migraine—current understanding and treatment. *N Engl J Med* 2002; 346(4):257–270.

Harooni H, Golnic KC, Geddie B, et al: Diagnostic yield for neuroimaging in patients with unilateral eye or facial pain. *Can J Ophthalmol* 2003;121(11):1633.

Hupp SL, Kline LB, Corbett JJ: Visual disturbances of migraine. *Surv Ophthalmol* 1989;33:221–236.

Paven-Langston D. Herpes zoster: antivirals and pain management. *Ophthalmology* 2008;115(suppl 2):S13–S20.

Riley FC Jr, Moyer NJ: Oculosympathetic paresis associated with cluster headaches. *Am J Ophthalmol* 1971;72:763–768.

Sanchez-Del-Rio M, Reuter U, Moskowitz MA: New insights into migraine pathophysiology. *Curr Opin Neurol* 2006;19(3):294–298.

CHAPTER 14

Neurovascular and Neurocutaneous Diseases

- ► CEREBROVASCULAR DISEASE 319
  - Carotid disease 319
  - Vertebrobasilar disease 324
  - Arteriovenous malformation 325
  - Arterial-cavernous sinus fistula 325
  - Aneurysms 327
  - Dolichoectatic arteries 327
- ► NEUROCUTANEOUS SYNDROMES 327
- Neurofibromatosis 328
- Encephalotrigeminal angiomatosis (Sturge-Weber syndrome) 330
- Retinal angiomatosis (von Hippel disease) 330
- Ataxia telangiectasia (Louis-Bar syndrome) 331
- Wyburn-Mason syndrome 331
- Tuberous sclerosis (Bourneville syndrome) 332
- ► KEY POINTS 333

The topic of neurovascular diseases is a broad one, and a number of the disorders discussed in earlier chapters belong in this category. The goal of this chapter is not to be all-inclusive, but rather to discuss the mechanisms of vascular disease that commonly affect the visual system. Inclusion of the phakomatoses in this chapter is appropriate because many of these diseases have neurovascular manifestations.

► CEREBROVASCULAR DISEASE

The vascular supply of the brain consists of the carotid system anteriorly and the vertebrobasilar system posteriorly. The circle of Willis is an anastomotic complex (of variable completeness) formed by the junction of the two systems (Figure 14-1). Common ischemic manifestations of cerebrovascular disease include transient neurological deficits and stroke. Seizures can also occur as a result of ischemia.

A *transient ischemic attack* (TIA) is an episode of transient neurological dysfunction that lasts less than 24 hours. Most TIAs last less than 20 minutes. The 24-hour time limit in the definition of a TIA is an arbitrary boundary; neurological episodes may last longer than 24 hours and still be reversible. *Stroke* occurs when ischemic events are of sufficient magnitude or duration to cause infarction. Vascular disease can cause a TIA or stroke in the carotid or the vertebrobasilar distribution (Table 14-1), producing signs and symptoms that help to localize the ischemic area of the brain and implicate specific arteries that supply the affected territory.

CAROTID DISEASE

TIAs or completed strokes in the distribution of the carotid system frequently involve the eye (Table 14-2).

Causes of Carotid Insufficiency

Causes of carotid insufficiency include emboli from the internal carotid arteries or more distant sources, stenosis of the internal carotid artery, internal carotid artery dissection, and thrombotic or vasculitic occlusion of the smaller terminal vessels in the carotid distribution (see Table 14-1).

Emboli to areas supplied by the carotid arteries may arise from carotid artery atheromas or from a more proximal source, such as the aortic arch or heart. Valvular heart disease, atrial myxoma, cardiac arrhythmia, patent foramen ovale with right to-left shunt, carotid dissection, and antiphospholipid antibody syndrome are all potential sources of emboli in the carotid distribution.

Critical *stenosis* or occlusion of the internal carotid artery can cause neurological events from hypoperfusion. A significant reduction in distal flow generally requires 50% to 90% stenosis of the carotid artery. The redistribution of perfusion at the circle of Willis (see Figure 14-1) and other cerebral anastomotic connections may preserve function even with complete carotid occlusion, but TIAs or stroke can occur with even small fluctuations in blood pressure in this tenuous situation.

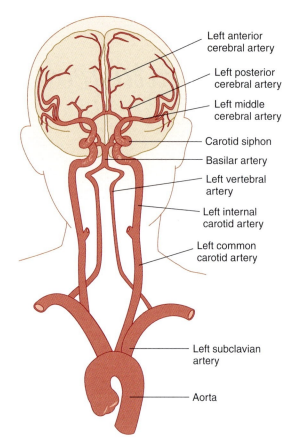

Figure 14–1. Cerebrovascular anatomy. The vascular supply to the brain consists of the carotid arteries anteriorly and the vertebrobasilar system posteriorly (see also Figure 5–11). (Reproduced, with permission, from Waxman SG: *Clinical Neuroanatomy*, 26th ed. New York: McGraw-Hill; 2010, Figure 12–1.)

Carotid dissection occurs when a break in the intimal lining of the carotid artery allows intraluminal blood to dissect into the arterial wall. The dissection can narrow the lumen, occlude branches in the area of the dissection, or produce emboli. Carotid dissection was discussed in Chapter 13. Arterial dissection can also occur in the basilar and vertebral arteries.

Thrombosis of the smaller distal supply arteries to the brain or eye can cause transient or permanent ischemic events. Damage to the small vessels from systemic hypertension (lipohyalinosis), vasculitis, and hypercoagulable states can lead to local occlusion from thrombosis (see Table 14–1). Subcortical lacunar infarcts and anterior ischemic optic neuropathy result from these thrombotic mechanisms rather than from emboli.

Signs and Symptoms

TIAs or stroke related to carotid disease manifest as *ipsilateral* monocular visual loss and/or *contralateral*

▶ **TABLE 14–1. MECHANISMS OF CEREBROVASCULAR ISCHEMIA**

EMBOLI
Atheromatous disease of any proximal artery
- Platelet-fibrin
- Cholesterol (Hollenhorst plaque)

Cardiac
- Atrial fibrillation, acute myocardial infarction
- Calcific emboli from diseased valve
- Septic emboli from bacterial endocarditis
- Atrial myxoma embolization
- Right-to-left shunts (paradoxical emboli)

Other
- Fat
- Amniotic fluid
- Coagulopathies

LARGE VESSEL STENOSIS
Atherosclerotic disease
Fibromuscular dysplasia
Arterial dissection
Congenital malformation

HYPOPERFUSION
Cardiac insufficiency
Massive blood loss
Anaphylaxis

SMALL VESSEL ATHEROTHROMBOSIS
Atherosclerosis
Hypercoagulable states
Hyperviscosity syndromes

VASOSPASM
Subarachnoid hemorrhage
Migraine

VASCULITIS

VENOUS THROMBOSIS
Hypercoagulable states
Hyperviscosity syndromes

▶ **TABLE 14–2. MANIFESTATIONS OF ISCHEMIA IN THE CAROTID DISTRIBUTION**

OPHTHALMIC ARTERY
Ocular ischemic syndrome, ophthalmic artery occlusion, PION

Posterior Ciliary Arteries
AION (not likely to be embolic)

Central Retinal Artery and Branches
CRAO, BRAO

MIDDLE CEREBRAL ARTERY
Contralateral hemiparesis, clumsiness, numbness, paresthesias, and aphasia

Abbreviations: AION, anterior ischemic optic neuropathy; BRAO, branch retinal artery occlusion; CRAO, central retinal artery occlusion; PION, posterior ischemic optic neuropathy.

hemiparesis, clumsiness, numbness, paresthesias, and aphasia (see Table 14-2).

Transient monocular visual loss (TMVL, also called *amaurosis fugax*) is a TIA involving the retinal circulation. Visual loss can occur as a result of emboli to the central retinal artery or its retinal branches, or when hypoperfusion results from high-grade carotid stenosis. Patients often describe visual loss as a curtain or shade that is pulled over the vision from above or below, or as a more generalized dark cloud obscuring vision. The visual loss usually reaches its greatest extent before 30 seconds, and usually resolves in less than 5 minutes (range: 2-30 min). Other causes of transient visual loss are listed in Table 1-3.

Emboli to the central retinal artery and its branches can often be seen and identified with the ophthalmoscope and include cholesterol (Hollenhorst plaque), fibrin, or platelet material originating from carotid atheromatous ulcerations, and less commonly calcific emboli from cardiac valves or fat emboli from long bone fracture.

Hollenhorst plaques are cholesterol crystals that appear similar to mica flakes on ophthalmoscopy. They appear as shiny, refractile orange-yellow crystals slightly larger than the blood column, lodged at bifurcations in the retinal arterial tree (Figures 14-2 and 14-3). Because they are flat, they do not always occlude the vessel and may be asymptomatic.

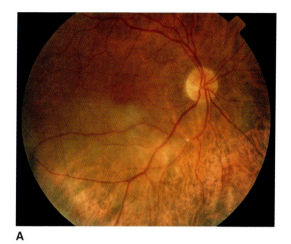

A

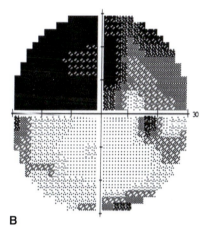

B

Figure 14-3. **Branch retinal artery occlusion.** A 62-year-old woman reported a sudden change in the vision of her right eye. **(A)** An embolus is seen, lodged at a bifurcation in the inferior vascular arcade. Retinal edema can be seen in the distribution of the occluded retinal artery. **(B)** Humphrey automated perimetry shows a superior altitudinal defect (mimicking an optic nerve-related visual field defect).

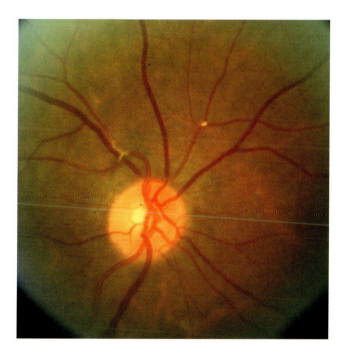

Figure 14-2. **Retinal emboli.** Two types of retinal emboli can be seen in this fundus photograph of a right eye: a fibrin-platelet embolus straddling the bifurcation of the superior temporal arteriole and a Hollenhorst plaque lodged at the trifurcation of a superior nasal arteriole.

Fibrin-platelet emboli form a dull, white material that fills the lumen and occludes the arterioles, causing transient visual loss or retinal infarct. This toothpaste-like material can occasionally be seen in long strands, slowly snaking through the retinal arterial tree (see Figure 14-2). Hollenhorst plaques and fibrin-platelet emboli typically originate from atheromatous disease of the carotid arteries or the aortic arch.

Calcific emboli are dull-white discrete emboli that suggest a cardiac source, such as a diseased valve. *Fat emboli* can occur in patients with long bone and flat bone fractures or with pancreatitis. Other retinal embolic sources include septic vegetations from bacterial endocarditis, cardiac myxoma, and amniotic fluid.

Transient monocular visual loss in patients <40 years old is unlikely to be related to atherosclerotic disease. Potential causes include cardiac abnormalities (right-to-left shunts, valvular disease), retinal migraine (see Chapter 13), or hypercoagulable states (see Table 4–4).

Central retinal artery occlusion (CRAO) produces sudden, profound, painless visual loss. Acutely, the retinal arteries are narrowed, and the infarcted retina is pale and edematous. Sludging and "box car" formation (separation of red blood cell clumps with intervals of plasma) may be evident in the retinal vessels. Because no inner retinal layers are present over the foveola, this area does not swell and the normal color of the intact choroidal circulation creates the characteristic foveolar "cherry red spot" surrounded by pale retina (see Figure 6–4). If there is a portion of the retina supplied by a cilioretinal vessel (arising from the choroidal circulation), it will be spared (Figure 14–4). An embolus can be seen in the central retinal artery at the disc in 10% to 20% of patients. Retinal edema generally dissipates over several days, and over time the disc develops a mild diffuse pallor along with global nerve fiber layer dropout, and the narrowed arteries may display sheathing.

The most common mechanism of a CRAO is atheroembolism. The emboli usually arise from a carotid source, but the heart, aortic arch, or other distal sites can be sources of emboli. Giant cell arteritis is a possible cause in patients older than 50 years and must be an urgent consideration (directed history, erythrocyte sedimentation rate, and C-reactive protein) because failure to diagnose this condition early can result in bilateral blindness. In addition, localized atheromatous stenosis, vasospasm, hypoperfusion, and hypercoagulable states can cause a CRAO.

The prognosis for visual recovery following an embolic central retinal artery occlusion is poor. Studies demonstrate irreversible retinal damage after 60 to 100 minutes of occlusion. Therapies aimed at lowering the intraocular pressure (IOP) (glaucoma medications, paracentesis) in the acute setting to increase the perfusion gradient have a sound theoretical basis but are rarely effective. Other modalities (usually equally disappointing) include ocular massage to dislodge emboli and carbogen therapy.

Branch retinal artery occlusion (BRAO) results when emboli lodge in the more distal parts of the retinal arterial tree, resulting in a focal retinal ischemic event with a corresponding focal visual field defect (see Figure 14–3). Similar to CRAO, emboli are the most common cause, but retinal vasculitis and ophthalmic migraine are other possible mechanisms.

Ophthalmic artery occlusion may be difficult to differentiate from a CRAO. However, a "cherry red spot" is not present because the choroidal circulation is also affected. This entity is far more likely than CRAO to cause NLP (no light perception) or LP (light perception) vision.

Ocular ischemic syndrome is produced when chronic hypoperfusion of the eye occurs. This condition is usually the result of vascular occlusive disease of the carotid artery or aortic arch, where few collateral arterial anastomoses are present. Unlike embolic events, the signs and symptoms are slow in onset (Table 14–3) and may be confused with other ocular disorders.

Venous stasis retinopathy (VSR) is a manifestation of carotid occlusive disease characterized by dot and blot hemorrhages and venous engorgement. The relationship between retinal venous changes and carotid insufficiency is unclear, but the cause is most likely related to ischemia at the microvascular

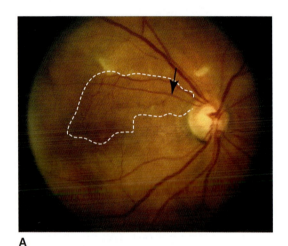

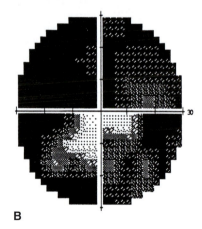

Figure 14–4. **Central retinal artery occlusion with cilioretinal artery sparing.**
(A) Retinal ischemia and edema are present throughout the fundus except for an area of the macula (enclosed by *dotted line*) supplied by a cilioretinal artery (*arrow*). **(B)** The visual field shows sparing of a portion of the visual field corresponding to the distribution of the cilioretinal artery and unaffected retina.

▶ **TABLE 14-3. OCULAR ISCHEMIC SYNDROME**

SYMPTOMS
Chronic eye pain and poor vision

SIGNS
Anterior Segment
- Conjunctival injection
- Corneal edema
- Aqueous flare
- Iris ischemia with atrophy and iridoplegia
- Neovascularization of the iris
- Cataract
- Low IOP (ciliary body ischemia)
- High IOP (neovascular glaucoma)

Fundus
- Midperipheral dot-blot retinal hemorrhages
- Microaneurysms
- Neovascularization
- Vitreous hemorrhage
- Venous engorgement
- Low perfusion pressure measured with ophthalmodynamometry
- Decreased filling and increased transit time on IVFA

Abbreviations: IOP, intraocular pressure; IVFA, intravenous fluorescein angiography.

---

level. The retinal findings may be confused with diabetic retinopathy or central retinal vein occlusion.

Curiously, carotid occlusive disease seems to have a protective effect with regard to the development of hypertensive and diabetic retinopathy: Retinal disease is less severe on the side ipsilateral to severe carotid stenosis. Long-standing unilateral carotid occlusive disease can also "protect" the cornea from deposits of serum lipids, hence a unilateral corneal arcus suggests carotid stenosis on the side without the arcus.

Patients with poor ocular perfusion may describe transient visual loss following exposure to a bright light, similar to a persistent afterimage following flash photography. This symptom likely results from an inability of the retina to quickly recover metabolically because of ischemia. These patients would be expected to have a markedly abnormal photo-stress test (discussed in Chapter 2).

Evaluation and Treatment

Carotid stenosis often produces an audible bruit, but this finding lacks sensitivity and specificity. Patients with total or near-total occlusion do not have a bruit (because there is little or no flow), and patients with bruits may have little or no carotid occlusion.

Carotid duplex ultrasound permits a noninvasive assessment of the extracranial carotid arteries. In skilled hands, this method is reasonably sensitive and specific. *Transcranial Doppler* uses ultrasound methods through specific acoustic windows in the skull to evaluate intracranial arteries but is less precise than carotid duplex studies. *Magnetic resonance angiography (MRA)* (see Figure 1–13) allows visualization of both extracranial and intracranial cerebral blood flow without injection of contrast material (though contrasted studies provide the best resolution). *Computed tomography angiography* (CTA) combines intravascular contrast injection with 3-D imaging, providing exquisite views of the vasculature and surrounding anatomy (see Figure 1–14).

However, at present, catheter cerebral angiography remains the gold standard for evaluation of the carotid arteries and the intracranial vessels. As discussed in Chapter 1, the procedure is invasive, requiring the insertion of an intravascular catheter and injection of contrast material, and is not without risk.

Carotid endarterectomy is the surgical removal of thrombus and stenotic material from the carotid lumen, restoring distal flow. The procedure has been shown to reduce the risk of stroke in patients with symptomatic atherosclerotic carotid stenosis who have a 70% to 99% carotid artery occlusion (Box 14–1). However, stroke is one of the potential risks of the procedure. Obviously, endarterectomy is helpful only if the risk of the procedure is less than the risk of stroke without surgical intervention. Currently, endarterectomy is considered an option for patients with symptomatic high-grade stenosis if performed in a medical center with a complication rate of less than 3%. Other factors, such as the patient's general medical health and age, are important in surgical decision making.

Many patients who are symptomatic from carotid embolic disease do not have significant carotid stenosis; surgical therapy may not be an option. Medical therapy includes antiplatelet agents (aspirin, dipyridamole-aspirin [Aggrenox], clopidogrel [Plavix]) and anticoagulants (Coumadin) to reduce the formation of emboli within the diseased carotid arteries.

The diagnosis of an ischemic process affecting the eye is often the "tip of the iceberg," and the ophthalmologist needs to be aware of the systemic implications. The risk of additional cerebrovascular events requires neurological or neurosurgical consultations. Patients with cerebrovascular disease are very likely to have coronary artery disease (which is the major cause of death in patients with cerebrovascular disease). Risk

> **BOX 14–1. CAROTID ENDARTERECTOMY: CLINICAL TRIALS**

The North American Symptomatic Carotid Endarterectomy Trial (NASCET, 1991) and the European Carotid Surgery Trial (ECST, 1995) compared medical treatment to carotid endarterectomy (CEA) in patients with symptomatic carotid stenosis (retinal or hemispheric transient ischemic attacks [TIAs]). Both studies showed that CEA was better than medical therapy in reducing the risk of ipsilateral stroke if the stenosis was severe (≥70% occlusion), but the benefit was not clear for moderate occlusion (50–69% occlusion).

In the subgroup of patients in the NASCET study who had transient monocular visual loss (amaurosis fugax), the risk of stroke was approximately 10%, regardless of the degree of carotid stenosis, However, the presence of additional risk factors for stroke suggested some benefit for CEA including male gender, age greater than 75 years, previous hemispheric TIAs or stroke, intermittent claudication, carotid stenosis of 80% to 94%, and absence of collateral vessels on angiography.

The complication rate for CEA in the NASCET study was 2.1%, but patients older than 80 years and those with severe concomitant systemic illnesses were excluded from this study. The decision to perform carotid endarterectomy must weigh the potential benefit of the surgery against the risk of the procedure.

factors such as diabetes mellitus, hypertension, hyperlipidemia, and cigarette smoking need to be evaluated by the patient's general medical physician. Also the potential systemic adverse effects of treatments, such as the risk of bleeding with anticoagulants, need to be considered in the initial treatment plan and monitored long term.

VERTEBROBASILAR DISEASE

The vertebrobasilar system (posterior cerebral circulation) is comprised of the paired *vertebral arteries* that merge to form the midline *basilar artery*, and distal branches including the posterior cerebral arteries (see Figure 14–1).

Causes of Vertebrobasilar Insufficiency

Similar to carotid artery disease, atheromatous disease in the vertebrobasilar system can result in emboli, or hypoperfusion from stenosis or thrombosis, causing TIAs or completed strokes (see Table 14–1). Emboli from other sources, such as the heart, and disorders of cardiac output can affect areas in the distribution of the vertebrobasilar system. Other causes of hypoperfusion in the vertebrobasilar system include migraine, vasospasm, hyperviscosity syndromes, hypercoagulable states, congenital malformations, subclavian steal syndrome, and vertebral or basilar artery dissection. Vertebral artery occlusion can occur from cervical trauma and has been reported following chiropractic manipulation of the cervical spine.

Signs and Symptoms

The basilar artery and its branches supply the brainstem and the vast majority of the primary visual cortex (via the posterior cerebral arteries). Transient or persistent motility disturbances and visual field defects are therefore common symptoms of vertebrobasilar disease.

Transient visual loss from vertebrobasilar insufficiency (VBI) is bilateral and usually briefer than transient monocular visual loss from carotid disease (usually lasting 1 minute or less), described by patients as blurred or "out-or-focus" vision. Other transient neurological symptoms (Table 14–4) commonly occur. Completed strokes are usually the result of emboli. Infarctions in the distribution of the posterior cerebral arteries frequently produce homonymous visual field defects without other neurological deficits ("silent stroke").

Brainstem ischemia can result in transient or lasting motility disturbances from a variety of causes: cranial

> **TABLE 14–4. SIGNS AND SYMPTOMS OF VERTEBROBASILAR INSUFFICIENCY**

Transient binocular visual loss (usually <1 min)
Homonymous hemianopia
Diplopia (supranuclear palsies, INO, rarely infranuclear)
Nystagmus and oscillopsia
Ataxia, imbalance, staggering
Vertigo
Tinnitus and deafness
Vomiting
Dysarthria
Dysphagia
Hemiparesis and hemiplegia
Hemisensory disturbances
"Drop attacks"
Headache
"Salt and pepper" facial pain

Abbreviation: INO, internuclear ophthalmoplegia.

nerve nuclei or fascicle involvement, horizontal or vertical gaze palsy, internuclear ophthalmoplegia (INO), or skew deviation. Nystagmus and central Horner syndrome can also occur.

Evaluation and Treatment

Vertebrobasilar atherosclerotic disease is often diagnosed based on clinical signs and symptoms in patients with known systemic atherosclerosis. Transcranial Doppler, MRA, and MRI are helpful ancillary studies. Because no surgical therapies are available for most patients, cerebral angiography is performed in only unusual cases, such as when subclavian steal syndrome is suspected. Antiplatelet therapy and anticoagulants are the main medical therapies.

Similar to carotid atheromatous disease, the presence of vertebrobasilar disease is evidence of more widespread vascular disease. The patient's general medical physician will need to address this larger problem in addition to the cerebrovascular disease by evaluating underlying systemic risk factors such as hypertension, diabetes, hypercholesterolemia, and cigarette smoking. These patients are more likely to have a myocardial infarction rather than a stroke as their major ischemic risk.

ARTERIOVENOUS MALFORMATION

Arteriovenous malformations (AVMs) are a developmental anomaly in which arteries and veins communicate directly without an intervening capillary bed. The tangle of blood vessels can cause signs or symptoms by exerting a mass effect on neighboring structures, by "stealing" arterial blood and causing ischemia, or by bleeding into the subarachnoid space or brain parenchyma. Seizure is a common presenting sign. Hemorrhage in the subarachnoid space causes sudden, severe headache with a stiff neck and depressed consciousness.

Not all AVMs become symptomatic. Those that do are most likely to present in patients in their 20s and 30s. Systemic hypertension, trauma, or coagulopathies may be important cofactors causing an AVM to become symptomatic.

Occipital lobe AVMs can cause occipital lobe seizures which present as unformed visual hallucinations that may be similar to the scintillating scotoma of migraine. However, an occipital AVM rarely fully mimics the timing and progression of the visual aura of classic migraine, especially the tendency of migraine to alternate side to side (see Table 13–4). In any case, patients with scintillating scotomas that are exclusively one-sided and that have features atypical for migraine may need to have neuroimaging to evaluate the possibility of an AVM.

Hemorrhage into the occipital lobe from an AVM causes severe headache and a homonymous visual field defect. An expanding hematoma from a bleeding supratentorial AVM can cause brain herniation.

Brainstem AVMs can cause internuclear ophthalmoplegia, skew deviations, and gaze palsies. These brainstem capillary angiomas are typically small and are better visualized with MRI than cerebral angiography.

AVMs that drain directly into the dural sinuses (*dural AVMs*) can cause elevation of the intracranial pressure by directly elevating superior sagittal sinus venous pressure or by causing dural sinus thrombosis (see Figure 4–17). These AVMs may not be visible with standard MRI. MRA and magnetic resonance venography (MRV) offer a more sensitive perspective, but selective cerebral angiography is currently the most sensitive and descriptive method of imaging dural AVMs. An occult dural AVM should be especially considered when intracranial hypertension without identifiable cause occurs in men or nonobese individuals.

The treatment of nonbleeding AVMs is controversial. The natural history of AVMs is difficult to know because asymptomatic individuals with AVMs do not come to medical attention. Options include observation, intravascular embolization techniques, direct surgical excision, and combined intravascular/surgical excision techniques.

ARTERIAL-CAVERNOUS SINUS FISTULA

The cavernous sinus is a unique intracranial structure because it is a dural venous sinus that surrounds the internal carotid artery. Arterial-cavernous sinus fistulas occur when high-pressure arterial blood communicates directly with the venous spaces constituting the cavernous sinus or its venous tributaries. There are two forms of arterial-cavernous sinus fistulas: direct (high-flow) fistulas and indirect (low-flow or dural) fistulas.

Direct carotid-cavernous sinus fistulas are produced when direct communication occurs between the high-pressure intracavernous carotid artery and the cavernous sinus. Direct fistulas are usually the result of trauma but rarely can arise from rupture of an intracavernous aneurysm. Because the venous drainage from the eye and orbit normally flows into the cavernous sinus, a carotid-cavernous sinus fistula causes sudden orbital vascular engorgement, often with high-pressure arterial blood reversing the normal venous flow in the superior ophthalmic vein. Signs and symptoms include the sudden onset of pulsatile exophthalmos, pulsatile bruit, conjunctival injection, and chemosis. The episcleral and conjunctival vessels become "arterialized," developing a peculiar corkscrew appearance

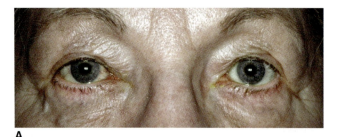

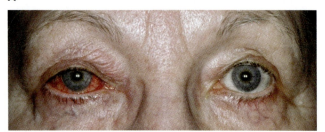

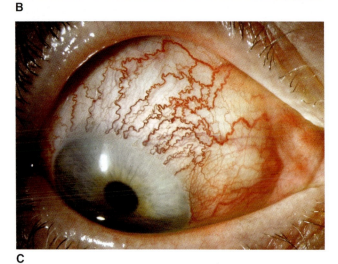

Figure 14–5. **Carotid-cavernous sinus fistula.** A 61-year-old woman complained of 4 months of horizontal double vision and 1 month of a red right eye. Angiography eventually revealed a right carotid-cavernous sinus fistula. **(A)** On presentation the right eye was minimally injected. **(B)** Two weeks later, conjunctival injection was prominent. **(C)** The conjunctival vessels are dilated and tortuous ("corkscrew" vessels) and characteristically extend to limbus as shown.

(Figure 14–5). Ophthalmoplegia occurs from ischemia and compression of the intracavernous cranial nerves or is caused by mechanical restriction imposed by engorged extraocular muscles. Elevated episcleral venous pressure can cause elevated IOP often with blood visible in Schlemm canal on gonioscopy. Central retinal vein occlusion can also occur. Posterior drainage through the superior and inferior petrosal sinuses may produce facial pain and a sixth cranial nerve palsy. Signs and symptoms may be bilateral (or contralateral) even when the fistula is unilateral because the right and left cavernous sinuses are anatomically connected across the diaphragm sellae.

Indirect or dural-cavernous sinus fistulas are abnormal communications between the smaller meningeal arterial branches of the internal or external carotid system and the cavernous sinus. These smaller vessels are "slow-flow" relative to the direct fistulas, and the signs and symptoms are slower to develop and usually less severe. Not uncommonly, patients may present with only conjunctival injection initially, which may be confused with chronic conjunctivitis or orbital Graves disease. Proptosis, only rarely pulsatile, may be absent or slight. Cranial nerve (CN) VI palsies often occur because this cranial nerve and an engorged inferior petrosal vein share the confines of Dorello canal (see Chapter 8). Indirect fistulas are associated with hypertension, collagen vascular disease, and atherosclerosis, and occur most commonly in postmenopausal women.

Signs suggestive of a direct or indirect carotid-cavernous sinus fistula with CT or MRI include a dilated superior ophthalmic vein, enlargement of the cavernous sinus or its intracranial connections, and mild symmetric enlargement of the extraocular muscles. Orbital ultrasound and MRA are also useful diagnostic tools. Cerebral angiography may be required if the diagnosis is uncertain or if intravascular treatment is anticipated. Selective injection of both the internal and external carotid artery on both sides is required to fully define the potential feeder arteries in indirect fistulas, even when the signs are unilateral. The risks of angiography must be weighed against potential benefits in each patient.

Unlike direct fistulas, up to 50% of patients with indirect dural-cavernous fistulas have spontaneous resolution, sometimes as a result of spontaneous cavernous sinus thrombosis. Spontaneous resolution may occur after diagnostic angiography.

Because spontaneous resolution can occur, indirect carotid-cavernous fistulas with tolerable symptoms may not require treatment. Treatment indications for the ophthalmic manifestations of both direct and indirect fistulas include progressive visual loss from venous stasis retinopathy or intractable glaucoma, exposure keratopathy from proptosis, unrelenting pain, or persistent diplopia. The treatment of carotid-cavernous fistulas is complex. Current techniques involve the use of arteriographically guided intravascular materials to embolize or thrombose vessels participating in the fistula. The goal is to close the fistula by obliterating the arterial feeder vessels. In some cases, causing thrombosis of the cavernous sinus or interconnecting venous structures is the only option. The placement of detachable balloons in the cavernous sinus is a treatment option in some direct fistulas. The risk of stroke and other neurological deficits from intravascular intervention must be weighed against the anticipated benefit of treatment and the natural course of the disease.

ANEURYSMS

Aneurysms are saccular outpouchings at weak points in the intracranial arterial system. Because of their appearance, they are also called *berry aneurysms*. Aneurysms typically form at arterial branch junctions, where the media of the arterial wall may be poorly developed. Because these aneurysms are thought to form as the result of a developmental abnormality, they are sometimes called congenital aneurysms, but they are not present at birth. Other factors associated with the formation of aneurysms include systemic hypertension, elastic tissue disorders such as Ehlers-Danlos syndrome, and polycystic kidney disease.

Progressive enlargement of an aneurysm can compress adjacent structures and produce clinical findings similar to any space-occupying intracranial mass. Rupture of an aneurysm is usually cataclysmic because blood under arterial pressure enters the subarachnoid space or ventricles, or dissects into the brain parenchyma.

Most saccular aneurysms arise at arterial junctions in the circle of Willis. Of these, 50% involve the anterior communicating artery, with 50% distributed evenly between the posterior communicating, internal carotid, and middle cerebral arteries. Although *anterior communicating artery* aneurysms are the most common, they rarely produce focal neurological signs before rupture. Aneurysms that arise at the origin of the *posterior communicating artery* can compress CN III, causing a CN III paresis and periocular pain (see Figure 9–11B). The importance of pupillary involvement in differentiating a compressive CN III palsy from an ischemic mononeuropathy was discussed in Chapter 9 (see Figure 9–14). Recognizing the signs and symptoms of a posterior communicating artery aneurysm is particularly important because this is one of the few situations when patients are symptomatic *before* an aneurysm ruptures. Following rupture of an aneurysm, the mortality is 50%, but the outcome is dramatically better when an aneurysm is diagnosed and treated before rupture. Posterior communicating artery aneurysms are often evident with MRI and MRA, and CTA, but cerebral angiography is currently the mainstay of diagnosis. Neurosurgical treatment includes a direct approach via craniotomy, or interventional radiological catheter techniques (eg, coiling).

Carotid-ophthalmic artery aneurysms can compress the adjacent intracranial optic nerve, resulting in slow, progressive visual loss. These aneurysms occur more commonly in women than in men and are often bilateral.

Aneurysms arising from the *intracavernous carotid artery* tend to slowly enlarge within the cavernous sinus, causing compression of CNs III, IV, V_1, and VI. CN VI is often the first nerve affected because it does not travel with the other cranial nerves in the relative protection of the lateral wall of the cavernous sinus. Rarely, superior extension of the aneurysm can cause visual loss from optic nerve compression. Pain is common but may not occur until late. As discussed above, the rare occurrence of an intracavernous aneurysm rupture results in a carotid-cavernous fistula, rather than a subarachnoid hemorrhage.

Giant aneurysms typically arise from the supraclinoid portion of the intracranial carotid artery. These aneurysms produce symptoms primarily from a mass effect, causing slowly progressive visual loss from compression of the chiasm or optic nerves.

The diagnosis of intracavernous and giant aneurysms can often be made with CT/CTA or MRI/MRA. Cerebral angiography currently offers the best definition and permits the use of intravascular techniques for treatment.

Less than 15% of intracranial aneurysms arise in the *vertebrobasilar system*. The vast majority of these aneurysms arise at the bifurcation of the basilar artery. In most cases, these aneurysms are asymptomatic unless they rupture. Occasionally, an aneurysm at the basilar bifurcation may become large enough to compress the brainstem or involve the third cranial nerves in the subarachnoid space before rupture.

DOLICHOECTATIC ARTERIES

Dolichoectasia is the development of atherosclerotic enlargement and tortuosity of arteries in the carotid or vertebrobasilar system. Dolichoectatic arteries (sometimes called *fusiform aneurysms*) are more common in men than in women and are associated with hypertension, atherosclerotic cardiovascular disease, abdominal aortic aneurysms, and advanced age. Dolichoectatic arteries cause symptoms by compression of adjacent structures and by vascular occlusion.

Fusiform enlargement of the intracranial carotid arteries can compress the optic nerves and cause slowly progressive visual loss with optic nerve pallor. Dolichoectasia of the basilar artery is common and can compress the brainstem or cause traction of the cranial nerves within the subarachnoid space. Slowly progressive multiple cranial neuropathies with long-tract motor and sensory signs can occur. Hemifacial spasm can result from compression or traction of CN VII by neighboring arteries. Some cases of trigeminal neuralgia are the result of vascular compression of the trigeminal root-entry zone by tortuous adjacent arteries.

▶ NEUROCUTANEOUS SYNDROMES

At least six neurocutaneous syndromes, or *phakomatoses*, are recognized. These multisystem disorders are characterized by hamartomas of skin, eye, central nervous system (CNS), and viscera (Table 14–5). A *hamartoma* is an abnormal tissue proliferation of

▶ TABLE 14–5. NEUROCUTANEOUS SYNDROMES

Disease Type	Inheritance Pattern	Skin	Eye	CNS	Other Findings
NF1 (von Recklinghausen disease)	Autosomal dominant (chromosome 17), complete penetrance	Café-au-lait, axillary/inguinal freckling, neurofibromas	Lisch nodules, plexiform neurofibromas of eyelid, retinal astrocytomas, congenital glaucoma	Optic nerve and chiasm gliomas; multiple tumors of brain, spinal cord, meninges, and nerves	Pheochromocytoma, osseous defects including dysplasia of the greater wing of the sphenoid
NF2	Autosomal dominant (chromosome 22)	As for NF1	Early cataract	Bilateral acoustic neuromas, other tumors	
Encephalofacial angiomatosis (Sturge-Weber)	Sporadic	Nevus flammeus in trigeminal distribution	Choroidal hemangioma, congenital glaucoma	Leptomeningeal hemangioma	
Klippel-Trenaunay-Weber	Sporadic	As for Sturge-Weber	As for Sturge-Weber	Intracranial angiomas	Somatic hemihypertrophy of limbs or digits
Angiomatosis retinae (von Hippel and von Hippel-Lindau)	Autosomal dominant (chromosome 3) or sporadic		Retinal capillary angioma	Cerebellar hemangioblastoma; brainstem and spinal cord angioma	Renal, pancreatic, hepatic, epididymal cysts; pheochromocytoma, renal cell carcinoma, and visceral angiomas
Ataxia telangiectasia (Louis-Bar syndrome)	Autosomal recessive (chromosome 11)	Cutaneous telangiectasia	Conjunctival telangiectasia	Cerebellar ataxia, gaze palsies	Thymic hypoplasia (IgA deficiency), malignant lymphoma, and leukemia
Wyburn-Mason syndrome	Sporadic		Racemose retinal angioma, orbital AVMs	AVMs in midbrain, frontal lobes, posterior fossa	AVMs of maxilla, pterygoid fossa, and mandible
Tuberous sclerosis (Bourneville syndrome)	Autosomal dominant (chromosome 9)	Adenoma sebaceum, periungual fibromas, café-au-lait spots, ash-leaf patches	Astrocytic hamartomas of the optic nerve and retina	Periventricular (brain stones) and cortical astrocytic hamartomas (seizures)	Cardiac rhabdomyomas, renal cysts, angiomyolipomata, and pulmonary fibrosis/cysts

Abbreviations: AVMs, arteriovenous malformations; CNS, central nervous system; IgA, immunoglobulin A.

normal-appearing mature cells, forming a mass that consists of elements that are normally found at the site. A hamartoma is not a neoplasm because it is a *malformation* of tissues, rather than a *transformation* of previously normal tissue.

An understanding of the neurocutaneous syndromes is important for two reasons: (1) These conditions may be first discovered on an eye or neuro-ophthalmic examination, and the examiner must know the significance of the findings and the importance of a systemic evaluation and appropriate consultations. (2) Patients with these diagnoses may require lifelong surveillance because of the risk of developing associated ophthalmic, neurological, or systemic complications over time.

NEUROFIBROMATOSIS

Neurofibromatosis is characterized by multiple neurofibromas, pigmented skin lesions, osseous malformations, and a propensity for tumors. *Neurofibromas* are benign hamartomas occurring as individual cutaneous fibroma molluscum on the face and body or as confluent cordlike *plexiform neurofibromas* on the eyelid. Multiple cutaneous pigmented macules (*café-au-lait spots*) are characteristic (Figure 14–6). Additional

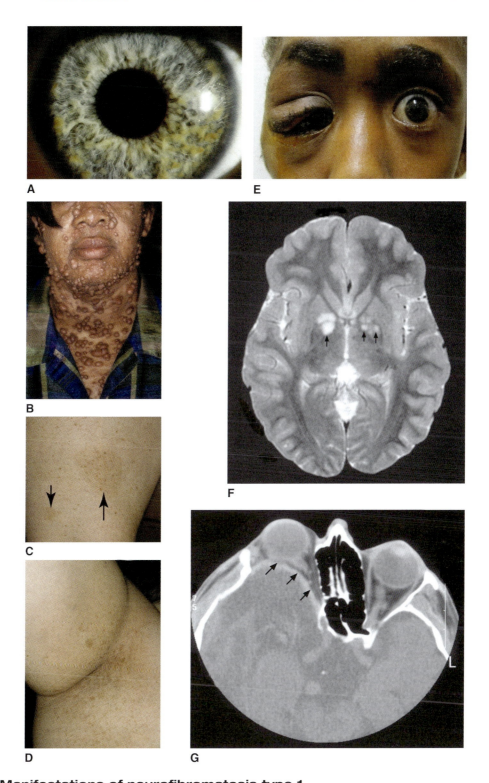

Figure 14–6. **Manifestations of neurofibromatosis type 1.**
Findings in patients with neurofibromatosis type 1 (NF1) are illustrated. **(A)** Iris Lisch nodules are present in virtually all adult patients with NF1. They are yellow-brown splotches that appear to be "stuck-on" the iris surface. **(B)** Cutaneous neurofibromas. **(C)** Café-au-lait spots. Two can be identified in this photograph (*arrows*), a large one on the right and a smaller patch on the left. **(D)** Axillary freckling (same patient as in **C**). **(E)** Plexiform neurofibroma of the right upper eyelid causing an S-shaped deformity. **(F)** Magnetic resonance imaging (axial T2-weighted image) shows neurofibromas in the thalamus and basal ganglia (*arrows*). This is the same patient with the optic nerve glioma in Figure 4–27. **(G)** Axial computed tomography scan of aplasia of the greater wing of sphenoid (*arrows*). This bony defect can result in pulsatile exophthalmos as the normal pulsations of brain are directly transmitted to the orbital contents. (**E** courtesy of Andrew Ting; **G** courtesy of RP Yeatts.)

clinical features define two genetically and clinically distinct types of neurofibromatosis: NF1 and NF2.

NF1 (von Recklinghausen neurofibromatosis) is an autosomal dominant disorder associated with chromosome 17. In addition to neurofibromas (see Figure 14–6B, E) and café-au-lait spots (see Figure 14–6C), the disorder is characterized by multiple tumors of brain, spinal cord, meninges, and peripheral nerves (see Figure 14–6F). Osseous abnormalities of the vertebral bodies or long bones and defects in the greater wing of sphenoid occur. The latter bony defect can result in an orbital encephalocele that may present as either an orbital mass or a pulsating exophthalmos (see Figure 14–6G).

Gliomas of the optic nerve or chiasm and meningiomas affecting the visual system are common in NF1 (see Figure 4–27). Additional ocular manifestations include congenital glaucoma, retinal astrocytomas, and iris (Lisch) nodules (see Figure 14–6A). Lisch nodules are both sensitive and specific for this disorder, occurring in greater than 95% of patients older than 6 years with NF1.

NF2 is an autosomal dominant disorder associated with abnormalities on chromosome 22, defined by the presence of bilateral acoustic (CN VIII) neuromas (schwannomas). Patients typically present as young adults with hearing loss (acoustic component of CN VIII), nystagmus (vestibular component of CN VIII), and/or facial weakness (compression of adjacent CN VII). Approximately 60% of patients have café-au-lait spots or neurofibromas. Other CNS tumors are rare, and Lisch nodules are not present. Juvenile cataracts are common in patients with NF2.

ENCEPHALOTRIGEMINAL ANGIOMATOSIS (STURGE-WEBER SYNDROME)

Sturge-Weber syndrome is characterized by a congenital unilateral cutaneous "port-wine stain" angioma (nevus flammeus), that approximates the distribution of the trigeminal nerve, and ipsilateral hemangiomas of the eye and brain (Figure 14–7). Leptomeningeal hemangiomas in the parietal-occipital area (usually ipsilateral to the port-wine stain, but can be bilateral) are common and cause seizures, contralateral hemiparesis, homonymous hemianopia, and learning disabilities. Calcification of the cortex under these hemangiomas gives a characteristic "railroad or tram track" appearance on CT neuroimaging.

Choroidal hemangiomas also occur. These lesions may be small and discrete or involve the entire uveal tract, giving the fundus a characteristic "tomato ketchup" appearance. Visual loss may result from an exudative maculopathy or retinal detachment. Glaucoma can develop at any point in the course of this disorder, due to iris/angle abnormalities and elevated episcleral venous pressure. The risk of glaucoma is greatest when the facial hemangioma involves the upper eyelid.

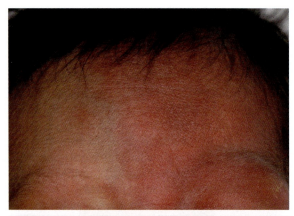
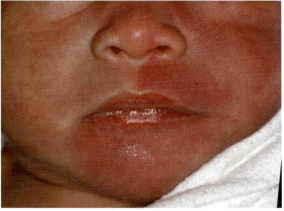

Figure 14–7. Sturge-Weber syndrome. This child with Sturge-Weber syndrome has an extensive unilateral facial hemangioma (nevus flammeus). This photograph demonstrates that although the lesions are generally in the distribution of the trigeminal nerve, they may cross the midline somewhat. (Courtesy of RG Weaver Jr.)

Klippel-Trenaunay-Weber syndrome is likely a variant of Sturge-Weber syndrome with additional characteristics including orbital and retinal varicosities and hemihypertrophy of limbs or digits.

RETINAL ANGIOMATOSIS (VON HIPPEL DISEASE)

Retinal angiomatosis is characterized by multiple retinal capillary angiomas, which are bilateral 50% of the time. The ophthalmoscopic appearance ranges from small vascular lesions of the disc or retina to fully developed angiomas with an enlarged feeder artery and draining vein (Figure 14–8). Because the lesions develop over time, patients with known or suspected retinal angiomatosis must have regular retinal examinations their entire lives. An exudative maculopathy, retinal detachment, proliferative retinopathy, and/or neovascular glaucoma may contribute to visual loss. Retinal angiomatosis may be an autosomal dominant or a sporadic condition.

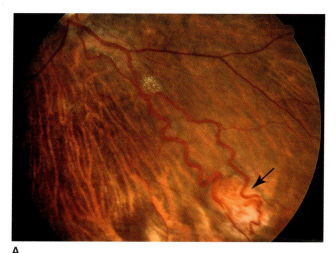

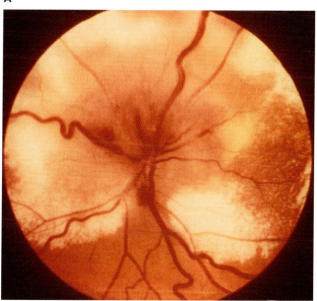

Figure 14–8. **Retinal angiomatosis (von Hippel disease).**
(A) Well-developed retinal lesions in this disorder appear as a discrete retinal angioma (*arrow*) with an enlarged feeder artery and draining vein, as seen in this photograph. **(B)** Retinal angiomas can cause an exudative retinopathy with severe visual consequences, as seen in a different patient with retinal angiomatosis. Note the retinal detachment above the optic disc and extensive subretinal and intraretinal exudates.

Cerebellar hemangioblastomas occur in approximately 25% of patients with von Hippel disease, and their presence changes the clinical designation to von Hippel-Lindau disease (VHL, or retinocerebellar angiomatosis). Hemangioblastomas in the brainstem and spinal cord can also occur. Other lifelong sporadically occurring manifestations of angiomatosis retinae include pheochromocytoma, renal cell carcinoma, and renal, pancreatic, hepatic, and epididymal cysts.

VHL is an autosomal dominant condition resulting from a mutation in the VHL tumor suppressor gene on chromosome 3.

ATAXIA TELANGIECTASIA (LOUIS-BAR SYNDROME)

Patients with ataxia telangiectasia usually present with progressive ataxia in childhood. Additional defining characteristics include conjunctival and skin telangiectasias. Oculomotor apraxia (loss of ability to generate saccades) is a common finding that frequently progresses to total ophthalmoplegia. Patients with ataxia telangiectasia have thymic hypoplasia and immunoglobulin A (IgA) deficiency, and as a result are susceptible to infection, particularly to frequent and often severe respiratory infections. Malignant lymphoma and leukemia are also associated with ataxia telangiectasia. The genetic defect is on chromosome 11, and the inheritance pattern is autosomal recessive.

WYBURN-MASON SYNDROME

Wyburn-Mason syndrome is a rare sporadic congenital condition with unilateral retinal and ipsilateral intracranial AVMs. The hallmark of Wyburn-Mason syndrome is the *racemose angioma* of the retina. This retinal AVM consists of a direct communication between retinal arteries and veins (without an intervening capillary bed), appearing as a sector of tortuous, dilated retinal vessels, sometimes causing hemorrhage and vision loss (Figure 14–9). AVMs of the optic nerve and chiasm also occur.

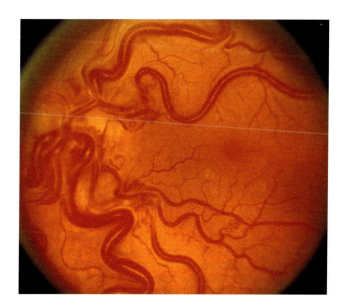

Figure 14–9. **Retinal racemose angioma in Wyburn-Mason syndrome.**

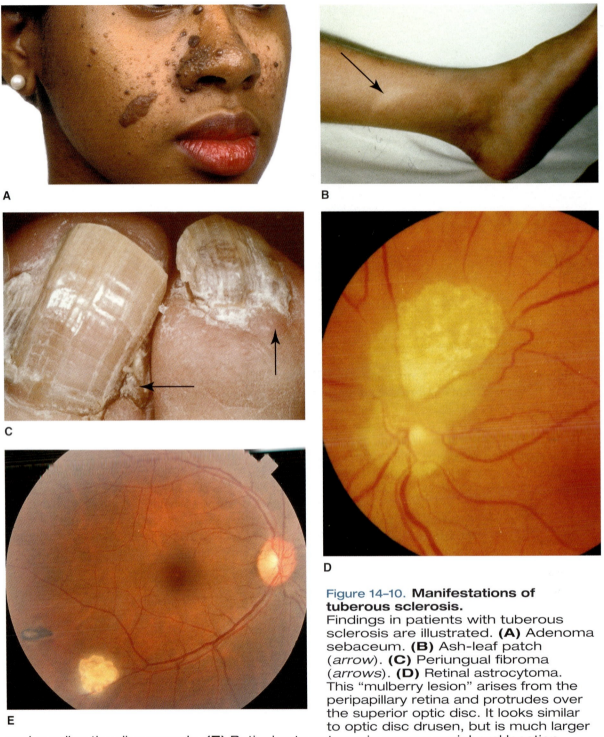

Figure 14-10. **Manifestations of tuberous sclerosis.**
Findings in patients with tuberous sclerosis are illustrated. **(A)** Adenoma sebaceum. **(B)** Ash-leaf patch (*arrow*). **(C)** Periungual fibroma (*arrows*). **(D)** Retinal astrocytoma. This "mulberry lesion" arises from the peripapillary retina and protrudes over the superior optic disc. It looks similar to optic disc drusen, but is much larger and overlies the disc vessels. **(E)** Retinal astrocytoma in a more peripheral location along the inferior vascular arcade.

AVMs occurring in the orbit can cause proptosis, conjunctival injection, or an orbital bruit. Seizure disorders and spontaneous intracranial hemorrhage can occur from AVMs in the midbrain and posterior fossa. AVMs can also occur in the maxilla, pterygoid fossa, and mandible (with the potential for complicating dental procedures and oral surgery).

TUBEROUS SCLEROSIS (BOURNEVILLE SYNDROME)

Tuberous sclerosis is characterized by adenoma sebaceum and astrocytic hamartomas of the retina and brain. Adenoma sebaceum (unlike the name suggests) are hamartomatous angiofibromas, distributed in a butterfly pattern over the nose and cheeks (Figure 14–10A). Other cutaneous manifestations include periungual fibromas of toenails (see Figure 14–10C) or fingernails, shagreen patches, and ash-leaf patches. Shagreen patches are large, elevated, hyperpigmented areas on the trunk. Ash-leaf patches are areas of skin depigmentation that fluoresce under a Wood lamp, and are considered pathognomonic for tuberous sclerosis (see Figure 14–10B). Most patients have multiple retinal astrocytic hamartomas in one or both eyes that generally do not affect vision. The hamartomas, composed of astrocytes arising from the retinal ganglion cell layer, are frequently located adjacent to the optic disc (see Figure 14–9D, E). Most children with tuberous sclerosis will not develop new retinal astrocytic hamartomas after one year of age. Calcified periventricular and cortical astrocytic hamartomas give a characteristic appearance on CT imaging ("brain stones"), but MRI is considered a better imaging test for this condition. Subependymal nodules along the ventricular surface can continue to proliferate over time, occasionally obstructing ventricular outflow and causing papilledema. Epilepsy and mental deficiency are common. Cardiac rhabdomyomas, renal cysts, and angiomyolipomas can also occur.

Tuberous sclerosis has an autosomal dominant pattern of inheritance, but two-thirds of cases are spontaneous mutations. Genetic defects occur in one of two distinct genes: the gene on chromosome 9 that encodes for hamartin or the gene on chromosome 16 that encodes for tuberin. Tuberin and hamartin form a heterodimer that is involved in inhibition of cell growth and proliferation; therefore, defects in either protein can affect this function, producing the many manifestations of tuberous sclerosis.

▶ KEY POINTS

- A transient ischemic attack (TIA) is an episode of reversible neurological dysfunction of less than 24-hour duration commonly caused by thromboembolism, thrombotic occlusion, or vasculitis of the cerebrovascular system.
- Amaurosis fugax (or transient monocular visual loss) is frequently caused by emboli to the retinal arteries, with visual loss typically lasting less than 5 minutes.
- Retinal emboli include Hollenhorst plaques (crystalline cholesterol) and fibrin-platelet emboli from atheromatous disease of the carotid arteries or aortic arch, or calcific emboli from calcified heart valves.
- Most central retinal artery occlusions are embolic, but vasculitis (GCA) and hypercoagulable states should also be considered.
- The presence of retinal emboli indicates systemic arteriosclerotic disease with an adverse survival rate often related to ischemic heart disease.
- A significant reduction in distal flow generally requires 50% to 90% stenosis of the carotid artery, whereas embolic phenomena can occur from minimal carotid artery plaque.
- Venous stasis retinopathy and ocular ischemic syndrome can result from chronic ischemia induced by carotid occlusive disease.
- Carotid duplex ultrasound and MRA are useful in evaluating the carotid system, but cerebral angiography remains the gold standard.
- Endarterectomy reduces the risk of stroke in patients with symptomatic carotid artery stenosis and 70% to 99% occlusion in centers where the operative risks are less than 3%.
- Transient or persistent motility disturbances and visual field defects are common symptoms of vertebrobasilar disease.
- Arteriovenous malformations (AVMs) cause symptoms by exerting a mass effect, by bleeding into the subarachnoid space or brain tissue, and occasionally by shunting blood away from normal structures.
- Occasionally, occipital lobe AVMs produce positive visual phenomena that resemble the scintillating scotoma of classic migraine, but with AVMs the visual changes do not alternate sides, and the clinical features are usually atypical for migraine.
- Occult dural AVMs are a potential cause of intracranial hypertension.
- Signs and symptoms of an arterial-cavernous sinus fistula include episcleral and conjunctival injection (arterialization), chemosis, proptosis, elevated IOP with blood in Schlemm canal, motility disturbances (typically CN VI palsy), and venous stasis retinopathy.
- Direct carotid-cavernous sinus fistulas result from a direct communication between the intracavernous carotid artery and the (venous) cavernous sinus and are usually the result of trauma.
- Indirect carotid-cavernous sinus fistulas are abnormal communications between meningeal branches of the carotid system and the cavernous sinus or its tributaries and are "slow flow," usually with less prominent signs than direct fistulas.
- Four-vessel cerebral angiography is required to define the complex flow in dural-cavernous sinus fistulas and to implement intravascular treatment techniques, but the risk of angiography must be weighed against benefits in each case.
- Aneurysms are saccular outpouchings at arterial branches that can compress adjacent structures; rupture causes subarachnoid hemorrhage.

- Recognizing the signs and symptoms of CN III compression from a posterior communicating aneurysm can be lifesaving because surgical repair before rupture carries a far better prognosis.
- Dolichoectasia of the basilar artery can cause compression of local structures, resulting in slowly progressive multiple cranial neuropathies with long-tract motor and sensory signs.
- The neurocutaneous syndromes (phakomatoses) are characterized by hamartias and hamartomas of the skin, eye, CNS, and viscera.
- Gliomas of the optic nerves and chiasm are common in NF1.
- Bilateral acoustic neuromas characterize NF2.
- Sturge-Weber syndrome is characterized by unilateral hemangiomas of the face, eye, and brain; glaucoma may be present when the facial hemangioma involves the upper eyelid.
- The retinal lesions in angiomatosis retinae (von Hippel disease) are bilateral in 50% of patients and continue to develop throughout life.
- Patients with ataxia telangiectasia have thymic hypoplasia and IgA deficiency, causing susceptibility to frequent and often severe respiratory infections.
- Wyburn-Mason syndrome is characterized by AVMs of the retina (racemose angioma); AVMs of the optic nerve, chiasm, orbit, posterior fossa, maxilla, pterygoid fossa, and mandible can also occur.
- Tuberous sclerosis is a disorder with autosomal dominant inheritance characterized by cutaneous adenoma sebaceum and astrocytic hamartomas of the retina, optic nerve, and brain.

SUGGESTED READING

Books

Biousse V: Cerebrovascular diseases, in Miller NR, Newman NJ, Biousse V, Kerrison JB. (eds): *Walsh and Hoyts' Clinical Neuro-ophthalmology*, Vol 2, 6th ed. Philadelphia, PA: Lippincott Williams and Wilkins; 2005:1967–2186.

Kerrison JB: The phacomatoses, in Miller NR, Newman NJ, Biousse V, Kerrison JB. (eds): *Walsh and Hoyts' Clinical Neuro-ophthalmology*, Vol 2, 6th ed. Philadelphia, PA: Lippincott Williams and Wilkins; 2005:1823–1898.

Kupersmith MJ, Berenstein A: *Neurovascular Neuro-ophthalmology*. Berlin: Springer-Verlag; 1993.

Lewis AR: The phacomatoses: neurocutaneous disorders, in Kline LB (ed): *Neuro-ophthalmology Review Manual*. 7th ed. Thorofare, NJ: Slack; 2013:257–268.

Articles

Treatment of Carotid Disease

Barnett HJM, Taylor DW, Eliasziw M, et al: North American symptomatic carotid endarterectomy trial collaborators: benefit of carotid endarterectomy in patients with symptomatic moderate or severe stenosis. *N Engl J Med* 1998;339:1415–1425.

Biousse V, Trobe JD: Treatment of monocular visual loss. *Am J Ophthalmol* 2003;140:7.

Chassin MR: Appropriate use of carotid endarterectomy. *N Engl J Med* 1998;339:1468–1471.

Kistler JP: The risk of embolic stroke, another piece of the puzzle. *N Engl J Med* 1994;331:1517–1519.

Kistler JP, Buonanno FS, Gress DR: Carotid endarterectomy—specific therapy based on pathophysiology. *N Engl J Med* 1991;325:505–507.

North American Symptomatic Carotid Endarterectomy trial collaborators: Beneficial effect of carotid endarterectomy in symptomatic patients with high-grade carotid stenosis. *N Engl J Med* 1991;325:445–453.

Tu JY, Hannan EL, Anderson GM, et al: The rise and fall of carotid endarterectomy in the United States and Canada. *N Engl J Med* 1998;339:1441–1447.

Ocular Manifestations of Cerebrovascular Disease

Brown GC, Magargal LE: The ocular ischemic syndrome. Clinical, fluorescein angiographic and carotid angiographic features. *Int Ophthalmol* 1988;11:239–251.

Bruno A, Corbett JJ, Biller J, et al: Transient monocular visual loss patterns and associated vascular abnormalities. *Stroke* 1990;21:34–39.

Carter JE: Carotid artery disease and its ocular manifestations. *Ophthalmol Clin NA* 1992;5:425–443.

Hayreh SS, Kolder HE, Weingeist TA: Central retinal artery occlusion and retinal tolerance time. *Ophthalmology* 1980;87:75–78.

Hollenhorst RS: Significance of bright plaques in the retinal arterioles. *JAMA* 1961;178:23–29.

Petzold A, Islam N, Hu HH, Plant GT. Embolic and nonembolic transient monocular visual loss: A clinicopathologic review. Surv Ophthalmol 2012;58:42–62.

Valesini G, Priori R, Luan FL, et al: Amaurosis fugax and antiphospholipid antibodies. *Lancet* 1990;336:374.

Vertebrobasilar Disease

Smoker WRK, Corbett JJ, Gentry LR, et al: High-resolution computed tomography of the basilar artery: 2. Vertebrobasilar dolichoectasia: clinical-pathologic correlation and review. *AJNR* 1986;7:61–72.

Neurocutaneous Syndromes

Dotan SA, Trobe JD, Gebarski SS: Visual loss in tuberous sclerosis. *Neurology* 1991;41:1915–1917.

Yohay K: Neurofibromatosis types 1 and 2. *Neurology* 2006;112:86–93.

INDEX

Note: Page numbers followed by *b*, *f*, or *t* indicate boxes, figures, or tables, respectively.

A

Abducens nerve (CN VI)
 clinical implications in anatomy for
  cavernous sinus, 220–222
  Gradenigo syndrome, 220
  nucleus and fascicles, 220, 221*f*, 236
  orbit, 222
  subarachnoid space, 220
 differential diagnosis and evaluation of, 222–223, 223*f*, 223*t*, 224*f*
 management of, 223–224
 signs and symptoms, 217, 219*f*
Abduction, 186*b*,
Aberrant regeneration of the oculomotor nerve, 231-233, 232*f*, 235*t*, 267, 268*t*, 272*t*, 278*f*
Acetazolamide, 108*f*, 112, 113, 115
Acquired ocular motor apraxia, 247–248
Acquired pendular nystagmus (APN), 256
 drugs used in treating, 257*t*
 location of lesion causing, 255*t*
Acromegaly, 145*f*
Action myotonia, 204
Acute inflammatory demyelinating polyradiculopathy (AIDP), 293, 293*t*
Acute posterior multifocal placoid pigment epitheliopathy (AMPPE), 166
Acute zonal occult outer retinopathy (AZOOR), 171
Adduction, 186*b*, 200
Adenoma sebaceum, 328*t*, 332–333, 332*f*
Adie pupil (Tonic), 9–10, 264, 268*t*, 272*t*, 283*f*

causes of, 280
differential diagnosis and evaluation of, 281
pathophysiology of, 278–279, 279*f*
signs and symptoms of, 279–280, 280*f*
Afferent visual system, 61*f*
Afterimages, 7*t*
Age-related macular degeneration (ARMD), 167
Agnosia
 finger, 153
 visual, 154–155, 159
Agraphia 153, 154*f*
AIBSE (acute idiopathic blind spot enlargement), 72*t*, 169
AIDP. *See* Acute inflammatory demyelinating polyradiculopathy
AION. *See* Anterior ischemic optic neuropathy
Alcoholism, 122, 123*f*
Alexander law, 252, 255
Alexia, 153, 154*f*, 158, 310
Alternate cover testing, ocular motility examination with, 190–191, 190*f*
Altitudinal visual field defect, 66*f*, 67, 67*f*
Amaurosis fugax, 6*t*, 198*f*, 309, 321, 333
Amblyopia, 173, 181
Amiodarone, 124, 124*t*
AMPPE. *See* Acute posterior multifocal placoid pigment epitheliopathy
Amsler grid testing, 38–39, 38*f*, 57, 181
Aneurysms, 327, 333
Angular gyrus, 151*f*, 15–154, 154*f*
Anhidrosis, 269–270, 272*t*, 284

Anisocoria, 9–10, 173*b*, 268–269, 269*f*
 clinical evaluation of, 283–284
Anomalous optic disc, 91*t*, 132–134, 133*f*
Anterior ischemic optic neuropathy (AION), 89*t*, 92. *See also* Nonarteritic anterior ischemic optic neuropathy
Anton syndrome, 156
Aplasia, 134
APN. *See* Acquired pendular nystagmus
Apraclonidine (Iopidine) test, 273, 274*f*, 275*f*, 275*t*, 276, 277*b*, 284
Apraxia, 153, 331
 acquired oculomotor, 247–248
 congenital oculomotor, 247, 247*f*
Arcuate scotoma, 66*f*, 67, 67*f*
Argyll Robertson pupil, 267, 268*t*
ARMD. *See* Age-related macular degeneration
Arterial-cavernous sinus fistula, 325–327, 326*f*
Arteriovenous malformation (AVM), 325, 333
Arteritic anterior ischemic optic neuropathy, 96–99
 causes of, 96, 97*f*
 clinical course for, 94–96
 differential diagnosis of, 95*t*, 97–98, 98*f*
 evaluation of, 98–99
 signs of, 96–97, 98*t*
 symptoms of, 96
 treatment of, 99
Asthenopia, 173*b*
Ataxia telangiectasia (Louis-Bar syndrome), 328*t*, 331
Aura (migraine), 6, 6*t*, 7*t*, 8, 157*b*, 308–310, 308*f*, 309*t*, 310*f*, 316, 325

INDEX

Auscultation of orbit, 198–200, 198f
Automated perimetry, 44–47, 57
   frequency doubling technique with, 47
   Humphrey Visual Field Analyzer II for, 44f
   increasing stimulus size in, 46f
   screening strategies test for, 47
   statistical analysis for, 47, 48f
   30-2 and10-2 comparison for, 46f
   threshold values for, 45–46, 45f
Autosomal dominant (Kjer) optic atrophy, 124–125, 125f
AVM. See Arteriovenous malformation
AZOOR. See Acute zonal occult outer retinopathy

B

B vitamins deficiency, 122–124, 124t
Balint syndrome, 153–154
Basilar-type migraine, 310, 317
Behçet disease, 204t
Bell palsy, 292, 292f, 298
Bell phenomenon, 291f, 295, 298
Benedikt syndrome, 229, 229f
BENEFIT study, 105b
Benign eyelid myokymia, 297–298
Benign intracranial hypertension (BIH), 107
Bielschowsky three-step test, ocular motility examination with, 192, 193f
Big blind-spot syndromes, 72t
BIH. See Benign intracranial hypertension
Bilateral bow-tie atrophy, 142f
Bilateral optic neuropathies, 72t
Bilateral temporal visual field defect, 71–72, 71f, 83
Blepharitis, 161
Blepharoptosis. See Ptosis
Blepharospasm
   facial nerve palsy with, 295, 298
   photophobia associated with, 10t
Blind spot, 42b, 42f
Botulism, 215
Bourneville syndrome. See Tuberous sclerosis
Bow-tie optic atrophy 77, 77f, 141, 143f, 147, 148f
Brainstem lesions, 234
Branch retinal artery occlusion (BRAO), 164, 165f

Branch retinal vein occlusion (BRVO), 166
BRAO. See Branch retinal artery occlusion
Brightness sense testing, 37, 57
Brown tendon sheath syndrome, 210–211, 211f, 215–216
BRVO. See Branch retinal vein occlusion

C

CADASIL. See Cerebral autosomal dominant arteriopathy with subcortical infarcts and leukoencephalopathy
Café-au-lait spots, 118f, 328t, 329f, 330
Caloric testing. See Oculovestibular testing
Cancer-associated retinopathy (CAR), 169–171, 181
Carotid disease, 319–324, 320t, 321f, 322f
Carotid dissection, 313
Carotid-cavernous fistula, 197, 198f, 209, 219t, 220, 234t, 235t, 271t, 278f, 326
Cataract, 164
Catheter angiography, 25, 26f
Cat-scratch neuroretinitis (CSD), 121–122, 121f
   evaluation of, 122
   signs of, 122
   symptoms of, 122
   treatment of, 122
Cavernous sinus
   abducens nerve with, 220–222
   oculomotor nerve with, 231
   trochlear nerve with, 224–226
Cecocentral scotoma, 66f, 68
Central retinal artery occlusion (CRAO), 164–166, 165f
Central retinal vein occlusion (CRVO), 166
Central serous chorioretinopathy, 167, 167f, 181
Cerebellar disease, 248
Cerebellopontine angle, 220, 232t, 235, 288, 290t, 296, 298, 306, 307t
Cerebral angiography, 24–26
   catheter, 25, 26f
   CT angiography (CTA), 25, 25f
   digital subtraction, 25
   MRA, 24, 24f

Cerebral autosomal dominant arteriopathy with subcortical infarcts and leukoencephalopathy (CADASIL), 166
Cerebrovascular disease, 319–327, 320f, 320t
   aneurysms, 327, 333
   arterial-cavernous sinus fistula, 325–327, 326f
   arteriovenous malformation, 325, 333
   carotid disease, 319–324, 320t, 321f, 322f
   dolichoectatic arteries, 327
   vertebrobasilar disease, 324–325
CHAMPS study, 105b
Charles Bonnet syndrome, 7b
Cherry red spot 164, 165f
Chiasm
   anatomy of
     occipital lobe, 155–156
     optic tracts, 147
     parasellar region, 140f
   parasellar region disorders with, 139–147
     bilateral bow-tie atrophy, 142f
     craniopharyngiomas, 144t, 145, 146f
     destination of axons passing through, 140b
     differential diagnosis of, 144t
     evaluation and management of, 147
     hemifield slide phenomenon, 141, 141f
     meningiomas, 144t, 145
     pilocystic astrocytoma, 143f
     pituitary adenoma, 144–145
     pituitary macroadenomas, 143, 144f, 145f
     RAPD, 141
     retrograde axonal atrophy, 141
     signs and symptoms of, 139–143, 141f–143f
   visual field defects of, 71–74
     bilateral temporal, 71–72, 71f, 72f, 72t, 73f, 83
     combination defects, 73–74
     incongruous homonymous, 71f
     junctional scotomas, 71f, 72–73, 74b, 74f, 75f
     paracentral bitemporal, 71f
Chief complaint, 3–11
   anisocoria, 9–10
   characteristics that help define, 4t

diplopia, 8–9, 8t, 27
hallucinations, 5–8, 5b
pain, 10
patient's degree of concern with, 3, 27
photophobia, 10, 10t
positive visual phenomena, 5–8, 6t, 7t, 27
ptosis, 9, 9b
visual loss, 4–5, 4f, 5f
Chronic progressive external ophthalmoplegia (CPEO), 201–203, 203f, 203t
Kearns-Sayre syndrome with, 203, 203t, 215
Ciliary ganglion 231, 278, 279f, 280
Cluster headache, 311, 317
CME. *See* Cystoid macular edema
CN III. *See* Oculomotor nerve
CN IV. *See* Trochlear nerve
CN V. *See* Trigeminal nerve
CN VI. *See* Abducens nerve
CN VII. *See* Facial nerve
CNs. *See* Cranial nerves
Cocaine test, 272–273, 273f, 282f
Cogan lid twitch sign, 212
Coloboma, 134, 135f
Color vision testing, 39–40, 39f, 40f
Comitance, 186b
Compressive optic neuropathies
optic nerve sheath meningiomas, 115–117, 116f
other causes of, 117–118
Compressive optic neuropathy, 98t, 208f
Computed tomography (CT), 20, 21f, 28
Confrontation perimetry, 43–44, 43f, 57
Confusion, 186b
Congenital fibrosis syndromes, 211
Congenital nystagmus, 253–254, 258
Congenital oculomotor apraxia, 247, 247f
Congenital ptosis, 196
Congruency
defined, 62b
retrochiasmal visual defects and, 76, 76f, 77f
Conjunctival injection, orbital Graves disease with, 209
Constriction, 62b
Contrast sensitivity testing, 35–37, 35f–37f, 37b, 56–57

Convergence insufficiency, 251
Convergence spasm, 173b, 222, 223f
Convergence-retraction nystagmus, location of lesion causing, 255t
Corneal curvature, 162, 163f
Corneal epithelial dystrophies, 162, 162f
Cortical blindness, 156, 156f
Counting fingers, 34b
CPEO. *See* Chronic progressive external ophthalmoplegia
Cranial nerve palsies
abducens nerve in
clinical implications in anatomy for, 220–222, 221f, 236
differential diagnosis and evaluation of, 222–223, 223f, 223t, 224f
management of, 223–224
signs and symptoms, 217, 219f
facial nerve in, 292–294, 292f, 293t, 294f
multiple cranial neuropathies in
clinical implications in anatomy for, 234, 234f, 234t
evaluation and management of, 235–236, 235f, 235t
oculomotor nerve in
aberrant regeneration with, 231–232, 232f, 236
clinical implications in anatomy for, 228–231, 229f–231f, 236
differential diagnosis of, 232
evaluation and management of, 232–233, 232t, 233f
signs and symptoms, 228, 228f
trochlear nerve in
clinical implications in anatomy for, 224–226, 225f, 226f, 236
differential diagnosis of, 226, 226t
evaluation and management of, 226–228, 227f
signs and symptoms, 224, 225f
Cranial nerves (CNs), 217. *See also specific cranial nerves*
anatomy of, 218f
causes of ocular motor neuropathies of, 219t
Craniopharyngiomas, 144t, 145, 146f
CRAO. *See* Central retinal artery occlusion
CRASH trial, 128
Critical flicker fusion, 41b
Crocodile tears, 290, 298

Crohn disease, 204t
Crowded optic discs, 134
CRVO. *See* Central retinal vein occlusion
CSD. *See* Cat-scratch neuroretinitis
CT. *See* Computed tomography
CT angiography (CTA), 25, 25f
CT venography, 25
CTA. *See* CT angiography
Cystoid macular edema (CME), 14, 89t, 120–121, 167, 170f, 171t

D

Dacryoadenitis, 204t
Delusions, 5b
Devic disease. *See* Neuromyelitis optica
Diabetic papillopathy, 99–100, 100f
Diamox. *See* acetazolamide
Diffuse orbital inflammation, 204t
Diffusion weighted imaging (DWI), 23t
Digital subtraction angiography (DSA), 25
Diplopia, 8–9, 27, 173b
causes of monocular, 8t
confusion with, 8
defined, 186b
Graves disease with, 8–9
Diplopic visual fields, ocular motility examination with, 191
Dissociated nystagmus with INO, 255t, 256
Divergence insufficiency, 222, 251
Dolichoectatic arteries, 327
Doll's head maneuver. *See* Oculocephalic maneuver
Dorsal midbrain syndrome, 189t, 229f, 243, 243t, 244f, 258, 267, 284
Double Maddox rod test, ocular motility examination with, 192
Downbeat nystagmus, 253–254, 258
drugs used in treating, 257t
location of lesion causing, 255t
Dry eye syndrome, 10t, 161
DSA. *See* Digital subtraction angiography
Duane syndrome, 222–223, 224f
Ductions, 186b
DWI. *See* Diffusion weighted imaging
Dysesthesias, 173b

E

Edinger-Westphal nucleus, 229, 240f, 242f, 243f, 246f, 266–267, 268f
Electronic medical record (EMR), 4
Electrophysiological tests, 53–57
    electroretinogram, 53–55, 54f, 57
    multifocal ERG, 55–56, 55f
    visual evoked potential, 56, 56f, 57
Electroretinogram (ERG), 53–55, 54f, 57
    functional visual loss testing with, 180
    multifocal, 55–56, 55f
Elevated discs without drusen, 134
Emboli, 319–321
    calcific, 320t, 321, 333
    cardiac, 320t
    fat, 320t, 321
    retinal, 321f, 333
    septic, 320t
EMR. See Electronic medical record
Encephalotrigeminal angiomatosis (Sturge-Weber syndrome), 330, 330f, 334
Endpoint nystagmus, 253
Epithelial defects, 162
Erdheim-Chester disease, 204t
ERG. See Electroretinogram
Erythrocyte sedimentation rate (ESR), 99, 135
ESR. See Erythrocyte sedimentation rate
Ethambutol toxicity 122, 123b, 124, 124t
ETOMS study, 105b
Euthyroid orbital Graves disease, 207f
Exposure keratopathy
    management of, 295
    risk factors for, 294–295
Extraocular muscles
    anatomy and function of, 201, 202f, 203t
    innervation for, 202f
    ocular motility disorders with, 201, 202f, 203t
    primary and secondary actions of, 203t
Eye examination, 12–13, 13b
Eye movement recording, ocular motility examination with, 194
Eyelid retraction
    differential diagnosis of, 197t
    Graves disease with, 197f, 197t
    orbital Graves disease with, 207
Eyelid spasms, 173b
Eyelids
    examination techniques for, 195–196, 195t, 196f
    eyelid retraction with, 197, 197f, 197t
    facial nerve disorders with, 197
    ptosis with, 196–197, 196f, 196t, 197f

F

Facial diplegia, 293t
Facial myokymia, 297, 297f
Facial nerve (CN VII)
    assessment of, 199, 199f
        facial motor function in, 291, 291f
        hearing in, 292
        taste in, 291–292
        tear function, 292
    disorders of
        benign eyelid myokymia, 297–298
        blepharospasm, 295, 298
        facial myokymia, 297, 297f, 298
        hemifacial spasm, 295–297, 296f, 297f
    exposure keratopathy with
        management of, 295
        risk factors for, 294–295
    neuroanatomy of
        facial nucleus and fascicles, 288, 289f, 290t
        subarachnoid space, 288
        supranuclear pathways, 287–288, 288f
        temporal bone and peripheral course, 288–291
    palsies with
        acute inflammatory demyelinating polyradiculopathy, 293, 293t
        Bell palsy, 292, 292f, 298
        herpes zoster oticus, 292–293, 298
        Melkersson-Rosenthal syndrome, 294
        Möbius syndrome, 294, 294f
        myasthenia gravis, 294
        other infectious diseases, 293
        sarcoidosis, 294
        trauma, 293–294
Facial nerve disorders, 197
Facial numbness, 305–306, 307t, 316
Family album tomography (FAT scan), 9b
Farnsworth D15 test, 40f
Farnsworth-Munsell 100 hue test (FM-100), 39, 39f
FAT scan. See Family album tomography
FDT. See Frequency doubling technique
Fixation, ocular motility examination with, 186–187, 187t
Fixation reflex, 245t, 251
FLAIR. See Fluid attenuated inversion recovery
Floaters, 7t
Fluid attenuated inversion recovery (FLAIR), 23t
FM-100. See Farnsworth-Munsell 100 hue test
Focal macular disease, 62, 66f
Folic acid deficiency, 122–124, 124t
Forced duction testing, ocular motility examination with, 192–194, 194f
Formal perimetry, 44
Fourth cranial nerve. See trochlear nerve
Foville syndrome, 220
Frequency doubling technique (FDT), 47
Frontal eye field, 241, 245, 245t, 246f, 247, 258
Frontal lobe lesions, 247
Functional neuroimaging, 26–27, 27f
Functional visual loss. See Nonorganic vision disorders

G

Gaze centers, internuclear. See Internuclear gaze centers
Gaze palsy, 241–242
Gaze-evoked nystagmus, 253, 256, 258
    location of lesion causing, 255t
Gaze-paretic nystagmus, 253
Gerstmann syndrome, 153
Giant cell arteritis (GCA), 96–99, 97f, 98t, 104t, 204t, 312
    AION due to, 92, 94, 96–98
    ischemic manifestations from, 95t
    optic disc elevation from, 89t
    optic disc swelling from, 90t
    optic perineuritis with, 105
    PION due to, 98, 98t
Glaucoma, 128–129, 129f, 130f
Glioma. See optic nerve glioma
Goldmann perimetry, 47–51, 49f, 50f, 57

automated perimetry compared to, 50f
patient positioning for, 47, 49f
subjective nature of, 49
visual field with, 50f
Gout, 204t
Gradenigo syndrome, 220, 234t, 293
Granulomatosis with polyangiitis, 119t, 204t
Graves disease. *See also* Orbital Graves disease
diplopia with, 8–9
eyelid retraction in, 197f, 197t
Graves orbitopathy, 89t
Guillain-Barré syndrome, 219t, 236, 290t, 293, 293t

H
Hallucinations, 5–8, 5b
occipital lobe chiasmal disorder with, 156, 157t
optic radiations with, 154
Hand movement, 34b
Hangover headache, 10t
Hardy-Rittler-Rand color plates, 40
Headache. *See also* Migraine
cluster, 311, 317
hangover, 10t
tension-type, 311, 317
Hemianopia, 62b
Hemifacial spasm, facial nerve palsy with, 295–297, 296f, 297f
Hemifield slide phenomenon, 141, 141f
Hereditary optic neuropathies
autosomal dominant optic atrophy, 124–125, 125f
Leber hereditary optic neuropathy, 125–127, 126f, 135
Herpes zoster ophthalmicus, 10, 304, 305, 307t, 313–314, 314f, 316, 317
Herpes zoster oticus, facial nerve palsy with, 292–293, 298
Heteronymous, 62b
High accommodative convergence-to-accommodation ratio, 251
Hill of vision, 42, 42f, 43b
Hirschberg test, ocular motility examination with, 191
History of present illness, 3–11, 4t
HIV (Human immunodeficiency virus), 4, 11, 293, 293t, 309t
Hollenhorst plaques, 14, 165f, 320t, 321, 321f, 333

Homonymous visual field loss, 156–157, 158b
Homonymous visual field patterns, 74
Horizontal gaze center disorders
gaze palsy, 241–242
internuclear ophthalmoplegia, 239–241, 240f, 241f
one-and-a-half syndrome, 242, 242f
Wernicke encephalopathy, 242, 242b
organization of, 239–242, 240f–242f, 242b
medial longitudinal fasciculus, 239, 240f, 257
paramedian pontine reticular formation, 239, 240f, 257–258
Horner syndrome. *See* Oculosympathetic paresis
Humphrey Visual Field Analyzer II, 44f
Hutchinson pupil, 231, 278
Hydroxyamphetamine. *See* Paradrine test
Hypoplasia, 134
Hypothalamus, 142–143

I
Idiopathic intracranial hypertension (IIH), 107–115, 108f, 109t
causes of, 109t, 110
clinical course for, 115
differential diagnosis of, 110–111, 112f, 113f
signs of, 108b, 109–110, 110f, 111f
symptoms of, 107–109, 108b
treatment of, 111–115, 112f
Idiopathic orbital inflammatory syndrome (IOIS), 204–205, 204t, 205f, 215
painful ophthalmoplegia related to, 234, 234t
IIH. *See* Idiopathic intracranial hypertension
Illusions, 5b
Incomitance, 186b
Incongruous homonymous visual field defect, 71f
Infectious optic neuropathies
cat-scratch neuroretinitis, 121–122, 121f
optic disc edema with macular star, 120–121

other infectious neuropathies, 122
Inflammatory optic neuropathies, 119–120, 120b, 120f
Internuclear gaze centers
horizontal gaze, 239–242, 240f–242f, 242b
vertical gaze, 242–244, 243f, 243t, 244f
Internuclear ophthalmoplegia, 239–241, 240f, 241f
Intracanalicular optic nerve course, 86f, 88
Intracranial optic nerve course, 86f, 88
Intraocular optic nerve course, 85–87, 86f, 87f
Intraorbital optic nerve course, 86f, 87–88
Intravenous fluorescein angiography (IVFA), 14–15, 28
performance of, 14, 14f
sequence using, 15f
Intrinsic neoplasms, 118–119
lymphoproliferative disorders, 119, 119f, 119t
melanocytomas, 119, 119f, 119t
optic nerve gliomas, 118–119
Involutional ptosis, 196–197, 197f
IOIS. *See* Idiopathic orbital inflammatory syndrome
Iris
anatomy of, 261–262, 262f
efferent disorders of visual system with, 269
Iritis, photophobia associated with, 10t
Ischemic mononeuropathy, 222–223, 223f, 223t, 224f
Ischemic optic neuropathies
arteritic anterior, 95t, 96–99, 97f, 98f, 98t
diabetic papillopathy, 99–100, 100f
nonarteritic anterior, 92–96, 93f, 95t, 96t
papillophlebitis, 100, 101f
radiation optic neuropathy, 100
Ishihara color plates, 40
IVFA. *See* Intravenous fluorescein angiography

J
Jaw claudication, 5, 96, 312, 315
Jerk nystagmus, 190, 241, 252–255
Junctional scotomas, 71f, 72–73, 74b, 74f, 75f
Juvenile xanthogranuloma, 204t

K

Kearns-Sayre syndrome (KSS), 203, 203t, 215
Keratoconus, 163f
Kinetic perimetry, 44, 57
Kjer dominant optic atrophy 124, 125f
KSS. See Kearns-Sayre syndrome

L

Lambert-Eaton syndrome (LES), 215
Lamina cribrosa, 86
Latent hyperopia, 164
Latent nystagmus, 253
Lateral geniculate nucleus (LGN), 76f, 78, 78f
   chiasmal disorders of, 148–150, 148f–150f
   layered structure of, 148f
   sectoranopia from, 150f
   vascular supply to, 149f
Leber hereditary optic neuropathy (LHON), 125–127, 126f, 135
   optic disc elevation from, 89t
LES. See Lambert-Eaton syndrome
Leukemia, 119t
LGN. See Lateral geniculate nucleus
LHON. See Leber hereditary optic neuropathy
Light perception vision, 34b
Light-near dissociation of pupil, 267, 267b, 268t
Lisch nodules, 12, 328t, 329f, 330
LogMAR acuity tests, 32, 33f
Louis-Bar syndrome. See Ataxia telangiectasia
Lyme disease, optic disc elevation from, 89t
Lymphoma, 119t
Lymphoproliferative disorders, 89t, 119, 119f, 119t

M

Macula, OCT imaging of, 16, 17f
Maculopathies, 167–168, 167f–170f, 171t
   cystoid macular edema causing, 167, 170f
   epiretinal membranes causing, 167, 168f
   niacin toxicity causing, 167, 170f
   retinal trauma causing, 168
   vitamin A deficiency causing, 168
   vitreomacular traction causing, 167, 169f

Maddox rod, 191–192. See also Double Maddox rod test; Single Maddox rod test
Magnetic resonance angiography (MRA), 24, 24f, 28
Magnetic resonance imaging (MRI), 20–21, 22f, 23t
   anatomic structures are identified in, 22f
   echo time of, 20
   functional, 26
   repetition time of, 20
   techniques of, 23t
Magnetic resonance spectroscopy, 26
Magnetoencephalography (MEG), 27
Magnocellular system, 37b, 41b, 148, 148f, 151f
Meckel cave, 304, 307t, 316
Medial longitudinal fasciculus (MLF), 239, 240f, 257
MEG. See Magnetoencephalography
Meibomian gland dysfunction, 161
Meige syndrome, 288, 296, 297f, 298
Melanocytomas, 89t, 119, 119f, 119t
Melanoma-associated retinopathy (MAR), 171
Melkersson-Rosenthal syndrome, 290t, 293t, 294
Meningiomas, 89t, 144t, 145
Meridian, 62b
MEWDS, 72t, 171, 181
Meyer loop, 78
Midbrain relative afferent pupillary defects, 267–268
Migraine, 307–311, 308f, 309t, 310f, 317
   photophobia associated with, 10t
Migraine
   basilar-type, 310, 317
   visual aura in, 6, 6t, 7t, 8, 157b, 308–310, 308f, 309t, 310f, 316, 325
Millar-Gubler syndrome, 220
Miller Fisher syndrome, 219t, 235t, 236, 293, 293t
Mitochondrial optic neuropathy, 123b
MLF. See Medial longitudinal fasciculus
Möbius syndrome, 223, 223t, 235t, 293t, 294, 294f
Monocular diplopia, 8, 8t, 27, 35b, 162, 164, 173b
Moore lightning streaks, 7t

MRA. See Magnetic resonance angiography
MRI. See Magnetic resonance imaging
Müller muscle, 262, 269, 272
Multifocal ERG, 55–56, 55f
Multiple cranial neuropathies
   clinical implications in anatomy for, 234, 234f, 234t
      brainstem lesions, 234
      painful ophthalmoplegia, 234, 234t
   evaluation and management of, 235–236, 235f, 235t
Multiple myeloma, 119t
Multiple sclerosis, optic neuritis with, 102f, 104b, 105b
Muscular dystrophies
   action myotonia with, 204
   myotonic dystrophy, 204, 204f, 215
   oculopharyngeal dystrophy, 204
   percussion myotonia with, 204
Myasthenia gravis, 211–215, 212f, 214b, 214f
   cause of, 212
   evaluation and differential diagnosis of, 213–214, 214b, 214f
   facial nerve palsy with, 294, 298
   signs and symptoms of, 212–213, 212f
   treatment options for, 214–215
Myelin sheath, 87
Myelinated retinal nerve fibers, 134
Myokymia
   benign eyelid, 297–298
   facial, 297, 297f, 298
   superior oblique, 257
Myopathies
   chronic progressive external ophthalmoplegia, 201–203, 203f, 203t
   muscular dystrophies, 204, 204f
   orbital inflammatory disorders, 204–205, 204t, 205f
Myopia, 72t, 73f
Myositis, 204t
Myotonic dystrophy, 204, 204f, 215

N

NAION. See Nonarteritic anterior ischemic optic neuropathy
Nasal step defects, 64, 66f
NASCET study, 324b
Near card, 32, 33f

Near synkinetic triad, 251, 258, 268
Necrobiotic xanthogranuloma, 204t
Nerve fiber layer defect, 63–68
  altitudinal visual field defect, 66f, 67, 67f
  arcuate scotoma, 66f, 67, 67f
  cecocentral scotoma, 66f, 68
  nasal step defects, 64, 66f
  organization of, 62–63, 66f
  temporal wedge, 66f, 68, 69f
Neurocutaneous syndromes, 327–333, 328t
  ataxia telangiectasia, 328t, 331
  encephalotrigeminal angiomatosis, 330, 330f, 334
  neurofibromatosis, 328–330, 328t, 329f
  retinal angiomatosis, 328t, 330–331, 331f, 334
  tuberous sclerosis, 328t, 332–333, 332f, 334
  Wyburn-Mason syndrome, 328t, 331–332, 331f, 334
Neurofibromatosis, 328–330, 328t, 329f
Neurogenic pain, 313–315, 314f, 317
Neuroimaging, 19–26
  brain in, 24
  cerebral angiography in, 24–26, 24f–26f
  computed tomography based, 20, 21f, 28
  functional, 26–27, 27f
  MRI in, 20–21, 22f, 23t, 28
  orbit in, 21–24, 28
Neuromuscular junction disorders
  botulism, 215
  Lambert-Eaton syndrome, 215
  myasthenia gravis, 211–215, 212f, 214b, 214f
Neuromyelitis optica (NMO), 98t, 105
Neuro-ophthalmic examination
  brain imaging in, 24
  cerebral angiography in, 24–26, 24f–25f
  chief complaint in, 3–11, 4f, 5b, 5f, 6t, 7t, 8t, 9b, 10t, 27
  clinical ancillary tests in, 13–19, 14f–20f
  components in, 12t
  computed tomography in, 20, 21f, 28
  eye exam in, 12–13, 13b
  function in, 11
  functional neuroimaging, 26–27, 27f
  guide for, 12t
  history of present illness in, 3–11, 4t
  intravenous fluorescein angiography in, 14–15, 14f, 15f, 28
  magnetic resonance imaging in, 20–21, 22f, 23t, 28
  neuroimaging in, 19–26, 21f, 22f, 23t, 24f–27f
  optical coherence tomography in, 15–19, 16f–19f, 28
  orbit exam in, 12–13
  orbit imaging in, 21–24, 28
  patient history in, 11
  photography in, 14, 27
  structure in, 11
  suggested sequence for, 12t
  ultrasonography in, 19, 19f, 20f
Neuroretinitis, 121, 121f, 135. See also Cat-scratch neuroretinitis
Neurovascular diseases
  cerebrovascular disease, 319–327, 320f, 320t
    aneurysms, 327, 333
    arterial-cavernous sinus fistula, 325–327, 326f
    arteriovenous malformation, 325, 333
    carotid disease, 319–324, 320t, 321f, 322f
    dolichoectatic arteries, 327
    vertebrobasilar disease, 324–325
Niacin deficiency, 122–124, 124t
NMO. See Neuromyelitis optica
Nonarteritic anterior ischemic optic neuropathy (NAION), 92–96, 93f
  causes of, 94
  clinical course for, 94–96
  differential diagnosis of, 94, 96t
  evaluation of, 94, 95t
  signs of, 93–94
  symptoms of, 92–93
  treatment of, 94
Nonorganic vision disorders, 173–181, 173b, 181
  electrophysiological testing for, 180
  evaluating patients with, 174b
  examining patients with, 175–180, 175t
  history of, 174–175, 175f
  relative afferent pupillary defect test for, 179–180
  spectrum of patients with, 174b
  treatment of, 180–181
  visual acuity with, 175t, 176–177
  visual fields with, 175t, 177–179, 177f–180f
Notation, 34f
Nutritional optic neuropathies. See Toxic/nutritional optic neuropathies
Nystagmus, 251–257
  acquired, 254–256, 255t
  acquired pendular, 255t, 256, 257t
  classification and terminology for, 252, 252f
  congenital, 253–254, 258
  convergence-retraction, 255t
  dissociated nystagmus with INO, 255t, 256
  downbeat, 253–254, 255t, 257t, 258
  endpoint, 253
  gaze-evoked, 253, 255t, 256, 258
  gaze-paretic, 253
  latent, 253
  nonpathological forms of, 253
  nystagmus-like oscillations, 256–257
  ocular bobbing, 255t, 256
  oculopalatal myoclonus, 255t, 256, 259
  optokinetic, 252
  periodic alternating, 253, 255t, 257t, 258
  physiological, 252–253
  rebound, 255, 255t
  see-saw, 255, 255t, 257t, 258
  spasmus nutans, 253, 258
  superior oblique myokymia, 257
  torsional, 257t
  treatment for, 257, 257t
  upbeat, 255t, 257t
  vestibular, 255–256, 255t, 256t
  vestibulo-ocular, 253
  voluntary, 253
  waveforms, 252f

O

Obliquely inserted optic discs, myopia with, 72t
Occipital lobe
  anatomy of, 155–156
  chiasmal disorders of, 155–156
    cortical blindness, 156, 156f
    hallucinations, 156, 157t
    Riddoch phenomenon, 155
    signs and symptoms for, 155–156, 155f, 156t

Occipital lobe (*continued*)
    vertebrobasilar insufficiency, 156
    visual field characteristics of, 79-83, 80f, 155
OCT. *See* Optical coherence tomography
Ocular alignment assessment, 187t, 190–192, 190f–193f
Ocular bobbing, location of lesion causing, 255t
Ocular bobbing nystagmus, 256
Ocular causes of pain, 311–312, 317
Ocular duction testing, 187
Ocular flutter, 248
Ocular motility, 187t
    alternate cover testing for, 190–191, 190f
    ancillary methods for, 189–190, 189b, 189f, 190b
    Bielschowsky three-step test for, 192, 193f
    diplopic visual fields for, 191
    double Maddox rod test for, 192
    eye movement recording in, 194
    fixation in, 186–187, 187t
    forced duction testing for, 192–194, 194f
    Hirschberg test for, 191
    nystagmus in, 194
    ocular alignment assessment for, 187t, 190–192, 190f–193f
    ocular duction testing in, 187
    ocular versions and ductions in, 187, 187t
    oculocephalic maneuver for, 189, 200
    oculovestibular testing for, 189–190, 190b
    optokinetic nystagmus testing for, 189, 189b, 189f
    primary and secondary deviation for, 191, 191f
    pursuits in, 187t, 188, 200
    red glass test for, 191
    saccades in, 187t, 188–189, 200
    single Maddox rod test for, 191–192, 192f, 200
    vergence in, 187–188, 188f
Ocular motility disorders
    anatomy and function of, 201, 202f, 203t
    cranial nerve palsies
        abducens nerve, 217–223, 219f, 221f, 223f, 223t, 224f, 236
        multiple cranial neuropathies, 234–236, 234f, 234t, 235f, 235t
        oculomotor nerve, 228–232, 228f–233f, 232t, 236
        trochlear nerve, 224–228, 225f–227f, 226t, 236
    extraocular muscles with, 201, 202f, 203t
    myopathies
        chronic progressive external ophthalmoplegia, 201–203, 203f, 203t, 215
        muscular dystrophies, 204, 204f, 215
        orbital inflammatory disorders, 204–205, 204t, 205f
    neuromuscular junction disorders
        botulism, 215
        Lambert-Eaton syndrome, 215
        myasthenia gravis, 211–215, 212f, 214b, 214f
    restrictive orbitopathies
        Brown tendon sheath syndrome, 210–211, 211f, 215–216
        congenital fibrosis syndromes, 211
        orbital Graves disease, 206–210, 207f, 208f, 209t, 215
        orbital trauma, 210, 211f
Ocular surface disease, 161–162, 162b
Ocular tilt reaction (OTR), 250
Ocular versions and ductions, 187, 187t
Oculocephalic maneuver, 189, 200
Oculogyric crisis, 248
Oculomotor nerve (CN III), 186b
    aberrant regeneration with, 231–232, 232f, 236
    clinical implications in anatomy for, 228–231, 229f–231f, 236
    cavernous sinus, 231
    fascicles, 229, 231f
    nucleus, 228–229, 229f–230f
    orbit, 231
    subarachnoid space, 229–231
    differential diagnosis of, 232
    evaluation and management of, 232–233, 232t, 233f
    parasympathetic efferent pupil disorders with, 277–278, 278f
    signs and symptoms, 228, 228f
Oculopalatal myoclonus, 255t, 256, 259
Oculopharyngeal dystrophy, 204
Oculosympathetic paresis (Horner syndrome)
    causes of, 270–272, 271f, 271t
    differential diagnosis for, 272, 272t
    evaluation and management of, 277
    pharmacologic testing for, 272–277, 273f–276f, 275t, 277b
    signs and symptoms of, 269–270, 270f
Oculovestibular testing, 189–190, 190b
ODEMS. *See* Optic disc edema with macular star
OKN. *See* Optokinetic nystagmus testing
Oligodendrocytes, 87
One-and-a-half syndrome, 242, 242f
ONTT. *See* Optic neuritis treatment trial
Ophthalmoplegia, 203f, 203t
OPN. *See* Optic perineuritis
Opsoclonus, 248–249
Optic atrophy, 147, 148f
Optic cup, 86, 86f
Optic disc
    anatomy of, 85–86, 86f
    cupping with pallor, 88
    cup-to-disc ratio for, 86, 86f
    "discs at risk," 86
    OCT of, 19
Optic disc–related visual field defect, 63–68
    altitudinal visual field defect, 66f, 67, 67f
    arcuate scotoma, 66f, 67, 67f
    cecocentral scotoma, 66f, 68
    nasal step defects, 64, 66f
    organization of, 62–63, 66f
    temporal wedge, 66f, 68, 69f
Optic disc drusen, 129–132, 135
    causes of, 132
    differential diagnosis of, 132
    evaluation of, 132
    optic disc elevation from, 89t
    peripapillary choroidal neovascular membrane with, 132f
    pseudopapilledema from buried, 131f
    signs of, 129–132, 131f, 132f
    symptoms of, 129
    treatment of, 132
    visual field loss with, 131f
Optic disc edema. *See* Optic disc swelling
Optic disc edema with macular star (ODEMS), 120–121
Optic disc swelling (edema), 89–90
    causes of, 89t, 90f

cottonwool spots with, 92f
features of, 91t
prelaminar, 89f
pseudopapilledema compared to, 91t
retinal hemorrhages with, 91f
severe, 91f
Optic nerve anatomy, 85–88
blood supply in, 87f
intracanalicular course in, 86f, 88
intracranial course in, 86f, 88
intraocular course in, 85–87, 86f, 87f
intraorbital course in, 86f, 87–88
lamina cribrosa in, 86
myelin sheath in, 87
optic cup in, 86, 86f
optic disc in, 85–86, 86f
optic nerve head in, 85
Optic nerve compression, 209
Optic nerve disorders, 85–135
anomalous optic disc, 132–134, 133f
aplasia, 134
coloboma, 134, 135f
crowded optic discs, 134
elevated discs without drusen, 134
hypoplasia, 134
myelinated retinal nerve fibers, 134
tilted optic discs, 134
clinical expression of, 88–90
accompanying signs, 90, 91f, 92f
optic disc swelling, 89–90, 89f, 89t, 90f, 91t
pallor and cupping, 88
compressive optic neuropathies, 115–118
optic nerve sheath meningiomas, 115–117, 116f
other causes of, 117–118
glaucoma, 128–129, 129f
hereditary optic neuropathies, 124–127
autosomal dominant optic atrophy, 124–125, 125f
Leber hereditary optic neuropathy, 125–127, 126f, 135
infectious optic neuropathies, 120–122
cat-scratch neuroretinitis, 121–122, 121f
optic disc edema with macular star, 120–121
other infectious neuropathies, 122

inflammatory optic neuropathies, 119–120, 120b, 120f
intrinsic neoplasms, 118–119
lymphoproliferative disorders, 119, 119f, 119t
melanocytomas, 119, 119f, 119t
optic nerve gliomas, 118–119
ischemic optic neuropathies, 92–100
arteritic anterior, 95t, 96–99, 97f, 98f, 98t
diabetic papillopathy, 99–100, 100f
nonarteritic anterior, 92–96, 93f, 95t, 96t
papillophlebitis, 100, 101f
radiation optic neuropathy, 100
optic disc drusen, 129–132, 131f, 132f, 135
optic neuritis, 100–105, 102f, 103t, 104b, 104t, 105b, 106f
optic perineuritis, 105
papilledema, 106–115
idiopathic intracranial hypertension, 107–115, 108b, 108f, 109t, 110f–114f
mechanism of, 106–107, 107f
other causes of, 107
toxic/nutritional optic neuropathies, 122–124, 123b, 123f, 124t, 135
traumatic optic neuropathies, 127–128, 128f, 135
Optic nerve gliomas, 118–119, 135
Optic nerve head, 85
Optic nerve sheath meningiomas, 115–117, 116f
causes of, 117
differential diagnosis of, 117
symptoms and signs of, 115–117
treatment of, 117
Optic neuritis, 100–105, 135
causes of, 103
clinical course for, 104–105, 104b, 104t, 105b
differential diagnosis of, 103
evaluation of, 103
multiple sclerosis with, 102f, 104b, 105b
optic disc elevation from, 89t, 90f
signs of, 101–103
symptoms of, 101
treatment of, 103–104, 103t
variations of, 105, 106f
Optic neuritis treatment trial (ONTT), 101, 103–104, 103t

Optic perineuritis (OPN), 105, 135, 204t
Optic radiations, 78, 150–155, 151f, 152t
Optic tract
anatomy of, 147
disorders of, 147
visual field defects with, 76f, 77, 77f, 83
Optic tract syndrome, 77f
Optical coherence tomography (OCT), 15–19, 16f–19f, 28
macular imaging with, 16, 17f
optic disc with, 19
retinal nerve fiber layer with, 16, 18f–19f
spectral domain, 16
time domain, 16
Optokinetic nystagmus testing (OKN)
ocular motility examination with, 189, 189b, 189f
parietal lobe signs with, 151–152, 252
Optokinetic reflex, 245t, 250
Optotypes, 32, 33f
Orbit
abducens nerve with, 222
auscultation of, 198–200, 198f
examination of, 12–13
imaging, 21–24, 28
inspection of, 197–198, 198f
oculomotor nerve with, 231
palpation of, 198
parasympathetic pathway in, 264f
trochlear nerve with, 224–226
Orbital and cavernous sinus disease, 312
Orbital apex syndrome, 219t, 222, 231, 234–235, 235t
Orbital cellulitis, 204t
Orbital Graves disease, 206–210, 207f, 208f, 209t, 215
compressive optic neuropathy with, 208f
conjunctival injection with, 209
defined, 206
differential diagnosis of, 209–210, 209t
euthyroid, 207f
evaluation of, 209–210
eyelid retraction with, 207
ocular misalignment in, 207f
optic nerve compression with, 209
signs and symptoms of, 206–209, 209t
treatment of, 210

Orbital inflammatory disorders, 204–205, 204t, 205f
Orbital trauma, 210, 211f
OTR. See Ocular tilt reaction

P
Pain and sensation
  causes of, for face and head, 306–315, 307t
    carotid dissection, 313
    cluster headache, 311, 317
    giant cell arteritis, 312
    intracranial disorders, 312–313, 313f, 317
    migraine, 307–311, 308f, 309t, 310f, 317
    neurogenic pain, 313–315, 314f, 317
    ocular causes of pain, 311–312, 317
    orbital and cavernous sinus disease, 312
    sinus and dental disease, 315
    tension-type headache, 311, 317
    unknown origin, 315
  facial numbness, 305–306, 307t, 316
  photophobia with, 10, 315–316, 316t
  trigeminal nerve with
    clinical testing of, 304–305
    neuroanatomy of, 303–304, 304f, 305f, 306t, 316
    symptoms of, 305
Painful ophthalmoplegia, 234, 234t
Palinopsia, 152, 157
Palpation of orbit, 198
Palsy, 186b
PAN. See Periodic alternating nystagmus
Papilledema, 106–115, 135. See also Optic disc swelling
  enlarged blind spots from, 72t
  idiopathic intracranial hypertension, 107–115, 108b, 108f, 109t, 110f–114f
  mechanism of, 106–107, 107f
  other causes of, 107
Papillophlebitis, 89t, 100, 101f
Paracentral bitemporal visual field defect, 71f
Paradrine (hydroxyamphetamine) test, 273–276, 274f, 276f, 277b, 282f, 284
Paralysis, 186b

Paramedian pontine reticular formation (PPRF), 239, 240f, 257–258
Paraneoplastic optic neuropathy, 98t
Parasellar region
  anatomy of, 140f
  chiasmal disorders of, 139–147, 140b, 140f
    bilateral bow-tie atrophy, 142f
    craniopharyngiomas, 144t, 145, 146f
    destination of axons passing through, 140b
    differential diagnosis of, 144t
    evaluation and management of, 147
    hemifield slide phenomenon, 141, 141f
    meningiomas, 144t, 145
    pilocystic astrocytoma, 143f
    pituitary adenoma, 144–145
    pituitary macroadenomas, 143, 144f, 145f
    RAPD, 141
    retrograde axonal atrophy, 141
    signs and symptoms of, 139–143, 141f–143f
Paresis, 186b
Parietal lobe
  parietal lobe signs and symptoms, 151–154
    Balint syndrome, 153–154
    dominant parietal lobe, 153, 154f
    nondominant parietal lobe, 152–153
    optokinetic nystagmus, 151–152
    visual field defects, 151, 153f
Parvocelluar system, 37b, 148, 148f, 151f
Paton lines, 91f, 91t, 92, 108f
Peduncular hallucinosis, 157b
Percussion myotonia, 204
Perimetry techniques, 43–52
  automated perimetry, 44–47, 44f–46f, 48f, 57
  confrontation perimetry, 43–44, 43f, 57
  formal perimetry, 44
  Goldmann perimetry, 47–51, 49f, 50f, 57
  interpreting results of, 52
  kinetic perimetry, 44, 57
  static perimetry, 44, 57
  tangent screen, 51–52, 51f
Periodic alternating nystagmus (PAN), 253, 258

drugs used in treating, 257t
location of lesion causing, 255t
PET. See Positron emission tomography
Phakomatoses. See Neurocutaneous syndromes
Phorias, 186b
Photography, 14, 27
Photophobia, 10, 10t, 28, 173b
  pain and sensation with, 315–316, 316t
  vision loss from, 173b
Photopsias, 7t
Photo-stress testing, 38, 57
Pilocystic astrocytoma, 143f
Pinhole acuity, 34, 35b
PION. See Posterior ischemic optic neuropathy
Pituitary adenoma, 144–145
Pituitary gland, 141
Pituitary macroadenomas, 143, 144f, 145f
  acromegaly and visual loss with, 145f
  bitemporal visual field loss from, 144f
Plasmacytoma, 119t
Plexiform neurofibroma, 328, 328t, 329f
Polyarteritis nodosa, 204t
Polymyalgia rheumatica, 90t, 96, 98t
Poor visual acuity, 34b
Positive visual phenomena, 5–8, 6t, 7t, 27
Positron emission tomography (PET), 26, 27f
Posterior commissure, 243, 266, 267
Posterior communicating artery aneurysm, 230f, 232, 232t, 233f, 234t
Posterior ischemic optic neuropathy (PION), 92, 98, 98t
Posterior scleritis, 204t
Postfixation scotoma, 141, 142f
Post-herpetic neuralgia, 293, 298, 313, 317
PPRF. See Paramedian pontine reticular formation
Primary and secondary deviation, 191, 191f
Progressive supranuclear palsy, 10t, 248
Proptosis, 204, 206–207, 209–210, 209t
Pseudoisochromatic color plates, 40, 40f

Pseudopapilledema, optic disc edema compared to, 91*t*
Pseudotumor cerebri. *See* Idiopathic intracranial hypertension
Psoriatic and rheumatoid arthritis, 204*t*
Ptosis (blepharoptosis), 9, 9*b*, 196–197
  congenital, 196
  dermatochalasis compared to, 196*f*
  differential diagnosis of, 196*t*
  involutional, 196–197, 197*f*
Pulfrich phenomenon, 41*b*
Punctate keratopathies, 162
Pupil, 194
  afferent disorders of, 266–267, 266*t*
  anatomy/pathophysiology of
    afferent pupillary pathway/midbrain connections in, 265–266, 265*f*
    iris in, 261–262, 262*f*
    parasympathetic innervation in, 262–265, 264*f*
    sympathetic innervation in, 262, 263*f*
  efferent disorders of visual system with
    anisocoria, 268–269, 269*f*, 283–284
    iris and local factors in, 269
    oculosympathetic paresis, 269–277, 270*f*, 271*f*, 271*t*, 272*t*, 273*f*–276*f*, 275*t*, 277*b*
    parasympathetic in oculomotor nerve, 277–278, 278*f*
    parasympathetic in tonic pupil, 278–281, 279*f*, 280*f*, 283*f*
    pharmacologically dilated pupil, 281
    pupil states without anisocoria, 268
    transient pupillary dilation, 281–283
  midbrain disorders affecting
    light-near dissociation, 267, 267*b*, 268*t*
    midbrain relative afferent pupillary defects, 267–268, 284
Purkinje images, 7*t*
Pursuits
  defined, 186*b*
  disorders, 249
  ocular motility examination with, 187*t*, 188, 200
  pathways, 249
  systems and pathways of, 245*t*

Q
Quadrantanopia, 62*b*, 67*t*, 80*f*, 81*f*, 82

R
Radiation optic neuropathy (RON), 100
Racemose angioma of the retina, 328*t*, 331, 331*f*
Ramsay Hunt syndrome, 292, 298
RAPD. *See* Relative afferent pupillary defect
Raymond syndrome, 220
Rebound nystagmus, 255, 255*t*
Red glass test, ocular motility examination with, 191
Relative afferent pupillary defect (RAPD), 52–53, 53*f*, 57, 147
  chiasmal disease with, 141
  ocular media and pupil disorders with, 266–267, 266*t*
  test, 179–180
Release visual hallucinations. *See* Charles Bonnet syndrome
Rest test (for myasthenia), 212*f*
Restrictive orbitopathies
  Brown tendon sheath syndrome, 210–211, 211*f*, 215–216
  congenital fibrosis syndromes, 211
  orbital Graves disease, 206–210, 207*f*, 208*f*, 209*t*
  orbital trauma, 210, 211*f*
Retina
  cross-section of, 61, 64*f*
  hemorrhages with, 91*f*
  disorders of, *See* retinal disorders
  organization of, 60–61, 64*f*
  rods and cones distribution in, 61, 64*f*
  visual field defects, 61–62, 65*f*, 66*f*
Retinal angiomatosis (von Hippel disease), 328*t*, 330–331, 331*f*, 334
Retinal artery occlusion, 98*t*
Retinal disorders, 164–172, 165*f*
  AMPPE, 166
  ARMD, 167
  AZOOR, 171
  BRAO, 164, 165*f*
  BRVO, 166
  CADASIL, 166
  cancer-associated retinopathy, 169–171
  central serous chorio retinopathy, 167, 167*f*
  CRAO, 164–166, 165*f*
  CRVO, 166
  maculopathies, 167–168, 167*f*–170*f*, 171*t*
  melanoma-associated retinopathy, 171
  photophobia associated with, 10*t*
  retinal vasculopathies, 164–167, 165*f*
  retinitis pigmentosa, 168
  Stargardt disease, 168–169, 172*f*
  vasculitis, 166, 166*f*
Retinal nerve fiber layer (RNFL), OCT of, 16, 18*f*–19*f*
  visual field defect associated with, 63-68, 66*f*, 68*f*
Retinal vasculopathies, 164–167, 165*f*
Retinitis pigmentosa, 10*t*, 62, 65*f*, 168
Retrobulbar inflammatory disorder, 98*t*
Retrobulbar optic neuritis, 98*t*
Retrochiasmal lesions, 98*t*
Retrochiasmal visual defects, 74–78
  congruous versus incongruous, 76, 76*f*, 77*f*
  homonymous visual field patterns, 74
  visual acuity affected by, 76–78
Retrograde axonal atrophy, 141
Riddoch phenomenon, 155
riMLF. *See* Rostral interstitial nucleus of MLF
RNFL. *See* Retinal nerve fiber layer
RON. *See* Radiation optic neuropathy
Rostral interstitial nucleus of MLF (riMLF), 242–243, 243*f*, 258

S
Saccades, 258
  defined, 186*b*
  disorders
    acquired ocular motor apraxia, 247–248
    cerebellar disease, 248
    congenital oculomotor apraxia, 247, 247*f*
    frontal lobe lesions, 247
    ocular flutter, 248
    oculogyric crisis, 248
    opsoclonus, 248–249
    progressive supranuclear palsy, 248

Saccades (continued)
   saccadic intrusions, 248–249, 248t
   spinocerebellar ataxias, 248, 248t
   square-wave jerks, 248, 249t
  ocular motility examination with, 187t, 188–189, 200
  pathways for horizontal, 245, 246f, 246t
  pathways for vertical, 245, 246f, 246t
  synthesis of, 244–245, 245f
  systems and pathways of, 245t
Saccadic intrusions, 248–249, 248t
Sarcoid optic neuropathy, 120b
Sarcoidosis, 119t, 120f, 204t
  facial nerve palsy with, 294
  optic disc elevation from, 89t
Scheerer phenomenon, 7t
Scintillating scotoma, 6, 7t, 8, 10, 308, 308f, 309t, 310f, 316
Sclerosing inflammation, 204t
Scotoma, 62b
Sectoranopia, 150f
See-saw nystagmus, 143, 255, 258
  drugs used in treating, 257t
  location of lesion causing, 255t
Self-induced eye trauma, 173b
Sensory visual function testing, 31–57
  clinical test for, 32–41
    Amsler grid testing, 38–39, 38f, 57, 181
    brightness sense testing, 37, 57
    color comparison, 40
    color vision testing, 39–40
    contrast sensitivity testing, 35–37, 35f–37f, 37b, 56–57
    critical flicker fusion, 41b
    Farnsworth-Munsell 100 hue test, 39, 39f
    photo-stress testing, 38, 57
    pseudoisochromatic color plates, 40, 40f
    Pulfrich phenomenon, 41b
    stereopsis testing, 40–41, 41f
    visual acuity testing, 32–35, 32f–34f, 34b, 35b
  perimetry techniques for, 43–52
    automated perimetry, 44–47, 44f–46f, 48f, 57
    confrontation perimetry, 43–44, 43f, 57
    formal perimetry, 44
    Goldmann perimetry, 47–51, 49f, 50f, 57
    interpreting results of, 52
    kinetic perimetry, 44, 57
    static perimetry, 44, 57
    tangent screen, 51–52, 51f
  physiological/electrophysiological responses in, 52–56
    electrophysiological tests, 53–56, 54f–56f, 57
    electroretinogram, 53–55, 54f, 57
    multifocal ERG, 55–56, 55f
    relative afferent pupillary defect testing, 52–53, 53f
    visual evoked potential, 56, 56f, 57
  visual field test for, 41–52
    blind spot in, 42b, 42f
    hill of vision in, 42, 42f, 43b
    size and shape in, 41–43, 42b, 42f, 43b
Shagreen patch, 333
Short T1 inversion recovery (STIR), 23t
Shortening test distance, 34, 34b
Simultanagnosia, 247
Single Maddox rod test, 191–192, 192f, 200
Single photon emission computed tomography (SPECT), 26–27
Sinus and dental disease, 315
Sixth cranial nerve. See abducens nerve
Skew deviation, 250
Slitlamp examination, 12t, 13b
Snellen visual acuity test, 32–35, 32f, 34f
  notation in, 34f
  optotypes used in, 32, 33f
  wall chart in, 32f
Spasm of near reflex, 251
Spasmus nutans, 253, 258
SPECT. See Single photon emission computed tomography
Spinocerebellar ataxias, 248, 248t
Square-wave jerks, 248, 249t
Stargardt disease, 168–169, 172f
Static perimetry, 44, 57
Stereopsis testing, 40–41, 41f
STIR. See Short T1 inversion recovery
Stroke. See cerebrovascular disease
Sturge-Weber syndrome. See Encephalotrigeminal angiomatosis
SUNCT, 311
Superior oblique myokymia, 257
Supranuclear visual motor system
  internuclear gaze centers
    horizontal gaze, 239–242, 240f–242f, 242b
    vertical gaze, 242–244, 243f, 243t, 244f
  supranuclear pathways and disorders
    fixation reflex, 245t, 251
    optokinetic reflex, 245t, 250
    pursuit, 245t, 249
    saccades, 244–249, 245f–247f, 245t, 246t, 248t, 249f, 258
    vergence, 245t, 250–251
    vestibulo-ocular reflex, 245t, 249–250
Susac syndrome, 166
Syphilis, 119t, 204t
  optic disc elevation from, 89t
  optic perineuritis with, 105
Systemic lupus erythematosus, 119t, 204t

T

Tadpole pupils, 281
Tangent screen, 51–52, 51f
Tear film disorders, 161–162, 162b, 162f
  blepharitis, 161
  corneal epithelial dystrophies, 162, 162f
  dry eye syndrome, 161, 181
  epithelial defects, 162
  meibomian gland dysfunction, 161
  punctate keratopathies, 162
Temporal crescent, 59, 60f
Temporal lobe
  temporal lobe signs and symptoms, 154–155
    occipitotemporal region, 154–155
    sensory hallucinations, 154
    visual field defects, 154
Temporal raphe, 63
Temporal wedge, 66f, 68, 69f
Tensilon test, 213, 214b, 214f, 235
Tension-type headache, 311, 317
Third cranial nerve. See oculomotor nerve
Tilted optic discs, 134
Titmus fly stereotest, 41f
Tolosa-Hunt syndrome, 234, 234t
TON. See Traumatic optic neuropathies
Tonic pupil. See Adie pupil
Torsional nystagmus, drugs used in treating, 257t

Toxic/nutritional optic neuropathies, 122–124, 135
  alcoholism, 122, 123f
  amiodarone, 124, 124t
  B vitamins deficiency, 122–124, 124t
  folic acid deficiency, 122–124, 124t
  mitochondrial optic neuropathy, 123b
  niacin deficiency, 122–124, 124t
Transient visual loss, duration, etiology, and characteristics of, 6t
Transient visual obscurations (TVO), 6t, 109
Traumatic optic neuropathies (TON), 127–128, 128f, 135
  causes of, 127–128, 128f
  differential diagnosis of, 128
  evaluation of, 128
  signs of, 127
  symptoms of, 127
  treatment of, 128
Trichinosis, 204t
Trigeminal nerve (CN V)
  assessment of, 199, 199b
  clinical testing for pain with, 304–305
  neuroanatomy of pain with, 303–304, 304f, 305f, 306t, 316
  symptoms of pain with, 305
Trigeminal neuralgia, 10, 306, 307t, 314, 314f, 317, 327
Trigeminovascular system, 303, 308
Trochlear nerve (CN IV)
  clinical implications in anatomy for, 236
    cavernous sinus, 224–226
    nucleus and fascicles, 224, 225f, 226f
    orbit, 224–226
    subarachnoid space, 224
  differential diagnosis of, 226, 226t
  evaluation and management of, 226–228, 227f
  signs and symptoms, 224, 225f
Tropias, 186b
Tuberculosis, 105, 119t, 204t
Tuberous sclerosis (Bourneville syndrome), 328t, 332–333, 332f, 334
Tumbling E card, 34b
TVO. *See* Transient visual obscurations

U

Uhthoff phenomenon, 101
Ulcerative colitis, 204t
Ultrasonography, 19, 19f, 20f
Uncal herniation, 264
Unexplained visual loss, 161–181
  anterior segment disorders causing, 161–164
    cataract, 164
    corneal curvature, 162, 163f
    latent hyperopia, 164
    ocular surface disease, 161–162, 162b, 162f, 181
    refractive states, 164
    tear film disorders, 161–162, 162b, 162f, 181
  elusive neuro-ophthalmic disorders causing
    amblyopia, 173, 181
    retrobulbar and intracranial disorders, 173
  nonorganic vision disorders causing, 173–181, 173b, 174b, 175t, 177–180f, 181
  ocular disease causing, 161–173
  retinal disorders causing, 164–172, 165f, 166f–170f, 171t, 172f, 181
Upbeat nystagmus
  drugs used in treating, 257t
  location of lesion causing, 255t

V

Vasculitis, 166, 166f
VBI. *See* Vertebrobasilar insufficiency
VEP. *See* Visual evoked potential
Vergence, 250–251
  disorders of, 251
  ocular motility examination with, 187–188, 188f
  organization of, 251
  systems and pathways of, 245t
Versions, 186b
Vertebrobasilar disease, 324–325
Vertebrobasilar insufficiency (VBI), 6t
Vertical gaze center
  disorders, 243–244, 243t, 244f
  organization of, 242–243, 243f
  rostral interstitial nucleus of MLF with, 242–243, 243f, 258
Vestibular nystagmus, 255–256, 255t, 256t
Vestibulo-ocular nystagmus, 253
Vestibulo-ocular reflex, 245t, 249–250

Visual acuity testing, 32–35, 32f–34f, 34b, 35b
  counting fingers in, 34b
  hand movement in, 34b
  light perception in, 34b
  LogMAR acuity tests, 32, 33f
  near card in, 32, 33f
  notation in, 34f
  optotypes used in, 32, 33f
  pinhole acuity in, 34, 35b
  poor visual acuity in, 34b
  shortening test distance in, 34, 34b
  Snellen visual acuity test, 32–35, 32f, 34f
  tumbling E card in, 34b
Visual aura in migraine, 6, 6t, 7t, 8, 157b, 308–310, 308f, 309t, 310f, 316, 325
Visual evoked potential (VEP), 56, 56f, 57, 180
Visual field
  afferent visual system, 61f
  binocular viewing, 60f
  defined, 62b
  organization, 59–60
    chiasm, 69–71, 70f, 71f
    lateral geniculate nucleus, 78
    nerve fiber layer/optic disc, 62–63, 66f
    occipital lobe lesions, 79, 79f
    optic radiations, 78
    retina, 60–61, 64f
  temporal crescent of, 59, 60f
Visual field defects, 59–83
  altitudinal visual field defect, 66f, 67, 67f
  arcuate scotoma, 66f, 67, 67f
  cecocentral scotoma, 66f, 68
  chiasm, 71–74
    bilateral temporal visual field defect, 71–72, 71f, 72f, 72t, 73f
    combination defects, 73–74
    incongruous homonymous visual field defect, 71f
    junctional scotomas, 71f, 72–73, 74b, 74f, 75f
    paracentral bitemporal visual field defect, 71f
  lateral geniculate nucleus, 78, 78f
  nasal step defects, 64, 66f
  nerve fiber layer/optic disc, 63–68, 66f, 67f, 67t, 69f
  occipital lobe lesions, 79–83
    bilateral homonymous defects, 81–82, 82t

Visual field defects (*continued*)
    horizontal meridian with respect to, 80–81, 81*f*
    macular sparing, 80
    quadrantanopia, 81*f*
    temporal crescent, 82, 83*f*
    watershed infarcts, 79–80, 80*f*, 81*f*
  optic radiations, 78
  optics and media with, 59–60
  optics tract, 76*f*, 77, 77*f*, 83
  retina, 61–62
    focal macular disease, 62, 66*f*
    retinitis pigmentosa, 62, 65*f*
  retrochiasmal, 74–78
    congruous versus incongruous, 76, 76*f*, 77*f*
    homonymous visual field patterns, 74
    visual acuity affected by, 76–78
  temporal wedge, 66*f*, 68, 69*f*
  terms used to describe, 62*b*
Visual loss, 4–5. *See also* Nonorganic vision disorders; Unexplained visual loss
  glaucoma with, 129
  homonymous, 156–157, 158*b*
  optic disc drusen with, 131*f*
  pituitary macroadenomas with, 144*f*, 145*f*
  severity of, 5
  time course of, 4*f*, 5*f*
  transient, 6*t*
Visual motor system
  eyelids of
    examination techniques for, 195–196, 195*t*, 196*f*
    eyelid retraction with, 197, 197*f*, 197*t*
    facial nerve disorders with, 197
    ptosis with, 196–197, 196*f*, 196*t*, 197*f*
  facial nerve assessment for, 199, 199*f*
  observation of, 186
  ocular motility of, 186–194, 187*t*, 188*f*–193*f*, 189*b*, 190*b*, 200
  orbit and adnexa of, 197–200, 198*f*
  pupils of, 194
  terminology used with, 185–186, 186*b*
  trigeminal nerve assessment for, 199, 199*b*
Voluntary nystagmus, 173*b*, 253
von Hippel disease. *See* Retinal angiomatosis
Von Recklinghausen. *See* Neurofibromatosis

W

Wallenberg lateral medullary syndrome, 271, 271*f*, 284
Weber syndrome, 229, 231*f*. *See also* Encephalotrigeminal angiomatosis
WEBINO, 241, 241*f*
Wernicke encephalopathy, 242, 242*b*
Wilbrand knee, 74*b*
Wyburn-Mason syndrome, 328*t*, 331–332, 331*f*, 334